Markham J. Geller, Strahil V. Panayotov
Mesopotamian Eye Disease Texts

Die babylonisch-assyrische Medizin in Texten und Untersuchungen

Begründet von Franz Köcher

Herausgegeben von
Robert D. Biggs und Marten Stol

Band 10

Markham J. Geller, Strahil V. Panayotov

Mesopotamian Eye Disease Texts

The Niniveh Treatise

DE GRUYTER

The work on this volume as part of the project BabMed – Babylonian Medicine has been funded by the European Research Council (ERC) under the European Union's Seventh Framework Programme (FP7/2007–2013; Project No. 323596).

European Research Council

Established by the European Commission

ISBN 978-1-5015-1527-9
e-ISBN (PDF) 978-1-5015-0655-0
DOI https://doi.org/10.1515/9781501506550

Library of Congress Control Number: 2020938883

Bibliographic information published by the Deutsche Nationalbibliothek
The Deutsche Nationalbibliothek lists this publication in the Deutsche Nationalbibliografie; detailed bibliographic data are available on the Internet at http://dnb.dnb.de.

Printing and binding: CPI books GmbH, Leck

www.degruyter.com

MIX
Papier aus verantwortungsvollen Quellen
FSC
www.fsc.org
FSC® C083411

Acknowledgments

This contribution to the *Babylonisch-assyrische Medizin* series was conceived as part of the original application to the European Research Council for an Advanced Grant on ancient Babylonian medicine, which developed into the project known as BabMed (2013–2018) at the Freie Universität Berlin and led by M. J. Geller.

A deep debt of gratitude must go to Irving Finkel and Eric Schmidtchen, who contributed their own texts to this volume, and to Marten Stol, who sent extensive corrections and comments on the work before being sent to press. Moreover, Dr. Annie Attia, a professional ophthalmologist, scrutinized the progress of the IGI edition from its begining to end, and offered invaluable suggestions and discussions on eye ailments.

Thanks are due to F. Badalanova-Geller, A. A. Fadhil, A. Giannese, M. Guichard, E. Jiménez, and E. Schmidtchen for providing joins and/or photos. Diverse comments from T. Kwasman, F. Wiggermann, and K. Simkó were also helpful.

This volume also owes thanks to those who helped design the original ERC application, in particular Cale Johnson, as well as administrators at the Freie Universität, Eva-Marie Silies, Michael Vallo, Sebastian Brocksch, Hauke Ziemssen, and Agnes Kloocke, among others, who advised and coordinated the ERC Project so efficiently and effectively.

Work on the present volume would not have been possible without European Research Council funding of the Advanced Grant Project No. 323596 BabMed, with the full title, 'Fragments of cuneiform medicine in the Babylonian Talmud: Knowledge Transfer in Late Antiquity'.

It is also important to acknowledge the Wellcome Trust, which awarded the sabbatical funding to allow Geller to spend the 2005–2006 academic year in Paris, as Visiting Professor at the EPHE. Funding for the indexing of the volume was provided by a grant from the Institute of Jewish Studies at University College London.

Thanks also go to colleagues from Walter de Gruyter who have seen this volume through to publication, in particular Albrecht Doehnert, Katrin Mittman, and especially to Florian Ruppenstein.

Thanks are due to J. Eule, M. Hilgert, and J. Marzahn, who facilitated work in the Vorderasiatisches Museum zu Berlin; to I. L. Finkel and J. Taylor for assistance in the British Museum, and to C. B. F. Walker and M. C. Ludwig for their hospitality. We acknowledge the Trustees of the British Museum for allowing reproductions of tablets in their collections.

Personal thanks must also be extended to Mancho Vekov, Daniel Vatchkov, Valery Stoyanov and the Bulgarian Academy of Sciences, which has funded Strahil Panayotov's research after the completion of BabMed, and especially to Florentina Badalanova Geller, who has supported this work continually and faithfully over many years.

Last but not least, gratitude is also due to Gergana Francis.

https://doi.org/10.1515/9781501506550-201

Table of Contents

Preface

Like all large text editions, the present work has a long and complex history. The plan for a comprehensive modern edition and translation of Mesopotamian eye disease texts began in 2005, when Geller was invited to spend a year in Paris as Visiting Professor at the École Pratique des Hautes Études, supported by a research grant from the Wellcome Trust. The decision to study eye disease texts was made jointly by Geller with Dr. Annie Attia and Dr. Gilles Buisson, editors of the *Journal des Médecines Cunéiformes* and practicing physicians. Eye disease was chosen because of the existence of an extensive corpus of texts in cuneiform script, and the study could take advantage of Dr. Attia's personal expertise as an ophthalmologist. The three collaborators met every Friday to read through eye disease texts in the library of the Collège de France, throughout 2005–2006. There was not much previous work to take advantage of, since the only modern study of Mesopotamian eye disease had been a Würzburg dissertation from Jeanette Fincke (2000), which was useful for its extensive discussion of relevant terminology and numerous excerpts, but her work did not edit eye-disease texts. By the end of 2006, a preliminary edition of the main eye-disease texts from Nineveh had taken shape, with a translation in both English and French, but much work remained to be done.

Eye disease became one of the key texts to be studied in the programme of the ERC Advanced Grant BabMed (2013–2018), in which Geller was the PI and Panayotov a postdoctoral researcher. With the earlier preliminary edition from Paris as a starting point, Panayotov assembled all exemplars of eye disease texts into an IGI corpus, with the crucial decision being made to have Nineveh manuscripts as the basic exemplars – i.e. duplicates – and parallel witnesses from other sites treated as secondary. This is an important methodological innovation for working with serialized Nineveh texts. Geller and Panayotov each collated IGI tablets, and they jointly read every line of every text together, agreeing on a translation and key points for an explanatory philological commentary on the texts. Panayotov collated every relevant text in the British Museum and the Vorderasiatisches Museum in Berlin and Geller collated tablets in Istanbul as well. In the few instances when a text could not be collated, photos were used instead. Panayotov was responsible for the text layout and for the transliteration and transcription of the eclectic text, and the basic draft of the translation and commentary was his work, with additions and corrections made by Geller. Panayotov took photos, assembled the plates, and composed a complete glossary of IGI as well as a list of Sumerian logograms, with reproductions of the cuneiform signs for each logogram, which was novel. He also composed the indicies. While the philological commentary was being written, Panayotov incorporated many references to further work on IGI carried out by Annie Attia, which appeared as a French translation and interpretation of IGI, in the *Journal des Médecines Cunéiformes* in 2015. Finally, each co-author wrote his own introduction to the volume, reflecting their individual interests in the material. Geller proofread and corrected the whole volume on several occasions.

https://doi.org/10.1515/9781501506550-202

Neither author would have been able to produce this edition of IGI working alone, and this text edition confirms the distinct advantages of collaborating in a large project, while incorporating the assistance and support of other colleagues over many years. The German capital proved to be an ideal working environment for the BabMed Project, with many opportunities for consultation and collaboration with colleagues in the Topoi Excellence Cluster, from the Freie Universität, Humboldt Universität, and Max Planck Institut für Wissenschaftsgeschichte. The broader context of ancient medicine often featured in these discussions, on Greek medicine and science with Philip van der Eijk, Markus Asper, and Gerd Grasshoff, on Chinese medicine with Paul Unschuld, on Mesopotamian intellectual culture with Eva Cancik-Kirschbaum, and on common sense science with Klaus Geus. Glenn Most's Anneliese Maier research colloquium addressing methodological issues of editing ancient texts proved useful. The various discussions and Topoi seminars all had an impact on the vision of Mesopotamian eye disease within ancient science proposed in this volume. Furthermore, members of the BabMed research team, together with students and visiting scholars such as Henry Stadhouders, Amar Annus, András Bacskay, and Frans Wiggermann, participated in the weekly Keilschriftmedizin Seminar, which advanced the work on cuneiform medicine and related texts. Frans Wiggermann shared his personal research archive and *Zettelkasten* on Mesopotamian medicine. In addition, many scholars associated with BabMed, in particular Irving Finkel, Marten Stol, Nils Heeßel, Daniel Schwemer, Martin Worthington, Annie Attia, and Gilles Buisson, participated in BabMed workshops and lent their considerable expertise to a fuller understanding of Babylonian medicine.

It is gratifying to know that the present volume is not the end of the road for work on eye disease texts within Babylonian medicine. A new project, NinMed, managed by Jon Taylor of the British Museum and funded by the Wellcome Trust, will continue the pioneering work of BabMed. The three-year project will create online editions and translations of the extensive medical treatises of the Nineveh Royal Library. Panayotov, who designed the original project proposal, will be a primary contributor to NinMed, with Geller and Irving Finkel as project collaborators. The transition from BabMed to NinMed has already proved to be productive for the present edition. The Electronic Babylonian Literature (eBL) tools, under the guidance of E. Jiménez, has proved to be particularly useful in catching small inconsistences in the transliteration of IGI, which is being digitalised by Panayotov for the NinMed project. The shift in venue from the Freie Universität Berlin to the British Museum will bring the editions of Babylonian medicine closer to the cuneiform tablets. Nevertheless, cross-border cooperation with colleagues in Berlin and elsewhere will continue to play an important role in deciphering, interpreting and contextualising ancient Babylonian medicine, and in particular its close associations with other systems of medicine in the ancient world.

Overview of Cuneiform Eye Disease Texts (Strahil V. Panayotov)

Cuneiform therapeutic prescriptions on eye disease form the largest surviving corpus of ophthalmology from the Ancient Near East, sharing numerous comparable features with medical practices from synchronic and diachronic neighbouring cultures. This volume is the first complete edition and commentary on Mesopotamian medicine from Nineveh dealing with diseases of the eye. This ancient work, languishing in the British Museum since the 19th century, is preserved on several large cuneiform manuscripts from the Royal Library of Ashurbanipal, from the 7th century BCE. In contrast to classical sources, the material edited in this volume derives from original manuscripts and not from later copies. Thus, the cuneiform texts in this volume are of utmost importance for the history of ancient medicine.

Eye disease texts written on cuneiform tablets are represented by therapeutic prescriptions and incantations, which are discovered mainly from the 1st millennium BCE. However, scattered vestiges of their forerunners are known from the 3rd and 2nd millennia BCE, showing that the textual production of the eye disease texts – most of which were edited in this volume – were transmitted, collected and edited over two millennia.

Important works from other scholars have to be briefly mentioned. The relevant Nineveh tablets from the British Museum were partially identified, copied and translated by the British scholar Reginald Campbell Thompson. Later on, the material was systematized, joined and copied by Franz Köcher and published by 1980 in *Die babylonisch-assyrische Medizin in Texten und Untersuchungen,* volume 6. The *Grossmeister*, Köcher, produced hand copies and indices of cuneiform manuscripts which are extremely valuable for the current book, but Köcher hardly ever published editions or translations of medical texts. Multiple therapeutic texts on eye disease were discussed in Fincke 2000: 6ff., which has a good introduction on textual history. Notably, Jeannette Fincke's dissertation concentrates on terminology, and does not edit entire texts. The IGI treatise from Nineveh was translated and commented on for the first time by Annie Attia in 2015. Dr. Attia's work is of importance, since it is the only treatment of IGI from a professional ophthalmologist. Thus, her work has been consulted together with our critical edition.

3rd Millennium BCE

Incantations

Sumerian incantations of the 3rd millennium BCE are the earliest witnesses to eye disease therapy.

VAT 12597 originates from Fāra-Šuruppak, dating to ED IIIa, 2600–2500 BCE. A passage from this tablet (r. X 7 – XI 9) contains an incantation, which is the earliest example

https://doi.org/10.1515/9781501506550-001

of an historiola on eye disease (Krebernik 1984: 54–63, No. 8; Cunningham 1997: 19, 37, 41; Rudik 2011: FSB 23). This genre is also known from the 2nd and 1st millennium BCE.

HS 1552 from Nippur is another incantation on eye disease, dating to the Ur III period, ca. 2100–2000 BCE (van Dijk and Geller 2003: 26; Rudik 2011: FSB 24).

Therapeutic prescriptions

Beside incantations, there are a few Sumerian prescriptions for eye complaints from the 3rd millennium BCE, which are worth being re-edited and translated here, since they were previously thought to be incantations.

CBS 6195

Origin and date: Nufar-Nippur. ED IIIb (2500–2340 BCE)
Copy: PBS 9/40
Photo: http://cdli.ucla.edu/dl/photo/P263932.jpg
Literature: van Dijk and Geller 2003: 77

1	x x ⌜še-bar⌝$^{?}$ utu	… (old reading [é]n ⌜é⌝-[nu-r]u / ⌜^{d}⌝utu)
2	7 […] gi	and 7 reeds$^{?}$
3	u$_4$-⌜ten⌝-ta	^{4}you put ^{3}in the evening
4	a-a ù-gar	in water.
5	ge$_6$-ba-a-ka	At midnight
6	igi ^{d}utu-šè	– before dawn –
7	igi-a gar-ra	apply (the salve) onto the eye.
r.1	eme-ni lú ì-ni-zu	The man who knows his language(-spell)
r.2	a-rá-7-àm	$^{r.3}$rubs his eye (with the salve) $^{r.2}$seven times.
r.3	igi-na bí-íb-ùr-e	

This prescription shares similarities with a therapeutic ritual, see Rudik 2011: FBS 102. FSB 82.

Another text with ‘defective’ Sumerian spellings exemplifies early therapeutic prescriptions of eye disease in combination with treating with lice.

HS 1357

Origin and date: Ur III (2100–2000 BCE)
Copy: TMH NF I 357
Photo: https://cdli.ucla.edu/dl/photo/P134667.jpg
Literature: van Dijk and Geller 2003: 75; Bauer 2007: 179; Attinger 2008: 10, 12

1	ì-nin	(for ì-nun)	
2	uh-uš-da ù-da-hi	(sandhi for uh-huš)	He mixes [1]ghee [2]with red louse.
3	igi gi$_6$-ga ù-gar ba-áš	(for igi gig)	He applies (the salve) on the sick eye (and) he anoints (the sick eye).
4	nam-en-li uh-uš-da ù-da-hi		He mixes prime quality juniper (resin) with red louse.
4	uh-huš ba-áš		He rubs on the red louse.

2nd Millennium BCE

Incantations

By this period Sumerian and Akkadian incantations were addressing eye complaints from different provenances. The evidence shows that incantations spread throughout Mesopotamia and its periphery, as an integral part of medical procedures. Notably, part of the material from the 2nd millennium BCE was transmitted into the 1st millennium BCE. Incantations portray etiology and implicit theory of harm through metaphorical language (see Panayotov 2017).

VAT 1413 is an Old Babylonian (1900–1600 BCE) incantation in Sumerian (CDLI P342906; Falkenstein 1931: 44. Cunningham 1997: 141, No. 198). This text features a divine dialogue between Enki and Asalluhi, which is a spiritual topic in incantations used in Mesopotamian magic and medicine for three thousand years (Annus 2019). VAT 1413: 15 shows the earliest example of the rubric [ka-in]im-ma igi-gi[g-ga-kam] (if reconstructed properly), which is common later on in Nineveh, e.g. IGI 1: 96', 108' and so on.

Ish. 35-T. 19 is an Old Babylonian forerunner in Akkadian of an historiola concerning the creation of the *merhu*-kernel. The etiology of this harmful agent is also known from the Nineveh eye disease treatise, which is briefly discussed with literature in the notes to IGI 1: 194'.

BM 122691 is an Old Babylonian tablet from Tel Duweihes. Its lower edge reads *ši-iptum ša i-ni* [(x)]. However, this incantation is directed against the 'evil eye' and is not therapeutic, although intended to avert evil (discussed with literature in Geller 2003; and SEAL 5.1.7.2).

BM 79022 rev. 19ff. (edited and discussed in Wasserman 2010) mentions a brief incantation similar to an historiola. Its content suggests that it has been used for therapeutic purposes.

YBC 4616 is another historiola describing a worm causing eye reddening. A later version of the very same incantation might have contained some of the broken parts of the Nineveh IGI treatise, as did Ish. 35-T. 19 (translation modified after SEAL 5.1.26.2):

> Anu begot the sky, the sky bore the earth, the earth bore the stench, the stench bore the mud, the mud bore the fly, the fly bore the worm. The worm is the daughter of Gula, clad in a garment, thick with blood – the devourer of child's blood is reddening his eyes. Damu cast the incantation and Gula slew the thick worm, slaughtered them for the (sake of the) child. He opened his mouth, took the breast, raised his eyes, (and began to) suck. The incantation is not mine, it is the incantation of Damu and Gula. Damu cast (it) and I (the medical practitioner) took (it).

In addition, several incantations from the Middle Babylonian period (1400–1100 BCE) could be recognized as forerunners to the Nineveh material. The comparable texts – under § I. 3 Related Manuscripts from Different Cities; Periphery – were found in Emar and Ugarit, and might be considered either as a Babylonian import or local production.

Therapeutic prescriptions

Old Babylonian therapeutic texts (1900–1600 BCE) are written almost exlusively in syllabic orthography and are welcome counterparts to the encrypted material from the first millennium BCE edited in this volume.

ASC 207 col. i has a passage on eye disease, which was initially transcribed during BabMed seminars in Berlin 2017–2018, mainly by H. Stadhouders. This remedy illustrates internal medication for *amurriqānu* 'jaundice' of the eyes. Healing this eye condition is also known from IGI 2: 115f'.

27 AŠ *a-wi-lum*	'If a man's
28 *i-na-šu a-wu-ri-qa-*	eyes [29]suffer
29 *-na-am ma-ar-ṣa*	[28-29]from 'jaundice'.
30 *zi-bi-bi-a-nam*	[31]You crush
31 *ta-ha-aš-ša-al-ma*	[30]*zibibiānum*-cumin [31]and
32 *a-na li-ib-bi*	[34]pour (it)
33 *ši-ka-ri-*⌜*im*⌝	[32]into

34 *ta-ša-ap-pa-[a]k*	[33]beer.
35 *ta-ša-aq-q[í]*	You give (to him) to drink (it).
36 *i-ne-⸢e-eš⸣*	He will get better.’

Notably, ASC 207 uses AŠ, either in place of the more common DIŠ for *šumma* (Fincke 2007: 134), or as a short hand for *ašar* used in HS 1883, see below and the notes to IGI 1: 55.

HS 1883 (BAM 393) is an Old Babylonian tablet from Nippur, which contains eye prescriptions among others (Attinger 2008: 14, fig. 2; Geller 2006). However, I.L. Finkel has suggested that this tablet might possibly be a later copy of an Old Babylonian text, see Abusch and Schwemer 2011: 66. For the incipit style see the notes to IGI 1: 55.

Old Babylonian Medicine from Ur by Irving L. Finkel

Worth noting are some unpublished Old Babylonian medical texts in the British Museum, which were excavated by H.R. Hall (Finkel 2004: 26). Selected passages on eye disease will be briefly presented below. The full edition of the tablets will follow in a separate publication.

BM 113967+ col. ii (part of a two-column tablet)
17’ [*šum-ma*] *a-wi-lum i-na-šu ṣí-i*[*l-la-am*]
18’ *me-e* ⸢*šur-ni*⸣*-im me-e am-ma-aš-tam*[?]-[*ka-al*(?)]
19’ *me-e pu-qú-ut-t*[*i-im* ....]
20’ *ši-zi-ib* [*musukkati* (?) ....]
21’ *i-ni-šu te-qì-*[*ma*]
22’ *i-*[*ne-e-eš*]
17’ If a man’s eyes (suffer) ‘shadow,’
18’ [21’]you daub his eyes [18’]with *šurnû* juice, *maštakal* juice
19’ *puquttu* juice [....................................]
20’ milk from [a woman in maternity (?), and ...]
22’ and he will get better.

BM 113935+ col. iv (part of a three-column tablet)
18’ *šum-ma a-wi-lum i-na-šu ši-ši-tum*
19’ *ma-ar-t*[*a-a*]*m ša ar-ab-b*[*i*?]-x
20’ [*t*]*e-le-eq-qí-ma*
21’ *a-na pu-ur-sí-ti-im wa-ru-*[*uq-ti-im*]
22’ [*ṭ*]*a-ab-ta-am za-ku-ta-a*[*m*]
23’ [*u*]*b-ta-al-la-*⸢*al*⸣-[*ma*]

24f.' fragmentary
18' If a man's eyes have a membrane
19' [20']you procure [19']gall of a doormouse? ...
21' [23']He shall mix (it) [21']in a green bowl
22' with pure salt.

BM 113938+ col. iii (?) (part of a three-column tablet)
3' [*šum-ma a-wi*]*-lum i-na-šu e-ši-a*
4' [....................]*-am hu-šu-ul-ma*
5' [....................] *pu-šu-uš-ma*
6' [....................] x *šu-ku-um-ma*
7' [(...) *n*]*i-iṭ-lam ú-ṣa-*⌜*ab*?⌝
3' If a man's eyes are blurred,
4' crush [....................], and
5' anoint him [...........], and
6' apply [...........], and
7' [...] will increase eyesight.

Therapeutic prescriptions (continued)

Mesopotamian eye disease texts were transmitted in Hattuša. They are conveniently collected on http://www.hethport.uni-wuerzburg.de /HPM/index.html, CTH 809. Passages paralleling the IGI treatise from Nineveh have been included in the present edition in § II.3 Related Manuscripts from Different Cities BoA (KUB 4/50) and in § III.3 Related Manuscripts from Different Cities BoB (KUB 37/2) and BoC (KUB 4/55).

More therapeutic texts on eye disease in the late Old Babylonian and/or Middle Babylonian period are still unknown, and their existence is acknowledged by the catalogue BM 103690, line 39: ⌜DIŠ NA⌝ [x x] x dam? pa ⌜IGI.MIN⌝-*š*[*ú*? *i*]*-bar-ru-ra* 'If a man ... his eyes flicker' (Finkel 2018).

Middle Babylonian therapeutic prescriptions are rare, but recently some tablets from Baghdad (IM 202631 and IM 202652, photos courtesy of Dr. A.A. Fadhil) show that the period witnessed an abundance of therapeutic material. The exemplar IM 202631 is faked to a great extent, although some original passages remain. The original signs of the tablet are written in Babylonian script, most likely of Middle Babylonian origin, since the shape of the signs is similar to BM 103690 (Finkel 2018). IM 202631 was a large six column tablet, similar to IM 202652, a forerunner to BRONCHIA 5 (Panayotov 2018a: 90, 102). Probably, both tablets (IM 202631 and IM 202652) originate from the same unknown provenance where fake text was added to the original tablets. Sadly, only a few genuine passages of IM 202631 are preserved. The last prescription from the first column of IM 202631 shows a remedy against blood in the eyes (DIŠ.NA IGI.MIN-*šú* MÚD DIRI-*ma*). Prescriptions against this condition are also known from IGI 1: 36', 45', 79' and so on.

Furthermore, on the reverse of IM 202631, there are fragmentary eye prescriptions mixed with fake passages.

Several Middle Assyrian prescriptions on eye disease are preserved from the city of Assur. The exact dating of the manuscripts from Assur is rather difficult, but paleographic and material observations suggest that there are more Middle Assyrian tablets from Assur in the *Vorderasiatisches Museum zu Berlin* than previously expected.

BAM 12 is a neatly written Middle Assyrian tablet, baked in antiquity, showing the typical contrast between the white slip and the reddish core, exemplified by the so-called Tiglath-Pileser I (1115–1076 BCE) tablets (see Lambert 1957/58: 39ff.; Lambert 1965: 283; Pedersén 1985: 31). Köcher's copy shows several miscopied signs, e.g.: i' 9' ^{giš}MI.PAR$_4$; i' 11' ^{giš}PÈŠ (which confused CAD Š/3 386b); i' 17' PA.

Another tablet from the same period is AmA (BAM 165) mentioned in § I. 3 Related Manuscripts from Different Cities, which is partly related to IGI. The dating of BAM 18 and BAM 159 (see § I. 3 Related Manuscripts from Different Cities) might be Middle or Late Assyrian.

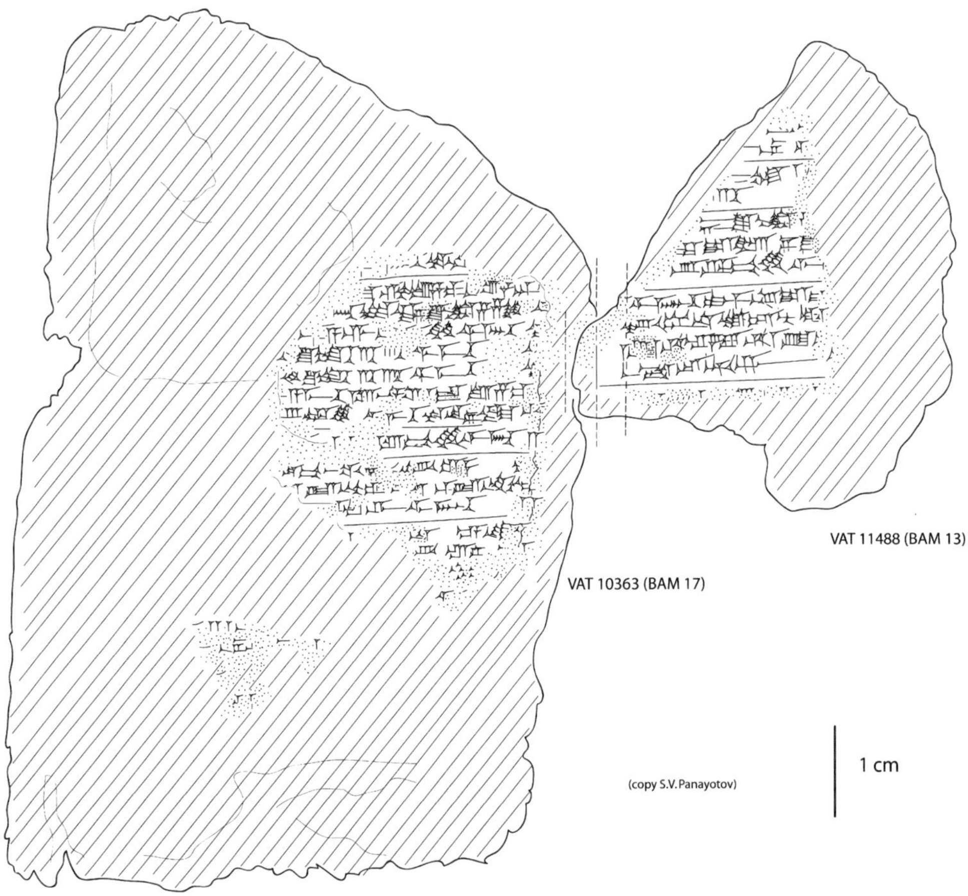

BAM 13, 17 and 25: according to Franz Köcher, VAT 11488 (BAM 13) probably belongs to VAT 11409+ (collated). But the shape of the signs, the thickness of the fragment as well as the colour of the clay are very different. VAT 10363 (BAM 17) can be tentatively dated as early Neo-Assyrian or late Middle Assyrian according to the shape of the sign LI [parameters: a2b4c5], l. 13', and also the shape of TU, col. i 3' (see Gottstein and Panayotov 2014). Furthermore, the same shape of the sign LI [a2b4c5] can be observed on VAT 11488 (BAM 13) at line ii 9', which also shows Middle Assyrian MEŠ [a1b5] at l. 8' and AH [a3b2c5] at l. 6'. The copy above shows a possible positioning of fragments BAM 13 and 17. Additionally, VAT 16464 (BAM 25) has the same colour clay, and shows Middle Assyrian sign forms of BA on lines 5', 8' [a1b1c2], DIM [a1b3c2], the HI-group with five wedges [c5], and MEŠ [a1b5 or a1b4]. The thickness of the fragments (BAM 17= 3,2 cm, also Köcher, BAM 1: XV) and their similar features suggest that BAM 13, 17 and 25 were originally part of a three column tablet on eye disease, which might have been serialized. Other serialized Middle Assyrian medical texts from Assur are known, see BAM 11 (series for ghost afflictions: $^{\text{rev: 36}}$18 *bu-ul-ṭú ša* SAG.KI.DAB.BA ^{37}IM.GÍD.DA 1.KAM.MA ^{38}*ša bīt*(É) *Ra-bi-a-ša-*^{d}AMAR.UTU (*pace* the reading of Heeßel 2009: 25), and BAM 36 (series for lung problems), l. 5': [... G]IŠ.GÀR MUR.MEŠ [GIG.MEŠ].

1st Millennium BCE

Incantations

It is probably by chance that most of the material is known only from Nineveh. All of the incantations on eye disease known to us were collected and revised in the IGI Nineveh treatise by Ashurbanipal's scholars and are edited in the present volume. There are rare IGI parallels from outside of Nineveh, like Ms. HA (STT 279) from Huzirina in § I. 3 Related Manuscripts from Different Cities.

A systematic study of the figurative language of medical incantations in general was produced by Collins 1999 and Geller 2007c. Attia 2015 and Panayotov 2017 took a closer look at the eye disease incantations, which are the best example so far of an implicit theory of causation and etiology of ophthalmological problems, expressed through allegories and metaphors.

Therapeutic prescriptions

Like with the incantations, the biggest collection of eye disease therapeutic texts is the IGI treatise from Nineveh itself. However, it is not the only systematized therapeutic corpus of eye disease from the first millennium BCE. The series on eye disease from Assur is known only from catch-lines, as with BAM 3, which was incidentally an import from Babylonia ($^{\text{col. iv 47}}$ *ina pu-ut* ^{giš}ZU URI^{ki} ZI-*ha*):

> *šumma*(DIŠ) *amēlu*(NA) *īnāšu*(⌜IGI.MIN-*šú*⌝) *ṣilla*(GISSU) *ár-ma arkīšu*(EGIR-*šú*)
> The (series) 'If a man's eyes are covered with a shadow' (is written) after it (this tablet).

Pace the translation in Worthington 2006: 32, *arkīšu*(EGIR-*šú*) is a short-hand for *arkīšu*(EGIR-*šú*) *iššaṭṭar*, designating the next tablet in a cuneiform collections, as shown by the catchline of the next relevant example, AO 11447 (Geller 2007b).

> *šumma*(DIŠ) *amēlu*(NA) *īnāšu*(⌜IGI.MIN⌝-*šú*) *dāma*(MÚD) *malâ*(DIRI) *maṭâma*(LAL-*ma*) *u i-bar-ru-*⌜*ra*⌝ ... *arkīšu*(EGIR-*šú*) *iš-šaṭ-tar*
> The (series) 'If a man's eyes are full of blood, and flicker, (and his eyesight) is diminished...' is written after it (this tablet).

Although the Assur series on eye disease are unknown, a number of therapeutic texts from Assur allude to their content, for instance AO 11447, BAM 3 (13, 17 and 25 see above), 14, 15, 16, 18, 19, 20, 21, 22, 23, 28, 50, 156, 159, 165, 183, 328 (BM 123362, Ms. XA, see § IV. 1. 3 Related Manuscripts from Different Cities). They all share common therapeutic texts with the IGI treatise from Nineveh, noted in the present edition. Isolated additional therapeutic material from Assyria is also known from Kalhu (CTN 4/123, Ms. KA in § II. 3 Related Manuscripts from Different Cities) and Huzirina (STT 279, Ms. HA in § I. 3 Related Manuscripts from Different Cities), but also STT 105.

As stated above, BAM 3 shows that some therapeutic eye disease texts in Assur were imported from Babylonia. Mainly I.L. Finkel and M.J. Geller have collected Late Babylonian unpublished tablets concerned with eye ailments in the British Museum. Other Late Babylonian texts on eye disease are scattered around the world. Presumably coming from Babylon are: VAT 17406 (BAM 382, Ms. bB, § II. 3 Related Manuscripts from Different Cities), BM 37119 (a copy of SVP to the left), BM 38483, BM 38673, BM 38679 (a copy by SVP on the next page), BM 39872, BM 39725, BM 40737 (Ms. xB in § III. 3 Related Manuscripts from Different Cities), BM 41173 + 41199, BM 41261, BM 41293 + 44866 (Ms. bA in § I. 3 Related Manuscripts from Different Cities), BM 45941, BM

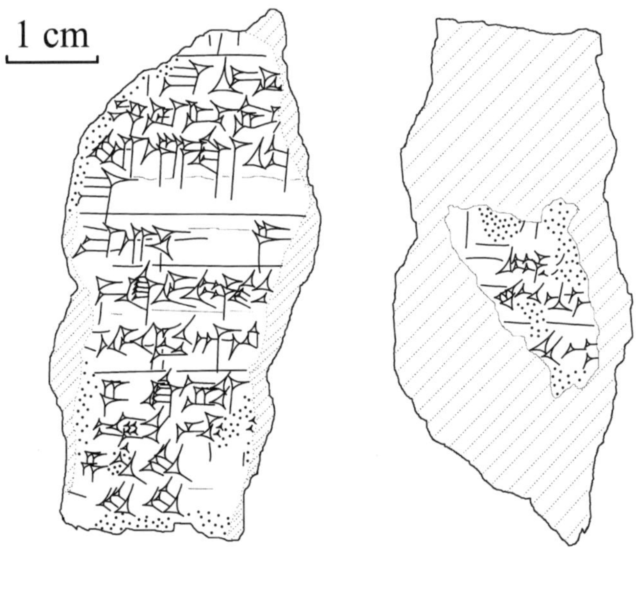

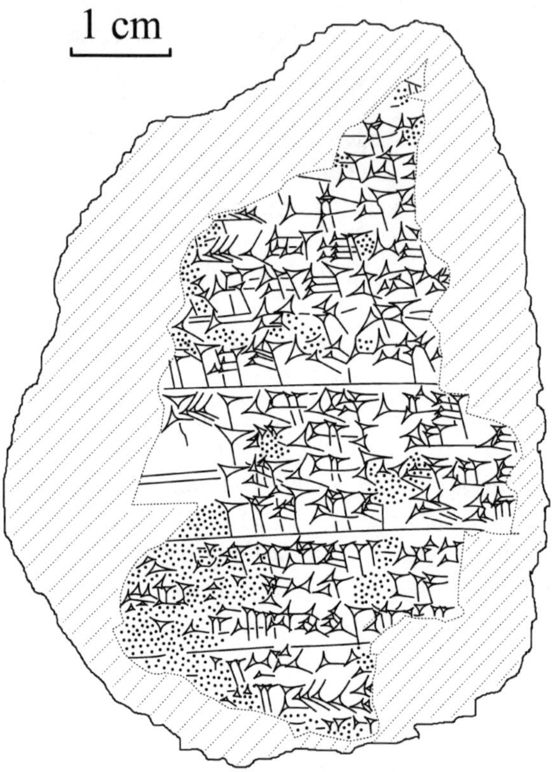

49133. The catchline of BM 35512 refers to relevant prescriptions as well, see Bácskay 2018c.

Presumably from Sippar are: BM 54641 + 54826 (Ms. xA §I.3 Related Manuscripts from Different Cities), BM 50508, BM 54808 + 54816, BM 70420 + 70436, BM 76023 + 83009, BM 73420, BM 109097a, BM 68373, BM 50508. Another important tablet from this city is IM 132670 (Ms. sA in § I. 3 Related Manuscripts from Different Cities). Presumably from Sippar is also CBS (Kh2) 1543, *PBS* 1/2, 121 in Abusch and Schwemer 2011, text 10.2, p. 405. *Pace* their transcription of the incipit we read SAG.KI.DAB.BA TUK.TUK.

Uruk has also yielded therapeutic texts on eye disease, like BAM 403, BAM 410, SpTU 50, and SpTU 22+85.

The provenance of BM 132097 (Geller 1988) is unclear, see Fincke 2000: 9 fn 59. Also, the Nineveh fragment, K 10535 edited in § IV. 9 NV (AMT 18/3) was a Babylonian import from an unknown city, if not written in Nineveh.

The Late Babylonian material on eye disease, although partly fragmentary, needs a proper edition and comparison with the Nineveh IGI treatise, which is beyond the scope of the present volume.

Eye Disease Texts meet Royal Letters in Nineveh

The IGI treatise from Nineveh is the second chapter of the Nineveh Medical Encyclopaedia (henceforth NME), created especially for the Royal Library of Ashurbanipal in Nineveh (Panayotov 2018a: 109ff.). Vestiges of the NME were discovered in the ancient mound of Kuyunjik, where the royal letters of Nineveh were also found. The letters reflect daily life of the King, his consort, and his scholars, who were dwelling and working inside the capital (on the next page see the reconstruction of the Nineveh vicinities by Reade 2016: 48 fig. 7). Royal letters contain abundant medical references and there is a good discussion of this material in Geller 2010a: 75ff.

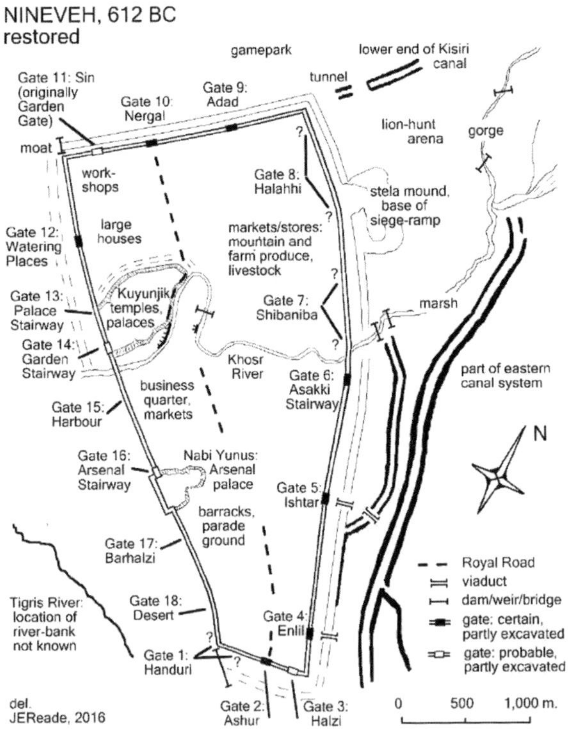

Information from the NME is reflected in royal letters but there are certain specifics which make comparisons difficult. The royal letters and NME employ stylistically different language while addressing the same medical issues. The royal letters were written mainly syllabically in an official Assyrian dialect, politely addressing the king in indirect speech, while therapeutic prescriptions of the NME were written mostly logographically in the technical language of medicine, but employing literary language in the therapeutic incantations. Let us observe how a common head therapy is addressed in the first chapter of the NME: (SAG.DU-*su*) SAR-*ab* LAL-*ma* 'you shave (his head and) bandage (it with bandages)' (see the edition in § V, NI i 4ff.), compared to the same statement from a royal letter: *ma-a* SAG.D[U-*su*] *nu-gal-li-*[*ib* ...] *ṣi-in-di* [...] *ni-ir-k*[*u-us*] 'let us shear [his] head and bind [it] with [...] bandages' (modified after SAA 10: no. 335: 2ff.). Logically, royal scholars must have had access to the NME and similar material from the Royal Library, since their letters allude to therapeutic material which existed in Nineveh, like the expression *ina bu-ul-ṭi gab-bu* 'among the entire therapeutic prescriptions' (modified after SAA 10: no 326: 3), implying most probably the content of the NME. This very same letter tells us about a remedy for a royal baby: [r.1]*ina pi-i-šú ù* DÚR-*šú* [r.2]*ú-še-šar-am-ma* [r.3]⌜*i*⌝*-ba-al-lu-uṭ* 'he purges through his mouth and his anus, and he will get better' (modified after SAA 10: no 326). Notably this looks like a direct citation from the eighth chapter of 'STOMACH' of the NME: *ina* KA-*šú u* DÚR-*šú* SI.SÁ *tu*-SUD-*šú-ma* TI-*uṭ* 'he purges through his mouth and his anus, you sprinkle him and he will get better' (modified after Cadelli 2000: 72: 30, see especially p. 352 fn. 347, and p. 397 fn. 121).

Similar, to the case addressed above, we can compare other ailments and treatments from the IGI treatise to royal letters. Let us look at the *hunṭu* condition (a kind of burning sensation in the eyes) of the Assyrian king Esarhaddon. The word *hunṭu*, as a kind of fever, described the poor health of the Assyrian king (Stol 2007a: 21; Parpola 1983). In one letter, the scholar Ikkaru refers to Esarhaddon as [17]*hu-un-ṭu* [18][*ina* ŠÀ *e*]*-na-a-te uk-ti-il*$_5$, '*hunṭu* lingered in (his) eyes' (modified after SAA 10: no 328). This letter also suggests that the *hunṭu* condition might be linked to warm weather (SAA 10: no 328 r.9ff.). In another letter, Esarhaddon complains in a statement reported by the scholar Marduk-šākin-šumi: [6]*ma-a a-hi-ia* [7]*še-pi-ia la-mu-qa-a-a* [8]*ù ma-a* IGI.MIN-*ia la a-pat-ti* [9]*ma-a mar-ṭak kar-rak* 'My arms and legs are weak and I cannot open my eyes, I am scratched and lie prostrate!' Then Marduk-šākin-šumi says: [10]*ina* ŠÀ *ša hu-un-ṭu* [11]*šu-ú ina* ŠÀ *eṣ-ma-a-ti* [12]*ú-kil-lu-u-ni* [13]*ina* ŠÀ-*bi šu-ú* [14]*la-áš-šú hi-ṭu* 'This is because *hunṭu* lingered inside the bones. It is therefore not serious' (modified after SAA 10: no 242). This complex medical condition was caused by *hunṭu*, which seems to occur often to various persons from the royal family and affecting different body parts, eyes included (also SAA 10: nos. 193, 243, 320). The chief physician Urad-Nanaya, who had difficulties identifying Esarhaddon's *hunṭu*, treated it with different salves and *ṣilbānu*-bandages (probably crosswise arranged, see Geller 2010a: 83 and Marsham 2011: 103), which caused the king to sweat (SAA 10: no. 315). The condition *hunṭu* also affected royal babies, but it was reported as not serious (SAA 10: no. 213: [8]*hi-ṭu la-áš-šú*).

Surprisingly, if we survey the therapeutic material on eye disease, we do not find the condition *hunṭu* referring to eyes, otherwise common in royal letters. This must be due to stylistic differences between letters and therapeutic texts. First, the word *hunṭu* (var. *humṭu*) is the Assyrian form of *himṭu* (Stol 2007a: 21). However, *himṭu* does not seem to appear in therapeutic texts in this form. Instead of the nominal form, therapeutic texts employ a stative form of *hamāṭu* 'to burn' (IGI 1: 14') describing a burning sensation of the eye, which might also suggest a reddish color, since the stative is also used in physiognomic omens (Alamdimmû tablet 8) to describe the color of the human face (Böck 2000: 112: 73ff.). Often, *hamāṭu* refers to inflamed eyes due to *ṣētu*-sun-heat (IGI 2: 9). One therapeutic prescription from IGI 3 is particularly descriptive: [49']If a man's eyes cannot see (*īnāšu lā inaṭṭalā*): that man is inflamed with sun-heat (*ṣēta hamiṭ*): [50']\[you pound\] [49']one shekel of bat guano, [50']half shekel of white plant, (and) one fourth shekel of *emesallu*-saline solution in mountain honey and ghee, (and) you daub his eyes (with it),' see also § IV.6 NS (AMT 18/4): 6'). The phrase *īnāšu lā inaṭṭalā* 'his eyes cannot see' is another way of saying IGI.MIN-*ia la a-pat-ti* 'I cannot open my eyes' cited in SAA 10: no 242 above. The prescription of IGI 3 mentions the warm weather suggested as a probable cause of *hunṭu* (SAA 10: no 328 r.9ff.), similar to the expression, 'inflamed with sun heat' (*ṣēta hamiṭ*) from therapeutic texts. Sun-heat (*ṣētu*) was a daily problem in Mesopotamia, and it was likely that it caused sunstroke. We suggest that *hunṭu* from the royal letters is equivalent to the stative of *hamāṭu* 'to burn', or to the expression *ṣēta hamiṭ* 'inflamed with sun heat' from therapeutic texts. Stol asks, 'Is it possible that the normal Assyrian word for fever *hunṭu* is an abbreviation of this Old Babylonian *himiṭ ṣēti*?' (Stol 2007a: 38, also 34 fn. 90). In other words, *hunṭu* from the royal letters represented a burning sensation (i.e. inflammation) caused by sun heat, corresponding to the stative of *hamāṭu* and the expression *ṣēta hamiṭ* from therapeutic prescriptions. The burning sensation could be recognised by its reddish color, but was nothing really to worry about, as royal physicians report.

Cuneiform Eye Disease Texts in Near Eastern and Greco-Roman Perspective

From the 5th century BCE onwards, Greco-Roman scholars argued about how visual perception functioned. Consequently, they developed extramissionist and intromissionist theories of vision and sight (Coughlin 2016: 56). Cuneiform medical texts are silent about the function of the human eyes and vision, although implicit eye-disease theory and etiological explanations can be recognized in medical incantations. The eye in Mesopotamia was conceived as a water source dating back to mythical time when the world was created (Panayotov 2017: 211f.). This metaphor reflects tears which flow from the eyes like a river from the ground.

Historical sources from the Ancient Near East occasionally mention ophthalmological drugs and doctors dispatched internationally. In the 13th century BCE, the Hittite king Hattušili III suffered from eye problems. He received particular drugs for his treatment from the Egyptian Pharaoh Ramses II. This case was recorded in diplomatic correspondence (Edel 1976: 44, 76; Ritner 2000: 112; Couto 2013: 405). Another case is reported by Herodotus: in the 6th century BCE a chosen eye-doctor of the Egyptian Pharaoh Amasis was unwillingly sent to Persia, in order to help with eye treatment for Cyrus (cf. Zaccagnini 1983: 255f.).

Ancient Egypt, prominent in eye-doctors and remedies, shares conceptual metaphors with Mesopotamia, ancient Greece and even modern languages. The Egyptian *pds.t* 'small ball' – describing an eye problem – is similar to the Akkadian term *merhu* 'kernel,' or Greek *krithè* 'barley grain,' or even German *Gerstenkorn* (Panayotov 2017: 214ff).

Medical prescriptions from Papyrus Ebers (16th century BCE) resemble material edited in this volume:

> Another (recipe) for removing cloudiness from the eye(s). Myrrh: 1 measure. "Great-protection" mineral/incense: 1 measure. šsy.t-mineral: 1 measure. Colocynth/carob (d3r.t): 1 measure. Lower Egyptian gy.t-plant: 1 measure. Green eye paint: 1 measure. Excrement(?) of a gazelle: 1 measure. Interior of a q3dy.t-animal/insect: 1 measure. White/bright oil. Place in water. Allow to spend the night in the dew. Strain. Bandage with it for four days. Otherwise said: Then you should pour it by means of a feather of a vulture (as an eyedropper). See Westendorf 1999: Ebers § 339.

Drugs in this prescription have precise measures, also found throughout Mesopotamian eye disease material; for references see SILA$_{4/x}$, *uṭṭatu*, *šiqlu* in the glossary. Furthermore, the Egyptian formulation 'allow to spend the night in the dew' is another way of saying 'let it stay under a star' (= stay overnight), frequent in Mesopotamian medicine as well (IGI 1: 81', IGI 3: 34'), see Ritner 2000: 112. Another comparable drug is 'excrement(?) of a gazelle,' reminiscent of the common 'gazelle droppings' (IGI 2: 177'; IGI 3: 72'). The duration of the eye bandage in Ebers is also known from IGI 2: 1–7. The alternative use of a vulture feather as an eye-dropper comes close to the drug application by bronze tube in IGI 1: 86f.', and although the medical instrument is different, the formulation, style and technology are comparable.[1]

A common practice in ancient Near Eastern medicine deserves to be mentioned – the treatment of blindness with animal liver (Stol 1986), as recorded in IGI 3: 75 (employing a donkey-liver), 81, 89. A chronological survey would be particularly telling for universal healing practices in the ancient Near East. In the 16th century BCE, Papyrus Ebers mentions the use of beef liver against blindness:

> Ein anderes (Heilmittel) für die Blindheit in beiden Augen: Leber des Rindes, gebraten (und) ausgepreßt; werde daran geben (=an das Auge). Wirklich vorzügliche (Methode). See Westendorf 1999: Ebers § 351.

Papyrus London from the 14th century BCE mentions a similar case:

> Ein anderes Heilmittel. Leber des Rindes, gegeben auf Feuer von Strohhalmen des Emmers oder Gerste, geräuchert in ihrem Rauch; werde ihr (der Leber) Wasser ausgedrückt an die beiden Augen. See Westendorf 1999: 40, 149, 612.

Papyrus London is useful for pointing out international medical relationships, since it contains references to Crete as Keftiu (Arnott 2004: 165f.), and the Near East as Samāna (see Beck 2015). Also, the first Semitic spell (27) from Papyrus London mentions 'another incantation against the strangulation-disease (*ḥmkt*) in the language of the foreigners' (Ritner 2000: 110). We suggest that *ḥmkt* derives from the Akkadian medical condition *hiniqtu*.[2]

The material on blindness from Hattuša has been noticed and discussed by Stol (1986: esp. 296f.), and included in the present edition to IGI 3: 81ff.'

IGI material from the 7th century BCE, edited in the present volume is also comparable to the Hippocratic Treatise on the Eye, 5th century BCE:

> As a medicaton for nyctalopia (night blindness) let the patent drink squirting-cucumber juice, have his head cleaned, and reduce his neck as much as possible, compressing it for a very long time. When remission occurs give him raw bull's liver dipped in honey, and have him drink down as much as he can, one or two. See Potter 2010: 385.

1 Akkadian recipes regularly employ a feather to induce vomiting. The Babylonian Talmud refers in several instances to drugs (such as goose fat) being applied with a feather.

2 In this respect, Semitc loanwords of medical plants employed in eye therapy are known in Mycenaean Greek: *Κύμινον* and *Σέλινον*, Akkadian *kamūnu* and *sahlānu* (Bourguignon 2012). Another case is *Sikillu* and *Σκίλλα* (Rumor, in press). Furthermore, a shared structural design exists between Akkadian drug lists (eye drugs included) and herbal descriptions in Theophrastus (Rumor 2018). The Mesopotamian drug list Irianna equates Akkadian drugs to those in the languages of *Kinahu*, *Muṣru*, *Šubria*, *Ahlamu*, *Kaššū*, *Elam* and *Meluhha* (forthcoming edition by J. Scurlock and J. Fincke), pointing to global Near Eastern medical terminology transfers.

Moreover, the Hippocratic Treatise on the Eye mentions copper as an ingredient used in eye therapy:

> When the eyelids become scabby, and itchiness is present: grind a lump of flower of copper against a wet stone, next rub off the eyelid with it, and then grind some scale of copper as fine as you can (= produce powder). Then add strained juice of unripe grapes, grind fine, and pour what is left into a red copper vessel, continuing to grind it a little at a time until it has the thickness of *mussotos*. Then, when this becomes dry, grind it fine and apply. See Potter 2010: 384f.

Diverse copper products are often found in Mesopotamian eye disease prescriptions; for references consult the present glossary under: *erû*, *erû labīru*, *erû zikaru*, *hīl erî*, *šuhtu*, *šuhtu ša tangussi*, *tangussu* (comparable to 'a red copper vessel' above).

In the first 1st century CE, Dioscorides, *De Materia Medica*, Book 2, mentions goat liver as a treatment for blindness:

> The watery fluid that drips from the liver of a goat whilst it is a roasting is good rubbed on for those troubled with night blindness. If anyone receives the smoke of it with open eyes whilst it is boiling he receives benefit from this. Eaten roasted it is good for the same purpose. They say that epilepsy may be discerned by eating the liver (especially) of the buck goat. See Osbaldeston and Wood 2000: 199.

Probably dating from the same century are the eye disease prescriptions found in Celsus 'De Medicina':

> There is besides a weakness of the eyes, owing to which people see well enough indeed in the day-time but not at all at night ... But such sufferers should anoint their eyeballs with the stuff dripping from a liver whilst roasting, preferably of a he-goat, or failing that of a she-goat; and as well they should eat some of the liver itself. But, we may also use with advantage the same remedies which dry up scars and trachoma. Some add honey to pound purslane seed until the mixture no longer drops from the end of a probe, and with it anoint the eyeballs. The same exercises, baths, rubbings and gargles are also used for their patients. See Spencer 1989: 225f.

The resemblances between the Mesopotamian treatment of blindness and those from the Babylonian Talmud (5th century CE) were pointed out by Stol 1986 and Geller 1991. Remarkably, the above-mentioned treatments have even commonalities with the much later Syriac Book of Medicine, a heterogeneous medical compilation:

> Another (prescription), which is to be used for those who cannot see in the twilight. Take the liver of a goat (or, stag), roast it until it is half-cooked, squeeze out the juice and catch the liquid which flowed from it in a glass vessel, and smear the eyes with it, and let the patient eat the liver. Now others stew the liver in a cooking pot, and order the patient to hold his head over the pot and to keep his head covered on all sides. The above medicines constitute the means which are to be used for dimness of sight, and effusion of the eyes, and nocturnal blindness. See Budge 1913: 96f.

Undoubtedly – via trade and diplomatic exchange – medical knowledge, doctors and drugs circulated in Egypt, Mesopotamia, Levant, Hatti, Mycenaean Greece and the

Greco-Roman World. The parallels in Ancient Near Eastern ophthalmological healing can be viewed as indirect borrowings and/or similarities in the light of a common prescription-based medical practice, rather than as a direct influence from one culture upon another. But a definitive view on this matter can only be based upon further research.

1 Introduction: Eye Disease in Mesopotamia (Mark J. Geller)

Eye disease is common to all systems of ancient medicine and its prominence among medical remedies may simply be explained by the prevalence and visibility of eye ailments in all ancient societies. This means that eye disease can offer useful comparative data for both diagnosis and pharmaceutical remedies, and even a cursory survey will show that certain types of medications were widely used throughout the Mediterranean and Near East. What is unusual about the Mesopotamian recipes in the present collection – drawn from the Nineveh Medical Encyclopaedia from the Royal Library of Ashurbanipal[1] as well as from duplicate and parallel texts from other sites – is the large number of incantations which accompany the medical recipes, and these provide clues to theories of eye disease and its treatment. Moreover, there is some similar medical data in the Syriac Book of Medicines and Babylonian Talmud, in Aramaic, which appear to betray some degree of awareness of the Akkadian treatments, and this provides important clues to the reception of Akkadian medicine into Late Antiquity.

1.1 Diagnosis of symptoms

Modern medicine distinguishes between signs and symptoms, the one referring to how the patient describes his or her own perceptions or pain, and the other referring to the observations by the physician based on examination and tests. Both types of notations appear in Babylonian medical and diagnostic texts, although usually restricted to external examination of the body without benefit of aids or instruments, which is why retrospective diagnoses are scarcely reliable.[2]

The usual pattern for all of Akkadian medicine is for symptoms to be introduced by the standard formulaic logograms DIŠ NA, understood to stand for *šumma amēlu*, 'if a man'.[3] Although this same formulaic notation also appears in the Diagnostic Hand-

1 For a description of the Nineveh Medical Encyclopaedia, see Panayotov 2018a.

2 Attia 2015: 4. See Fincke 2009: 99–101, in which she offers an abbreviated scheme for the sequence of symptoms within IGI, as well as (for comparison) the incipits of a single LB tablet dealing with eye disease (BM 54641 + 54826). Her categories of symptoms include: bloodshot eyes, foreign bodies in the eye, dysfunction of lachrymal glands, eyelids, internal eye pathologies, and 'shadow', as well as general categories of vision and eyesight.

3 The identification of the logogram DIŠ for *šumma* 'if' is likely to be correct and can be argued on the basis of older medical texts from the Old Babylonian period (c. 1700 BCE), which begin with the word *šumma* spelled out syllabically. However, Akk. *šumma* has other logograms in divination texts, such as BAD, and the DIŠ could be used to denote a separate entry, as in accountancy, rather than the word 'if'.

https://doi.org/10.1515/9781501506550-002

book,[4] it does not appear that the symptoms described in the therapeutic corpus were simply copied or drawn from the symptoms noted in the Diagnostic Handbook.[5] The first encountered (and most common notation of eye disease) is a straightforward statement that the patient's eye is 'sick' (*marṣu*);[6] while this may appear to be generic, this sparse symptom designation (like all others) nevertheless called for specific kinds of treatments,[7] suggesting a nosology not indicated by the text but obvious to the practitioner.

Treating the prescriptions and their associated symptoms in sequence within IGI, we turn now to a symptom with both a primary and secondary description,[8] in which the eyes are 'sick' (*marṣā*) and 'inflamed' (*hanṭā*),[9] with the latter term usually describing feverish conditions. The symptom is distinctive enough to warrant its own specific treatment, although the exact nature of the pathological condition is not adequately indicated (which is true of most of the symptom notations).

The next stage of symptoms is another two-clause description, beginning with the general condition of eyes being 'sick' (*marṣā*) and also 'closed' (*katmā*),[10] or additionally, that the patient cannot open his eyes for a period of time, lit. 'he cannot open (them) for many days'.[11] This recipe also includes a tertiary description, that his head is hot (with *ummu*-fever) and his eyes contain a film (*ṣillu*), which could indicate a variety of pathologies. The 'closing' of the eyes can be an indication of swelling, which, combined with fever and a filmy eye, provided the essential symptoms of this pathology.

In fact, there are some remarkable similarities between Hippocratic texts dealing with prognosis and Akk. diagnostic texts, if one assumes that DIŠ is not read as *šumma* or 'if', but rather as a new entry.

4 For the Diagnostic Handbook, see Labat 1951, Heeßel 2000, Scurlock 2014, and the unpublished dissertation of E. Schmidtchen, Freie Universität Berlin, 2018, now in press.

5 See the discussion below. The eye-symptoms in the Diagnostic Handbook are in the first instance associated with a condition of the temples of the head, as a secondary symptom affecting the eyes, while symptoms of the eyes as primary ailment usually describe the colour or condition of the eyes (e.g. crossed, uncoordinated, dilated, etc.). These are quite different from symptoms in the therapeutic corpus, although there are some common features, such as whether the eyes contain blood.

6 IGI 1 10' and 12', *šumma amēlu īnāšu marṣā,* 'if a man's eyes are sick.'

7 See IGI 1: 10–13, which involve daubing the eyes with a selection of minerals (including copper) and plant substances, and these treatments are not duplicated elsewhere for more specific symptoms.

8 This distinction between symptom notations which consist of a single clause or those which have a follow-up secondary notation is known from the Hippocratic Corpus, as noted in Langholf 1990 and discussed in Akk. recipes by Geller 2001/2002: 66.

9 IGI 1: 14': *šumma amēlu īnāšu marṣāma u hanṭa,* 'if a man's eyes are sick and burn.' This term *hanṭu* for feverish is unusual in this context, since the more usual terms are either *ummu* ('heat') or *ṣētu* ('sun-fever'), while the term *hunṭu* is more typical of private Neo-Assyrian letters between the king and his court physicians (see Parpola 1993: 336 and the discussion by Panayotov in his introduction above).

10 Lit. 'covered', cf. IGI 1: 21' *šumma amēlu īnāšu marṣāma u katmā,* 'if a man's eyes are sick and closed.'

11 IGI 1: 23' *šumma amēlu īnāšu marṣāma ūmē ma'dūti lā ipetti ina ummi qaqqadīšu īnāšu ṣilla malâ,* 'if a man's eyes are sick and then he cannot open (them) for many days, while having *ummu*-fever of his head (and) his eyes are filled up with a film.'

The text now returns to a single-clause description, moving away from the general category of the eyes being 'sick', but providing the single symptoms of the eyes being 'sick' (*marṣā*) specifically from 'dryness' (*tābīlu*),[12] for which rather elaborate treatments are recommended, applied through daubing or bandaging the eyes. The single-clause pattern continues for the next two prescriptions, again relying upon the general description of the eyes being 'sick' (*marṣā*),[13] but each with distinctive recipes, involving daubing and bandaging the eyes. These *marṣā*-prescriptions may serve as sub-headings for a new sequence of recipes, indicating a type of division between recipes of different categories.

The pattern introduced by the next three sets of prescriptions involves blood in the eyes. The first of these is a compound symptom with two separate if-clauses (*šumma*), the first describing the eyes as 'filled' (*malâ*) with blood, preventing the patient from sleeping, while the second clause describes the middle of the eye as 'red', with the eyes again being 'closed' (*katmā*), as above (IGI 1: 21').[14] The follow-up prescription with this theme is a single-clause entry that the eyes are 'suffused' (lit. 'blocked < *šanā'u*) with blood, which differs from eyes being filled with blood.[15] The interesting feature of this set of prescriptions is the use of Dreckapotheke (bat guano, lizard droppings, etc.). The third prescription in this series returns to the simple condition of the eyes being 'filled' (*malâ*) with blood, while offering no less than four different remedies for this condition.[16]

We cannot be certain about the specific symptoms which follow, since the introductory clauses are damaged, except that the very next prescription returns to the default incipit, 'if the man's eyes are sick' (*marṣā*).[17] This may, in fact, introduce a new type of symptom, as indicated by the succeeding prescription, 'if a man's eyes are found to have a deposit of blood' (*šikna ša dāmi*),[18] and at this point the text introduces no less than three incantations and accompanying medical rituals, and these form a block of text which concludes the recipes which precede it. This division makes sense in the light of what comes next, namely a prescription with an elaborate array of symptoms arranged over five descriptive clauses, beginning with the eyes being sick (*marṣā*).[19] In this case,

---

12 IGI 1: 26' *šumma amēlu īnāšu tābīla marṣā*, 'if a man's eyes suffer from dryness.'

13 IGI 1: 32', 34' *šumma amēlu īnāšu marṣā*, 'if a man's eyes are sick.'

14 IGI 1: 36'–37' *šumma amēlu īnāšu dāma malâma urra u mūša lā iṣallalma šumma libbi īnīšu sām īnāšu katmā*, 'if a man's eyes are full of blood and he cannot sleep day and night, if the inner part of his eyes is red, (and) his eyes are closed.'

15 IGI 1: 40' *šumma amēlu īnāšu dāma šunnu'*, 'if a man's eyes are suffused with blood.'

16 IGI 1: 45' *šumma amēlu īnāšu dāma malâ*, 'if a man's eyes are full of blood.'

17 IGI 1: 57', 59' *šumma amēlu īnāšu marṣā*, 'if a man's eyes are sick.'

18 IGI 1: 61' *šumma amēlu īnāšu šikna ša dāmi šaknā* (*var. inaṭṭal*), 'if a man's eyes have a blood deposit (var. but he is still able to see).'

19 IGI 1: 79'–80' *šumma amēlu īnāšu marṣāma dāma malâ baluhhī dāma ultatanni'ā dāmu dimātu ina libbi īnīšu ittaṣâ ṣillu lamassat īnīšu unakkap ašītu ana ṣilli itūr digal ikabbitūšu*, 'if a man's eyes are sick and then full of blood. They (= the eyes) are suffused with *baluhhu*-granules and blood, blood (and) tears

blood and tears emerge from the eyes, with a film (*ṣillu*) covering the eye's pupil; this medical condition also has four alternative recipes, followed by thirteen incantations and corresponding medical rituals, emphasising the seriousness of the problem, and bringing the reader to the end of the tablet.

The second tablet of IGI is thematically quite different, lacking the general observation that the eye is 'sick', which was a key *Leitmotif* of Tablet 1. What is of primary concern to Tablet 2 is the appearance of eye pathologies, with *murdinnu*-'brambles' appearing in the eye (1),[20] or *giddagiddû*-fibers (12),[21] which are not known from elsewhere, or a flesh-like lesion (or perhaps growth) in the eye (16).[22] None of these can be identified with modern diagnoses. The next symptom follows thematically with a description of hair (perhaps an eyelash) growing out of the eye causing blurred vision (17).[23] A group of subsequent prescriptions share variations of the same symptom of the eye being 'full' of moving tissue, perhaps indicating some type of tumour (19),[24] with variations being that the tissue (or flesh) keeps moving (*illak*, 22),[25] or that the diseased eye is full of tissue and blood (25).[26] The final symptom is that the eye is full of *qūqānu*-worms (27).[27] These worms are usually associated with the digestive tract, but this description is likely to be metaphoric for observable patterns of eye lesions, similar to the presence of 'brambles' in the eye mentioned above.

The prescriptions adopt a new direction (54'), featuring the patient's own report of his or her vision, with some part of the eyes (perhaps the pupils) being characterised as progressively becoming 'dark' (*īteneṭṭâ*), with a secondary remark that this condition is likely to persist and that the eyes will be 'cloudy' (*ippâ*), referring to the patient's vision rather than to the eye itself.[28] The subsequent sequence of eye symptoms reflect what the patient relates, that the eyes feel 'inflamed' (56')[29] or 'pressed' (*ṣuhhutā*, 63'),[30] or his

---

come out from within his eyes. A film pushes away the pupil of his eyes. The blurred vision has turned into a film, and (the eyes) make seeing burdensome for him.'

20 IGI 2: 1 *šumma amēlu īnāšu murdinnī malâ*, 'if a man's eyes are full of *murdinnu*-brambles.'

21 IGI 2: 12 *šumma amēlu īnāšu giddagiddâ ukallā*, 'if a man's eyes contain *giddagiddû* fibers.'

22 IGI 2: 16 *šumma amēlu ina īnīšu lipištu*, 'if there is a fleshy substance in a man's eyes.'

23 IGI 2: 17 *šumma amēlu ina īnīšu šārtu aṣât u īnāšu ašâ*, 'if a hair protrudes from a man's eyes, and his vision is blurred.'

24 IGI 2: 19 *šumma amēlu īnāšu šīra ālika malâ*, 'if a man's eyes are full of loose flesh.'

25 IGI 2: 22 *šumma amēlu īnāšu šīra ālika malâma u illak*, 'if a man's eyes are full of loose flesh and it moves.'

26 IGI 2: 25 *šumma amēlu īnāšu šīra u dāma malâ*, 'if his eyes are full of flesh and blood.'

27 IGI 2: 27 *šumma amēlu īnāšu qūqānī malâ*, 'if a man's eyes are full *qūqānu*-'worms.'

28 IGI 2: 54' *šumma ina īni* [...] *īteneṭṭâ amēlu šū šipiršu ilabbirma īnāšu ippâ*, 'if in the eye [his pupils(?)] keep darkening, the effect on that man will be long-lasting and his eyes will be cloudy.'

29 IGI 2: 56' *šumma amēlu īnāšū nuppuhā*, 'if a man's eyes are inflamed.'

30 IGI 2: 63' *šumma amēlu īnāšu ṣuhhutā*, 'if a man's eyes are under pressure.'

vision is 'dimmed' (*barrā*, 58')[31] or 'dark' (*arpā*, 61').[32] The next symptoms portray what can be seen by the physician, that the eyes are 'closed' (*katmā*),[33] probably reflecting external swelling which blocks the vision. The next two symptoms which can be identified refer to yellowness in the eye (*amurriqānu*), which might be jaundice, and this also reflects an external observation from the practitioner.[34]

A thematic change can now be seen in the prescription incipits, which return to the general theme of Tablet 1 in describing the eyes as being 'sick' (*marṣā*, IGI 2: 117', 121', 124'), but in this case more details are provided by secondary symptoms within additional clauses. It is difficult to gauge the precise meaning of 'sick', whether this might refer specifically to pain or discomfort, or simply that the eye was in an abnormal state. The first secondary clauses provide more precise information, stipulating that the eyes in this condition would not open over several days and would be affected by a 'film' (*ṣillu*), and that the patient's head would be hot;[35] it is difficult to know whether these symptoms occur concurrently or would have been alternative symptoms for 'sick' eyes. The second set of symptoms for 'sick' eyes is also quite specific, that a 'membrane' (*šišītu*) covers the pupil, tears flow, and a 'film' (*ṣillu*) fills the eyes;[36] the distinction between an ophthalmic 'membrane' and a 'film' cannot be precisely determined. The third symptom of sick eyes provides additional information, since the membrane covering the eye is described as a white spot (*pūṣu*, IGI 2: 124'), which causes the patient's vision to be 'difficult' (*kabit*, lit. 'heavy'),[37] again adopting a subjective report from the patient.

After a long gap with either no symptoms or only fragments of *šumma*-clauses, we encounter more objective descriptions of eyes, such as the eyes being 'rotten' (*madirā*, a term with Aramaic cognates referring to eggs),[38] and a series of prescriptions referring to the eyes being 'thickened' (*šamhā*) by the presence of a film (*ṣillu*), with the right and

31 IGI 2: 58' *šumma amēlu īnāšu barrā dimta ukallā*, 'if a man's eyes are dim and contain tears.'

32 IGI 2: 61' *šumma amēlu īnāšu arpā*, if a man's eyes grew *dark*.'

33 Lit. 'covered', cf. IGI 2: 76' *šumma amēlu īnāšu katmā*, 'if the man's eyes are closed.'

34 IGI 2: 115'–16' *šumma amēlu īnāšu amurriqāna malâ*, 'if a man's eyes are full of yellowness (jaundice).'

35 IGI 2: 117' *šumma amēlu īnāšu marṣāma ūmē ma'dūti lā ipetti ina ummi qaqqadīšu īnāšu ṣilla malâ*, 'if a man's eyes are sick and he cannot open (them) for many days, with his head being feverish, (and) his eyes are filled with a film.'

36 IGI 2: 121' *šumma amēlu īnāšu marṣāma šišītu muhha lamassat īnīšu armat dimta illak īnāšu ṣilla malâma*, 'if a man's eyes are sick, and a membrane covers the surface of the pupil of his eyes, tears flow, (and) his eyes are filled with a film.' See also IGI 2: 139'.

37 IGI 2: 124' *šumma amēlu īnāšu marṣāma šišītu muhha lamassat īnīšu armat digalšu kabiti*, 'if a man's eyes are sick, and [a membrane covers the surface of the pupil of his eyes], (and) his vision is "heavy".' Similar expressions occur in IGI 1: 80' (*digal ikabbitūšu*), IGI 2: 126' (*digalšu kabit*), and IGI 2: 137' (*kabit*), all indicating difficulty in seeing.

38 IGI 2: 196' *šumma amēlu īnāšu madirā*, 'if a man's eyes are rotten.'

left eye being treated individually.[39] This brings us towards the end of IGI Tablet 2, returning once again to the standard symptom that the patient's eyes are 'sick' (*marṣā*) but adding a second description of being 'shiny' (*namrā*),[40] followed by a variation of an earlier symptom, that the pupil of the eye or the eye itself is 'filled' by a film (*ṣillu*) and inflammation (*ṣirihtu*), indicating observations made by the practitioner.[41] The end of the tablet is fragmentary and no further symptoms can be recovered.

Tablet 3 of IGI features another type of symptom which attempts to establish causal factors which also serve as diagnoses. The initial short recipe provides a general description of the eyes as 'troubled', meaning 'blurred' (*dalhā*, IGI 3: 1), reflecting a patient's report on lack of clarity of vision.[42] The second prescription combines a subjective description of the symptoms with a putative diagnosis: while the patient continually sees a 'flash of light' (*burṣu*), his eyes are affected by a condition labelled as the 'Hand of a Ghost'.[43] It seems likely the eyes are affected by a Hand-of-the-Ghost medical syndrome rather than assuming an actual ghost as the disease vector.[44] The prescription itself is entirely pharmaceutical with no magical or ritual components to counter the activity of ghosts. More detailed information appears in the following recipe (IGI 3: 9) in a series of primary and secondary clauses, affirming that the patient has been 'seized' by the 'Hand of a Ghost'; it is important to note that the *primary* symptom is that the patient has been

---

39 IGI 2: 199'–202' *šumma amēlu īnāšu ṣilluma šamhā*, 'if a man's eyes have grown bulky with a film.' The verb *šamāhu* usually means to be 'lush' or 'luxuriant' in a positive sense (also 'prosperous'), which would hardly apply to a diseased or filmy eye, but one synonym list (Malku-šarru 4: 209) gives the term *kubburu* 'thick' as a synonym for *šamhu*, which could apply to a condition of the eyes.

40 IGI 2: 204' *šumma amēlu īnāšu marṣā namrā*, 'if a man's eyes are sick and shiny.' This incipit could possibly mark another subdivision of prescriptions.

41 IGI 2: 207' *šumma amēlu lamassāt īnāšu ṣilla malâ*, 'if the man's eyes pupils [are full] of a film,' and IGI 2: 209' *šumma īnu amēlu ṣillu ṣirihta mali*, 'if a man's eye is full of a film (and) has inflammation.'

42 IGI 3: 1 *šumma amēlu īnāšu dalhā*, a similar symptom of eye disease occurs in BAM 522 6', *šumma amēlu īnīšu dāma ṭiri dalhā*, 'if blood oozed from a man's eyes (and) they are 'troubled' (i.e. "blurred"),' providing a physical explanation for the meaning of *dalhu*.

43 IGI 3: 2 *enūma īnāšu burṣa iddanaggalā šugidimmakku*, 'when his eyes repeatedly see a flash of light, Hand of a Ghost.'

44 The term ŠU.GIDIM.MA ('hand of a ghost') is given in logographic form suggesting that the phrase might represent a disease label rather than the actual presence of a ghost. If a ghost was personally involved in causing the patient's illness, somewhere within the IGI texts one would expect to find an incantation or ritual against ghosts; this does not appear to be the case. A similar problem occurs in prescription incipits in BAM 520 (IGI Tablet 4?) 19' and 25', *šumma amēlu mukīl rēš lemutti iṣbassu*, 'if a Supporter-of-evil seized a man', which looks at first like the personal involvement of a *mukīl-rēš-lemutti*-demon, also known from incantation literature (see Farber 1974); in this latter case, the demonic name is given syllabically, not as the usual logogram SAG.HUL.HA.ZA. However, there is no other symptom mentioned other than the 'supporter-of-evil', suggesting that this term served as a label for some kind of medical syndrome which required no further elaboration, without any associated incantations aimed at countering a personal demonic attack (see BAM 520 11', No. IV.8 (p. 147).

attacked by this condition, with the eye symptoms themselves only occurring in the secondary clauses. These affirm that this Hand-of-the-Ghost pathology manifests itself in front of the patient's eyes (*ina pāni īnīšu*) like a lamp, a distant lightning-flash, or like a 'goat' (probably referring to the goat-star Lyra).[45] There is no clear suggestion of a ghost personally presenting itself to the patient, but a pathology which causes the patient to see light in various intensities, presumably at night.[46] This type of disease attribution occurs elsewhere in IGI Tablet 3, in unfortunately broken contexts, in which one finds references to the Hand of Šulpaea (IGI 3: 62') and Hand of Ištar (IGI 3: 63' and 66'); the hands of these gods are rarely found in other therapeutic texts, but are more typical of the Diagnostic Handbook and occasional Šumma ālu omens.[47] These particular attributions to the hands of these gods may also have been impersonal, since Šulpaea's name is glossed with a remark identifying this god with the destructive storm god Adad,[48] indicating an environmental influence on the symptoms. In any case, the atypical nature of these attributions suggests that they represent citations from another genre, most likely being the Diagnostic Handbook.[49]

The next legible incipit in Tablet 3 also provides a diagnostic remark, that the patient is blinded by 'sun-heat' (a type of fever, *ṣētu*); a more detailed description of how sun-heat affects the eyes is not given, except that the eye is 'inflamed' (*hamiṭ*).[50] The following prescription follows suit with a simple symptom that the patient's eyesight (*digil īnīšu*) is diminished,[51] without specifying a cause, but the complex nature of the prescription itself suggests some kind of topical cause for poor vision. More details are to found

---

45 IGI 3: 9 *šumma amēla* ŠU.GIDIM.MA *iṣbassuma ina pāni īnīšu kīma nūri lū kīma berqi rūqi ... lū kīma enzi ištanakkan amēlu šū šugidimmakku iṣbassu*, 'if "Hand of the Ghost" afflicts a man and appears in front of man's eyes like a lamp-light, like distant lightning ..., or like a goat, Hand of the Ghost has seized him.'

46 Marten Stol (personal communication) refers to a general pattern in Nineveh tablets of initial treatments reflecting *asûtu* while subsequent treatments respond to *āšipūtu* or 'supernatural' clauses (as in the Diagnostic Handbook). The point is that attributing symptoms to a 'supernatural' clause (like ghosts) may reflect what the patient sees or thinks but does not alter the pathology of the symptoms, which are essentially the same as those attributed to natural causes.

47 The 'hands' of various deities also occur in the Diagnostic Handbook entry for eyes, see Section VI of the Edition. Regarding the interpretation of such phrases within medical texts, see the discussion in Geller 2015a: 201–203, which disagrees with Heeßel 2007, and Böck 2014: 47, as well as with a recent opinion expressed in Heeßel 2018.

48 See IGI 3: 62', with a gloss *Adad rāhiṣ*, 'Adad causing flooding'.

49 Citations from the Diagnostic Handbook within therapeutic recipes are known (see Stol 1991). Since the Diagnostic Handbook belonged to the bailiwick of the exorcist (*āšipūtu*), such personal attributions of disease to the activities of gods are not out of place within that particular genre, although such references might be relics from prototype symptom-lists from the Old Babylonian period (see George 2013: 85–89).

50 IGI 3: 49' *šumma amēlu īnāšu lā inaṭṭalā amēlu šū ṣēta hamiṭ*, 'if a man's eyes cannot see: that man is inflamed with sun heat.'

51 IGI 3: 51' *šumma amēlu digil īnīšu maṭi*, 'if a man's eyesight is diminished.'

in the next available symptom (unfortunately damaged), which refers to something remiss with the 'hole' or 'perforations' (or perhaps simply 'cavity') of the eye(lids), resulting (in a secondary clause) in the patient being unable to sleep (presumably because of eye pain), and a third general observation that the eyes are abnormal (lit. 'heavy', *ikabbitā*) in regard to their anatomical structures (*minâtē*).[52] A similar description (iii 70') refers to the 'perforations' (or cavity) of the eye(lids) as 'elongated' or 'taut' (*šaddū*), resulting in the patient not being able to rise from bed,[53] which indicates a far more extensive pathology than an ophthalmic problem. It is also possible that these symptoms are not primarily caused by an eye disorder *per se* but rather reflect a condition in which the patient feels like his eye sockets are stretched or drawn tight, perhaps because of severe headaches which deprive the patient of sleep or cause extreme lethargy.

The next recipes in sequence refer to day and night blindness respectively,[54] which have two exceptional features. First, the prescription which follows from the symptom-incipit is not actually a medical recipe but consists of a medical procedure and incantation, without the usual labels of DÙ.DÙ.BI or KÌD.KÌD.BI and ÉN. However, the present reconstruction of IGI Tablet 3 assumes that the incantation and medical application elements are afterwards repeated with their appropriate labels (ÉN and DÙ.DÙ.BI, see IGI 3: 85'–90'). Second, it may not be coincidental that this particular prescription, unique in both form and content, has a parallel in in the Babylonian Talmud (Gittin 69a); the Talmud text is not similar in all respects, but it is similar enough to warrant comparison. Whereas the Akkadian prescription calls for children to be assembled to recite something (now lost), the Talmud has children beating potsherds behind the patient and reciting the phrase, 'be off, dog, depart, rooster!' In the Akkadian text, both the *mašmaššu*-exorcist and patient lift up seven loaves of bread and respectively recite the same phrase in dialogue form, 'accept (the bread)', addressing each other as one with a 'shining eye' or one with a 'staring eye' (i.e. sighted and blind). By contrast, the Talmud passage has seven pieces of meat (rather than loaves of bread) which are to be deposited at the patient's doorstep, to be consumed at the local garbage dump with an appropriate recitation for the night blindness to be removed. Nevertheless, IGI 3: 87'–88' gives an alternative ritual with seven lobes of animal lung to be eaten by the patient at his doorstep, which rounds out the comparison. This is not the only eye-disease prescription with a *Nachleben*: IGI 2: 105'–106' contains a fragmentary reference to piercing the eye of a

52 IGI 3: 68' *šumma amēlu šīli īnīšu ...-ma lā iṣallal eli minâtēšina ikabbitā*, 'if the perforations of a man's eyes .... and he cannot sleep, the (eyes) are 'heavy' in regard to their components.'

53 IGI 3: 70' *šumma amēlu šīlī īnīšu šaddūma mayyāla lā inašši*, 'if perforations of a man's eye(lids) are lengthened, and he cannot 'lift his bed' (get out of bed).'

54 IGI 3: 73'–74' *šumma amēlu ūma kalāma lā immar mūša kalāma immar sîn-lurmâ šumma amēlu ūma kalāma immar mūša kalāma lā immar sîn-lurmâ*, 'if a man cannot see during the whole day, (but) sees during the night: (it is) a day blindness. If a man sees during the whole day, (but) cannot see during the night: (it is) a night blindness.' Also, IGI 3: 75' and 81' *šumma amēlu īnāšu sillurmâ*, 'if a man's eyes (have) a day/night blindness.'

raven with a needle to see which plant the mother raven brings to heal its young, which has an almost exact parallel in the Syriac Book of Medicines, already noted by R. Campbell Thompson.[55] The Syriac Book of Medicines reads as follows:

> *sb prwg' dsnwnyt'*[56] *wᶜqwr ᶜynwhy w'swr bh 't' wšbwq lh bwnh tlt' ywmyn w'tyn 'mh wḥzyn lh d'ytwhy smy' w'zl' wmytyn ḥd mn ᶜqr' wsym' ᶜl ᶜynwhy wmtpthn*
> Take the chick of a swallow and pull out its eyes and bind a sign on it and leave it for three days. When its mother comes and sees it that it is blind, she goes and brings a certain root and places it on its eyes and they open.

As Thompson long ago noted, this matches up well with IGI 2: 105'–106':

> ... *īnīšunu ina ṣillî tutakkap* ... *šammī ša āribu ana ṣehrīšu ilqâ*
> ... you prick their eyes with a needle ... the plants which the raven took to its young.

The legendary healing knowledge of the mother bird may have circulated widely, since Celsus also remarks that the blood of a pigeon, dove, or swallow is an ideal medicament, because the vision of these birds, when injured from without, returns after an interval to its original state, most speedily in the case of a swallow. This also has given rise to the fable that old birds restore vision by a herb, when it returns spontaneously (Loeb Celsus, translation Spencer 1989: II 227).

The end of IGI Tablet 3 is fragmentary and no further symptoms can be recovered. BAM 520 may possibly represent IGI Tablet 4, but in any case, this tablet preserves some unusual symptom notations. In the first example (BAM 520 i 13'–14'), if the patient sees flashes of light, he should simply recite an incantation-like phrase and he will immediately recover: 'I belong to Enlil and Ninlil, I belong to Ištar and Nanaya.' Since there is no additional recipe with this inscription, it appears to belong either to folklore or magic. A second prescription (ibid. 19'–24') is aimed at a patient seized by a 'supporter-of-evil'-demon, which is a symptom in itself; no additional information was required. In this instance, the prescription calls for a 'man or woman' (an unusual combination in prescriptions) to go up to the roof and perform some type of flour ritual. Another prescription immediately follows this one (ibid. 25'–27'), which also gives the 'supporter-of-evil' (demon) as the primary symptom, but a second clause is added which gives further symptoms, that the patient suffers from fever, groans loudly, and sweats profusely; this combination of symptoms is not repeated in other tablets of IGI.

Another key source for eye symptoms can be found in texts comprising the medical series UGU, which appears to be a separate compendium of medical recipes (beginning with the head) which parallels other medical treatises devoted to specific anatomically-

55 See Thompson 1924: 32, Budge 1913: 662, Gottheil 1899: 193, 202.
56 Cf. Akk. *sinuntu*, 'swallow'.

based diseases. The relevant symptoms (from BAM 480, see p. 151) describe a collection of eye-symptoms drawn from individual IGI recipes, such as that the eyes 'blink' (*iṣap-parā*) and present blurred and clouded vision and dimness (*birratu, ipītu, išītu*), excessive tears, as well as the metaphoric 'brambles' and worms mentioned in other IGI recipes. The pattern appears to be that the text of UGU assembles a large number of separate recipes designed to treat a variety of head and eye ailments, all collected within a conglomerate single symptom notation. The eye symptoms in this text, however, are all secondary, following upon primary clauses describing fever in the cranium (or brain) and temples, etc., and the eye symptoms in UGU tend to be general, such as the eyes being inflamed or giving off excessive tears. It seems clear that UGU is not intended specifically for ophthalmic conditions, but in these instances for perceived diseases affecting the head in general.

The final crucial source for eye disease symptoms is the Diagnostic Handbook itself (see Section VI), and the descriptions of eye disease in this compendium follows the same pattern as noted with other pathologies, namely that symptom descriptions show a different character and vocabulary than those usually found in the therapeutic corpus (see Geller 2005: 11, 19). The differences are striking. In the Diagnostic Handbook, much more attention is paid to individual eyes, whether on the right or left, as presenting the primary symptoms, with those referring to both eyes being secondary. The Diagnostic Handbook usually focuses upon colour as a major criterion of disease, in this case describing the eye as 'dark' (*tarkat*),[57] 'dark-red' (*du''umu*)[58], 'black' (*ṣalmu*),[59] giving off a yellowish secretion (*kalû*),[60] or full of red silt (*qadūtu*).[61] Other eye descriptions are unique to the Diagnostic Handbook, such as the eyes 'moving in circles' (*ilawwi*), squinting (*kapṣat*),[62] or sunken (*maqtā*).[63] Some symptoms are standard, such as the eyes being 'full of blood' (*dāma malâ*),[64] or giving off tears (*dimāti ittanaddâ*),[65] or even that the eyes are simply 'sick' (*marṣā*), but in this latter case, an additional secondary symptom explains the general sense, e.g. that the eye is held fast (*kalât*) and cannot be raised (*lā inašši*).[66] In at least one instance, the eyes are described as 'staring' (*balṣā*),[67] which is

57 See VI Diagnostic Medical Omens ...: 11ff.'
58 See VI Diagnostic Medical Omens ...: 129ff.'
59 See VI Diagnostic Medical Omens ...: 124ff.'
60 See VI Diagnostic Medical Omens ...: 7ff.'
61 See VI Diagnostic Medical Omens ...: 71ff.'
62 See VI Diagnostic Medical Omens ...: 54ff.'
63 See VI Diagnostic Medical Omens ...: 93ff.'
64 See VI Diagnostic Medical Omens ...: 71ff.'.
65 See VI Diagnostic Medical Omens ...: 84ff.', along with *ibakkâ*, 'cry'.
66 See VI Diagnostic Medical Omens ...: 59'.
67 See VI Diagnostic Medical Omens ...: 89f.'

the same term appearing in a baroque medical ritual for day or night blindness, in which the ritual actor is described as 'staring of eyes' (*balṣā*), probably no coincidence.[68]

In general, one can easily notice that descriptions of eye-disease symptoms in the Diagnostic Handbook are much richer and more detailed than in the therapeutic texts, employing a very different choice of technical terms than in recipes, and this supports an earlier observation that the Diagnostic Handbook and therapeutic texts originated in very different scholarly ateliers.

1.2 Comparative material

Eye disease in the sole Hippocratic treatise devoted to ophthalmology, *On Sight*, provides some useful comparative data. One ailment is 'eyelids thicker than normal' (Loeb Hippocrates IX.5), or scabby and itchy eyelids (ibid. 6), which might resemble the IGI symptoms of pustules on the eyelids (IGI 2: 108'ff.). Other conditions appearing in this short treatise are night blindness (*nyctalopia*, Loeb Hippocrates IX 385.7), poor vision (ibid. 8), and references to the pupils of the eye being 'blue' or 'aquamarine' (ibid. 379.1), which might indicate a kind of film covering the eyes, similar to Akk. *ṣillu*. It is not possible to diagnose cataract, trachoma, papilloma, or even conjunctivitis, based upon the symptoms described in *On Sight* (pace Craik 2015: 260).

In contrast to the rather poor quality of the Hippocratic data, the Roman writer Celsus has much more detailed information to offer on the topic of ophthalmology, and because of the cosmopolitan nature of Rome in the first century, it is not impossible that some of Celsus' observations come from wider afield, both in areas of diagnosis and therapy. For instance, Celsus reports on conditions such as dimness of vision associated with pain in the head and bloodshot eyes (Loeb Celsus I 139 = II 8.18), or with a disease which he refers to by its Greek name *kephalaia* (ibid. 363 = IV.2.2).[69] Of particular interest to us is Book VI of Celsus, which offers a rich variety of treatments (mostly salves and ointments) against eye ailments, many of which can be identified in IGI. It is clear from Celsus, however, that these remedies were not inherited from earlier Hippocratic medicine (ibid. VI.6.E).

> According to Hippocrates, the oldest authority, the treatment of the eyes includes bloodletting, medicaments, the bath and wine, but gave little explanation of the proper times and reasons for these remedies, things of the highest importance in the art of medicine (Loeb Celsus, II 189).

---

68 It is possible that this medical ritual (see below) originated in *āšipūtu* rather than in classic *asûtu*.

69 The symptoms of the acute disease *kephaliaia* are all known from recipes as 'hot shivering' (*horror calidus*), paralysis, blurred vision, an altered mental state (*mentis alienatio*), vomiting, nosebleed, and with the body becoming cold and weak.

The primary disease-symptom is *lippitudo* (Gr. *ophthalmia*), characterised by excessive tears and mucous and swelling of the eyelids, which can take a variety of forms, such as pain and dryness, ulcerations, sleeplessness, as well as ruptures and inflammation (Loeb Celsus VI.6.B–E).[70] The symptoms described by Celsus resemble those in Akkadian eye-disease prescriptions.

Dioscorides offers significant comparative data on ophthalmic disease, both in terms of identifying ailments and the use of eye ointments as a treatment. As John Riddle points out, in the first two books alone, Dioscorides named twenty-eight different ophthalmological actions, e.g. diseases of the eyes, swollen eyes, pain of the eyes, itchy eyes, crossed eyes (our strabismus), scabs on the eyes, hardening of the eyes, fungus growth on eyelids,[71] wet humours of eyes (emphysema?), misting over of the eyes, sharpening of the eyesight, black eye, and corrosion of the eyelids (Riddle 1985: 49). Many of the descriptions of eye conditions in this list are reminiscent of IGI symptoms affecting the eyes, such as darkening or filmy eyes, but there is no mention in this list of bloodshot eyes or jaundice.

Parallels to the symptoms in IGI can also be found in the Syriac Book of Medicine,[72] which preserve the following symptoms of the eye.[73] Nos. 1–8 refer to diseases of the head.

No. 9. *lk'b' d*^{c}*yn'*, 'for eye-disease.'[74] This statement corresponds to the frequent Akkadian symptom, 'if a man's eyes are sick' (*šumma amēlu īnāšu marṣā*).

No. 10. *ltmr' d*^{c}*'ylyn l*^{c}*yn'*, 'for eyelashes which enter the eyes.' Cf. IGI 2: 98', *ana ... kappi inīšu šūṣi*, 'to remove his eyelash'.

---

70 Inflammation of the eye was distinguished by Methodists from inflammation of the liver or womb, which required different choices of remedies. Eye inflammation was treated by Methodists with poppy-juice, which was also favoured by Celsus, although oil as an eye treatment was considered as troublesome (see Tecusan 2004: 699).

71 Perhaps similar to *kurāru*-pustules on the eyelids in IGI 2: 108.

72 R. Campbell Thompson attempted to relate the Syriac Book of Medicine to Akkadian medicine in the notes to his translations of Akkadian medical texts (see Thompson 1924 and 1926 on eye disease texts), but he did not see general structural similarities in the third part of Budge's monumental 1913 study, which has no parallels with Galenic medicine (as in earlier sections of the S. B. M.).

73 The list of prescription incipits from the Syriac Book of Medicine are known from two late (19th century) manuscripts published in Budge 1913 and Gottheil 1899. Fortunately, the section which Gottheil edited covers diseases of the eyes, and hence its relevance for the present study. We follow Gottheil's numbering of the prescriptions. I am grateful to Stefanie Rudolf for corrected readings.

74 Syriac *k'b* 'grief, pain, disease' is roughly equivalent to Akk. *murṣu* also on the pattern of *k'b krs'* for a digestive disease and *k'b t*^{c}*l'* for 'baldness'; Syriac *k'b* also corresponds to Akk. *marṣu*, 'suffering, sore, sick'.

No. 11. *lʿyn' dʿyr' wl' dmk'*, 'for an eye which is awake (or: watches) and does not sleep.' Cf. IGI 1: 36', if a man's eyes are full of blood and 'he cannot sleep day and night' (*urra u mūša lā iṣallalma*), as well as IGI 3: 68', *lā iṣallal*, 'he (or his eye) does not sleep'.

No. 12. *lʿyn' d'yt bhyn bsr'*, 'for eyes which have flesh in them.' Cf. IGI 2: 16, *ina īnīšu lipištu*, if there is 'a fleshy substance in (a man's) eyes,' as well as a similar symptom (ibid. 19), *īnāšu šīra ālika malâ*, 'if a man's 'eyes are full of loose flesh.'

No. 13. *lmn' dsʿr' dyʿyn bʿyn'*, 'for whatever of hair growing in the eyes.' A similar symptom is found in IGI 2: 17, *ina īnīšu šārtu aṣât*, if 'a hair protrudes from (a man's) eyes.'

No. 14. *lʿyn' dnplyn tlpyhyn*, 'for eyes the eyelashes of which fall out.'

No. 15. *lʿyn' dntnṭrn mn tlg' wqryrwt'*, 'for eyes which refrain from snow and cold.'[75]

No. 16. *lʿyn' dp'š bhyn ḥl'*, 'for eyes in which dust remains behind.'[76]

No. 17. *lk'b ʿyn' ybyš' lʿyn' dkybn w'kln*, 'for dry eye-disease for eyes which are sick and hurt.'[77]

No. 18. *lʿyn' d'kln*, for eyes which hurt.[78]

No. 19. *lʿyn' dṭly' dkyb' wl' ptḥn*, 'for eyes of children which are sick and do not open'. In a non-pedriatic symptom in IGI 2: 117', a patient's eyes are ill and *ma'dūti lā ipetti*, 'he cannot open them for many days.'[79]

No. 20. *lʿyn' swmqt'*, 'for red eyes.' See IGI 1: 37', 'if the interior of a man's eyes are red' (*šumma libbi īnīšu sām*).

No. 21. *lmḥwt' w'šydwt' dʿyn'*, 'for a blow[80] and giving off (fluid)[81] of the eyes.'

---

75 Although 'snow' and frost do not appear in IGI as symptoms, the pair of terms *šuruppû* and *hurbāšu* for 'chills' and 'shivers' are commonplace in medical and magical texts, with the former word cognate to *šurīpu*, 'ice'.

76 This refers to a topos in eye-disease texts, in which specks of dust from the street, or algae, or a kernel of barley remains in the eye and needs to be washed out by tears; see IGI 1: 187'–189'.

77 Syr. *'kl* is a calque on Akk. *akālu*, 'to consume', but in medical contexts 'to be in pain'. Budge (1913: 660) translates this entry as, 'for the pain of eyes which are dry; for eyes which are weak and are being eaten away'; Budge separates the symptoms of dry eyes and 'weak' and painful eyes into two separate prescriptions, which appear as a single entry in Gottheil 1899: 191, 199.

78 Budge translates, 'For eyes which have gangrene,' but cf. CAD U/W 64, 'outbreak (of disease)'.

79 In a non-canonical LB eye-disease tablet (Fincke 2009: 93), a pediatric eye-disease clause is inserted into a collection of prescriptions meant for adults.

80 The eye being 'struck' (*mahiṣ*) or damaged occurs in eye symptoms of the Diagnostic Handbook (see Section VI Diagnostic Medical Omens ...: 55', and 57'.

81 Syr. *my' 'šydwt'* refers to an eye complaint (see S.B.M. 75:9). The term (< *'šd*, to 'pour') in a medical context is a calque on Akk. *nadû*, which refers in medical texts to an organ 'throwing off' liquids (blood, pus, tears, etc.). The usual expression in eye prescriptions is that the eyes throw off tears (*dimta ittanaddâ*), see BAM 521 5'.

No. 22 *lᶜyn' ddmᶜn*, 'for eyes which produce tears,' see IGI 1: 79', *dimātu ina libbi īnīšu ittaṣâ*, 'tears come out from the middle of his eyes'.

No. 23. *lzwq' dᶜyn'*, 'for *inflammation* of the eyes.'[82]

No. 24. *lnqwš' dᶜyn'*, 'for pulsating (lit. knocking) of the eyes.'

No. 25. *lk'b' rwrb' dᶜyn'*, 'for acute (lit. amplified) diseases of the eye.'

No. 26. *lᶜwbyn' wlrwḥ' dᶜyn'*, 'for swelling and wind of the eye,' cf. BAM 518 6', if a man's eyes are 'swollen and affected by wind' (*nuppuhāma šāra leqâ*).[83]

No. 27. *lyrqn' dᶜyn'*, 'for yellowness (jaundice) of the eye,' for which see IGI 2: 115'–16', 'if a man's eyes are 'full of yellowness' (or jaundice, *amurriqāna malâ*).'

No. 28. *lḥšwkn' dᶜyn'*, for darkening of the eyes,[84] which is similar to the symptom IGI 2: 61', 'if a man's eyes are 'dark' or 'cloudy' (*arpā*).'[85]

No. 29. *lᶜmṭn' dᶜyn'*, for obscurity of the eyes,[86] which corresponds to the condition in IGI 2: 54', *šumma ina īni* [...] *īteneṭṭâ*, 'if in the eye (the pupils?) become progressively darkened.'

No. 30. *lmn dmḥyl nwhrh*, 'for one who is weak in regard to light (scil. vision).'

No. 31. *lmn dl' ḥz' blly'*, 'for one who does not see at night,' corresponding to IGI 3: 75' and 81', *šumma amēlu īnāšu sillurmâ*, 'if a man's eyes have day (or) night blindness (*sillurmû*).'

No. 32. *lᶜyn' dnḥtyn ᶜlyhyn my' ḥly' w'wkm'*, 'for eyes into which a bright[87] or black liquid[88] descends.'

---

82 The meaning of Syr. *zwq'* is uncertain but it could be cognate to Akk. *zīqu*, 'blast' (of wind), since the idea of wind blowing foreign objects into the eye is a motif of IGI. See the incantation incipit in IGI 1: 163', *ina šamê šāru izīqamma ina īn amēli simmē ištakan*, 'Incantation: The wind blew in the sky and thus caused lesions in a man's eye.'

83 An incantation (IGI 1: 174') effectively explains this as, *šāru ša īn amēli uddupu ina īnīšu littaṣi*, 'may the wind which has inflated the man's eye depart from his eye(s)!'

84 This may be a hapax (Budge 1913: 557:18).

85 This condition might be caused by a 'film' (*ṣillu*) which frequently covers the eyes in IGI prescriptions (see IGI 2: 117', 121', 139', etc.).

86 The two terms *ḥšwkn'* and *ᶜmṭn'* are synonyms ('darkening') for limited vision, but the latter term would correspond to a film obscuring vision.

87 Although Aramaic *ḥly* denotes 'sweet', Akk. *helû* for 'bright' (referring to the colour of urine) is more appropriate in this context, see CAD H 169 (courtesy M. Stol).

88 This may be a calque on Akk. *adamatu*, 'black blood', which can emanate from the mouth or lungs, see CAD A/1, 94.

No. 33. *lḥwr' dʿyn'*, 'for whiteness[89] in the eyes,' probably referring to a white spot in the eye, corresponding to IGI 2: 124', *ana pūṣi ša muhhi lamassat īnīšu nasāhi*, 'in order to remove the white (spot) from the surface of the pupil of his eyes.'

A further study of the Syriac Book of Medicine in relation to earlier Babylonian medicine is an obvious desideratum, but even this preliminary survey of symptoms suffices to show how similar these medical genres can be.

1.3 Materia Medica

Medical recipes appear to be largely adapted to the particular medical problem they are designed to address, which means that *materia medica* ought in theory to be specific to each condition being treated. On the other hand, it is also clear that certain standard drugs appear frequently in recipes and in a fixed sequence, and this is sometimes reflected as well in drug lists.[90]

The first question is what were the typical drugs used in eye treatments? The usual recipe ingredients were either *simplicia* (a single drug for a single disease), or compound recipes with a combination of minerals and plants, as well as other organic ingredients (often Dreckapotheke); some of these were ordinary kitchen-like substances, others more exotic requiring complicated procedures for extraction. The *simplicia* can either be quite common medical ingredients, such as 'white plant' (IGI 1: 34', 44'), flour (IGI 2: 52'), crumbled bread (IGI 2: 67'), alum (IGI 1: 35'),[91] fox-grape (IGI 2: 63', 86'), pomegranate peel (IGI 2: 115'), or even bat guano (IGI 1: 44', IGI 2: 92', 141' probably a Deckname). More exotic *simplicia* include a kind of paste (*dāmātu*),[92], antimony mixed with sheep bone-marrow (IGI 2: 70', also IGI 3: 46'), or copper patina (or dust)[93] pulverised in gazelle fat (IGI 2: 147'). Other exotic *simplicia* are based upon animal organs, e.g. turtle gall bladder pounded in oil and copper (IGI 2: 71'), blood from a pig's belly (IGI 1: 48'), black snake fat (IGI 3: 68'), or a lizard's head similarly pounded in either oil (IGI 2: 73') or coals (IGI 2: 74'). Other animal organs include lamb ribs (IGI 2: 75') and mixture of cow and pigeon brains (IGI 2: 77'–78'), or eagle brains in mother's milk (IGI 2: 205'). IGI Tablet 3 (IGI 3: 37'–40') contains a series of *simplicia* to treat what is probably a Hand-of-the-

89 cf. Akk. *pūṣu*, see CAD P 539–40, but as a symptom this differs from the description of the eye, *pūṣ īni*, 'white of the eye' (ibid. 541).

90 See Geller 2005: 2–3. This particular aspect of therapy has not yet been fully researched, partly because the list Irianna remains unpublished.

91 a frequent ingredient in mouth-disease remedies

92 See the note to IGI 1: 42'. This paste, represented by the logogram ŠIM.BI.SIG$_7$.SIG$_7$, is not generally well attested outside of lexical lists.

93 Akk. *šuhtu*, also found as a simplicium in IGI 1: 16', IGI 2: 147', § V.1 (BAM 480) 44 and 60. Often *šuhtu* is a substance in which ingredients are mixed, e.g. IGI 2: 103'-104', 154'.

Ghost ailment, and each alternative recipe is based upon a single mineral ingredient: a 'red stone', 'discharge'-stone,[94] a black-coloured glass, as well as pulverised lapis, sardonyx, galena, and obsidium-stones.

Ordinary ingredients found in IGI 1: 10'–11' include 'horned' alkali (salicornia), sprouted grain, and *kasû*-sap to use in bandages for the eyes, while the eyes are then daubed with two mineral substances, *ashar* and *tuškû*, mixed in fat and ghee. Substances like *kasû* occur fairly regularly in eye recipes, often together with *sahlû*, but these two drugs are quite standard in all kinds of medical prescriptions and may not have played a distinctive role in treating eye ailments. Other drugs include *kammu*, thought to be a fungus but was an important tanning agent.

One of the unusual features of eye recipes is the relatively frequent presence of metal-based ingredients, especially copper and lead, as well as minerals such as *kohl* or antimony. This may not be coincidental, considering the fact that lead played a major role in eye-treatments in Roman medicine. Among such ingredients is *šuhtu* or copper dust / patina (IGI 1: 12'–16'; 2: 51', 61'–64', 71', 95', 101'–104', 147', 154', 157'–158'; 3: 53', BAM 439 6', BAM 480 44, 56, 60, 67), or a lead-spoon-salve (IGI 2: 166'; 3: 31', 54', 93', 105', BAM 480 71).

Ophthalmic *materia medica* rarely employ certain common drugs in eye recipes in comparison with other medical genres, such as kidney and rectal disease; examples of popular drugs are *tarmuš, imhur-līm* and *imhur-ešrā*, which hardly occur in IGI. Similarly, the frequent use of ostrich shell in internal medicine is so far lacking, although replaced by a single reference to raven egg (*pel āribi*, see IGI 2: 79'). Occasionally unique drugs appear in eye prescriptions, such as *mirqu*-powder (IGI 3: 41'), which might be a type of glass or mineral (CAD M/2, 108). Eye disease recipes did not attract the widespread use of Dreckapotheke in comparison with treatments for other ailments, although one single manuscript (Ms. NK = BAM 518: 4') defies this pattern by recommending the use of the 'bowl of a human skull' (*kalli gulgul amēli*). Otherwise, the few sporadic references to ox or sheep dung (*kabūt alpi / Šeriš / immeri*) or gazelle droppings (*piqan ṣabīti*) are atypical, with two of these references appearing in the same line of text (IGI 3: 72'). Of particular interest, however, is the use of the term *muhhu*, which in some instances clearly indicates the 'brain' of certain animals (*muhhu ša summati zikari*, 'brain of a male pidgeon', IGI 2: 77'; *muhhu ša rīmti*, 'brain of a wild cow', IGI 2: 77'; *muhhu ša erî*, 'brain of an eagle', IGI 2: 205'), but in another case *muhhu* is bone marrow (*muhhu ša eṣemti kurīti immeri*, 'marrow of a short sheep's bone', IGI 3: 46'). It seems clear from

---

94 This is probably a calculus or bladder stone which was re-used as a medical ingredient (see KADP 4 57, ed. Geller 2015b: 42, 44), also known from the Talmud (b. Gittin 69b). The calculus (*mūṣu*-stone) is recorded elsewhere in the drug list Irianna III 171 as medicinal (see MSL 10, 70: 32, cf. CAD P 107 s.v. *pappaltu*).

these references that Mesopotamian anatomy had no concept of the brain as a functioning sensory organ or associated it with cognition, a later discovery which remained disputed well into Late Antiquity.

1.4 Treatments

In contrast to internal diseases (e.g. *suālu* or digestive diseases, urinary-tract and rectal disease, and gynaecology), which usually call for potions and ingested substances, eye-disease tends to rely upon externally applied treatments. The predominant ophthalmic therapeutic applications consist of bandages or poultices, and daubing the eyes with various substances, often mixed with fats, oils, ghee, or animal, which served as a medium for the drugs. Apart from daubing, drugs could be blown into the patient's eyes through a reed or copper tube (IGI 1: 56', etc.). The various means of treatments can be found in the synopses of prescriptions at the beginning of each edition of IGI tablets in the present volume.[95]

1.5 Comparative material

Some, but by no means all, treatments find similar applications in the short Hippocratic Corpus, *On Sight*, a predominantly surgical manual which may have been composed by a non-Greek author, judging by its clumsy Greek (see Craik 2015). The Hippocratic text recommends purging the body, in addition to salves and poultices, with a reliance upon a copper substance identified as copper sulphate,[96] all of which resemble treatments recommended in the IGI tablets (see Craik 2015: 259–261). Here is an example from the Hippocratic treatise *On Sight* (Loeb Hippocrates IX = Potter 2010: 383, 6):

> Grind a lump of flower of copper against a whetstone, next rub off the eyelid with it, and then grind some scale of copper as fine as you can. Then add strained juice of unripe grapes, grind fine and pour what is left into a red copper vessel.

All of the elements in this recipe have equivalents (copper patina, 'fox-vine', and the use of a copper *tangussu*-kettle), which is hardly coincidental. Otherwise, there is only a brief reference to applying poultices and salves against pain and swelling (Loeb Hippocrates IX = Potter 2010: 385–86.9), and the treatise ends with an abrupt statement, that 'if there is no flux, it helps to apply ointments together with a dry medication.'

95 These synopses were composed by S. Panayotov.
96 See Loeb Hippocrates IX = Potter 2010: 383, translating 'flower of copper,' Gr. *anthos xalkou*.

Eye surgery is more difficult to identify among ancient sources, since the famous example of inserting a needle into the eye to remove a cataract is known only from Hammurapi's Law Code (Attinger 2008: 50), but is not prescribed in any known medical treatises for eye disease, and therefore subject to serious doubt. There is little in common with the methods advocated in the Hippocratic treatise *On Sight*, which recommends the use of cauterisation of blood vessels and scraping of the eyelids, in addition to general bloodletting and cutting of the scalp (see Craik 2015: 260).

The Latin medical compendium attributed to Celsus also offers much more in the way of comparative prescription data than does the Hippocratic treatise, with Celsus' rich descriptions of eye salves and treatments. Pharmacological treatments in Celsus are applied externally as compresses, to be spread either on linen or on wool,[97] and of special interest are the salves (*collyria*),[98] which Celsus notes come in many varieties and blends (Celsus VI.6.2). Unlike in Mesopotamia, these salves mentioned by Celsus are all associated with the names of Greek healers, such as Philo, Dionysius, Cleon, Attalus, Theodotus, and Euelpides, a famous oculist (Celsus VI.6.3–7).[99] The recipes cannot be effectively compared with Akkadian ones because of difficulties in identifying the respective *materia medica*, but nevertheless some general similarities can be noted. Celsus' drug regime regularly contains a mixture of organic (often gums) and metallic substances (usually copper and tin but also zinc as well as antimony). Eye salves similarly tend to mix plant and mineral substances which may have been applied with a lead-based ointment or a lead spoon (*itqur abāri*).[100] Another parallel might be Celsus' recommended recipe of rubbing the eye with the liver of a goat for night blindness (Celsus VI.6.38), which may reflect the various uses of goat milk and goat kidney in IGI recipes. The salient fact is that Celsus' medical work has never been compared with Akkadian medicine, although these were both ancient systems of treatment which clearly had some approaches in common.

1.6 Medical incantations: etiology, not magic

Before discussing details of the IGI medical incantations, it is worth considering the general role and function of 'medical incantations' within medical therapy in general. As

---

97 This is reminiscent of Akk. instructions that linen is to be used in the summer and wool in the winter, also known from the Babylonian Talmud (b. Gittin 69b).

98 See Loeb Celsus = Spencer 1989: II 154, noting that collyrium was administered in the form of 'a glutinous paste which was rolled and formed into sticks shaped like vermicelli (*collyra*).' This shape explains the reason for identifying Akk. *passu*, 'gaming piece', with collyrium, since this might represent the form in which the salve was administered.

99 Also mentioned are salves attributed to one Nileus, Philalethus (Celsus VI.6.10–12), Andrias (ibid. VI.6.15B) and to Hermon (ibid. VI.6.24).

100 See Thompson 1924: 16, suggesting an association between this ingredient and collyrium.

has been previously noted (Geller 2007c), incantations within medical recipes differ considerably in form and contact from formal incantations in Sumerian and Akkadian, which usually have a defined structure. Standard exorcistic incantations traditionally refer to the interference of a demon, ghost, or witchcraft, creating a situation featured in a dialogue between gods conveying the best method of dealing magically with the problem at hand, with the understanding that the exorcist himself is involved in this process; he is the recipient of a divine magical or ritual remedy which can resolve the problem or neutralise the demonic forces. The magic then usually relies upon a formal adjuration of the demons while invoking the names of powerful deities, asserting that the demon or ghost depart from its victim. It is fair to point out that virtually none of these characteristic features of exorcistic incantations are to be found within 'medical incantations', such as those preserved in IGI. In fact, the main similariy between incantations within therapeutic medicine and exorcistic incantations is the label ÉN ('incantation'), which appears before and often after a 'medical incantation' (also as TU_6.ÉN), designating this part of the medical work as a non-recipe text with a purpose other than providing drugs and treatments. These labels alone are the principal shared features with exorcistic incantations, along with the fact that the recitations in both genres may be recited by the healer or patient.

In effect, it is technically incorrect to refer to these Akkadian medical incantations as 'magic', which is itself a problematic term and concept. There is no term for 'magic' in Mesopotamia, and even Greeks and Romans borrowed this term from the Persians; Fritz Graf defines magic 'as the art of the *magos, magus*' (Graf 1997: 20), which is uncanny in terms of Mesopotamian terminology. The closest one comes to this concept is *mašmaššūtu* or *āšipūtu*, the job description of the 'exorcist' (*mašmaššu* or *āšipu*), which is the same type of *Teufelskreis* which Graf attributes to the Greek and Latin terms. The term *šiptu* for 'incantation' or 'spell' (equivalent to the logogram ÉN) belongs to this same semantic field. The problem is that as time progressed, many concepts and ideas within scholastic circles developed and changed while at the same time adhering to traditional vocabulary and terminology, and instead of inventing neologisms, Babylonian scholars were content to give new meanings to conventional terms. A good example of this is the term *šiknu*, which was adapted to mean 'properties' of plants or stones rather than merely their appearance.[101] The term *šiptu* within the context of medical therapy could have also adopted a more suitable connotation of 'etiology' rather than 'spell', since the ÉN passages within the prescriptions generally attempt to explain the origins or characteristics of a particular disease. This alteration in meaning may be reflected in a medical commentary from the noted Uruk scholar Anu-ikṣur, expounding a medical recipe for a stiff neck, with one cause of the symptoms being a ghost shouting into the

101 E.g. in texts dealing with the nature of plants and stones, etc. (e.g. *Šammu šikinšu* and *Abnu šikinšu*). For the argument that Babylonians (like other non-Greek thinkers) lacked the term for and concept of 'nature', see Rochberg 2016.

patient's ear (SBTU 3, 100).[102] The medical commentary remarks about this recipe, *lib-bu-u ki-ma sah-le-e li-iq-qa-lu ki-ma* MUN *li-'u-up šá ina* ÉN *u tu-e*, 'the (hermeneutic) meaning is: let it be roasted like *sahlû*, let it be dried out like salt – as in an incantation or spell.'[103] The idea is that the treatment is to be handled in the same fashion as ordinary *materia medica* (i.e. roasted and dried), although within an etiological 'incantation.'

Another important difference between exorcistic and medical incantations is the involvement of the practitioner himself within the process. The usual understanding of 'magic' is that the exorcist is intimately part of the transmission of a higher procedural knowledge, since he declares himself to be the exorcist of Ea and messenger of Marduk (see UH 3: 82–83). How different is the viewpoint in medical incantations: the *asû*-physician declares that the 'incantation is not mine, it is the incantation (of various healing gods, most often the healing goddess Gula and her consort Damu).'[104] The *asû* casts himself as a technician rather than divine agent; in one incantation (in IGI 1: 100'), he modestly claims to be the one who 'checks Gula's words' (*sāniq qabû ša Gula*), but takes no responsibility for her commands.[105] The point is that the tendency of the *asû*-physician to distance himself from the incantation, even as an etiological text, is in contrast to the role of the exorcist within magical healing, who characterises himself as personally involved in the magical procedures.

1.7 IGI 'incantations'

The inference to be drawn from this evidence is that the amount of 'magic' within IGI prescriptions is virtually negligible. The only attempt so far to analyse medical incantations within IGI can be found in an unpublished doctoral thesis (Collins 1999: 91–95), while a brief note by Marten Stol (Stol 1989a: 165) limited the discussion to whether trachoma might be reflected in an Old Babylonian recension of an IGI incantation. Collins has argued that medical incantations within IGI either describe general eye symptoms or specifically portray a 'sty' in the eye. Of particular relevance are his remarks on IGI incantations featuring two sisters separated either by a mountain or a wall (IGI 1: 98'–

102 It is telling that while ghosts are mentioned as vectors of disease within therapeutic recipes (perhaps allegorically), these same therapeutic texts never appear to have anti-ghost incantations.

103 see Frahm 2011: 97–98, although interpreting this line as referring to the patient, 'may he be parched like cress, may he wither up as if (affected) by salt' – (that is) what is (attested) in incantation(s) and spell(s).' The argument against this interpretation is that it is unlikely that the patient would be 'roasted' (*qalû*).

104 This is already a feature of OB incantations dealing specifically with diseases, as Goetze 1955: 11 [JCS 9], *ši-ip-tum úl-ul ia-a-tum ši-pa-at* ^{d}*ni-gi-ri-ma*, etc. 'the incantation is not mine, it is an incantation of Ningirimma'....

105 A similar phrase occurs in a parallel incantation in IGI 1: 134', but this time checking the words of Anu.

126'), metaphoric for the nose separating the two eyes; Collins infers from the metaphor that tearing or red eyes results from sisters crying because they cannot meet. Other details in these IGI incantations, that the eyes are invaded by foreign matter brought by the wind, such as chaff or dirt or algae, are explained by Collins as 'allergens', and that eye disease can be self-inflicted (Collins 1999: 94). None of this is very convincing, although innovative at the time when it was written.

Part of the incantation repertoire of *asûtu* consisted of incantations which had a long history and were known from Old Babylonian incantations. One of the most notable of these is the incantation against the *merhu* or a kernel of barley (or 'ergot', see Landsberger and Jacobsen 1955, with parallels in IGI 1: 194'–199'), explaining that the speck which enters the eyes and causes pain was part of some original design of creation. Once agriculture progressed through new technologies (irrigation, ploughing, etc.), the inevitable consequence was harm to humans caused by environmental factors, such as the kernel produced through harvesting grain. One key *Leitmotif* of the Old Babylonian *merhu*-incantation was the phrase, *mannum lušpur ana mārāt Ani ša šamê*, 'whom shall I send to the Daughters of Anu of Heaven?', a phrase which gets repeated in Middle Babylonian and later IGI incantations, as well as with other divine figures apart from Anum.[106] The precise identification of this puzzling nomenclature, used to introduce ritual acts, remains unresolved, since the celestial 'daughters of Anu' (often enumerated as 'seven and seven') remain anonymous, while at the same time this designation frequently refers to the notorious baby-strangling Lamaštu-demon.[107]

Let us revisit the incantations referring to the eyes as 'sisters' (see IGI 1: 98'–126'). The key aspects of these texts need to be reconsidered, namely why the eyes should be called 'sisters', and why being separated by a mud-brick wall or mountain (the nose) should cause eye ailments. There is obviously more than one level of allegory here. It is clear that facial physiognomy is being cast in landscape imagery, with the eyes as two 'sides' (*ahātu* = banks or shores) of canals or river, separated by either a natural or man-made border; natural elements may impact on either one or both sides of the divided

106 See Farber 1990: 301.

107 For the celestial Daughter of Anu as a standard epithet for the demon Lamaštu, see Farber 2014: 290–291, 298–299, 362, and see also Farber's observation distinguishing the 'benevolent daughters from their obnoxious sister Lamaštu' (Farber 1990: 301 n. 12). But who are these 'benevolent daughters'? A general category of supernatural opponents, the 'daughters of Anu', also appears in Maqlû Tablet 3, in two diametrically opposed roles, the first being when two or three Daughters of Anu arrive to counteract the activities of witches (3: 31–38), while the second passage (3: 62–63) declares that 'my sorcerers are the Sages of the Apsû, my sorceresses are the Daughters of Anu of Heaven, they hex me, they keep hexing me ', (*ēpišū'a apkallū ša apsî epišētū'a mārāt ^{d}Ani ša šamê eppušūni īteneppušūni*), see Abusch 2015: 72–75. According to this unusual declaration, the Daughters of Anu, like *apkallu*-sages, appear to be esteemed or at least respectable but nevertheless indulge in witchcraft. A new perspective on this question has recently been offered in Schwemer 2018: 176–183, showing how figurines of the patient were entrusted to Lamaštu (as Daughter of Anu) as part of an anti-witchcraft practice, hence employing one evil against another evil.

landscape.[108] The assumption is that just as the elements would affect individual properties on both sides of a boundary, so the eyes as independent organs could also suffer from the same medical condition. The allegory is reinforced by the statement in *Enūma eliš* identifying the source of the Tigris and Euphrates as the eyes of Tiamat.[109] The gender of 'sisters' is a result of the grammatical gender of 'eye' as a feminine noun; the underlying meaning is that the eyes are 'colleagues' (referring to the masculine equivalent *ahu*) in concert with each other when they move, although at the same time being entirely separate and independent entities; eye disease can affect either eye separately or both together.

At the same time, the eyes are also personified as sisters, with one eye not being able to cross over to the 'cheek' (*lētu*) of the other eye. On this personal level, the incantation then alludes to older incantations featuring the 'Daughters of Anu' bringing cold pure sea water to soothe fever or sore eyes; W. Farber refers to these daughters as a 'divine fire brigade' (see Farber 1990: 301–304).[110] Within IGI, however, an attempt is made to identify these 'daughters of Anu' (this time not heavenly) with the patient's eyes (IGI 1: 120'). Whomever is sent to these 'daughters' (in this case, the eyes) brings restorative waters in expensive exotic vessels made of onyx and lapis lazuli, which also casts the entire narrative into the realm of poetry and folklore.[111] This standard incantation motif works well as an allegory, as a way of depersonalising the magic, since the emphasis is on treating the feverish eyes with cool sea-water untouched by any unclean woman. This is far from the approach of incantations known from magical texts, which rely upon the power and authority of named gods.

IGI incantations describing the eyes as 'sisters' (or perhaps 'borders') share a Sumerian incipit (igi bar igi bar-bar igi bar-ra, etc.) with another etiological incantation (IGI 1: 89'–96'), describing the eyes as 'reddish' and 'crimson' (although 'angry' is a possible translation), as well as the eye being 'lazy', 'weak', or simply damaged. The incantation goes on to describe various pathologies of the eyes, such as being filled with blood or spotted, with appropriate allegorical comparisons (to the blood of slaughtered sheep, algae, or vinegar in a jar). The more interesting explanatory detail within the incantation, however, refers obliquely to the nose, which is described as a mud-brick wall upon which the patron god of wild beasts, Šakkan, seated himself, thereby preventing easy breathing (*lā napāše*). The double-metaphor is taken from the simple observation that a nose blocked by the grippe can feel like a mud-wall weighed down by a wild animal

108 See IGI 1: 128'–129', which refers to winds afflicting the eyes collectively, in another parallel incantation.

109 Cf. El. el. V 55: 100–101, *ip-te-ma i-na* IGI^{II}-*šá pu-r*[*a-at-at*] *i-di-ig-lat* 'He (Marduk) let flow (lit. opened) the Euphrates and Tigris from her (Tiamat's) eyes,' see Lambert 2013: 192–193.

110 IGI 1: 120', 'the two of them are the daughter(s) of Anu', referring to the IGI HUL or evil eye in this case.

111 As suggested previously (Farber 1990: 305).

perched upon it, a condition which can also affect the eyes. The incantation adds a figurative dimension to the rather arid diagnoses of the prescriptions, often based on analogies from the natural world.

The igi-bar incipit appears yet again in another incantation within the same context (IGI 1: 111'–115'), but this time asking rhetorically *why* the eyes are suffering from being bloodshot and blurry and in pain. The answer to the question is drawn from the natural environment, that pollen, chaff, or dust is being blown into the eyes, providing yet another colourful allegory to expand the diagnoses of the prescriptions.

Etiological incantations take on various other forms. One of these concerns eye disease affecting the 'lad' (Sum. GURUŠ, Akk. *eṭlu*) and 'maiden' (Sum. KI.SIKIL, Akk. *ardatu*), who appear in magical contexts as innocent victims who have not yet reached puberty (UH 4: 132'–133', see Geller 2016: 156). The incantation itself takes the form of a medical procedure not found in any prescription or medical ritual. In a recipe-like mode, the practitioner (exorcist or physician) is instructed, that 'you' request the offshoot (*libbu*, lit. 'heart') of a date palm, which 'you' soften by chewing and applying it to the young patient's temples. According to the incantation, this should do the trick, since the incantation reports that the eye of either lad or girl should improve (*iballuṭ*). The significant point is that this type of prediction – that the condition should recover – is *not* typical of magical incantations but is a signature feature of medical prescriptions. There is virtually no difference in this case between the incantation and prescription, except that the former is recited while the latter is not, but in any case, the ÉN passage hardly qualifies as a classically formulated magical spell.

However, not all IGI incantations are devoid of incantation characteristics. IGI 1: 163'–175' invokes the goddess Nammu under novel circumstances, which at first glance appear to be traditionally magical. The 'problem' is that the victim cries, suffering from lesions in the eye, and his troubles are noticed by Nammu, the primordial goddess of the Apsû (the subterranean source of all sweet waters); the pattern of a god or goddess noticing the patient's plight is typical of magical incantations, in which the younger god (Marduk) takes notice and reports the problem to his father Ea.[112] Nammu recommends a bandage of crushed *kasû*-plant (a standard example of *materia magica*)[113] combined with reciting the 'incantation of the Apsû', a common magical trope. The incantation also ends in a frequently encountered magical doxology, that the cause of the patient's

---

112 See Falkenstein 1931: 54–55. Variations on this theme occur within Udug-hul, with the usual pattern being that this divine dialogue is most commonly found in bilingual incantations (see Geller 2016: 20). There is a rather free parody of the Marduk-Ea dialogue within Lamaštu incantations, in which Marduk (under his magical cognomen of Asalluhi) sees Lamaštu and reports to his father Ea, 'My Father, I have seen the Daughter of Anu that she is gathering babies (*ušabbašu la'ûti*).' Ea replies in the usual fashion, 'Go, my son Marduk', then recommending an appropriate magical ritual against Lamaštu (Farber 2014: 178–179). This dialogue is one of the signatures of magical texts, but typically not rendered in its fullest form in Akkadian incantations.

113 The common recipe ingredient *kasû* has recently been identified as tamarind, see Eypper 2019.

'problem' should depart (*littaṣi*), in this case with the help of Nammu's touch. This structure looks convincingly magical, until one examines the fine print. First, there is no demon or ghost, since the cause of the patient's 'problem' is wind, which is responsible for infecting the diseased eye. Second, there is no invocation to Nammu or adjuration, but only a brief narrative explaining Nammu's involvement, and in fact the mythological association of Nammu with healing waters of the Apsû is allegorical for physical cleansing of a diseased eye. Finally, apart from external winds infecting his eye, the patient 'weeps bitterly by himself' (*ina rāmānišu marṣiš ibakki*), indicating that his own behaviour is partly responsible for his blurred vision.[114] In effect, despite the veneer of standard motifs, there is little in the way of magic in this incantation.

The patient's own tears are invoked in the incantation which immediately follows (IGI 1: 187'–193'), for a specific reason. The text describes the eyes as porous vessels (*šuharratu*, known from magical rituals), which have attracted the unwanted presence of particles of chaff, pebbles, twigs, dust, or algae, reflecting an earlier theme identifying the causes of eye discomfort. On this occasion, however, the incantation calls upon the eyes to use their tear ducts to wash away the debris before Gula arrives with her scalpel and uses surgery on the eye, always best to be avoided. This threat of surgery (without anaesthesia or antiseptics) was enough to make the patient hope for a cure. The prospect of the healing goddess Gula arriving with her scalpel and medicaments was hardly to be welcomed, and this no doubt reflects the general absence of surgery within medical treatises.

The etiological incantations provide meta-information which cannot be acquired from the prescriptions themselves, nor from medical narratives or anecdotes which might have been known to local physicians or healers. A good example of extraneous but relevant data is found in IGI 1: 159'–162', which responds to the open question of whether eye disease was considered to be a result of ageing and consequently a progressive loss of eyesight.[115] This incantation is addressed to the 'lad' and 'maiden' suffering from eye disease (*īni eṭli marṣat īni ardati marṣat*), followed by the rhetorical question, 'who could heal (this)' (*mannu uballiṭ*)? The most obvious frame of reference for this kind of question is the competition between exorcist (*āšipu* / *mašmaššu*) and physician (*asû*), with their respective methods and approaches. The answer to this question is somewhat ambivalent from our modern perspective, since the unspecified practitioner is told – in a standard 2.p.s. recipe form – that 'you' should chew a date palm shoot, twist it, and bind it on the temples and eyes of either the lad or maiden, to have the condition im-

---

114 The motif of the patient weeping occurs again in the incantation in IGI 1: 176'–179', with the two eyes weeping to the goddess Mami, their 'mother', complaining about their vision being affected by excess blood and wind.

115 An interest in the patient's age appears in Tablet 29 of the *Diagnostic Handbook*, which describes symptoms appearing in various stages of a patient's life (e.g. from birth through age fifty), see Heeßel 2000: 318–338 and Scurlock 2014, 216–222.

prove. Typically, this remedy is hardly medical or magical but something of a compromise between the two, and it was probably intentionally meant to represent a generic practice of healing which could have belonged to either sphere of *Heilkunde*.

It appears to be the case that some incantations are borrowed from another genre of medicine and somewhat arbitrarily inserted into eye-disease prescriptions. For instance, the incantation appearing in IGI 1: 65'–68' is gynaecological, taken from the standpoint of the 'seed' (probably the embryo) who calls out for its life to be saved. But the administering healer (midwife, exorcist, doctor?) judges that the woman cannot give birth and refrains from treatment. The 'invocation'-label (KA.INIM.MA) for this incantation associates it with eyes being full of blood (IGI.MIN-*šú* MÚD DIRI.MEŠ), which could tenuously be seen as related to menstrual bleeding, but the likelihood is that the incantation was intended to illustrate what happens when a condition is considered to be untreatable.

The etiological nature of medical incantations is apparent from other medical treatises, such as incantations against *būšānu*-disease, which affects the nose and mouth. The relevant incantations personify the disease as strong in its grasp (*dān ṣibissu*) like a lion which seizes the uvula (*napšāru*) and head (*qaqqadu*) or like a wolf which seizes the throat (*nurzu*) and gullet (*lu'u*), etc. We need to take special note of the refrain in this incantation, which tells us that the disease has set up its 'seat' among the relevant body's organs which the disease attacks: 'it (the disease) set its 'seat' (*ittadi kussišu*) in the windpipes (*ina imbub hašê*), between the teeth (*ina birīt šinnī*), or in the soft throat (*ina nurzi narbati*)' (Collins 1991: 90–91). The significant etiological point is that the text identifies the localised 'seat' of the disease, comparable to a statement in the Hippocratic treatise *Internal Affections*. This stipulates that while a few diseases have a 'seat' (*keimena*) in the body which can easily be seen, most diseases have a 'seat' internally which can only be detected by analysis of symptoms being hard, moist, hot or cold (see Jones 1998: 206–207, and Geller 2001/2002: 62). The fact that that this form of disease theory in the Hippocratic treatise could apply equally well to both Greek and Babylonian medicine is worthy of note.

Finally, not all incantations are in Akkadian, but at least three incantations for sick eyes appear in Sumerian (IGI 1: 155'–158' and BAM 520, 29'–36'), which is also typical of other medical genres, but one wonders why this is the case. Apart from the fact that Sumerian was the traditional language of formal magic, this was hardly an idiom which would have been understood by a patient, or perhaps even by the physician, and the relevance to eye disease is not obvious. A good example is the short incantation of IGI 1: 155': i-gi ti-la a-ga ti-la, which is hardly 'correct' Sumerian but phonetic for igi til-a aga til-a, 'the front is healthy, the back is healthy' (contrasting /igi/ and /aga/); the association with the previous prescription is only based on the homonym of the term /igi/ for both 'front' and 'eye'. A better example of the genre of a Sumerian medical incantation occurs in BAM 520 (which may in fact be IGI Tablet 4), which retains the signature features of a magical incantation, including a not-so-subtle gibe at the *asû*-physician! Even in this case, however, the text appears to be a parody of Sumerian magic rather than a genuine spell drawn from magical texts. For example, the incantation incipit states, ur-sag ^{d}asal-lú-hi igi-bi hé-pà sag-hul-ha-za hé-pà, 'May the hero Asalluhi adjure that eye, may he adjure the *mukīl-rēš-lemutti* (lit. 'Supporter-of-evil)-demon', which is based on a standard incantation phrase invoking Marduk as a hero (ur-sag ^{d}asal-lú-hi).[116] The problem occurs at the end of the phrase, igi-bi hé-pà ('may its eye be adjured'), since an eye cannot be adjured, but only evil demons, with heaven and earth or gods invoked as witnesses (zi an-na hé-pà, 'be adjured by heaven', etc.).[117] The phraseology of this medical incantation makes little sense as a spell, since the correct formula is zi – hé-pà, to be adjured by a benevolent power. The next clause is equally anomalous from a traditional standpoint, since it appears to be a corruption of the famous Marduk-Ea dialogue, in which Marduk approaches his father Ea in his temple and seeks advice. In the case of this incantation, the dialogue is muddled: ad-da-mu (var. ^{d}da-mu) dumu-sag ^{d}ag-ke$_4$ gù mu-un-na-an-dé-e, 'Damu, the first-born son of Nabû, speaks to him: 'my father'', and he receives an answer, dumu-mu nam ba-si-in-tal/tar igi nu-un-bar-ra, 'My son, the fate has been decided, the (patient) cannot see'. That this is a poor imitation of the Marduk-Ea dialogue would have been obvious to any learned practitioner, since the divine consultation provides a negative result: the matter is decided and the patient will remain blind. Furthermore, the incantation ends with the remark that the 'physician as judge cannot decide this case', that is, he cannot work out the diagnosis (^{lú}a-zu di-ku$_5$ inim-bi nu-mu-un-un-tar-ra), which hardly inspires confidence in the proficiency of the healer's knowledge.[118] In any case, what appears at first glance to be a standard type of Sumerian magical incantation turns out to be something of a satirical version of a Sumerian spell, which offers little support to the common idea that Babylonian medicine was heavily influenced by magic. As in previous cases, there is little actual magic to be seen in these texts.

---

116 The first c. 45 lines of a spell (Udug-hul Tablet 10, see Geller 2016, 324–331) also makes the connection between Marduk and the Supporter-of-Evil demon. See ibid. 328 (UH 10: 20), ur-sag ^{d}asal-lú-hi sag-hul-ha-za dab-ba me-en // MIN MIN *mukīl rēši lemutti kamû anāku*, 'I am the hero Marduk who binds the 'Supporter-of-evil'-demon'; see also ibid. 330 (UH 10: 35), ur-sag ^{d}asal-lú-hi sag-hul-ha-za igi-bar-ra // *qarradu* ^{d}*marduk mukīl rēš lemutti ippalisma*, 'the hero Marduk noticed the 'Supporter-of-evil'-demon.' The epithet is also applied to Ninurta, see Angim II 22 (= 81), ^{d}Ninurta ur-sag me-en, 'you, Ninurta, are a hero', as well as in Lugale 96 (ur-sag ^{d}nin-urta), and it was Ninurta who made fateful decisions (Lugale 437), ^{d}nin-urta dumu ^{d}en-líl-lá-ke$_4$ nam im-mi-ib-tar-re, 'Ninurta son of Enlil has decided the fate'; see van Dijk 1983 II 58 and 123).

117 Another idiomatic usage of this term would be mu pà-da, 'named' (lit. 'name being invoked').

118 Either the physician's knowledge of medicine or knowledge of Sumerian. An alternative interpretation could be that the human physician cannot do the job of the gods. A novel view of this incantation (Zomer 2018) argues that the healing god Damu (representing the *asû*) forbids the exorcist-god Nabû (representing the *āšipu*) to interfere with the patient's treatment. Zomer understands Damu telling Nabû, 'don't impose yourself upon him (the patient)' (nam-ba-ši-in-ri), but this is unconvincing when compared to the variants. In any case, the unorthodox character of the incantation is clear.

1.8 Medical 'rituals' or magical application

As is often mentioned but not explained, therapeutic prescriptions comprise three different genres, characterised by an incipit which typically begins DIŠ NA ..., often followed by a passage beginning with ÉN, and finishing with a third extract beginning either DÙ.DÙ.BI or KÌD.KÌD.BI, usually translated as 'its ritual'. The present work prefers to translate this latter label as '(its) medical application', referring back to the original prescription, with the assumption that the DÙ.DÙ.BI passage adds additional therapeutic information but is not actually a 'ritual' in the formal sense. What is a (magical) ritual? These are usually characterised by fairly standard procedures which involve setting up a censer, a torch, a holy water-container, an altar, and a brazier, often accompanied by making figurines and serving up various grains, confection, and legumes as offerings.[119] Not a single one of these paraphernalia occurs in IGI texts. It is clear from the start that DÙ.DÙ.BI passages in IGI have a different function and typology.

One of the key features of DÙ.DÙ.BI within IGI is the making of knots from various bits of *materia medica* to be tied to the patient, accompanied by reciting an associated incantation (e.g. IGI 1: 69'). On the surface this appears to be a magical act without any obvious medical utility, since knots and bonds are often associated with magic.[120] On the other hand, the distinctive pattern appears to be that magic is utilised to untie the harmful knots or bonds of demons or witches, while, by way of contrast, medical prescriptions tend to engage in knotting and binding either the patient or the *materia medica* for protective or therapeutic usage. It appears, in fact, that the act of untying is magical while the act of tying is (medical) therapeutic. From a modern perspective, there may not be any great distinction between these two acts, but from the psychological viewpoint of an ancient patient, this difference may have been quite significant. Magic serves the purpose of releasing the patient from demonic or witchcraft-induced restraints, while medicine offers the prospect of binding healing substances to the patient's body, for either protective or healing purposes. This may be the reason why medical applications regularly refer to *materia medica* being bound seven times together, with incantations being recited at each binding (e.g. IGI 1: 97', 109', etc.).[121]

Just as medical incantations afford an opportunity for the practitioner to explain (either to himself or to the patient) the nature of the illness or procedures, the medical applications provide additional instructions for how substances are to be applied. A good example are eye prescriptions (IGI 1: 58', 60') which call for daubing the patient's eyes with *ashar*-stone in ghee. Some twelve lines later, the DÙ.DÙ.BI text reminds the

---

119 See, for example, Abusch and Schwemer 2011: 263–264.

120 CAD K 437 goes so far as to define *kiṣru* as a 'knot' made for magical purposes.

121 Apart from spinning and twining red and white cords, making seven knots and applying these to the patient's eyes, occasionally exotic additional ingredients are also added, such as the knee of a sheep (IGI 1: 185').

practitioner that he needs to apply the *ashar*-stone to the interior of the patient's eye (*ana libbi īnīšu tanaddi*) rather than simply daub it, hence providing either additional or alternative information regarding the treatment. The third tablet of IGI employs a different type of medical application which involves leaving *materia medica* overnight on the roof and daubing the patient's eyes with it on the following morning (IGI 3: 27'–31').[122] This appears to be an elaboration of the standard prescription formula, *ina kakkabi tušbat*, 'you leave (the ingredients) out under the stars', presumably so that the mixture could cool overnight.

This survey shows that the DÙ.DÙ.BI passages accompanying the prescriptions are not essentially magical, even if they involve procedures which are unrelated to the direct applications of recipe ingredients. The IGI prescriptions with accompanying 'incantations' and 'rituals' offer important insights into what could be labeled (somewhat inaccurately) as 'secular' medicine. This seeks to establish non-supernatural (i.e. divine or demonic or sorcery-induced) involvement in therapy, distinguishing between the disciplines of medicine and magic. However, these same texts could potentially be interpreted differently by various 'readers', so that an *āšipu* may have applied these same prescriptions and incantations differently from an *asû*, offering alternative explanations to a patient for the efficacy of these remedies. This reminds us that the medical literature from Nineveh chiefly provides information regarding the discipline but not the practice of medicine.

122 The presumption is that the medical ingredients were listed in the preceding prescription.

§ I The Nineveh Manuscripts of Chapter One (IGI 1)

TITLE	IF A MAN'S EYES ARE SICK *šumma*(DIŠ) *amēlu*(NA) *īnāšu*(IGI.MIN-*šú*) *marṣā*(GIG) = Assur Medical Catalogue l. 8.

Sigla notations:
N = Nineveh, Neo-Assyrian. A, B, C, ... designate the different manuscripts.
Translation in italics are tentative reconstructions based on parallels.

Base Manuscript:	**NA (BAM 510)**, collated.
Museum number:	British Museum, K 2573 + 3465 + 6950 + 7241 + 8368 + 8997 + 10321 + 10613 + 10891 +12000p + 12831 + 13393 + 13482 + BU 89-4-26, 155 + Rm 264 + Sm 1464 (+) K 11847 [col. iii 17ff.] (+) K 13465 [AMT 18/1 = bot. col. iii].
Origin and date:	Nineveh, 7th century BC.
Type of tablet:	Two-column, portrait-oriented tablet. The two dividing rulings were made by a twisted thread and several round holes are visible at empty spaces.
Measurements:	ca. 25 × 16,8 × 2,9 (upper edge) – 3,6 (towards the middle) cm.
Copy:	BAM 510, AMT 18/1.
Photo/CDLI nr.:	Plates 1–7/P394523.
Literature:	Köcher 1980b: ix-xi, BAM 510; Geller 1984: 293ff.; Collins 1999: 94 note 39, 203ff., 206ff., 208ff., 210ff. 214ff., 216ff., 218ff., 220ff., 222ff., 225ff.; Fincke 2000: 330. Scurlock and Andersen 2005: 793; Foster 2005: 969f.; Fincke 2009; Geller 2007c: 392; Geller 2009: 5. Geller 2010a: 92ff., 107; Geller 2010b: 61ff.; Lambert 2013: 399f.; Scurlock 2014: 756; Attia 2015.

Duplicate 1:	**NB (BAM 513)**, collated.
Museum number:	British Museum, K 2570 + 3425 + 5000 + 7105 + 11683 + 13389 + BM 98942 + DT 172 + DT 371 + Rm 2, 381 + Sm 821 + 79-7-8, 192 + 82-3-23, 41 (+) 79-7-8, 156 [AMT 8/3].
Origin and date:	Nineveh, 7th century BC.
Type of tablet:	Two-column, portrait-oriented tablet. The two vertical dividing rulings were done with an instrument, presumably with the stylus. There are numerous round holes visible at empty spaces and the sides of the tablet.
Measurements:	ca. 25 × 16,6 × 2,4 (lower edge) – 2,8 (towards the middle) cm.
Copy:	BAM 513; Farber 1998: 68; AMT 8/3.
Photo/CDLI nr.:	Plates 7–12/P394520.

https://doi.org/10.1515/9781501506550-003

Literature:	Köcher 1980b: xi, BAM 513; Geller 1984: 293ff.; Farber 1998: 65ff.; Collins 1999: 203ff., 206ff., 208ff., 210ff. 213ff., 218ff., 220ff., 222ff.; Fincke 2000: 330. Scurlock and Andersen 2005: 793; Foster 2005: 969; Geller 2007c: 392; Fincke 2009; Geller 2009: 5. Geller 2010a: 107; Geller 2010b: 61ff.; Scurlock 2014: 756; Attia 2015.

Duplicate 2:	**NC (BAM 514)**, collated. (The line numeration does not always follow BAM 514).
Museum number:	British Museum, K 2456 [AMT 20/2] + K 2970 + K 2980 + Sm 1897 (+) K 8824 (+) K 2979 (+) K 14879 (courtesy E. Jiménez). K 8824 is a direct join, but cannot be physically attached due to the rough gypsum, which holds the other pieces together.
Origin and date:	Nineveh, 7th century BC.
Type of tablet:	Two-column, portrait-oriented tablet. The two vertical dividing rulings of the tablet were done with an instrument, presumably with a stylus. Occasionally, round holes are visible at empty spaces and on the sides of the tablets.
Measurements:	ca. 25 × 16,3 × ca. 2,8 (lower edge) – 3,1 (towards the middle) cm.
Copy:	BAM 514; AMT 20/2; Plate 18.
Photo/CDLI nr.:	Plates 12–18/P394759 (K 14879, P401052).
Literature:	Köcher 1980b: xi, BAM 514; Geller 1984: 293ff.; Farber 1998: 65; Collins 1999: 203ff., 206ff., 208ff., 210ff. 213, 214f., 216ff., 218, 219, 220ff., 222ff., 225ff.; Fincke 2000: 330f.; Scurlock and Andersen 2005: 793; Foster 2005: 968f.; Geller 2007c: 392; Fincke 2009; Geller 2009: 5. Geller 2010a: 107; Geller 2010b: 61ff.; Attia 2015.

§ I.1 Related Manuscripts containing IGI 2 and 3 from Nineveh

The texts included represent parallels and partial parallels from the other tablets of the IGI treatise.

Manuscript:	**ND (BAM 515)**, see **§ II.1**, parallels: 23ff.', 184', 200'.
Manuscript:	**NE (BAM 516)**, see **§ III.1**, parallels: 32f.', 184'.

§ I.2 Related other Manuscripts from Nineveh

The texts included represent parallels and partial parallels which are considered important for the compilation of the IGI-treatise. They come from other tablets and fragments from Nineveh containing prescriptions for sick eyes or from the UGU-treatise.

Manuscript:	**NJ (AMT 12/5)**, collated, parallels: 61ff.'.
Museum number:	British Museum, K 5852.
Origin and date:	Nineveh, 7th century BC.
Type of tablet:	The two-column portrait-oriented tablet is too fragmentary to judge but might be a fourth duplicate to IGI Tablet One.
Measurements:	ca. 2,3 × 3 × 1,4 cm
Copy:	AMT 12/5.
Photo/CDLI nr.:	Plate 42/P396208.

Manuscript: **NQ (BAM 521)**, see **§ IV. 4**, parallels: 35'

Manuscript: **NU (AMT 14/3)**, see **§ IV.8**, parallels: 81'.

§ I.3 Related Manuscripts from Different Cities

The texts included here represent parallels and partial parallels which are considered important for the compilation of the IGI-treatise. These are manuscripts coming from other periods and from cities other than Nineveh.

Sigla notations:

A = Assur, Late Assyrian. A, B, C, ... designate the different manuscripts.
Am = Assur, Middle Assyrian. A, B, C, ... designate the different manuscripts.
b = Babylon, Late Babylonian. A, B, C, ... designate the different manuscripts.
E = Emar, Middle Babylonian. A, B, C, ... designate the different manuscripts.
H = Huzirina, Late Assyrian. A, B, C, ... designate the different manuscripts.
s = Sippar, Late Babylonian. A, B, C, ... designate the different manuscripts.
U = Ugarit, Middle Babylonian. A, B, C, ... designate the different manuscripts.
u = Uruk, Late Babylonian. A, B, C, ... designate the different manuscripts.
x = unknown provenance, Late Babylonian. A, B, C, ... designate the different manuscripts.
Initial capital letters designate tablets in Assyrian script or northern scripts, and small letters tablets in Babylonian script.
Parenthesis [()] on a siglum designate a parallel text and not a duplicate.

Assyrian

Manuscript:	**AmA (BAM 165),** collated, parallels: 32f.'.
Museum number:	Vorderasiatisches Museum, Berlin, VAT 9467 + 10300 + 10414 + 12261 (+) 11824.
Origin and date:	Assur, Middle Assyrian.
Type of tablet:	Fragments of a multi-column tablet.
Measurements:	VAT 9467 + ca. 11,3 × 7,3 × 3,2 cm. // VAT 11824 ca. 3,1 × 3,9 × 2 cm.

Copy:	BAM 165; KAL 4/52; Copy of VAT 11824 in notes to IGI 1 32’.
CDLI nr.:	P281813.
Literatur:	Köcher 1963b: xvii; secondary literature in Maul and Strauß 2011: no. 52; Geller 2011: 340ff.

Manuscript:	**AA (BAM 20)**, collated, parallels: 23ff.’, 32ff.’.
Museum number:	Vorderasiatisches Museum, Berlin, VAT 8281.
Origin and date:	Assur, Neo-Assyrian.
Type of tablet:	Poorly preserved narrow, one-column, portrait-oriented tablet.
Measurements:	ca. 8,1 × 4,2 × 1,1–1,9 (towards the middle) cm.
Copy:	BAM 20, KAR 183.
CDLI nr.:	P285122.
Literature:	Köcher 1963a: xv; Fincke 2000: 329; Böck 2004: 38; Scurlock and Andersen 2005: 784. Scurlock 2014: 753; Attia 2015: 9, 10, 38, 45, 72.

Manuscript:	**AB (BAM 159)**, collated, parallels: 23ff.’, 41’.
Museum number:	Istanbul, A 198.
Origin and date:	Assur, Late Assyrian.
Type of tablet:	Three-column tablet.
Copy:	BAM 159;
Photo/CDLI nr.:	Plates 42–43/P285254.
Literature:	Köcher 1963b: xivff.; edition and literature in Parys 2014; Scurlock 2014: 754; Attia 2015: 9, 11, 31, 45.

Manuscript:	**AC (BAM 19)**, collated with a photo by M. Guichard, parallels: 32ff.’.
Museum number:	École Pratique des Hautes Études, Paris, EHE 330.
Origin and date:	Assur, Late Assyrian? However, the copy shows some signs (like BA in ^{lú}MAŠ.TAB.BA) in more Middle Assyrian palaeography.
Type of tablet:	Fragment of presumably one-column tablet.
Copy:	BAM 19.
Photo/CDLI nr.:	Plates 49/P285121.
Literature:	Scheil, V. 1921: 6ff. Köcher 1963a: xv; Fincke 2000: 329; Scurlock and Andersen 2005: 784; Attia 2015: 9f.

Manuscript:	**AD (BAM 22)**, collated, parallels: 61ff.’.
Museum number:	Vorderasiatisches Museum, Berlin, VAT 13732.
Origin and date:	Assur, Late Assyrian.
Type of tablet:	Lower half of a one-column, portrait-oriented tablet.
Measurements:	7 × 6,4 × 1,8–2,7 (towards the middle) cm.
Copy:	BAM 22.
CDLI nr.:	P285124.

Literature:	Köcher 1963: xv; Hannen 2014; Scurlock 2014: 753. Attia 2015: 13, 32, 39, 40, 44.

Manuscript:	**AE (BAM 18),** collated, parallels: 41'.
Museum number:	Vorderasiatisches Museum, Berlin, VAT 9896 + 10895 + 12399.
Origin and date:	Assur, Late Assyrian.
Type of tablet:	One-column, landscape-oriented tablet.
Measurements:	ca. 6,9 × 12,5 × 1,4–2,3 (towards the middle) cm.
Copy:	BAM 18.
CDLI nr.:	P285120.
Literature:	Köcher 1963: xv; Fincke 2000: 329; Scurlock and Andersen 2005: 779; Scurlock 2014: 753. Attia 2015: 11, 31.

Manuscript:	**AX (KAL 7/12),** collated, parallels: 100ff.'.
Museum number:	Vorderasiatisches Museum, Berlin, VAT 11096.
Origin and date:	Assur, Late Assyrian.
Type of tablet:	Fragment from the middle part of a two- or more column tablet. Some signs suggest also earlier dating (Meinhold 2017: 53 fn. 15'). There are tiny round holes made presumably by a straw.
Measurements:	7,8 × 7,4 × 1,0 cm.
Copy:	KAL 7/12
Literature:	Meinhold 2017: no. 12.

Manuscript:	**HA (STT 279),** photo collated, parallels: 159ff.'.
Museum number:	Anadolu Medeniyetleri Müzesi, Ankara, 51/72+83.
Origin and date:	Huzirina, Late Assyrian.
Type of tablet:	One-column, elongated portrait oriented tablet.
Measurements:	11,5 × 4,5 cm.
Copy:	STT 279.
CDLI nr.:	P338597.
Literature:	Fincke 2000: 335f.; Foster 2005: 969. Scurlock and Andersen 2005: 806; Attia 2015: 19f., 55.

Babylonian

Manuscript:	**bA (BM 41293 +),** collated, parallels: 41'.
Museum number:	British Museum, London, BM 41293 + 44866
Origin and date:	Babylon, Late Babylonian.
Type of tablet:	Upper part of two-column, portrait or landscape-oriented tablet.
Measurements:	13,4 × 9,8 × 2,6 cm
Copy:	Geller 2010a: 16, fig. 1.1; Plate 43.

Photo:	Plate 42.
Literature:	Geller 2010a: 16.

Manuscript:	**sA (Iraq 65),** collated with a photo, parallels: 32f.'.
Museum number:	National Museum of Iraq, Baghdad, IM 132670.
Origin and date:	Sippar, Late Babylonian.
Type of tablet:	Two-column, portrait oriented tablet.
Measurements:	21,5 × 13,3 cm.
Copy:	Iraq 65: 223, 229.
Photo/CDLI nr.:	Heeßel and al Rawi 2003: 222, 224, 228, 230/P404959.
Literature:	Heeßel and al Rawi 2003; Scurlock 2014: 760; Attia 2015: 23, 37, 41, 64.

Manuscript:	**uA (SpTU 50),** not collated, parallels: 184'.
Museum number:	National Museum of Iraq, Baghdad, Excavation no. W 22664.
Origin and date:	Uruk, Late Babylonian.
Type of tablet:	One-column, portrait oriented tablet.
Measurements:	6,5 × 5,1 cm.
Copy:	SpTU 50.
CDLI nr.:	P348655.
Literature:	von Weiher 1983: no. 50; Fincke 2000: 335; Scurlock and Andersen 2005: 803f.; http://oracc.org/cams/gkab/P348655; Scurlock 2014: 762. Attia 2015: 8, 71, 79.

Manuscript:	**xA (CM 37),** collated, parallels: 36ff.', 61ff.', 184'.
Museum number:	British Museum, BM 54641 + 54826
Origin and date:	Provenance Sippar (according to the British Museum Collection online), or Borsippa (according to Fincke 2009: 84). Late Babylonian.
Type of tablet:	One-column, portrait oriented tablet.
Measurements:	7,3 × 8,2 × 2,9 cm.
Copy:	Fincke 2009: 87, 89.
Photo:	Fincke 2009: 102f.
Literature:	Leichty 1986: 152, 157; Fincke 2009; Scurlock 2014: 759; Attia 2015: 6, 10, 13, 29, 37, 39, 71, 79.

Periphery

Emar

Manuscript:	**EA (EMAR 6/4),** not collated, parallels: 91', 94f.', 103', 136'.
Museum number:	National Museum of Syria, Aleppo? Msk 731030
Origin and date:	Emar, Middle Babylonian.
Type of tablet:	One-column, portrait oriented tablet.
CDLI nr.:	P271301.
Literature:	Arnaud 1987: 345f.; Viano 2016: 417; SEAL 5.3.8.1.

Ugarit

Manuscript:	**UA (AuOrS 23/27),** photo collated, parallels: 73', 89'.
Museum number:	National Museum of Syria, Damascus, RS 25.418.
Origin and date:	Ugarit, Middle Babylonian.
Type of tablet:	Too fragmentary for certainty.
Copy:	Arnaud 2007: plate xiii no. 27.
Photo/CDLI nr.:	del Olmo Lete 2014: plate XVIII.
Literature:	Arnaud 2007: 98f.; del Olmo Lete 2014: 69ff.; Viano 2016: 406.

Manuscript:	**UB (Ugaritica 5),** photo collated, parallels: 91', 136'.
Museum number:	National Museum of Syria, Damascus, RS 20.006.
Origin and date:	Ugarit, Middle Babylonian.
Type of tablet:	One-column, landscape-oriented tablet.
Copy:	Nougayrol 1968: no. 19
Literature:	Nougayrol 1968: 64f.; Fincke 2000: 338; Foster 2005: 967; Westenholz 2010: 389; del Olmo Lete 2014: 69ff.; SEAL 5.3.8.2.

Manuscript:	**UC (AuOrS 23/14),** not collated, parallels: 93', 98', 110'.
Museum number:	National Museum of Syria, Damascus, RS 94.2178.
Origin and date:	Ugarit, Middle Babylonian.
Type of tablet:	One-column, landscape-oriented tablet.
Literature:	Arnaud 2007: plate xif. no. 14; del Olmo Lete 2014: 59ff.; Viano 2016: 406.

§ I.4 Synopsis of the Prescriptions of Chapter One (IGI 1)

1ff.' Fragmentary prescriptions: preparation of medication in a bowl, daubing the eyes.

6f.' No diagnosis (but presumably as the previous one): medication with minerals, bat guano, bones, bone marrow, all pounded and blown into the eyes.

8f.' Medical application prescription for tying braided wool on the head containing sesame oil and plants, repeated over three days, daubing[?].

10f.' Prescription for sick eyes: plants, minerals and ghee, pounded in the sap of a *kasû*-plant, bandaging; minerals drenched in fat and pounded and mixed in ghee, daubing.

12f.' Prescription for sick eyes: sesame oil smeared on the temples; bandage with copper patina on the head temples; exudation of copper and minerals mixed in ghee, daubing the eyes: prognosis for recovery.

14f.' Prescription for sick and burning eyes: copper patina mixed in ghee, daubing; cutting garlic with a bronze knife, three times daubing; plant kneaded in beer dregs, bandaging.

16f.' Prescription for sick and burning eyes: parched and crushed copper patina, pounded in ghee, daubing.

18ff.' No diagnosis (but presumably same as the previous one): plant boiled in beer dripped into the eyes; preparation of plant mixture, bandaging; salve from condensed reddish kidney fat pounded on a spoon, daubing.

21f. Prescription for sick and closed eyes: rinsing seeds and plants, bandaging; medication of plants, daubing.

23ff. Prescription, known from numerous sources, for sick eyes, which cannot be opened for many days, being accompanied with fever: shaving the head, cooling it with dough; salve of plants and ghee on spoon, daubing.

26' Prescription for dry eyes: onion being chopped by the patient, drunk in beer, sprinkling oil into eyes: prognosis for recovery.

27' No diagnosis (but presumably same as the previous one): swallowing a pill on an empty stomach, consisting of powder of date stones kneaded in the sap of a *kasû*-plant.

28' No diagnosis (but presumably same as the previous one): salve of frog's bile mixed in ghee, daubing.

29' No diagnosis (but presumably same as the previous one), mixture of plant powder and flour kneaded in the sap of a *kasû*-plant, bandaging eyes and temples.

30f.' Fragmentary incantation for activating substances.

32f.' Prescription for sick eyes, known from numerous sources: plants roasted over charcoal, stirred in ghee, a sheep's kidney fat, wax, daubing.

34' Prescription for sick eyes: daubing the eyes with simplicia: plant and bat guano mixed in ghee, daubing.

35' Prescription for sick eyes: daubing the eyes with simplicia: a mineral pounded in ghee, a plant boiled in milk, bandaging.

36ff.' Prescription for eyes full of blood, including sleepless state with closed eyes: mixture of parched plant, a sheep's dung in the milk from a woman in maternity, bandaging. In the morning loosening the bandage, daubing the eyes with salve from pounded mineral in ghee, plant medication, bandaging the eyes with the plant wrapped in red and white wool, daubing.

40ff.' Prescription for eyes suffused with blood: mixture of plants and paste in honey, daubing; mixture of bat guano, plant and saline solution, daubing.

42' No diagnosis (but presumably same as the previous one): dryed plant spattered into the eyes, paste in ghee, presumably daubing.

43' No diagnosis (but presumably same as the previous one): lizard excrement in bone marrow, no consumption, presumably daubing or oral intake.

44' No diagnosis (but presumably same as the previous one): simplicia in oil and ghee, daubing.

45' Prescription for eyes full of blood: salve of simplicium in ghee, daubing.

46' No diagnosis (but presumably same as the previous one): salve of plants in ghee, daubing.

47' No diagnosis (but presumably same as the previous one): daubing with simplicia: pounded mineral in spittle, pounded mineral in the milk from a woman in maternity, daubing

48' No diagnosis (but presumably same as the previous one): dripping pig blood into the eyes.

49ff.' Fragmentary prescriptions for different seasons, plants mixed in different solvents depending on the season, daubing; blowing medication into the eyes.

57' Prescription for [sick eyes]: plants and powder mixture, drunk in wine.

58' No diagnosis (but presumably same as the previous one), salve of plants and stones pounded in ghee, daubing.

59f.' Prescription for sick eyes: bandaging; a mineral pounded in ghee, daubing.

61ff.' Prescription for bloody eyes: mixture of bat guano, saline, plants ground together in a sheep's bile, seasonal application, the mixture dissolved in different solvents depending on the season, daubing.

64' No diagnosis (but presumably same as the previous one): mixture of bat guano in mountain honey, daubing. This is a drug which is to be used for twenty days.

65ff.' Incantation for blood in the eyes.

69' Medical application with plants, knotted together, accompanying the previous incantation and recited over the fourteen plant knots.

70f.' Incantation for blood in the eyes.

72' Medical application accompanying the previous incantation: a mineral pounded in ghee, applied into the eyes.

73ff.' Incantation for blood in the eyes.

78' Medical application accompanying the previous incantation: pounded plant, resin, lizard excrement stirred in goat's milk, bandaging.

79ff.' Prescription for sick eyes with blood, tears, and film, accompanied by blurred vision: plant sap, dissolved in vinegar, macerated overnight under stars, processed in the morning, mixed with minerals, copper exudation and plants. All stirred together in rinsed vessel, kneaded in ghee and (pounded) mineral. The upper part of the eyes opened with the healer's finger and the medication applied onto the eyes. Then eyes must be kept closed and rubbed with the mixture for nine days.

86' Prescription for the same case: plant simplicium mixed in saline solution, and blown via a bronze tube into the eyes.

87' Alternative prescription for the same case: pounded exudation of copper and white plant blown into the eyes via a bronze tube.

88' Alternative prescription for the same case: pounded plants blown into the eyes via a bronze tube.

89ff.' Incantation for sick eyes.

97' Medical application accompanying the previous incantation recited over seven knots of white wool.

98ff.' Incantation for sick eyes.

109' Medical application accompanying the previous incantation recited over seven knots of red wool.

110ff.' Incantation for sick eyes.

117f.' Medical application accompanying the previous incantation recited over seven knots of red and white wool. Tying cords of red wool on the sick eye, and cord of white wool on the healthy eye: prognosis for recovery.

119ff.' Incantation for sick eyes with the same medical application as the previous one.

125ff.' Incantation for sick eyes with the same medical application as the previous one.

132ff.' Incantation for sick eyes with the same medical application as the previous one.

136ff.' Fragmentary incantations and medical applications.

150ff.' Incantation for sick eyes.

154' Medical application accompanying the previous incantation recited over seven knots of red and white wool: prognosis for recovery.

155f.' Incantation for sick eyes with the same medical application as the previous one.

157f.' Incantation for sick eyes with the same medical application as the previous one.

159ff.' Incantation for sick eyes with the same medical application as the previous one: prognosis for recovery.

163ff.' Bilingual incantation for sick eyes, without accompanying medical application.

176ff.' Incantation for sick eyes.

180f.' Medical application accompanying the previous incantation recited over tampons of red and white wool, red wool tampon applied on the sick eye, and the white one on the healthy: prognosis for recovery.

182ff.' Incantation for murky eyes.

185f.' Medical application with a sheep's knee, accompanying the previous incantation recited over seven knots: prognosis for recovery.

187ff.' Incantation for removing foreign objects from the eye as chaff, sherd or anything, without accompanying medical application.

194ff.' Incantation for removing the foreign object/disease (*merhu*) from the inside of the eyes.

200ff.' Catchline of chapter (tablet) two, name of chapter one, and not preserved Ashurbanipal colophon.

Edition of IGI 1

1’ [...] x [...] **2’** [...] *teqqi*	1’[...] x [...] 2’[...] you daub [(his eyes)].

1’ NC i 1’ [..] x [...]

2’ NC i 2’ [..] x *te-q*[*í*]

3’ [... *ana*] *pursīti taṣahhat* **4’** [...] *īnīšu teqqi*	3’[...] you press (their saps) out [into] a *pursītu*-bowl. 4’[... (and)] you daub his eyes.

3’ NC i 3’ [.. *ana* ^{du}]^{g}⸢BUR⸣.ZI ⸢SUR⸣

4’ NC i 4’ [..IGI.MI]N-⸢*šú*⸣ *te-qí*

5’ [...] ... **6’** *lulâ rikibti arkabi lipi eṣemti kurīti ša* [*immeri ... tasâk ...*]	5’[...] ... 6’[You pound] *lulû*-antimony, bat guano, marrow of a short bone of [a sheep ...]

5’ NC i 5’ [..] x-⸢*ma*?⸣

6’ NA i 1’ [KÙ.G]AN ⸢U_5.ARGAB^{mušen} Ì⸣.UDU GÌR.PAD.DA LÚGUD.DA *ša* [UDU ... SÚD ...]

NC i 6’ [..] x

NO DIVIDING LINE TO BE SEEN AFTER NC I 6’! PLACE TOO BROKEN.

7’ *šīpa tasâk ina* [*takkussi ana libbi īnīšu tanappah*]	7’You pound *šīpu*-paste, (which) [you blow into his eyes] through a reed-[straw].

7’ NA i 2’ [Š]IM.BI.KÙ.GI SÚD *ina* ^{g}[^{i}SAG.KUD *ana* ŠÀ IGI.MIN-*šú* BÚN]

NC i 7’ [..] x

NO DIVIDING LINE TO BE SEEN AFTER NC I 7’! PLACE TOO BROKEN.

Overview of IGI 1 Manuscripts and Parallels: **AA**=BAM 20; **AB**=BAM 159; **AC**=BAM 19; **AD**=BAM 22; **AE**=BAM 18; **AmA**=BAM 165; **AX**=KAL 7/12; **bA**=BM 41293+; **EA**=EMAR 6/4; **HA**=STT 279; **NA**=BAM 510; **NB**=BAM 513; **NC**=BAM 514; **ND**=BAM 515; **NE**=BAM 516; **NJ**=AMT 12/5; **NQ**=BAM 521; **NU**=AMT 14/3; **sA**=IRAQ 65; **UA**=AuOrS 23/27; **uA**=SpTU 50; **UB**=Ugaritica 5; **UC**=AuOrS 23/14; **xA**=CM 37

https://doi.org/10.1515/9781501506550-004

8' *kunša qaqqassu tarakkas ešeret* SILA$_4$!(KISAL) *šamna mišil* SILA$_4$!(KISAL) [... *ana*] *qaqqadīšu tašappak* [...] **9'** UD.3.KAM *tēteneppuš sahlê turrar tasâk* [...] ...	[8']You tie a wool braid on his head. You pour 10 SILA-measure sesame oil (and) one-half SILA-measure [... onto] his head (and) [...] [9']For three days, you do it again and again, you parch (and) pound *sahlû*-plant [...] ...

8' NA i 3' ⌜*kun*⌝-*ša*$_{25}$ SAG.DU-*su* KEŠDA 10 SILA$_4$!(KISAL) Ì+⌜GIŠ 1/2 SILA$_4$!(KISAL)⌝ x [...]

NC i 8' [.. *ana* SA]G$^?$.⌜DU$^?$-*šú*$^?$⌝ DUB-*a*[*k*$^?$ ....] x

9' NA i 4' UD.3.KAM* DÙ.DÙ-*uš* ZÀ.HI.LI ⌜*tur-ár*⌝ SÚD [..................................] x

NC i 9' [.................................ZÀ.HI.LI *t*]*ur-ár* SÚD x [................................] x

10' *šumma amēlu īnāšu marṣā habbur še'i arqūssu uhūla qarnānâ tasâk ina mê kasî talâš īnīšu taṣammid* **11'** *ashar tuškâ tasâk ina lipî tutahhah malmališ tasâk ina himēti taballal īnīšu teqqi*	[10']If a man's eyes are sick: you pound grain-sprout while still green, (and) horned *uhūlu*-alkali, you knead (them) in the sap of a *kasû*-plant, (and) bandage his eyes. [11']You pound *ashar*-stone (and) *tuškû*-mineral, drench (them) in fat, pound (them) in equal measure (and) mix (them) in ghee. You daub his eyes (with it).

10' NA i 5' DIŠ NA IGI.MIN-*šú* GIG HÉNBUR ŠE.AM ⌜SIG$_7$-*su*⌝ NAGA.SI SÚD *ina* A GAZI^{sar} SILA$_{11}$-⌜*aš*⌝ [............................]

NC i 10' [................................. HÉ]NBUR$^?$ ⌜ŠE.AM⌝ SIG$_7$-*su* NAGA.SI SÚD *ina* A GAZI^{sa}[^{r} SILA$_{11}$-*aš* IGI.MIN-*š*]*ú* ⌜LAL-*id*⌝

11' NA i 6' ^{na4}*às-har* ^{na4}*tu-uš-*⌜*ka-a*⌝ SÚD *ina* Ì.UDU *tu-tah-ha-ah mal-ma-liš* SÚD *ina* Ì.NUN H[E.HE ....]

NC i 11' [^{na4}*às-har* ^{n}]^{a4} ⌜*tuš-ka-a* SÚD *ina* Ì.UDU *tu*⌝-*tah-ha-ah mal-ma-liš* SÚD *ina* Ì.NUN H[E.HE IGI.M]IN-⌜*šú*⌝ MAR

Overview of IGI 1 Manuscripts and Parallels: **AA**=BAM 20; **AB**=BAM 159; **AC**=BAM 19; **AD**=BAM 22; **AE**=BAM 18; **AmA**=BAM 165; **AX**=KAL 7/12; **bA**=BM 41293+; **EA**=EMAR 6/4; **HA**=STT 279; **NA**=BAM 510; **NB**=BAM 513; **NC**=BAM 514; **ND**=BAM 515; **NE**=BAM 516; **NJ**=AMT 12/5; **NQ**=BAM 521; **NU**=AMT 14/3; **sA**=IRAQ 65; **UA**=AuOrS 23/27; **uA**=SpTU 50; **UB**=Ugaritica 5; **UC**=AuOrS 23/14; **xA**=CM 37

12’ *šumma amēlu īnāšu marṣā ešeret* SILA$_4$!(KISAL) *šamna ana nakkapātīšu tattanaddi šuhta ša aškāpi ina nādi tesêr* **13’** *ina nakkapātīšu taṣammid hīl erî ashar šīpa tasâk ina himēti taballal īnīšu tēteneqqīma iballuṭ*	12’If a man’s eyes are sick: you keep on applying 10 SILA-measure of sesame oil on his temples. You spread copper patina from a leatherworker onto a waterproof leather. 13’You bandage his temples (with the leather). You pound exudation of copper, *ashar*-stone (and) *šīpu*-paste, you mix (them) in ghee, you keep daubing his eyes, then he should recover.

12’ NA i 7’ ⌜DIŠ⌝ NA IGI.MIN-*šú* GIG 10 GA[ZI$^?$ .... *an*]*a* ⌜SAG⌝.KI.MEŠ-*šú* ŠUB.MEŠ *šu-uh-ta ša* AŠGAB *ina* KUŠ.EDIN [*te-ser*]

NC i 12’ ⌜DIŠ NA⌝ [IGI.MIN]-⌜*šú* GIG 10 SILA$_4$!(KISAL)$^?$ Ì.GIŠ *ana* SAG⌝.KI.MEŠ-*šú* ŠUB.MEŠ *šu-uh-ta ša* AŠ[GAB .... *t*]*e*$^?$-⌜*ser*$^?$⌝

13’ NA i 8’ [*ina* SA]G.KI.MEŠ-*šú* L[AL-*id* .... ^{n}]^{a4}*áš-har* ŠIM.BI.KÙ.GI SÚD *ina* Ì.NUN HE.HE IGI.MIN-*šú* MAR.⌜MEŠ⌝-*m*[*a*$^?$ T]I$^?$

NC i 13’ ⌜*ina*⌝ S[AG.K]I$^?$.[MEŠ-*š*]*ú* LAL-⌜*id* ILLU URUDU ^{na4}*ás-har*⌝ ŠIM.BI.KÙ.GI SÚD *ina* Ì.NUN HE.HE [..] x

14’ *šumma amēlu īnāšu marṣāma u hanṭā šuhta ša tangussi ina himēti tasâk īnīšu teqqi patar siparri* **15’** *ina mê temessi šūmī tasâk ištiššu šinīšu šalāšīšu īnīšu teqqi sahlê ina šuršummē šikari talâš taṣammid*	14’If a man’s eyes are sick and burn: you pound patina of a copper *tangussu*-kettle in ghee (and) daub his eyes. 15’You wash 14’a bronze knife 15’in water, you pound (with it) garlic (and) daub his eyes (with the paste) once, twice, three times. You knead *sahlû*-plant in beer dregs (and) you bandage (his eyes).

14’ NA i 9’ [.. SAH]AR.URUDU *ša* ŠEN.TUR *ina* Ì.NUN SÚD IGI.MIN-*šú* MAR GÍR.ZABAR

NC i 14’ ⌜DIŠ NA IGI.MIN-*šú* GIG-*ma u ha-an*⌝-*ṭa* SAHAR.URUDU *ša* ŠEN.TUR *ina* Ì.NUN SÚD IGI.M[IN-*šú* ....]

15’ NA i 10’ [..] ⌜1-*šú*⌝ 2-*šú* 3-*šú* IGI.MIN-*šú* MAR ZÀ.HI.LI *ina šur-šum-me* KAŠ SILA$_{11}$-*aš* LAL

Overview of IGI 1 Manuscripts and Parallels: **AA**=BAM 20; **AB**=BAM 159; **AC**=BAM 19; **AD**=BAM 22; **AE**=BAM 18; **AmA**=BAM 165; **AX**=KAL 7/12; **bA**=BM 41293+; **EA**=EMAR 6/4; **HA**=STT 279; **NA**=BAM 510; **NB**=BAM 513; **NC**=BAM 514; **ND**=BAM 515; **NE**=BAM 516; **NJ**=AMT 12/5; **NQ**=BAM 521; **NU**=AMT 14/3; **sA**=IRAQ 65; **UA**=AuOrS 23/27; **uA**=SpTU 50; **UB**=Ugaritica 5; **UC**=AuOrS 23/14; **xA**=CM 37

NC i 15' ⌜*ina* A LUH-*si* SUM[sar]⌝ *t*[*a-sàk*[?]] ⌜1-*šú*⌝ 2-*šú* 3-*šú* IGI.MIN-*šú* MAR ZÀ.HI.LI *in*[*a* ....]

16' *šumma* ... [... *šuhta*] *ša tangussi turrar tahaššal ina himēti damiqte tasâk* **17'** *enūma tēpušu* [...] *īnīšu teqqi*	[16']If ... [...] you parch (and) crush [patina] from a copper *tangussu*-kettle, (and) you pound (it) in a good quality ghee. [17']When you have made it [... (and)] you daub his eyes.

16' NA i 11' [...SAHAR.URUDU *š*]*a* ⌜ŠEN⌝.TUR *tur-ár* GAZ *ina* Ì.NUN SIG$_5$-*te ta-sàk*

NB i 1' [DIŠ] x x x (x) [...]

NC i 16' D[IŠ[?]... ŠEN.TU]R[?] ⌜*tur*[?]-*ár*[?]⌝ [...]

17' NA i 12' [...] IGI.MIN-*šú te-qí*

NB i 2' UD-*ma* DÙ-⌜*šú*⌝ [..]

NC i 17' too broken

18' *aktam tasâk ina šikari tušabšal* [...] *ana libbi īnīšu tunattak maštakal tasâk taṣammid* **19'** *papparhâ tasâk taṣammid sīha argāna barīrāta ina šizbi talâš taṣammid* **20'** *lipi kalīti sāma ina ṣēti tanaddi ina itqūr abāri tasâk īnīšu teqqi*	[18']You pound *aktam*-plant (and) boil it in beer [...]. You drip (the mixture) into his eyes. You pound *maštakal*-plant and bandage (his eyes). [19']You pound *papparhû*-purslane (and) bandage (his eyes). You knead *sīhu*-artemisia, *argānu*-plant, (and) *barīrātu*-sagapenum in milk (and) you bandage (his eyes). [20']You put reddish kidney fat in the sun-heat (and) pound (it) into a lead spoon(salve) (and) you daub his eyes.

18' NA i 13' [.. *an*]*a* ⌜ŠÀ⌝ IGI.MIN-*šú tu-na-ták* [ú]IN$_6$.ÚŠ SÚD LAL

NB i 3' [ú]*ak-tam* SÚD *ina* KAŠ ŠEG$_6$ x [...]

NC i 18' too broken

Overview of IGI 1 Manuscripts and Parallels: **AA**=BAM 20; **AB**=BAM 159; **AC**=BAM 19; **AD**=BAM 22; **AE**=BAM 18; **AmA**=BAM 165; **AX**=KAL 7/12; **bA**=BM 41293+; **EA**=EMAR 6/4; **HA**=STT 279; **NA**=BAM 510; **NB**=BAM 513; **NC**=BAM 514; **ND**=BAM 515; **NE**=BAM 516; **NJ**=AMT 12/5; **NQ**=BAM 521; **NU**=AMT 14/3; **sA**=IRAQ 65; **UA**=AuOrS 23/27; **uA**=SpTU 50; **UB**=Ugaritica 5; **UC**=AuOrS 23/14; **xA**=CM 37

19’ NA i 14’ [.. *ba-r*]*i-ra-ta*$_5$ *ina* GA *ta-là-aš* LAL

NB i 4’ BABBAR.HI^{sar} *ta-sàk* LAL ^{giš}*si-ha* ^{giš}*a*[*r-ga-nu* ....]

NC i 19’ too broken

20’ NA i 15’ [.. *i*]*na* DÍLIM A.BÁR SÚD IGI.MIN-*šú* MAR

NB i 5’ Ì.UDU ⌜ÉLLAG⌝ SA$_5$ *ina* UD.DA ŠUB ⌜*i*⌝-*n*[*a*$^?$ ....]

NC i 20’ [..M]AR

21’ *šumma amēlu īnāšu marṣāma u katmā kikkirâna* [...] *supāla arqūssu* **22’** *ina mê temessi taṣammid inib errî šamma peṣâ* [*tasâk* ... *īnī*]*šu teqqi*	[21’]If a man’s eyes are sick and closed: [22’]you wash *kikkirânu*-aromatic [..., and] [21’]*supālu*-juniper while still green in water, [22’](and) you bandage (his eyes). You [pound] fruit of *errû*-colocynth, white plant [...], (and) you daub his [eyes].

21’ NA i 16’ [..^{š}]^{im}⌜ŠE⌝.L[I........ *s*]*u*-⌜*pa-la*⌝ SIG$_7$-*su*

NB i 6’ DIŠ NA IGI.MIN-*šú* GIG-*ma ù* DUL ^{šim}⌜ŠE⌝.L[I$^?$......................................]

NC i 21’ [..] ⌜SIG$_7$-*su*⌝

22’ NA i 17’ [*ina* A.M]E[Š$^?$ .... ÚKU]Š.LAGAB Ú.BABBAR x [.. *t*]*e*-⌜*qí*$^?$⌝

NB i 7’ *ina* A.MEŠ LUH-*si* LAL-*id* GURUN ^{ú}ÚKUŠ.LAGAB ⌜Ú⌝ [.BABBAR SÚD ....]

NC i 22’ [.. IGI.MIN-*š*]*ú* ⌜*te-qí*⌝

Overview of IGI 1 Manuscripts and Parallels: **AA**=BAM 20; **AB**=BAM 159; **AC**=BAM 19; **AD**=BAM 22; **AE**=BAM 18; **AmA**=BAM 165; **AX**=KAL 7/12; **bA**=BM 41293+; **EA**=EMAR 6/4; **HA**=STT 279; **NA**=BAM 510; **NB**=BAM 513; **NC**=BAM 514; **ND**=BAM 515; **NE**=BAM 516; **NJ**=AMT 12/5; **NQ**=BAM 521; **NU**=AMT 14/3; **sA**=IRAQ 65; **UA**=AuOrS 23/27; **uA**=SpTU 50; **UB**=Ugaritica 5; **UC**=AuOrS 23/14; **xA**=CM 37

23’ *šumma amēlu īnāšu marṣāma ūmē ma’dūti lā ipetti ina ummi [qaqqadīšu īnāšu ṣilla malâ]*	[23’]If a man’s eyes are sick and then he cannot open (them) for many days, while having *ummu*-fever [of his head (and) his eyes are filled up with a film.]
24’ *qaqqassu tugallab ina ūme šalāšīšu līša tukaṣṣa zēr [maštakal] turrar*	[24’]You shave his head (and) three times a day, you cool off (his head) with dough. You parch seeds [*of maštakal-plant*].
25’ *ina himēti itqūr abāri tasâk īnīšu teqqīma*$^{?}$ *ina’eš*$^{?}$	[25’]You pound (them) in the ghee of a lead spoon(salve), (and) daub$^{?}$ his eyes, and he should get better$^{?}$.

23’ NA i 18’ [......... IGI.M]IN-*šú* GI[G .... *ma-’-d*]*u-ti* NU BAD *ina* KÚM [.....]
NB i 8’ DIŠ NA IGI.MIN-*šú* GIG-*ma* UD.MEŠ *ma-’-du-ti* NU BA[D ....]
NC i 23’ [.. -*š*]*ú*$^{?}$
(ND) ii 45f.’ [DIŠ NA IGI.MIN-*šú* G]IG-⌜*ma* UD *ma*⌝-’-*du-ti* NU ⌜BAD⌝ *ina* KÚM SAG-*šú* IGI.MIN-*šú* GIS[SU DIRI$^{?}$] / [... M]I$^{?}$
(AA) 11f.’ ⌜DIŠ$^{?}$⌝ NA IGI.MIN-*šú* GIG-*ma* UD-*me* ME[Š] / NU BAD-*te ina* KÚM SAG.DU-*šú* ⌜IGI⌝.MI[N-*šú*] / ⌜GISSU DIRI⌝ →
(AB) iv 3f.’ DIŠ NA IGI.MIN-*šú* GIG-*ma* UD.MEŠ *ma-’-du-te* NU BAD-⌜*te*⌝ / *ina* KÚM SAG.DU-*šú* IGI.MIN-*šú* GISSU DIRI

24’ NA i 19’ [SAG.D]U-*su* SAR-*a*[*b* .... N]ÍG.SILA$_{11}$.GÁ *tu-kàṣ-ṣ*[*a* ....]
NB i 8f.’ [....................] / SAR-*ab ina* UD-*me* 3-*šú* NÍG.SILA$_{11}$.GÁ *tu-kàṣ-ṣa* NU[MUN ....]
NC i 24f.’ [.. *tu*]-⌜*kàṣ*$^{?}$-*ṣa*$^{?}$⌝ / [..] x ⌜*tur*$^{?}$-*ár*$^{?}$⌝
(ND) ii 46 SAG.DU-*su tu-gal*-⌜*lab ina* UD-*me* 3-*šú* NÍG⌝.SILA$_{11}$.GÁ *tu-kàṣ*-⌜*ṣa* NUMUN ^{ú}IN$_{6}$.ÚŠ *t*[*ur-ár*]
(AA) 13f.’ SAG.⌜DU-*su*⌝ SA[R] / *ina* UD-*me* 3-*šú* NÍG$^{?}$⌝.SILA$_{11}$.GÁ *tu-kà*[*ṣ-ṣa*] / [NU]MUN ^{ú}IN$_{6}$.ÚŠ *tur-ár* →
(AB) iv 5f.’ SAG.DU-*su* SAR.SAR *ina* UD-*me* 3-*šú ša* NÍG.⌜SILA$_{11}$.GÁ⌝ / *tu-kàṣ-ṣa* NUMUN ^{ú}IN.NU.UŠ *tur*-⌜*ár*⌝

25’ NA i 20’ [*ina*] ⌜Ì⌝.NUN DÍLIM A.⌜BÁR⌝ *t*[*a-sà*]*k* IGI.MIN-*šú t*[*e*$^{?}$-*qí*$^{?}$-*ma*$^{?}$ *ina*$^{?}$-*eš*$^{?}$]
NB i 9f.’ [.................] / DÍLIM A.BÁR *ta-sàk* IGI.MIN-*šú* [.............................]

Overview of IGI 1 Manuscripts and Parallels: **AA**=BAM 20; **AB**=BAM 159; **AC**=BAM 19; **AD**=BAM 22; **AE**=BAM 18; **AmA**=BAM 165; **AX**=KAL 7/12; **bA**=BM 41293+; **EA**=EMAR 6/4; **HA**=STT 279; **NA**=BAM 510; **NB**=BAM 513; **NC**=BAM 514; **ND**=BAM 515; **NE**=BAM 516; **NJ**=AMT 12/5; **NQ**=BAM 521; **NU**=AMT 14/3; **sA**=IRAQ 65; **UA**=AuOrS 23/27; **uA**=SpTU 50; **UB**=Ugaritica 5; **UC**=AuOrS 23/14; **xA**=CM 37

NC i 26' [.. *in*]*a*$^{?}$-⸢*eš*$^{?}$⸣
THE DIVIDING LINE IS NOT VISIBLE!

(ND) ii 47 [*ina* Ì.NUN DÍLIM] ⸢A⸣.BÁR SÚD MAR A LUH-*si* GAZI^{sar} UGU ⸢IGI.MIN-*šú* GAR$^{?}$ EN$^{?}$ *ú-za-ku*⸣-*ú* GUR.G[UR]

(AA) 15ff.' *ina* Ì.⸢NUN$^{?}$⸣ / [DÍLIM] ⸢A$^{?}$⸣.BÁR SÚD IGI.MIN-*šú* MAR.M[E(Š)] / [*bul-ṭ*]*u*$^{?}$ *lat-k*[*u*$^{?}$]

(AB) iv 7f.' *ina* Ì.NUN DÍLIM A.BÁR SÚD IGI.MIN-*šú* / [M]AR.MEŠ-*ma bul-ṭu lat-ku*

26' *šumma amēlu īnāšu tābīla marṣā šamaškilla uhašša ina šikari išatti šamna ana libbi īnīšu tazarru*[*ma*$^{?}$ *ina'eš*$^{?}$]	[26'] If a man's eyes suffer from 'dryness': he (the patient) should chop *šamaškillu*-onion (and) drink it in beer. (Then) you sprinkle$^{?}$ sesame oil into his eyes [and and he should get better$^{?}$.]
Alternative prescription 1	**Alternative prescription 1**
27' *qēm aban suluppī turrar tasâk ina mê kasî talâš tukappat lām patān u'allat*	[27']You parch (and) pound powder of date stones, you knead (this flour) in the sap of a *kasû*-plant, you roll it (into a pill, which) he swallows before eating.
Alternative prescription 2	**Alternative prescription 2**
28' *muṣa''irāna arqa taṣallip marassu ina himēti taballal īnīšu teqqi*	[28']You dissect a yellow-green *muṣa''irānu*-frog (and) you mix its bile in ghee. You daub his eyes (with it).
Alternative prescription 3	**Alternative prescription 3**
29' *hamšat* SILA$_4$!(KISAL) *qēm hallūri šeššet* SILA$_4$!(KISAL) *qēm kasî hamšat šiqil sahlê ina mê kasî talâš nakkaptāšu īnīšu taṣammid*	[29']You knead 5 SILA-measure chickpea powder, 6 SILA-measure powder of *kasû*-plant, (and) 5 shekels of *sahlû*-plant in the sap of a *kasû*-plant. You bandage his temple (and) his eyes.

26' NA i 21' [............ I]GI.MIN-*šú ta-bi-la*$_{12}$ GIG SUM.SIKI[L-*l*]*a* ⸢*ú*⸣-*haš-šá ina* KAŠ NAG Ì+GIŠ *ana* ŠÀ ⸢IGI.MIN-*šú*⸣ M[AR-*ru-ma*$^{?}$ ....]

NB i 11' DIŠ NA IGI.MIN-*šú ta-bi-la*$_{12}$ GIG SUM.SIKIL-⸢*la*⸣ *ú-haš-šá ina* KAŠ NAG Ì.GIŠ *ana* Š[À...]

NC i 27' [..] x

Overview of IGI 1 Manuscripts and Parallels: **AA**=BAM 20; **AB**=BAM 159; **AC**=BAM 19; **AD**=BAM 22; **AE**=BAM 18; **AmA**=BAM 165; **AX**=KAL 7/12; **bA**=BM 41293+; **EA**=EMAR 6/4; **HA**=STT 279; **NA**=BAM 510; **NB**=BAM 513; **NC**=BAM 514; **ND**=BAM 515; **NE**=BAM 516; **NJ**=AMT 12/5; **NQ**=BAM 521; **NU**=AMT 14/3; **sA**=IRAQ 65; **UA**=AuOrS 23/27; **uA**=SpTU 50; **UB**=Ugaritica 5; **UC**=AuOrS 23/14; **xA**=CM 37

27’ NA i 22’ [.... N]A$_4$ ZÚ.LUM.MA *tur-ár* SÚD *ina* A ⸢GAZI^{sar} *ta*⸣*-la-aš tu-kap-pat la-a-am pa-*⸢*tan ú*$^{?}$⸣*-a*[*l-lat*$^{?}$]

NB i 12’ ZÌ NA$_4$ ⸢ZÚ.LUM.MA *tur-ár* SÚD *ina* A GAZI^{sar} *ta*⸣*-la-aš tu-kap-pat l*[*a-a-am* ....]

NC i 27’ too broken

28’ NA i 23’ [BIL.ZA.Z]A ⸢SIG$_7$⸣ *ta-ṣa-lip* ZÍ-⸢*su ina*⸣ Ì.NUN HE.HE IGI.MIN-*šú* ⸢*te-qí*⸣

NB i 13’ BIL.ZA.ZA S[IG$_7$ ....] ZÍ-⸢*su*⸣ *ina* ⸢Ì⸣.[NUN ....]

NC i 28’ too broken

29’ NA i 24’ [............ GÚ.G]AL 6 SILA$_4$!(KISAL) ZÌ GAZI^{sar} 5 GÍN ZÀ.H[I.LI *ina*] ⸢A GAZI^{sar} SILA$_{11}$-*aš* SAG.KI-*šú* IGI.MIN-*šú*⸣ LAL

NB i 14’ 5 SILA$_4$!(KISAL) ZÌ [..GÍ]N ZÀ.HI.⸢LI⸣ *in*[*a* A G]AZI^{sar} SI[LA$_{11}$-*aš*...]

NC i 29’ too broken

30’ *šiptu* [...] ... *ērupū egûma*	[30’]Incantation ... they cloud over, they become lazy$^{?}$. [31’]You say [...] ... three times over water.
31’ [...] ... *eli mê šalāšīšu taqabbi*	

30’ NA i 25’ [ÉN x x x (x)] x LAL A SAR NUMUN Ú x [x] x *e-ru-pu e-gu-ma*
NB i 15’ É[N$^{?}$ ....] x x *i-ru-p*[*u e-gu-ma*]
NC i 30’ too broken

31’ NA i 26’ [x x] x ⸢*e*⸣-[*l*]*i*$^{?}$ A 3-*šú* DUG$_4$.GA

NB i 16’ [............ *e-l*]*i*$^{?}$ ⸢A$^{?}$⸣ [.................]

NC i 31’ too broken

32’ *šumma amēlu* [*īnāšu marṣā nīnû atā’išu kasû*] *sahlê māš*(*t*)*u lipi kanakti zēr burāši*	[32’]If a man’s [eyes] are [sick: *nīnû*-mint, *atā’išu*-plant, *kasû*-plant,] *sahlû*-plant, *māš*(*t*)*u*-twin plant, *kanaktu*-aromatic pith, seed of juniper, [33’]*kammu*-tanning-fungus [of a leather worker. (These)

Overview of IGI 1 Manuscripts and Parallels: **AA**=BAM 20; **AB**=BAM 159; **AC**=BAM 19; **AD**=BAM 22; **AE**=BAM 18; **AmA**=BAM 165; **AX**=KAL 7/12; **bA**=BM 41293+; **EA**=EMAR 6/4; **HA**=STT 279; **NA**=BAM 510; **NB**=BAM 513; **NC**=BAM 514; **ND**=BAM 515; **NE**=BAM 516; **NJ**=AMT 12/5; **NQ**=BAM 521; **NU**=AMT 14/3; **sA**=IRAQ 65; **UA**=AuOrS 23/27; **uA**=SpTU 50; **UB**=Ugaritica 5; **UC**=AuOrS 23/14; **xA**=CM 37

33' *kammu [ša aškāpi samānat šammī ribku ša īnī ina pēmti] taqallu ina himēti lipî kalīti immeri iškūri tuštabbal īnīšu teqqi*	eight$^{?}$ drugs (are used) as an infusion for the eyes which you] roast [over charcoal]. (Then) you stir (them) in ghee, sheep's kidney-fat, and wax, (and) you daub his eyes.

32' NA i 27' DIŠ N[A .... GAZI^{s}]^{ar} *sah-lé-e* ^{ú}MAŠ.TAB Ì.UDU ^{šim}GIG NUMUN ^{šim}LI

NB i 17' too broken

NC i 32' too broken

(NE) iv 10 ^{ú}KUR.RA ^{ú}KUR.KUR GAZI^{sar} ^{ú}MAŠ.TAB.BA ^{šim}SES NUMUN ^{šim}LI

(AA) 1ff.' [DIŠ N]A ⌜IGI⌝.[MIN]-⌜*šú* GIG ^{ú}KUR⌝.R[A (^{ú}KUR.KUR)] / ⌜Ú *he-pí eš-šú sah-lé-e* ^{ú}⌝MA[Š.TAB.BA] / [Ì.UD]U ⌜^{šim}GIG NUMUN ^{šim}⌝ [LI]

(AC) 3ff.' [DIŠ NA IGI.MIN]-*šú* GIG ^{ú}KUR.RA ^{ú}KUR.KUR GA[ZI^{sar} / *sah-l*]*é-e* ^{ú}MAŠ.TAB.BA Ì.UDU ^{šim}G[IG / NUMU]N ^{šim}LI →

(AmA) ii' 9ff.' ⌜^{ú}KUR.RA ^{ú}⌝KUR.KUR / ⌜^{ú}⌝GAZI^{sar} ZÀ.HI.LI.A^{sar}

(AmA) ii' 11' ^{ú}MAŠ.TAB Ì.UDU ^{šim}⌜GIG⌝

(AmA) ii' 12' ^{ú}NUMUN ^{šim}LI →

(sA) ii 15ff. DIŠ NA IGI.MIN-*šú* GIG.MEŠ ^{ú}KUR.RA ^{ú}KUR.KUR / GAZI^{sar} *sah-lé-e* ^{ú}MAŠ.TAB.BA Ì.UDU ^{šim}GIG / NUMUN ^{šim}LI →

33' NA i 28' *kam-m*[*u* .... *ta-qàl-l*]*u ina* Ì.NUN Ì.UDU ÉLLAG UDU.NÍTA GAB.LÀL *tuš-tab-bal* IGI.MIN-*šú* MAR

NB i 18' too broken

NC i 33' too broken

(NE) iv 10 *kam-mu šá* AŠGAB 7 Ú.HI.A

(NE) iv 11 *rib-ku ša* IGI.MIN *ina* NE *ta-qal-lu ina* Ì.UDU GAB.LÀL *u* Ì.NUN SÚD IGI.MIN-*šú* MAR

(AA) 4f.' [*kam*]-⌜*mu šá* $^{\text{lú*}}$AŠGAB 8 Ú⌝ *r*[*ib-ki*] / [*šá* I]GI.⌜MIN *ina* NE BÍL-*lu*$_4$ *ina* Ì⌝.[UDU]

(AA) 6' [ÉLL]AG ⌜UDU.NÍTA GAB.LÀL *u* Ì.NUN⌝ SÚ[D MAR]

(AC) 5f.' *kám-mu šá* ^{lú}AŠGAB 8 Ú *rib-*⌜*ki*⌝ / [*šá* I]GI.MIN.MEŠ *ina* NE BÍL-*lu*$_4$ *u* Ì.UDU ÉLLAG UD[U NÍ]TA

(AC) 6' [GAB.LÀ]L *u* Ì.NUN SÚD IGI.MIN-*šú* ⌜MAR⌝

Overview of IGI 1 Manuscripts and Parallels: **AA**=BAM 20; **AB**=BAM 159; **AC**=BAM 19; **AD**=BAM 22; **AE**=BAM 18; **AmA**=BAM 165; **AX**=KAL 7/12; **bA**=BM 41293+; **EA**=EMAR 6/4; **HA**=STT 279; **NA**=BAM 510; **NB**=BAM 513; **NC**=BAM 514; **ND**=BAM 515; **NE**=BAM 516; **NJ**=AMT 12/5; **NQ**=BAM 521; **NU**=AMT 14/3; **sA**=IRAQ 65; **UA**=AuOrS 23/27; **uA**=SpTU 50; **UB**=Ugaritica 5; **UC**=AuOrS 23/14; **xA**=CM 37

(AmA) ii' 12' *kám-ma šá* ⸢^{lú}AŠGAB⸣

(AmA) ii' 13' 8 Ú *rib-ku ša* IGI.MIN ⸢BIL⸣
(AmA) ii' 14' *ina* Ì.UDU GAB.LÀL Ì.NUN.NA HE.HE

(sA) ii 17f. KÙ.GAN 8$^{?}$ Ú.HI.A / *rib-ki* DÙG.GA *šá* IGI.MIN *ta-qal-lu ina* Ì.NUN.NA
(sA) ii 19 Ì.UDU ÉLLAG GAB.LÀL SÚD IGI.MIN-*šú* MAR

34' *šumma amēlu īnāšu [marṣā šamma peṣâ ina himēti tasâk teqqi : šumma amēlu] īnāšu marṣā rikibti arkabi ina himēti tasâk teqqi*	34'If a man's eyes [are sick you pound white plant in ghee and daub (the eyes): If a man's eyes] are sick: you pound bat guano in ghee (and) daub (his eyes).

34' NA i 29' DIŠ NA IGI.MI[N-*šú* .... : IGI.MI]N-*šú* GIG U$_5$.ARGAB^{mušen} *ina* Ì.NUN SÚD MAR

NB i 19' too broken
NC i 34' too broken
(AC) 11f.' [DIŠ N]A ⸢IGI.MIN-*šú*⸣ GIG Ú.BABBAR *ina* Ì.NUN SÚD MAR / [DIŠ$^{?}$ KIMIN$^{?}$] ⸢U$_5$.ARGAB^{mušen}⸣ *ina* Ì.NUN SÚD MAR

35' *šumma amēlu īnāšu [marṣā aban gabî ina himēti tasâk teqqi : šumma amēlu] īnāšu marṣā sahlê ina šizbi tušabšal taṣammid*	35'If a man's eyes [are sick: You pound alum in ghee (and) daub (his eyes): If a man's] eyes are sick you boil *sahlû*-plant in milk (and) bandage (his eyes with it).

35' NA i 30' DIŠ NA IGI.MIN-⸢*šú*⸣ [GIG .... : DIŠ NA] ⸢IGI.MIN-*šú* GIG *sah-lé*⸣-*e ina* GA ŠEG$_6$-*šal* LAL

NB i 20' too broken
NC i 35' ⸢DIŠ NA IGI.MIN-*šú*⸣ [...]

(NQ) 8' [DIŠ NA IGI.MIN]-*šú* GIG *sah-lé*-⸢*e*⸣ [...]
(AC) 13' [DIŠ KIMIN N]A$_4$ ⸢*ga-bi-i ina* Ì⸣.NUN SÚD MAR
(AC) 14' [DIŠ$^{?}$ KIMIN$^{?}$ *sa*]*h*-⸢*lé*⸣-*e ina* GA SÚD MAR

Overview of IGI 1 Manuscripts and Parallels: **AA**=BAM 20; **AB**=BAM 159; **AC**=BAM 19; **AD**=BAM 22; **AE**=BAM 18; **AmA**=BAM 165; **AX**=KAL 7/12; **bA**=BM 41293+; **EA**=EMAR 6/4; **HA**=STT 279; **NA**=BAM 510; **NB**=BAM 513; **NC**=BAM 514; **ND**=BAM 515; **NE**=BAM 516; **NJ**=AMT 12/5; **NQ**=BAM 521; **NU**=AMT 14/3; **sA**=IRAQ 65; **UA**=AuOrS 23/27; **uA**=SpTU 50; **UB**=Ugaritica 5; **UC**=AuOrS 23/14; **xA**=CM 37

36’ *šumma amēlu īnāšu dāma* [*malâma urra u mūša lā iṣallalma* ...] ... *šumma libbi īnīšu sām* **37’** *īnāšu katmā kasâ turrar* [...] *kabūt immeri ina šizbi musukkati talâš taṣammid* **38’** *ina šēri tapaṭṭaršuma ashar ina himēti tasâk īnīšu teqqi* [(...)] *šuruš šammi rapādi ina patar siparri tanakkis* **39’** *ṭurri nabāsi u šīpāti peṣâti taṭammi talammi tarakkas nakkapātīšu kilaltān tarakkasma*[?] ... *tušeṣṣēma īnīšu* [*teqqi*]	36’If a man’s eyes are [full of] blood [and he cannot sleep day and night ...], if the inner part of his eyes is red, 37’(and) his eyes are closed: you parch *kasû*-plant [...], you knead sheep dung in the milk from a woman in maternity (and) bandage (his eyes). 38’In the morning you loosen it (the bandage), and then you pound *ashar*-stone in ghee, (and) daub his eyes [(...)]. You cut with a bronze knife the root of *rapādu*-disease-plant. 39’You spin a cord of red and white wool, you wrap and bind up (the root of *rapādu*-plant with the wool, and) tie (it) on his both temples, and ... you remove (it), and then [daub] his eyes.

36’ NA i 31’ DIŠ NA IGI.MIN-*šú* MÚ[D ....] x RI *šum*$_4$-*ma* ŠÀ IGI.MIN-*šú* SA$_5$

NB i 21’ [..] [........... Š]À[?] ˹IGI[?].MIN[?]˺-*š*[*ú*[?] ...]

NC i 36f.’ ˹DIŠ NA IGI.MIN-*šú* MÚD DIRI-*ma ur-ra u* GE$_6$ *la i*˺-*ṣa*[*l-lal-ma* ....] / ˹*šum*$_4$-*ma* ŠÀ IGI.MIN-*šú* SA$_5$˺ →

(xA) 8f.’ ˹DIŠ NA IGI˺.M[IN-*šú* MÚD] ˹DIRI.MEŠ-*ma ur-ri u* GE$_6$ *la i-ṣa-lal-ma* ...... x x IGI.MIN-*šú*˺ x [...] / ˹ŠÀ˺ I[GI.MIN-*šú*] ˹SA$_5$.MEŠ˺ →

37’ NA i 32’ IGI.MIN-*šú* DUL-*m*[*a* .... [munus]] ˹Ú˺.ZÚG SILA$_{11}$-*aš* LAL-*id*

NB i 22’ [.. ŠU]RUN ˹UDU˺ *ina* GA [munus]Ú.ZÚ[G ....]

NC i 37f.’ ˹IGI.MIN-*šú* DUL-*ma* GAZI[sar] *tur-ár* KI˺ x [.. ....] / ˹SILA$_{11}$-*aš* LAL-*id*˺ →

(xA) 9f.’ ˹IGI.MIN-*šú* DUL-*ma* GAZI[sar] *tur-ár*˺ .... / SILA$_{11}$-*aš* ˹LAL˺ →

38’ NA i 33’ *ina še-rì* DU$_8$-*šú-m*[*a* .... *ina* GÍR ZAB]AR KUD-[*iṣ*[?]]

Overview of IGI 1 Manuscripts and Parallels: **AA**=BAM 20; **AB**=BAM 159; **AC**=BAM 19; **AD**=BAM 22; **AE**=BAM 18; **AmA**=BAM 165; **AX**=KAL 7/12; **bA**=BM 41293+; **EA**=EMAR 6/4; **HA**=STT 279; **NA**=BAM 510; **NB**=BAM 513; **NC**=BAM 514; **ND**=BAM 515; **NE**=BAM 516; **NJ**=AMT 12/5; **NQ**=BAM 521; **NU**=AMT 14/3; **sA**=IRAQ 65; **UA**=AuOrS 23/27; **uA**=SpTU 50; **UB**=Ugaritica 5; **UC**=AuOrS 23/14; **xA**=CM 37

	NB i 23'	[.. SUHU]Š$^{?}$ ⌜Ú *ra-pa-di*⌝ *ina* GÍR ZA[BAR ....]
	NC i 38'	⌜*ina še-rì* DU$_{8}$-*šú-ma* ^{na4}*às-har ina* Ì.NUN SÚD IGI.MIN-*šú*⌝ MA[R ....]
	(xA) 10f.'	[*ina še-r*]*ì* ⌜DU$_{8}$-*šú-ma* <*ana*> TIN-*šú* $^{na4?}$*as-har ina* Ì.NUN SÚD IGI.MIN-*šú* MAR SUHUŠ⌝ Ú *ra*$^{?}$-*pa*$^{?}$-*di*$^{?}$⌝ / ⌜*ina* GÍR$^{?}$.ZABAR$^{?}$ KUD$^{?}$⌝ →
39'	NA i 34'	DUR ^{síg}HÉ.ME[D...]
	NB i 24f.'	[............................ SÍ]G ⌜BABBAR NIGIN⌝-*m*[*i*$^{?}$ *tar*]*a*-⌜*kàs*⌝ SAG.KI.MEŠ-*šú ki-lál-t*[*an*$^{?}$ ... / ...] È-⌜*ma*$^{?}$⌝ IGI.MIN-*šú t*[*e*$^{?}$-(*eq*)-*qí*]
	NC i 39f.'	⌜DUR ^{síg}HÉ.MED *u* SÍG BABBAR NU.NU NIGIN-*mi tara-kás*⌝ SA[G.KI ....] / ⌜*tara*$^{?}$-*kás*$^{?}$-*ma*$^{?}$ x x È-*ma*⌝ I[GI.MIN-*šú* ....]
	(xA) 11f.'	⌜^{síg}HÉ⌝.[MED.D]A SÍG BABBAR NU.NU NIGIN-*mi tara-kás* SAG.KI.MIN-*šú ki-lat-t*[*an*] / ⌜*tara-kás-m*[*a*] x$^{?}$ È-*ma* IGI.MIN-*šú* x

40' *šumma amēlu īnāšu dāma šunnuʾā zēr egemgīri dišip šadê lēra taballal* [*tasâk* (*īnīšu*) *teqqi*]	[40']If a man's eyes are suffused with blood: you mix seeds of *egemgīru*-plant, mountain honey, (and) *lēru*-paste, [you pound (them) and daub (his eyes)].
Alternative prescription 1 **41'** *ištēn šiqil rikibti arkabi mišil* SILA$_{4}$!(KISAL) *šamma peṣâ šušši emesalli ina* [*himēti tasâk īnīšu teqqi*]	**Alternative prescription 1** [41'][You pound] one shekel of bat guano, half SILA-measure of white plant (and) one-sixth (SILA-measure) *emesallu*-saline solution in [ghee and daub his eyes with (it)].
Alternative prescription 2 **42'** *šamma peṣâ tābīla ana libbi īnīšu tazarru dāmāta ina himēti* [...] **43'** *zê ṣurāri ina lipî eṣemti kurīti tasâk lā patān* [...]	**Alternative prescription 2** [42']You spatter white plant in a dry state into his eyes, [you pound] *dāmātu*-paste in ghee [and ...] [43']You pound lizard's excrement in the marrow of a short bone, without (him) eating, [...].

Overview of IGI 1 Manuscripts and Parallels: **AA**=BAM 20; **AB**=BAM 159; **AC**=BAM 19; **AD**=BAM 22; **AE**=BAM 18; **AmA**=BAM 165; **AX**=KAL 7/12; **bA**=BM 41293+; **EA**=EMAR 6/4; **HA**=STT 279; **NA**=BAM 510; **NB**=BAM 513; **NC**=BAM 514; **ND**=BAM 515; **NE**=BAM 516; **NJ**=AMT 12/5; **NQ**=BAM 521; **NU**=AMT 14/3; **sA**=IRAQ 65; **UA**=AuOrS 23/27; **uA**=SpTU 50; **UB**=Ugaritica 5; **UC**=AuOrS 23/14; **xA**=CM 37

Alternative prescription 3	**Alternative prescription 3**
44' *hamiš uṭṭat šamma peṣâ ina šamni tasâk īnāšu teqqi rikibti arkabi ina himēti tasâk īnāšu*$^?$ *teqqi*$^?$	44' You pound five grain measure of white plant in sesame oil, you daub his eyes. You pound bat guano in ghee, (and) you daub his eyes (with it).

40' NA i 35' DIŠ NA IGI.MIN-*šú* MÚD *šu-u*[*n-nu-'a* ....
....]

NB i 26' [.................................... *šu-u*]*n-nu-'a* NUMUN ^{giš}NÍG.⸢GÁN⸣.GÁN LÀL.KUR.RA SAHAR.KÙ.GI HE.H[E ....]

NC i 41' ⸢DIŠ NA IGI.MIN-*šú* MÚD *šu-un-nu-'a* NUMUN ^{giš}NÍG.GÁN.GÁN LÀL⸣.KU[R.RA ....]

(xA) 14' DIŠ N[A .... *šu-u*]*n-n*[*u-'a* .... ^{giš}NÍG.GÁ]N.GÁN$^{sar!(di)}$ LÀL.KUR.⸢RA SAHAR.KÙ⸣.GI 1-*niš* HE.HE S[ÚD (IGI.MIN-*šú*) MAR]

41' NA i 36' 1 GÍN U$_5$.ARGAB^{mušen} 1/[2 ....]

NB i 27' [1 GÍN U$_5$.AR]GAB^{mušen} 1/2 SILA$_4$!(KISAL) Ú.⸢BABBAR⸣ IGI.6.GÁL.LA ^{mun}*eme-sal-* ⸢*lì*⸣ *i*[*na*$^?$ ....]

NC i 42' ⸢1 GÍN U$_5$.ARGAB^{mušen} 1/2 GÍN Ú.BABBAR IGI.6.GÁL.LA ^{MUN}⸣*em*[*e-sal-lì* ....]

(AB) iv 25f.' 1 GÍN U$_5$.ARGAB^{mušen} 1/2 G[ÍN/GA]ZI ⸢Ú.BABBAR⸣ / 15 ŠE ^{mun}*eme-sal-lì* *ina* Ì.NUN SÚD ⸢IGI.MIN-*šú* MAR⸣

(AE) 3f. [DIŠ] ⸢Ú⸣ 1 SILA$_4$!(KISAL) U$_5$.ARGAB^{mu}[^{šen} 1/]2$^?$ SILA$_4$!(KISAL) ⸢Ú.BABBAR IGI.6.GÁL.LA⸣ / [^{mu}]^{n}*me$_5$-sal-lì ina* L[ÀL$^?$] *ta-sàk te-*⸢*qí*⸣

(bA) i' 2 ⸢1 GÍN U$_5$.AR[GAB^{mu}]^{šen} 1/2 GÍN ⸢Ú.BABBAR⸣ 15$^?$ ŠE *he-pí* : *eme-sal-lì* *ina* Ì.NUN SÚD *te-qí*

42' NA i 37' Ú.BABBAR *ta-bi-la*$_{12}$ *ana* ŠÀ IGI.MI[N-*šú*...
.......................]

NB i 28' [Ú.BABBAR *ta-b*]*i*$^?$*-la*$_{12}$ ⸢*ana* ŠÀ IGI.MIN-*šú*⸣ MAR-*ru* ŠIM.BI.SIG$_7$.SIG$_7$ *ina* ⸢Ì⸣ [.NUN ...]

NC i 43' ⸢Ú.BABBAR *ta-bi-la*$_{12}$ *ana* ŠÀ IGI.MIN-*šú* MAR-*ru* ŠIM.BI⸣.SI[G$_7$.SIG$_7$
.......................]

Overview of IGI 1 Manuscripts and Parallels: **AA**=BAM 20; **AB**=BAM 159; **AC**=BAM 19; **AD**=BAM 22; **AE**=BAM 18; **AmA**=BAM 165; **AX**=KAL 7/12; **bA**=BM 41293+; **EA**=EMAR 6/4; **HA**=STT 279; **NA**=BAM 510; **NB**=BAM 513; **NC**=BAM 514; **ND**=BAM 515; **NE**=BAM 516; **NJ**=AMT 12/5; **NQ**=BAM 521; **NU**=AMT 14/3; **sA**=IRAQ 65; **UA**=AuOrS 23/27; **uA**=SpTU 50; **UB**=Ugaritica 5; **UC**=AuOrS 23/14; **xA**=CM 37

43’	NA i 38’	ŠE$_{10}$ EME.ŠID *ina* Ì.UDU GÌR.PAD.DU LÚGUD.DA [.............................. ....]
	NB i 29’	[ŠE$_{10}$ EME.ŠID] *ina* ⸢Ì.UDU⸣ [GÌ]R$^{?}$.⸢PAD.DU LÚGUD⸣.DA SÚD *la pa-tan* [...]
	NC i 44’	⸢ŠE$_{10}$ EME.ŠID *ina* Ì.UDU GÌR.PAD.DU LÚGUD.DA SÚD⸣ *l*[*a*................ ...]
44’	NA i 39’	5 ŠE Ú.BABBAR *ina* Ì.GIŠ SÚD IGI.MIN-*šú* MA[R ....]
	NB i 30’	[.................................... S]ÚD IG[I.MIN-*šú*] ⸢MAR⸣ [U]$_5$.⸢ARGAB⸣^{mušen} *ina* Ì.NUN S[ÚD ....]
	NC i 45’	⸢5 ŠE Ú.BABBAR *ina* Ì.GIŠ SÚD IGI.MIN-*šú* MAR U$_5$.ARGAB⸣ ^{muš}[^{en} .... IGI.MIN]-⸢*šú*$^{?}$ MAR$^{?}$⸣

45’ *šumma amēlu īnāšu dāma malâ dāmāta ina himēti tasâk teqqi*	45’If a man’s eyes are full of blood: you pound *dāmātu*-paste in ghee, you daub (his eyes).
Alternative prescription 1 **46’** *maštakal tarmuš malmališ taballal ina himēti nikipta [zikar u sinniš] tasâk īnīšu teqqi*	**Alternative prescription 1** 46’You mix in equal measure *maštakal*-plant and *tarmuš*-lupine, you pound [male and female] *nikiptu*-plant in ghee, (and) daub his eyes.
Alternative prescription 2 **47’** *aban tašrīti ina ru’ti tasâk teqqi* : *šimbizidâ*$^{?}$ (...) *ina šizbi musukkati [tasâk ...] hašhūra tasâk teqqi*	**Alternative prescription 2** 47’You pound *tašrītu*-stone in spittle (and) daub (his eyes with it) : [You pound] *šimbizidû*-galena$^{?}$ (...) in the milk from a woman in maternity, you pound ... (and) an apple, (and) daub (his eyes).
Alternative prescription 3 **48’** *dāma ša libbi šahî ana libbi īnīšu [tunattak ...] ... īnīšu taṣammid*	**Alternative prescription 3** 48’You [drip] into his eyes blood from a pig’s heart ... you bandage his eyes.

Overview of IGI 1 Manuscripts and Parallels: **AA**=BAM 20; **AB**=BAM 159; **AC**=BAM 19; **AD**=BAM 22; **AE**=BAM 18; **AmA**=BAM 165; **AX**=KAL 7/12; **bA**=BM 41293+; **EA**=EMAR 6/4; **HA**=STT 279; **NA**=BAM 510; **NB**=BAM 513; **NC**=BAM 514; **ND**=BAM 515; **NE**=BAM 516; **NJ**=AMT 12/5; **NQ**=BAM 521; **NU**=AMT 14/3; **sA**=IRAQ 65; **UA**=AuOrS 23/27; **uA**=SpTU 50; **UB**=Ugaritica 5; **UC**=AuOrS 23/14; **xA**=CM 37

45’ NA i 40’ DIŠ NA IGI.MIN-*šú* MÚD DIRI [... ....]

NB i 31’ [... ŠI]M.BI.SIG₇.⸢SIG₇ *ina* Ì.NUN⸣ SÚD MAR :

NC i 46’ ⸢DIŠ NA IGI.MIN-*šú* MÚD DIRI ŠIM.BI.SIG₇⸣.[SIG₇ *ina* Ì].⸢NUN SÚD MAR⸣

46’ NA i 41’ ᵘIN₆.ÚŠ ᵘ*tar-muš mal-ma-li*[*š* ....]

NB i 31’ : ⸢ᵘIN.NU.UŠ⸣ ᵘ*tar-muš₈ mal-ma-liš* HE.HE *i*[*na* ....]

NC i 47’ ⸢ᵘIN₆.ÚŠ ᵘ*tar*⸣-*m*[*uš*? .... HE.H]E ⸢*ina* Ì.NUN *ni-kip-tu₄*⸣ [NÍTA? *u*? MUNUS? S]ÚD ⸢IGI.MIN⸣-*šú* ⸢MAR⸣

47’ NA i 42’ NA₄ BAL *ina* ÚH SÚD MAR : *ši*[*m*?-*bi*?-*zi*?-*da₄*? ....]

NB ii beginning of col. ii

NC i 48’ ⸢NA₄ BAL⸣ [....] ⸢*ina* GA⸣ munus ⸢Ú.ZÚG⸣ [SÚD? x] ⸢x HAŠHUR SÚD MAR⸣

48’ NA i 43’ MÚD *ša* ŠÀ ŠAH *ana* ŠÀ IGI.MIN-*š*[*ú tu-na-tak/ták* ....]

NC i 49’ [...] x x [... IG]I.MIN-*šú* LAL

49’ [... *īnīšu*] *teqqi*	49’[...] you daub [his eyes.]

49’ NB ii 1’ [.. IGI.MIN-*šú*] MAR?

50’ [... *ana libbi īnīšu*] *tazarri*	**50’** [...] you spatter [... into his eyes.]

50’ NB ii 2’ [.. *ana* ŠÀ IGI.MIN-*šú t*]*a*-⸢*zar*⸣-*ri*

51’ [...] *sahlâ šammi ašî* **52’** [...] ... *ina ummāti ina mê kasî temessi*	51’[...you pound] *sahlû*-plant, *ašû*-disease-plant, 52’[...] ... In the summer, you wash (the ingredients) in the sap of a *kasû*-

Overview of IGI 1 Manuscripts and Parallels: **AA**=BAM 20; **AB**=BAM 159; **AC**=BAM 19; **AD**=BAM 22; **AE**=BAM 18; **AmA**=BAM 165; **AX**=KAL 7/12; **bA**=BM 41293+; **EA**=EMAR 6/4; **HA**=STT 279; **NA**=BAM 510; **NB**=BAM 513; **NC**=BAM 514; **ND**=BAM 515; **NE**=BAM 516; **NJ**=AMT 12/5; **NQ**=BAM 521; **NU**=AMT 14/3; **sA**=IRAQ 65; **UA**=AuOrS 23/27; **uA**=SpTU 50; **UB**=Ugaritica 5; **UC**=AuOrS 23/14; **xA**=CM 37

53' [...] *tābīla taṭeppi*	plant. 53'[...] (and) you apply (it on the eyes) in dry state.

51' NB ii 3' [...] ZÀ.HI.L]I⸢sar⸣ Ú *a-ši-i*

52' NB ii 4' [...] x *ina um-ma-tu ina* A GAZI^{sar} LUH

53' NB ii 5' [...] *ta-bi-l]*a_{12} *ta-ṭe-ep-pi*

NC ii 1' x [...]

54' *šumma amēlu* [...] *u šamni tasâk tēteneqqi* **Alternative prescription 1** **55'** *ana ašri šanîmma* [...] *tasâk tēteneqqi* **Alternative prescription 2** **56'** *ana ašri šanîmma* [... *šamma peṣâ*] *tābīla ana libbi īnīšu tanappah*	54'If a man's [...], you pound (drug(s)) [in ...] and sesame oil, (and) keep daubing (his eyes). **Alternative prescription 1** 55'Alternatively: you pound [...], you keep daubing (his eyes). **Alternative prescription 2** 56'Alternatively: [...] you blow white plant in a dry state into his eyes.

54' NB ii 6' [...] x ⸢*u* Ì.GIŠ SÚD *te-te*⸣*-né-eq-qí*

NC ii 2' DIŠ NA x [...]

55' NB ii 7' [..] x [x SÚ]D ⸢MAR⸣.MEŠ

NC ii 3' DIŠ ⸢KIMIN⸣ [...]

56' NB ii 8' [.......................... Ú.BABBAR *ta-b]i-la*$_{12}$ ⸢*ana* ŠÀ IGI.MIN-*šú* MÚ⸣*-ah*

NC ii 4' DIŠ KIMIN x [...]

57' *šumma amēlu īnāšu* [*marṣā*? ... *lišān*] *kalbi maštakal ina isqūqi taballal ina karāni išatti*	57'If a man's eyes are [sick ...] 'dog's [tongue]' plant (and) *maštakal*-plant you mix in coarse flour, (then) he drinks (it) in wine. 58'You pound in ghee white

Overview of IGI 1 Manuscripts and Parallels: **AA**=BAM 20; **AB**=BAM 159; **AC**=BAM 19; **AD**=BAM 22; **AE**=BAM 18; **AmA**=BAM 165; **AX**=KAL 7/12; **bA**=BM 41293+; **EA**=EMAR 6/4; **HA**=STT 279; **NA**=BAM 510; **NB**=BAM 513; **NC**=BAM 514; **ND**=BAM 515; **NE**=BAM 516; **NJ**=AMT 12/5; **NQ**=BAM 521; **NU**=AMT 14/3; **sA**=IRAQ 65; **UA**=AuOrS 23/27; **uA**=SpTU 50; **UB**=Ugaritica 5; **UC**=AuOrS 23/14; **xA**=CM 37

58’ *šamma peṣâ* [...] *ashar ina himēti tasâk teqqi*	plant, [...] x (and) *ashar*-stone (and) daub (his eyes).

57’ NB ii 9’ [..^{ú}EME.U]R.GI$_7$ ^{ú}IN$_6$.UŠ *ina* ZÌ.KUM HE.HE *ina* GEŠTIN N[A]G$^?$

NC ii 5’ DIŠ NA IGI.⸢MIN-*šú*⸣ [GIG$^?$ ... ^{ú}EME.UR.G]I$_7$ ⸢^{ú}IN$_6$.UŠ⸣ *i*[*na*$^?$ ....]

58’ NB ii 10’ [... $^{\text{na4}}$*a*]*s-har ina* Ì.NUN SÚD *te*-⸢*qí*⸣

NC ii 6’ Ú.BABBAR ŠI[M ....] ⸢*ina* Ì.NUN⸣ S[ÚD ...]

59’ *šumma amēlu īnāšu marṣā* [...] ...-*šu pāna pāni tašakkan tarakkas* **60’** [...] *ashar ina himēti tasâk teqqi*	[59’]If a man’s eyes are sick: you make his [...] ... face forwards, and bind (it). [60’][...] you pound *ashar*-stone in ghee (and) daub (his eyes).

59’ NB ii 11’ [...] x-⸢*šú*⸣ *pa-na pa-ni* GAR-*an tara-kás*

NC ii 7’ ⸢DIŠ NA IGI.MIN⸣-*šú* GI[G .... *p*]*a-na* ⸢*pa-ni* GAR⸣-*a*[*n tara-k*]*ás*

60’ NB ii 12’ [...^{n}]$^{\text{a4}}$*as-har ina* Ì.NUN SÚD MAR

NC ii 8’ [.................] x [...] *ina* ⸢Ì⸣.NUN SÚD MAR

61’ [*šumma amēlu īnāšu šikna*] *ša dāmi* [*šaknā* (var. *inaṭṭal*) *šamma peṣâ*] *rikibti arkabi emesalli nīnâ* **62’** [*atā’iša kukra lipi kanakti*] *šammī annûti tamarraq ina marat immeri* **63’** [*taballal passa teppuš šumma kūṣu ina mê šumma ummātu*] *ina mê kasî tasappan īnīšu teqqi*	[61’][If a man’s eyes have a blood deposit (var. but he is still able to see): white plant], bat guano, *emesallu*-saline solution, *nīnû*-mint, [62’][*atā’išu*-plant, *kukru*-aromatic, *kanaktu*-aromatic pith]; you grind these drugs together (and) [[63’]mix (the ingredients)] [62’]in bile of a sheep. [63’][You make a collyrium stick (out of it). You soften (it) in water when winter] (and) in the sap of a *kasû*-plant [when summer], (and) you instil his eyes (with the ‘liquid’).

Overview of IGI 1 Manuscripts and Parallels: **AA**=BAM 20; **AB**=BAM 159; **AC**=BAM 19; **AD**=BAM 22; **AE**=BAM 18; **AmA**=BAM 165; **AX**=KAL 7/12; **bA**=BM 41293+; **EA**=EMAR 6/4; **HA**=STT 279; **NA**=BAM 510; **NB**=BAM 513; **NC**=BAM 514; **ND**=BAM 515; **NE**=BAM 516; **NJ**=AMT 12/5; **NQ**=BAM 521; **NU**=AMT 14/3; **sA**=IRAQ 65; **UA**=AuOrS 23/27; **uA**=SpTU 50; **UB**=Ugaritica 5; **UC**=AuOrS 23/14; **xA**=CM 37

61' NB ii 13' [.. U$_5$.A]RGAB^{mušen} ^{mun}*eme-sal-lì* ^{ú}KUR.RA

NC ii 9f.' [...................................... *š*]*á* M[ÚD .... U$_5$.ARGAB^{mu}]^{šen} ^{mun}*eme-sal-lì* / [^{ú}KUR.RA]

(NJ) 2f.' DIŠ NA IGI.MIN-*šú ši*[*k-na* ......] x [..] / ⸢^{ú}⸣KUR.RA →

(AD) r.8f.' DIŠ NA IGI.MIN-*šú šik-na šá* MÚD *šak-*⸢*na* IGI⸣-*al* ⸢Ú⸣.BABBAR / U$_5$.⸢ARGAB⸣^{mušen} ^{mun}*eme-sal-lì* ⸢^{ú}⸣ KUR.⸢RA⸣ →

(xA) 16f.' [DIŠ NA] ⸢IGI.MIN-*šú šik-na šá* MÚD⸣ *š*[*ak-n*]*a* ⸢Ú.BABBAR U$_5$⸣.[ARGAB^{mu}]^{šen} ⸢^{mun}⸣*em*[*e-sal-lì*] / ⸢^{ú}KUR.RA⸣ →

62' NB ii 14' [.. Ú HI].⸢A⸣ *an-nu-ti* 1-*niš ta-mar-raq ina* ZÍ UDU.NÍTA$^{?}$

NC ii 10f.' [^{ú}KU]R.K[UR ....] Ú.MEŠ ⸢ŠEŠ⸣ 1-*niš ta-*⸢*mar-raq*⸣ / [*ina* ZÍ UDU.NÍTA]

(NJ) 3' ⸢^{ú}⸣K[UR.KUR ....]

(NJ) 4' [...................................... UD]U.NÍTA

(AD) r.9ff.' ⸢^{ú}KUR⸣.KUR / ^{šim}GÚR.GÚR Ì.UDU ^{šim}GIG 7 ⸢Ú⸣.HI.A ŠEŠ 1-*niš* ⸢SÚD⸣ / *ina* ZÍ UDU.NÍTA →

(xA) 17f.' ⸢^{ú}⸣ [KUR.KUR ^{šim}G]ÚR.⸢GÚR GAZI^{sar}⸣ [x x x] ⸢x⸣ 8 ⸢Ú⸣.HI.A Š[EŠ ....] / ⸢*ina* ZÍ UDU.NÍTA⸣ →

63' NB ii 15' [.. GAZ]I^{sar} *ta-sa-pan* IGI.MIN-*šú* MAR

NC ii 11' [...] x [............................] x ⸢*ina* A GAZI^{sar}⸣ *ta-sa-*⸢*pan* IGI.MIN-*šú* MAR⸣

(NJ) 4' HE.HE ⸢ZA⸣.N[A ....]

(AD) r.11f.' HE.HE ZA.NA DÙ-*uš* ⸢*šum*$_4$⸣-*ma* É.MEŠ *ina* A.MEŠ / *šum*$_4$-*ma* EN.TE.NA *ina* A.GEŠTIN.NA *t*[*a*]-*sa-pan* MAR

(xA) 18' H[E.HE ZA.N]A ⸢DÙ-*uš šum*$_4$-*ma* EN.TE⸣.[NA *ina*] ⸢A⸣.[M]EŠ ⸢*šum*$_4$-*ma* AMA.MEŠ *ina* A GAZI^{sar} *ta*⸣-*s*[*a-pan* MAR]

64' *šalāšat šiqil rikibti arkabi mišil šiqil šamma peṣâ ina dišip šadê tasâk īnīšu teqqi annû šammu* UD.20.KAM	64'You pound 3 shekels of bat guano, half shekel of white plant in mountain honey, daub his eyes; this is a drug (which is to be used) for twenty days.

Overview of IGI 1 Manuscripts and Parallels: **AA**=BAM 20; **AB**=BAM 159; **AC**=BAM 19; **AD**=BAM 22; **AE**=BAM 18; **AmA**=BAM 165; **AX**=KAL 7/12; **bA**=BM 41293+; **EA**=EMAR 6/4; **HA**=STT 279; **NA**=BAM 510; **NB**=BAM 513; **NC**=BAM 514; **ND**=BAM 515; **NE**=BAM 516; **NJ**=AMT 12/5; **NQ**=BAM 521; **NU**=AMT 14/3; **sA**=IRAQ 65; **UA**=AuOrS 23/27; **uA**=SpTU 50; **UB**=Ugaritica 5; **UC**=AuOrS 23/14; **xA**=CM 37

64'	NA ii 1'	3 GÍN ⌜U₅⌝.[ARGABmušen ....]
	NB ii 16'	[.. *in*]*a* LÀL.KUR.RA SÚD IGI.MIN-*šú* MAR *an-nu-u šam-mi* UD.20.KÁM
	NC ii 12'	⌜3⌝ G[ÍN ....] ⌜1/2? GÍN Ú⌝.[BABBAR .... SÚ]D IGI.MIN-*šú* MAR ⌜*an*⌝-*nu* Ú UD.20.KÁM

65' *šiptu* ib-da-gub numun [... *ina*] *kīri balāṭi* **66'** *balātī napšir balātī napšir* **67'** *ba'lat ina itti amallik* [...] *sinništu ul ullad akla mēṣa mādu tê šipti* **68'** *ka'inimma īnāšu dāma malâ*	65'Incantation: the seed stays with it [........ in the] 'kiln of life', 66''My life be saved; my life be saved!' 67'She is too large; I can judge from the symptom [... (this)] woman cannot give birth. I hold back (treatment) completely. Incantation spell. 68'Invocation (for the case if) his eyes are full of blood.

65'	NA ii 2'	ÉN ib-da-g[ub ....]
	NB ii 17'	[.. *k*]*i*?-⌜*i*⌝-*ri ba-la-ṭi*
	NC ii 13'	ÉN ib-⌜da-gub numun?⌝ [................................ *in*]*a*? ⌜*ki-i*⌝-*ri ba*-⌜*la-ṭi*⌝
66'	NA ii 3'	*ba-la-ṭi n*[*a-ap-ši-ir ba-l*]*a*-⌜*ṭi na*⌝-[*ap-ši-ir*]
	NB ii 18'	[............................ *ba-la*]-*ṭi* ⌜*na*⌝-*ap-ši-ir*
	NC ii 14'	*ba-la-ṭi na-ap-ši-i*[*r* .... *na-a*]*p*-⌜*ši-ir*⌝
67'	NA ii 4'	*ba-'-la-at ina it-ti* [.... MU]NUS? ⌜NU⌝ Ù.TU *ak-lá me-ṣa ma*-⌜*a*⌝-[*du* TU₆.ÉN]
	NB ii 19'	[..] x ⌜NU⌝ Ù.TU ⌜*ak+lá me*⌝-*ṣa ma-a-du* TU₆.ÉN
	NC ii 15'	*ba-'-la-at ina it-ti a-ma-li*[*k*? .... TU₆.É]N
68'	NA ii 5'	KA.INIM.[MA IG]I.MIN-*šú* MÚD DI[RI.MEŠ]
	NB ii 20'	[......................................] MÚD DIRI.MEŠ

Overview of IGI 1 Manuscripts and Parallels: **AA**=BAM 20; **AB**=BAM 159; **AC**=BAM 19; **AD**=BAM 22; **AE**=BAM 18; **AmA**=BAM 165; **AX**=KAL 7/12; **bA**=BM 41293+; **EA**=EMAR 6/4; **HA**=STT 279; **NA**=BAM 510; **NB**=BAM 513; **NC**=BAM 514; **ND**=BAM 515; **NE**=BAM 516; **NJ**=AMT 12/5; **NQ**=BAM 521; **NU**=AMT 14/3; **sA**=IRAQ 65; **UA**=AuOrS 23/27; **uA**=SpTU 50; **UB**=Ugaritica 5; **UC**=AuOrS 23/14; **xA**=CM 37

NC ii 16' ˹KA˺.INIM.MA ˹IGI.MIN-*šú*˺ [........................]

69' *dudubi šuruš urâni ... uqnâta tarakkas erbēšeret kiṣrī takaṣṣar ēma takaṣṣaru šipta tamannu ina nakkaptīšu tarakkas*	69'Its medical application: you bind (together) root of *urânu*-plant, [...], and *uqnâtu*-blue-plant, (and) make fourteen knots. Wherever you make a knot you shall recite the incantation (see ll. 65ff.' above), (and) you bind it on his temple.

69' NA ii 6' DÙ.DÙ.BI SUHU[Š 14
K]A.KEŠDA KEŠDA *e-ma* KEŠDA ÉN ŠID-*nu ina* SAG.K[I-*šú* ....]

NB ii 21' [... 14
K]A.˹KEŠDA˺ KEŠDA *e-ma* KEŠDA ÉN ŠID-*nu ina* ˹SAG˺.KI-*šú tara-kás*

NC ii 17' DÙ.DÙ.BI SUHUŠ ^{ú}˹HA SAHAR$^{?}$ x $^{ú?}$˺ZA.GÌN.NA *tara-kás* 14
KA.KE[ŠDA ....]

70' *šiptu huhahi lā bāmâ huhahi lā bāmâ u agašgû uqatta agašgû uqatta tê šipti*	70'Incantation: (The syllables) hu-ha-hi: not by halves! hu-ha-hi: not by halves! Even a novice can complete it (the syllabary). A novice can complete it! Incantation spell.
71' *ka'inimma šumma amēlu īnāšu dāma malâ*	71'Invocation: if a man's eyes are full of blood.

70' NA ii 7' ÉN *h*[*u-ha-hi* ....
TIL.L]A A.GA.ÁŠ.GA TIL.LA TU$_6$.É[N]

NB ii 22' [... A.G]A.˹ÁŠ˺.GA
TIL.LA A.GA.ÁŠ.GA TIL.LA ˹TU$_6$.ÉN˺

NC ii 18' ÉN *hu-*˹*ha*˺*-h*[*i la b*]*a-*˹*ma hu-ha*˺*-hi la ba-ma* ˹*u* A$^{?}$˺.G[A$^{?}$.ÁŠ.GA
....]

71' NA ii 8' [...] MÚD DIRI.M[EŠ]

NB ii 23' [................................] IGI.MIN-*šú* ˹MÚD DIRI.MEŠ˺

NC ii 19' ˹KA.INIM.MA DIŠ NA IGI.MIN˺-*šú* [........................]

Overview of IGI 1 Manuscripts and Parallels: **AA**=BAM 20; **AB**=BAM 159; **AC**=BAM 19; **AD**=BAM 22; **AE**=BAM 18; **AmA**=BAM 165; **AX**=KAL 7/12; **bA**=BM 41293+; **EA**=EMAR 6/4; **HA**=STT 279; **NA**=BAM 510; **NB**=BAM 513; **NC**=BAM 514; **ND**=BAM 515; **NE**=BAM 516; **NJ**=AMT 12/5; **NQ**=BAM 521; **NU**=AMT 14/3; **sA**=IRAQ 65; **UA**=AuOrS 23/27; **uA**=SpTU 50; **UB**=Ugaritica 5; **UC**=AuOrS 23/14; **xA**=CM 37

72' *dudubi ashar ina himēti tasâk ana libbi īnīšu tanaddi*	72'Its medical application: you pound *ashar*-stone in ghee and apply (it) into his eyes.

72' NA ii 9' [... SÚ]D$^{?}$ *ana* ŠÀ IGI.MIN-*šú* Š[UB]

NB ii 24' [... SÚ]D ⸢*ana* ŠÀ IGI.MIN-*šú* ŠUB⸣

NC ii 20' ⸢DÙ.DÙ⸣.BI ⸢$^{\text{na4}}$*ás*⸣-*har ina* Ì.NUN ⸢SÚD⸣ [....................................]

73' *šiptu* igi ti-la a-ga ti-la geštu kún-na a-ga kún-na ú-⸢hu⸣-ur-sag-gi-na-ta **74'** *šahī šurrāta kušrīn kušrinni šēru šēra ekkal dāmu* **75'** *dāma inaṣṣab šer'ānu šer'ānu uqannan liddi Gula tê balāṭi enqūti* **76'** *ṣimdēti liqerribū attī taškunī balāṭ bulṭi* TU$_6$.ÉN.É.NU.RU **77'** *ka'inimma šumma amēlu īnāšu dāma malâ*	73'Incantation: The eye is healthy, the back is healthy, the ear is shining, the back is shining by means of the 'real mountain plant'. 74'You (the patient) have been leaning (over) my pig! (You Gula) fix me, fix me here! (Because) flesh consumes flesh, blood 75'sucks blood, sinew twists sinew. May Gula cast the life incantation! May the (medical) experts 76'produce the bandages! You (Gula) set the healing-efficacy of the remedy! Incantation spell. 77'Invocation: if a man's eyes are full of blood.

73' NA ii 10' [.. kún-n]a ú-⸢hu-ur-sag⸣-g[i-na-ta]
NB ii 25' [.. kún-n]a ⸢ú-hu-ur-sag-gi⸣-na-ta
NC ii 21' ÉN igi ti-la a-ga ti-la geštu kún$^{?}$-na a-ga kún-na ú-⸢hu⸣-[ur-sag-gi-na-ta]
(UA) r.7f. [ÉN igi t]i-la a-ga ti-[la] / [...] x x [...] / [...] gi-na-ta [...]

74' NA ii 11' [..] *še-e-ru še-e-ra e-k*[*al* ....]
NB ii 26' [.. *še*]-⸢*e*⸣-*ru še-e-ra e-kal da-mu*
NC ii 22' *ša-hi šur-ra-ta kuš-ri-in kuš-ri-in-ni še-e-ru še-e-r*[*a* ....]

75' NA ii 12' [... Š]UB-*di* ^{d}*gu-la* TU$_6$ ⸢TI⸣.[LA ....]

Overview of IGI 1 Manuscripts and Parallels: **AA**=BAM 20; **AB**=BAM 159; **AC**=BAM 19; **AD**=BAM 22; **AE**=BAM 18; **AmA**=BAM 165; **AX**=KAL 7/12; **bA**=BM 41293+; **EA**=EMAR 6/4; **HA**=STT 279; **NA**=BAM 510; **NB**=BAM 513; **NC**=BAM 514; **ND**=BAM 515; **NE**=BAM 516; **NJ**=AMT 12/5; **NQ**=BAM 521; **NU**=AMT 14/3; **sA**=IRAQ 65; **UA**=AuOrS 23/27; **uA**=SpTU 50; **UB**=Ugaritica 5; **UC**=AuOrS 23/14; **xA**=CM 37

NB ii 27' [.. *ú-qa-an-n*]*a-an* ŠUB-*di* ^{d}*gu-la* TU$_6$ TI.LA ⸢*en*⸣-*qu-ti*

NC ii 23' *da-ma i-na-ṣab* SA-*a-nu* SA-*a-nu ú-qa-an-na-an* ŠUB-*di* ^{d}*gu-la* TU$_6$ ⸢TI⸣.L[A ....]

76' NA ii 13' [.. *b*]*a-laṭ bu-ul-ṭi* TU$_6$.ÉN [............]

NB ii 28' [... *taš-ku*]*n*$^{?}$ *ba-laṭ bu-ul-ṭí* TU$_6$.ÉN.É.NU.RU

NC ii 24' *ṣi-im-de-ti li-qer-*⸢*ri*⸣-*bu at-ti taš-ku-ni ba-laṭ bu-ul-ṭi* TU$_6$.ÉN.É.N[U.RU]

77' NA ii 14' [......................... N]A IGI.MIN-*šú* MÚD DI[RI.MEŠ]

NB ii 29' [..............................] IGI.MIN-*šú* MÚD DIRI.MEŠ

NC ii 25' KA.INIM.MA DIŠ NA IGI.MIN-*šú* MÚD DIRI.[MEŠ]

78' *kidkidbi šalāš uṭṭat uhūli qarnānî šalāš uṭṭat hīl abukkati šalāš uṭṭat zê ṣurāri ištēniš tasâk ina šizbi enzi tarabbak īnīšu taṣammid*	[78']Its medical application: you pound together three grains of horned *uhūlu*-alkali, three grains of gummy resin of *abukkatu*-plant (and) a three grain-measure of lizard's excrement. You make an infusion from (them) in goat's milk, bandage his eyes (with it).

78' NA ii 15' [... LI.TA]R ⸢3 ŠE ŠE$_{10}$ EME.ŠID 1-*niš* SÚD *ina* GA UD$_5$⸣ [*tara-bak* IGI.MIN-*šú* LAL]

NB ii 30' [... SÚ]D [*ina* G]A UD$_5$ *tara-bak* IGI.MIN-*šú* ⸢LAL⸣

NC ii 26' ⸢KÌD⸣.KÌD.BI 3 ŠE NAGA.SI 3 ŠE ILLU LI.TAR 3 ŠE ŠE$_{10}$ EME.ŠID 1-*niš* SÚD *ina* GA UD$_5$ *tara-bak* IGI. ⸢MIN-*šú*⸣ LA[L]

79' *šumma amēlu īnāšu marṣāma dāma malâ baluhhī dāma ultatanni'ā dāmu dimtu ina libbi īnīšu ittaṣâ*	[79']If a man's eyes are sick and then full of blood. They (= the eyes) are suffused with *baluhhu*-granules (and) blood, blood (and) tear(s) come out from the middle of his eyes. [80']A film pushes away

Overview of IGI 1 Manuscripts and Parallels: **AA**=BAM 20; **AB**=BAM 159; **AC**=BAM 19; **AD**=BAM 22; **AE**=BAM 18; **AmA**=BAM 165; **AX**=KAL 7/12; **bA**=BM 41293+; **EA**=EMAR 6/4; **HA**=STT 279; **NA**=BAM 510; **NB**=BAM 513; **NC**=BAM 514; **ND**=BAM 515; **NE**=BAM 516; **NJ**=AMT 12/5; **NQ**=BAM 521; **NU**=AMT 14/3; **sA**=IRAQ 65; **UA**=AuOrS 23/27; **uA**=SpTU 50; **UB**=Ugaritica 5; **UC**=AuOrS 23/14; **xA**=CM 37

80' *ṣillu lamassat īnīšu unakkap ašītu ana ṣilli itūr digal ikabbitūšu bīna arqūssu tuhassa*	the pupil of his eyes. The blurred vision has turned into a film, with seeing being burdensome to him. You squeeze *bīnu*-tamarisk while still fresh (and) [81']soak (it) in strong vinegar and let it stay under a star (= stay overnight). In the morning, you press it out into a funnel (lit. *huliam*-vessel). [82']You pound separately *alluharu*-mineral, white plant, *emesallu*-saline solution, fat, *tuškû*-mineral, black cumin (and) exudation of copper. [83']You take in equal amounts, stir (them) together. You pour (them) into the funnel (lit. *huliam*-vessel), which you have (earlier) rinsed. [84']You knead (it) in ghee and *šumēnu*-mineral, then you open the upper part of his eyes with a finger (and) put (the medication) into his eyes. [85']He keeps his eyes closed (while) you rub his eyes (i.e. the eyelids and surroundings) and continuously do this for nine days.
81' *ina ṭābāti dannāti tarammuk ina kakkabi tušbât ina šēri ana libbi huliam taṣahhat*	
82' *alluhara šamma peṣâ emesalli lipâ tuškâ zība hīl erî ahennû tasâk*	
83' *malmališ teleqqe ištēniš tuštemmid ana libbi huliam ša tašhutu tašappak*	
84' *ina himēti u šumēni talâšma rēš īnīšu ina ubāni tepette ana libbi īnīšu tašakkan*	
85' *īnāšu katmā ukâl īnīšu takârma* UD.9.KAM *annâ tēteneppuš*	
Alternative prescription 1	**Alternative prescription 1**
86' *ana ašri šanîmma murra šamma peṣâ emesalli ina uppi siparri ana libbi īnīšu tanappah*	[86']Alternatively: you blow bitter-plant, white plant (and) *emesallu*-saline solution with a bronze tube into his eyes.
Alternative prescription 2	**Alternative prescription 2**
87' *šumma amēlu šanîš hīl erî šamma peṣâ tasâk ina uppi siparri ana libbi īnīšu tanappah*	[87']If a man: alternatively, you pound exudation of copper (and) white plant, you blow it with a bronze tube into his eyes.

Overview of IGI 1 Manuscripts and Parallels: **AA**=BAM 20; **AB**=BAM 159; **AC**=BAM 19; **AD**=BAM 22; **AE**=BAM 18; **AmA**=BAM 165; **AX**=KAL 7/12; **bA**=BM 41293+; **EA**=EMAR 6/4; **HA**=STT 279; **NA**=BAM 510; **NB**=BAM 513; **NC**=BAM 514; **ND**=BAM 515; **NE**=BAM 516; **NJ**=AMT 12/5; **NQ**=BAM 521; **NU**=AMT 14/3; **sA**=IRAQ 65; **UA**=AuOrS 23/27; **uA**=SpTU 50; **UB**=Ugaritica 5; **UC**=AuOrS 23/14; **xA**=CM 37

Alternative prescription 3	**Alternative prescription 3**
88' *šumma amēlu šanîš urnê šamma peṣâ tasâk ina uppi siparri ana libbi īnīšu tanappah*	88'If a man: alternatively, you pound *urnû*-plant (and) white plant, you blow (them) with a bronze tube into his eyes.

79' NA ii 16' DIŠ NA IGI.⸢MIN⸣-*š*[*ú* .... *ul-ta-t*]*a-ni-ʾa* MÚD ÉR *ina* ŠÀ IGI.MIN-*šú* ⸢È⸣-[*a*]

NB ii 31' [.......... .... Š]À IGI.MIN-*šú* ⸢È-*a*⸣

NC ii 27' [DIŠ N]A IGI.MIN-*šú* GIG-*ma* MÚD DIRI ^{šim}BULUH.HI.A MÚD *ul-ta-ta-ni-ʾa* MÚD ÉR *ina* ŠÀ IGI.MIN-*šú* ⸢È⸣-[*a*]

80' NA ii 17' GISSU ^{d}⸢LAMA⸣ IG[I.MIN-*šú* .... GISSU GU]R *di-gal*$_{9}$ DUGUD-*šú* ^{giš}ŠINIG SIG$_{7}$-*su tu-*[*ha-sa*]

NB ii 32' [.......... .... ^{giš}ŠI]NIG ⸢SIG$_{7}$-*su tu-ha-sa*⸣

NC ii 28' [GIS]SU ^{d}LAMA IGI.MIN-*šú ú-na-kap a-ši-tu ana* GISSU GUR ⸢*di*⸣-*gal*$_{9}$ ⸢DUGUD⸣-*šú* ^{giš}ŠINIG SIG$_{7}$-*su tu-ha-s*[*a*]

81' NA ii 18' *ina* A.GEŠTIN.NA KALA.GA *tar*[*a-muk* .... Á.G]Ú.ZI.GA *ana* ŠÀ *hu-li-ia-am* ⸢SUR⸣-[*at*]

NB ii 33' [.......... Á.GÚ.ZI.G]A *ana* ŠÀ *hu-li-ia-am* SUR-*at*

NC ii 29' [*ina* A.GE]ŠTIN.NA KALA.GA *tara-muk ina* UL *tuš-bat ina* Á.GÚ.ZI.GA *ana* ŠÀ *hu-li-ia-am* SUR-⸢*at*⸣

(NU) 7' [.......... S]IG$_{7}$-*su* SÚD A.MEŠ-*šú* SUR-*at ina* UL *tuš-bat* KIMI[N]

82' NA ii 19' IM.SAHAR.BABBAR.KUR.RA Ú.BABBAR ^{mu}[^{n} .... Ì.UD]U *tuš-ka-a* ^{ú}*zi-ba-a* ILLU ⸢URUDU *a-he*⸣-[*nu-ú* ...]

NB ii 34' [.......... .... ^{ú}*z*]*i-ba-a* ILLU URUDU *a-he-nu-ú* SÚD

NC ii 30' [IM.SAHAR].BABBAR.KUR.RA Ú.BABBAR ⸢^{mun}*eme-sal-lì* Ì.UDU *tuš-ka-a*⸣ ^{ú}*zi-ba-a* ILLU URUDU *a-he-nu-u* SÚD

83' NA ii 20' *mál-ma-liš* TI-*qé* 1-*niš tuš-te-mid an*[*a* ŠÀ *hu-li-ia-a*]*m ša ta-áš-hu-tu* DUB-[*ak*]

Overview of IGI 1 Manuscripts and Parallels: **AA**=BAM 20; **AB**=BAM 159; **AC**=BAM 19; **AD**=BAM 22; **AE**=BAM 18; **AmA**=BAM 165; **AX**=KAL 7/12; **bA**=BM 41293+; **EA**=EMAR 6/4; **HA**=STT 279; **NA**=BAM 510; **NB**=BAM 513; **NC**=BAM 514; **ND**=BAM 515; **NE**=BAM 516; **NJ**=AMT 12/5; **NQ**=BAM 521; **NU**=AMT 14/3; **sA**=IRAQ 65; **UA**=AuOrS 23/27; **uA**=SpTU 50; **UB**=Ugaritica 5; **UC**=AuOrS 23/14; **xA**=CM 37

	NB ii 35’	[... *hu-l*]*i-*⸢*ia*⸣*-am ša ta-áš-hu-tu* DUB-*ak*
	NC ii 31’	[.............] TI-*qé* 1-*niš tuš-te-mid ana* ŠÀ *hu-li-ia-am* ⸢*ša*⸣ *ta-áš-hu-tu* DUB-*ak*$^{?}$
84’	NA ii 21’	*ina* Ì.NUN *u* ^{na4}ŠU. ⸢MÌN SILA$_{11}$-*aš*$^{?}$(text NU)-*ma* SAG⸣ I[GI.MIN-*šú*] *ina* ŠU.SI BAD-*te ana* ŠÀ IGI.MIN-*šú* GAR-[*an*]
	NB ii 36’	[.. IGI.MIN-*š*]*ú* *ina* ŠU.SI BAD-*te ana* ŠÀ IGI.MIN-*šú* GAR-*an*
	NC ii 32’	[... Ì.NU]N ⸢*u*⸣ ^{na4}ŠU.MÌN SILA$_{11}$-*aš*$^{?}$(text NU)-*ma* ⸢SAG IGI⸣.MIN-*šú* *ina* ŠU.⸢SI BAD-*te*⸣ *ana* ŠÀ IGI.MIN-*šú* GAR-*an*
85’	NA ii 22’	IGI.MIN-*šú* DUL-*ma ú-kal* IGI.MIN-*šú ta-kar-*⸢*ma* UD⸣.9.KÁM *an-na-a* DÙ.[MEŠ]
	NB ii 37’	[......................................IGI.MI]N-*šú ta-kar-ma* UD.9.KAM* *an-na-a* DÙ.MEŠ
	NC ii 33’	[.............. DU]L-*ma ú-kal* IGI.MIN-*šú* ⸢*ta-kar-ma*⸣ UD.9.KÁM *an-na-a* DÙ.MEŠ
86’	NA ii 23’	DIŠ KIMIN ⸢^{šim}⸣SES Ú.BABBAR ^{mun}*eme-sal-lì* [*ina* MU]D ZABAR *ana* ŠÀ IGI.MIN-*šú* B[ÚN$^{?}$]
	NB ii 38’	[... ^{mu}]^{n}*eme-sal-lì ina* MUD Z[ABAR *ana* ŠÀ IGI].MI[N-*šú* BÚN]
	NC ii 34’	[........................SE]S Ú.BABBAR ^{mun}*eme-sal-lì ina* MUD ZABAR *ana* ŠÀ IGI.MIN-*šú* BÚN
87’	NA ii 24’	DIŠ NA MIN ILLU URUDU Ú.BABBAR SÚD [*ina* MU]D ⸢ZABAR⸣ *ana* ŠÀ IGI.MIN-*šú* [BÚN]
	NB ii 39’	[... SÚ]D$^{?}$ [...................................... ....]
	NC ii 35’	[................ ILL]U$^{?}$ ⸢URUDU Ú⸣.BABBAR SÚD *ina* MUD ZABAR *ana* ŠÀ IGI.MIN-*šú* BÚN

88' NA ii 25' ⌜DIŠ⌝ NA MIN [ú]*úr-né-e* Ú.BABBAR SÚD ⌜*ina* MUD ZABAR⌝ *ana* ŠÀ IGI.MIN-*šú* [BÚN]

NB ii 40' [... S]ÚD ⌜*ina* MUD⌝ ZABA[R ....]

NC ii 36' [...............................] ⌜Ú⌝.BABBAR SÚD ⌜*ina* MUD ZABAR⌝ *ana* ŠÀ IGI.MIN-*šú* BÚN

89' *šiptu* igi bar igi bar-bar igi bar-ra bar-bar igi huš igi huš-huš igi bar-ra huš-huš	[89']Incantation: the open eye is a staring eye, the opened eye stares, the reddish eye is a crimson eye, the opened eye is crimson.
90' igi bar ná-a igi bar da-a igi bar hul-a *īnā abâtu īnā ašâtu*	[90']The open eye is drowsy, the open eye is weak, the open eye is harmed. O cloudy eyes, blurred eyes (vision).
91' [*pursīt*] *dāmi šuharratu īnā kīma niksi immeri dāma šenâ*	[91'][The (eye)] blood [vessel] is porous. The eyes are suffused with blood like a slaughtered sheep,
92' *kīma mê ša agalapê alapâ nadâ kīma karpat ṭābāti nadâ ṣilla*	[92']they (= the eyes) are spotted like the (muddy) water of a lagoon with *alapû*-algae, they (= the eyes) are spotted like a vinegar-jar with a film.
93' *ina berīšina pitiqtu patqat īrub Šakkan ina berūšina ittadi kussâšu*	[93']In between them (= the eyes), a mud-brick wall is constructed (= nose). (The god) Šakkan entered between them (= the eyes) and installed his seat.
94' *aššum annītu ina libbi annīte lā napāše šiptu ul yā'uttun šipat Ea u Asalluhi*	[94']Therefore, one can not breathe in the middle of this (nose). The incantation is not mine; it is the incantation of Ea and Asalluhi,
95' *šipat Dāmu u Gula šipat Ningirimma bēlet šiptī Gula bulliṭīma qīštaki liqī tê šipti*	[95']the incantation of Dāmu and Gula, the incantation of Ningirimma, mistress of incantations. O Gula keep (me) healthy and accept your fee. Incantation spell.
96' *ka'inimma īni marušti*	[96']It is an invocation for a sick eye.

89' NA ii 26' ÉN igi bar igi bar-bar igi bar-ra bar-bar ⌜igi huš⌝ igi huš-huš igi bar-ra h[uš-huš]

Overview of IGI 1 Manuscripts and Parallels: **AA**=BAM 20; **AB**=BAM 159; **AC**=BAM 19; **AD**=BAM 22; **AE**=BAM 18; **AmA**=BAM 165; **AX**=KAL 7/12; **bA**=BM 41293+; **EA**=EMAR 6/4; **HA**=STT 279; **NA**=BAM 510; **NB**=BAM 513; **NC**=BAM 514; **ND**=BAM 515; **NE**=BAM 516; **NJ**=AMT 12/5; **NQ**=BAM 521; **NU**=AMT 14/3; **sA**=IRAQ 65; **UA**=AuOrS 23/27; **uA**=SpTU 50; **UB**=Ugaritica 5; **UC**=AuOrS 23/14; **xA**=CM 37

	NB ii 41’	[.................................... b]ar-ra bar-bar igi huš igi huš-huš igi bar-ra h[uš-huš]
	NC ii 37’	[.....................................bar-r]a bar-bar igi huš igi huš-huš igi bar-ra ⸢huš-huš⸣
	(UA) 5’	[én igi h]uš igi huš-huš igi bar-ra hu[š-huš ....]
90’	NA ii 27’	[igi b]ar ⸢ná-a igi bar da-a igi bar hul⸣-a IGI.MIN *a-ba-tu* IGI.MIN *a-*[*ša-tu*]
	NB ii 42’	[.............................. d]a-a igi bar hul-a IGI.MIN *a-ba-tu* IGI.MIN *a-*⸢*ša*⸣-[*tu*]
	NC ii 38’	[............................. da]-⸢a⸣ igi bar hul-a IGI.MIN *a-ba-tu* IGI.MIN *a-*⸢*ša*⸣-[*tu*]
91’	NA ii 28’	[.................. *šu-h*]*ar-ra-tú* IGI.MIN ^{ERASURE} GIN$_7$ *nik-si* UDU.NÍTA MÚD [............]
	NB ii 43’	[.......................... *šu-h*]*ar-ra-te* IGI.MIN GIN$_7$ *nik-si* UDU.⸢NÍTA MÚD *še-en-a*⸣
	NC ii 39’	[........] ⸢MÚD$^?$ *šu*$^?$*-har*$^?$⸣-[*ra-t*]*e* ⸢IGI.MIN⸣ GIN$_7$ *nik-si* UDU.NÍTA ⸢MÚD⸣ *š*[*e-en-a*]
	(NC) iii 39’	⸢ÉN⸣ [.................................... IGI.MIN *pur-s*]*i-*⸢*it*⸣ MÚD *šu-har-ra-tu*
	(UB) 4f.	IGI.MEŠ *pur-sí-it* ⸢MÚD⸣.ME[Š] / *šu-har-re-tu*$_4$
	(EA) 3	*pur-si-it da-mi i-na-š*[*u*]
92’	NA ii 29’	[.....................................] ⸢*a*⸣*-la-pa-a* ŠUB-*a ki-ma* DUG A.GEŠTIN.NA ŠUB-*a* [.......]
	NB ii 44’	[.. *a-la-p*]*a-a* ŠUB-*a ki-ma* DUG A.GEŠTIN.NA ⸢ŠUB-*a*⸣ *ṣil-la*
	NC ii 40’	⸢GIN$_7$ A.MEŠ *šá*⸣ *a-gala-pe-e a-l*[*a-pa-a* .... *ki-m*]*a* DUG ⸢A.GEŠTIN.NA⸣ [....................]
93’	NA ii 30’	[................................. *pat-qa*]*t*$^?$ ⸢KU$_4$-*ub*⸣ ^{d}GÌR *ina be-ru-ši-na it-ta-*[*di* ....]
	NB ii 45’	[...................... *pi-ti-i*]*q-tu*$_4$ *pat-qat* KU$_4$-*ub* ^{d}GÌR *ina be-ru-ši-na it-ta-di* ^{giš}GU.ZA-*šú*
	NC ii 41’	*ina be-ri-ši-na pi-ti-iq-tu*$_4$ *pat-q*[*at* .... *be-ru-š*]*i-n*[*a* ....]

Overview of IGI 1 Manuscripts and Parallels: **AA**=BAM 20; **AB**=BAM 159; **AC**=BAM 19; **AD**=BAM 22; **AE**=BAM 18; **AmA**=BAM 165; **AX**=KAL 7/12; **bA**=BM 41293+; **EA**=EMAR 6/4; **HA**=STT 279; **NA**=BAM 510; **NB**=BAM 513; **NC**=BAM 514; **ND**=BAM 515; **NE**=BAM 516; **NJ**=AMT 12/5; **NQ**=BAM 521; **NU**=AMT 14/3; **sA**=IRAQ 65; **UA**=AuOrS 23/27; **uA**=SpTU 50; **UB**=Ugaritica 5; **UC**=AuOrS 23/14; **xA**=CM 37

(UC) r.14 x *i-na be-ri-šu pí-ti$_4$-ik-tu$_4$ pa-at-ka-at* TU$_6$.ÉN.É.NU.⸢RU⸣

94’ NA ii 31’ [.. É]N ⸢*ul*⸣ *ia-at-tú-un* ÉN ^{d}*e-a* ⸢*u*⸣ [..............]

NB ii 46’ [..] *la na-pa-še* ÉN *ul* ⸢*ia-at-tu-un*⸣ ÉN ^{d}*e-a u* ^{d}*asal-lú-hi*

NC ii 42’ *áš-*⸢*šúm*⸣ *an-ni-tu ina* ŠÀ *an-ni-te la na-pa-še* É[N$^{?}$ ....]

(EA) 13 *ši-ip-tu ú-ul i-ia-tù*

95’ NA ii 32’ [..] ⸢*be-let*⸣ ÉN ^{d}*gu-la* TI.LA-*ma* NÍG.BA-*k*[*i* ....]

NB ii 47’ [....................... ^{d}*gu-l*]*a* ÉN ^{d}*nin-gìrima be-let šip-te* ^{d}*gu-la* TI-*ma* NÍG.BA-*ki* TI TU$_6$.ÉN

NC ii 43’ ÉN ^{d}*da-mu u* ^{d}*gu-la* ⸢ÉN ^{d}*nin-gìrima*⸣ [.. ....]

(EA) 13f. *ši-pa-at* ^{d}*da-mu* / *u* ^{d}*gu-la*

96’ NA ii 33’ [........................] IGI GIG.GA.[.........]

NB ii 48’ [.......................] IGI GIG.GA.A.KÁM

NC ii 44’ KA.INIM.MA [..................................]

97’ *dudubi annû ša šīpāti peṣâti ṭurra taṭammi sebet kiṣrī takaṣṣar ēma takaṣṣaru šipta tamannu ina īnīšu balitti tarakkassu*	97’Its medical application: you spin this which is a cord of white wool. You shall tie (on) seven knots. Whenever you make a knot, you shall recite the (above) incantation, and bind it on his healthy eye!

97’ NA ii 34’ [.. KE]ŠDA *e-ma* KEŠDA ÉN ŠID-*nu ina* IGI-*šú* ⸢TI⸣.L[A-*ti* ....]

Overview of IGI 1 Manuscripts and Parallels: **AA**=BAM 20; **AB**=BAM 159; **AC**=BAM 19; **AD**=BAM 22; **AE**=BAM 18; **AmA**=BAM 165; **AX**=KAL 7/12; **bA**=BM 41293+; **EA**=EMAR 6/4; **HA**=STT 279; **NA**=BAM 510; **NB**=BAM 513; **NC**=BAM 514; **ND**=BAM 515; **NE**=BAM 516; **NJ**=AMT 12/5; **NQ**=BAM 521; **NU**=AMT 14/3; **sA**=IRAQ 65; **UA**=AuOrS 23/27; **uA**=SpTU 50; **UB**=Ugaritica 5; **UC**=AuOrS 23/14; **xA**=CM 37

NB iii 1	[.............. *an-nu*]-⌜*ú ša* SÍG BABBAR DUR NU.NU 7 KA.KEŠDA KEŠDA⌝ *e-ma* KEŠDA ÉN ŠID-*nu ina* IGI-*šú* ⌜TI.LA-*ti* KEŠDA-*su*⌝
NC ii 45f.'	⌜DÙ.DÙ⌝.BI *an-nu-u ša* SÍG BABBAR DUR NU.NU ⌜7⌝ [.......................... ....] / *ina* IGI-*š*[*ú* ....]

98' *šiptu* igi bar igi bar-bar igi bar-ra bar-bar igi huš igi huš-huš igi bar-ra huš-huš **99'** [igi bar ná-a igi] bar da-a igi bar hul-a *īnā ap/bâtu īnā ašâtu īnā ša dāma malâ* **100'** [*anāku* ...] ... *sāniq qabû ša Gula* **101'** *šittama šinama ahhātu ina berūšina parik šadû* **102'** *manna lušpur ana mārat Ani ša šamê* **103'** *liššâni tallīšina hulāli karpātīšina uqnî ebbi lisāpāni mê ayabbi* **104'** *tâmti rapašte ša harištu lā ūridu ana libbi musukkati lā imsû qātīša* **105'** *lislânimma/limlânimma likeṣṣâ umma ṣirihta ša libbi īnīšu* **106'** *šiptu ul yā'uttun šipat Ea u Asalluhi šipat Dāmu u Gula* **107'** *šipat Ningirimma bēlet šipte Gula bulliṭīma qīštaki liqī tê šipti* **108'** *ka'inimma īni marušti*	[98']Incantation: The open eye is a staring eye, the opened eye stares, the reddish eye is a crimson eye, the opened eye is crimson. [99'][The open eye is drowsy], the open [eye] is weak, the open eye is harmed (lit. evil). O, cloudy eyes, O blurred eyes, eyes which are full of blood. [100'][I am ...] ... the one who executes the command of Gula. [101']They are two, the two are sisters (= the eyes), between whom a mountain is parked! [102']Whom shall I send to the celestial daughter of Anu? [103']May they bring forward their flasks (made) from banded agate (onyx), their vessels (made) from pure lapis lazuli, and draw water of the sea [104']and ocean, into which no woman in confinement plunged (and) no woman in maternity washed her hands! [105']May they sprinkle (var. fill water) and cool off the *ummu*-fever (and) the hotness midst of his (patient) eyes. [106']The incantation is not mine. It is the incantation of Ea and Asalluhi, the incantation of Dāmu and Gula, [107']the incantation of Ningirimma, mistress of incantations. O, Gula keep me healthy and accept your fee. Incantation spell. [108']It is an invocation for a sick eye.

98'	NA ii 35'	[..igi h]uš-huš igi bar-ra [..........]

Overview of IGI 1 Manuscripts and Parallels: **AA**=BAM 20; **AB**=BAM 159; **AC**=BAM 19; **AD**=BAM 22; **AE**=BAM 18; **AmA**=BAM 165; **AX**=KAL 7/12; **bA**=BM 41293+; **EA**=EMAR 6/4; **HA**=STT 279; **NA**=BAM 510; **NB**=BAM 513; **NC**=BAM 514; **ND**=BAM 515; **NE**=BAM 516; **NJ**=AMT 12/5; **NQ**=BAM 521; **NU**=AMT 14/3; **sA**=IRAQ 65; **UA**=AuOrS 23/27; **uA**=SpTU 50; **UB**=Ugaritica 5; **UC**=AuOrS 23/14; **xA**=CM 37

	NB iii 2	[ÉN igi bar igi b]ar-bar igi bar-ra bar-bar igi huš igi huš igi bar-ra huš-huš
	NC iii	begins.
	(UC) r.10	TU$_6$.ÉN.É.[NU.RU ....] igi huš igi huš-huš igi bar-ra huš-huš
99’	NA ii 36’	[.. *a-p]a-tú* IGI.MIN *a-šá-tú* IGI.MIN *ša* MU[D ....]
	NB iii 3	[igi bar ná-a igi] bar da-a igi bar hul-a IGI.MIN *a-ba-a-tu* ⌜IGI.MIN⌝ ⌜*a*⌝*-ša-tu* IGI.MIN *ša* MUD DIRI-*a*
100’	NA ii 37’	[.. *qá-b]u-ú šá* ^{d}*gu-*⌜*la*⌝
	NB iii 4	[..] x 50 NA 50 *sa-niq qá-bu-ú šá* ^{d}*gu-la*
	(AX) ii’ 1’	*ana-*⌜*ku*⌝$^{?}$ x [..]
101’	NA ii 38’	[.. *p]a-rik* KUR-*ú*
	NB iii 5	⌜*2-ma ši-na*⌝*-m[a ah]-ha-a-tu*$_4$ *ina bé-ru-ši-na pa-rik* KUR-⌜*ú*⌝ →
102’	NA ii 39’	[.. *a-ni]m*$^{?}$ *šá* AN-*e*
	NB iii 5	*man-na lu-uš-pur ana* DUMU.MUNUS ^{d}*a-nim šá* AN-*e*
	(AX) ii’ 2’	*man-na* [...]
103’	NA iii 1	*liš-šá-a-ni tal-l[i-ši]-na* ^{na4}NÍR DUG.MEŠ-*ši-na* ^{na4}ZA.GÌN *eb-bu li-sa-pa-a-ni* A.MEŠ A.AB.BA
	NB iii 6	*liš-šá-ni*$^{?}$ *tal-l[i-š]i-na* ^{na4}NÍR DUG.MEŠ-*ši-na* ^{na4}ZA.GÌN *eb-bu li-sa-pa-a-ni* A.MEŠ A.AB.BA →
	(AX) ii’ 3ff.’	*liš-šá-*⌜*a*⌝*-[ni* ....] / *kar-p[a-ti-ši-na* ....] / *li-s[a*$^{?}$*-pa-a-ni* ....] / *i-n[u* ....]
	(EA) 11	*li-ši-a-ni ú-ša-ba-ni me-e* A.BA DAGAL-*ti*
104’	NA iii 2	*tam-tì* DAGAL-*te ša* ⌜*ha-riš*⌝*-tu la ú-ri-du ana lìb-bi mu-suk-ka-tú la* LUH-*u qa-ti-šá*
	NB iii 6f.	*ta-ma-ti* DAGAL-*ti / ša ha-riš-t[u*$^{?}$ *l]a*$^{?}$ *ú-ri-du a-na lìb-bi mu-suk-ka-tu la* LUH-*u qa-te-šá*
105’	NA iii 3	*lis-la-ni-im-ma* ⌜*li*⌝*-ke-eṣ-ṣa-a* KÚM *ṣi-ri-ih-tú šá* ŠÀ IGI.MIN-*šú*
	NB iii 8	*lim-la-ni-im-m[a*$^{?}$ *l]i-ke-eṣ-ṣa-a* KÚM *ṣi-ri-ih-tu šá* ŠÀ IGI.MIN-*šú*
	(AX) ii’ 7’	*ana* IGI.M[IN-*šú* ....]

Overview of IGI 1 Manuscripts and Parallels: **AA**=BAM 20; **AB**=BAM 159; **AC**=BAM 19; **AD**=BAM 22; **AE**=BAM 18; **AmA**=BAM 165; **AX**=KAL 7/12; **bA**=BM 41293+; **EA**=EMAR 6/4; **HA**=STT 279; **NA**=BAM 510; **NB**=BAM 513; **NC**=BAM 514; **ND**=BAM 515; **NE**=BAM 516; **NJ**=AMT 12/5; **NQ**=BAM 521; **NU**=AMT 14/3; **sA**=IRAQ 65; **UA**=AuOrS 23/27; **uA**=SpTU 50; **UB**=Ugaritica 5; **UC**=AuOrS 23/14; **xA**=CM 37

106’ NA iii 4 ÉN *ul ia-at-t*[*u*]*-un* ÉN ^{d}40 *u* ^{d}*asal-lú-hi* ÉN ^{d}*da-mu u* ^{d}*gu-la*
NB iii 9 ÉN *ul ia-a*[*t-tu-un* É]N ^{d}40 *u* ^{d}*asal-lú-hi* ⌜ÉN ^{d}*da*⌝*-mu u* ^{d}*gu-la*
(AX) ii’ 8f.’ É[N ....] / ⌜^{d}⌝ [..]

107’ NA iii 5 ÉN ^{d}*nin-*⌜*gìrima*⌝ *be-let šip-te* ^{d}*gu-la* TI.LA-*ma* NÍG.BA-*ki* TI-*i* TU$_6$.ÉN

NB iii 10 ÉN ^{d}*nin-gì*[*rima* ... *šip-t*]*e* ⌜^{d}*gu-la* TI.L[A-*ma* NÍG.BA-*k*]*i*? [TI]-⌜*i* TU$_6$.ÉN⌝

NC iii 10’ [ÉN] ⌜^{d}*nin-gìrima be-let šip-te* ^{d}*gu*⌝-[*la* ....]

(AX) ii’ 10’ E[N? ....]

108’ NA iii 6 KA.INIM.MA IGI GIG.GA.A.KÁM

NB iii 11 KA.INIM.MA [...............................]

NC iii 11’ KA.INIM.MA [.................................]

(AX) ii’ 11f.’ K[A.INIM.MA ....] / *u* x [......]

109’ *dudubi annû ša šīpāti sāmāti ṭurra taṭammi sebet kiṣrī takaṣṣar ēma takaṣṣaru šipta tamannu ina īnīšu maruštī tarakkas*	109’Its medical application: you spin that which is a cord of red wool, you shall tie seven knots (on it). Whenever you make a knot, you shall recite the incantation (see above). You shall bind (it) on his sick eye!

109’ NA iii 7 DÙ.DÙ.BI *an-nu-u ša* [SÍG S]A$_5$ DUR NU.NU 7 KA.KEŠDA KEŠDA *e-ma* ⌜KEŠDA ÉN⌝ ŠID-*nu ina* IGI-*šú* GIG-*tì* KEŠDA

NB iii 12 DÙ.DÙ.BI *an-nu-ú š*[*a* ....
....]

NC iii 12’ DÙ.DÙ.BI *an-nu-u ša* SÍG SA$_5$ ⌜DUR⌝ NU.NU 7 KA.KE[ŠDA
....]

(AX) ii’ 13’ D[Ù.DÙ.BI ....
....]

Overview of IGI 1 Manuscripts and Parallels: **AA**=BAM 20; **AB**=BAM 159; **AC**=BAM 19; **AD**=BAM 22; **AE**=BAM 18; **AmA**=BAM 165; **AX**=KAL 7/12; **bA**=BM 41293+; **EA**=EMAR 6/4; **HA**=STT 279; **NA**=BAM 510; **NB**=BAM 513; **NC**=BAM 514; **ND**=BAM 515; **NE**=BAM 516; **NJ**=AMT 12/5; **NQ**=BAM 521; **NU**=AMT 14/3; **sA**=IRAQ 65; **UA**=AuOrS 23/27; **uA**=SpTU 50; **UB**=Ugaritica 5; **UC**=AuOrS 23/14; **xA**=CM 37

110' *šiptu* igi bar igi bar-bar igi bar-ra bar-bar igi huš igi huš-huš igi bar-ra huš-huš **111'** igi bar ná-a igi bar da-a igi bar hul-a *īnā apâtu īnā ašâtu* **112'** *īnā pursīt dāmi šuteṣlipātu ammīn tabbâ ammīn taššâ* **113'** *ammīn ikkalkināši bāṣu ša nāri taltallû ša gišimmari* **114'** *ša titti niqqāša ša ari tibnīšu alsīkināši alkāni* **115'** *ul alsīkināši ul tallakāni lām itbâkkināši šūtu iltānu šadû amurru šiptu* **116'** *ka'inimma īni marušti*	110'Incantation: The open eye is a staring eye, the opened eye stares, the reddish eye is a crimson eye, the opened eye is crimson. 111'The open eye is drowsy, the open eye is weak, the open eye is harmed (lit. evil). O cloudy eyes, O blurred eyes, 112'O eyes intersected by blood vessels! Why are you cloudy? Why are you blurry? 113'Why does the sand of the river, the pollen of the date palm 114'(or) the fig, (or) chaff of its straw 113'cause you pain? 114'I called to you, come here (to hide)! 115'Did I not call you? Will you not come here, before the south, north, east (and) west wind rise up against you? (This is) the incantation. 116'It is an invocation for a sick eye.

110'	NA iii 8	ÉN igi bar ig[i .... bar-r]a ⸢bar⸣-bar igi huš igi huš-⸢huš⸣ igi bar-ra huš-huš
	NB iii 13	ÉN igi bar igi bar-bar i[gi ....]
	NC iii 13'	ÉN igi bar igi bar-bar igi bar-ra bar-bar igi huš igi h[uš-hu]š ⸢igi bar⸣-ra ⸢huš⸣-huš
	(AX) i' 1f.'	[.................................. bar]-bar / [...]-⸢huš⸣
	(UC) r.10	TU$_6$.ÉN.É.[NU.RU...............................] igi huš igi huš-huš igi bar-ra huš-huš
111'	NA iii 9	igi bar n[á-a ....] igi bar hul-a IGI.MIN *a-pa-tu* IGI.MIN *a-ša-tu*
	NB iii 14	igi-bar ná-a igi-ba[r ....]
	NC iii 14'	igi-bar ná-a igi-bar da-a igi-bar hul-a IGI.MIN ⸢*a-pa*⸣-*tu* IGI.MIN *a-ša-*⸢*tu*⸣
	(AX) i' 3f.'	[.. h]ul-a / [......................] *šá* MÚD DIRI-*a*
112'	NA iii 10	IGI.MIN *pur-*[*sít* MÚD *šu-te-eṣ-li-p*]*a-*⸢*a*⸣*-tu am-mìn tab-ba-a* ⸢*am-mìn*⸣ ⸢*taš-šá-a*⸣

Overview of IGI 1 Manuscripts and Parallels: **AA**=BAM 20; **AB**=BAM 159; **AC**=BAM 19; **AD**=BAM 22; **AE**=BAM 18; **AmA**=BAM 165; **AX**=KAL 7/12; **bA**=BM 41293+; **EA**=EMAR 6/4; **HA**=STT 279; **NA**=BAM 510; **NB**=BAM 513; **NC**=BAM 514; **ND**=BAM 515; **NE**=BAM 516; **NJ**=AMT 12/5; **NQ**=BAM 521; **NU**=AMT 14/3; **sA**=IRAQ 65; **UA**=AuOrS 23/27; **uA**=SpTU 50; **UB**=Ugaritica 5; **UC**=AuOrS 23/14; **xA**=CM 37

	NB iii 15	⸢IGI.MIN *pur-sít* MÚD⸣ [.................................... *tab-b*]*a-*⸢*a am-mìn taš-šá-a*⸣
	NC iii 15'	IGI.MIN *pur-sít* MÚD *šu-te-eṣ-li-pa-a-tu am-mìn tab-ba-a am-mìn taš-šá-a*
	(AX) i' 5f.'	[.................................... *šu-har*]*-ra-a-te* / [............................]-⸢*ni*$^{?}$ *taš*⸣*-šá-a*
113'	NA iii 11	*am-mì-n*[*i* .... *ba-a-ṣ*]*u ša n*[*a-a-ri* ....]
	NB iii 16	[.. *t*]*al-tal-lu-ú šá* ^{giš}GIŠIMMAR
	NC iii 16'	*am-mì-ni ik-kal-ki-na-ši ba-a-ṣu ša na-a-ri tal-tal-lu-ú šá* ^{giš}⸢GIŠIMMAR⸣
	(AX) i' 7f.'	[..........................]-⸢*ši ba*⸣*-a-ṣu šá na-a-ri* / [.................................... ....]
114'	NA iii 12	*šá ti-*[*it-tu ni-iq-qa-š*]*a* [...]
	NB iii 17	[.. IN.NU-*š*]*u al-si-ki-na al-ka-n*[*i*]
	NC iii 17'	*šá ti-it-tu ni-iq-qa-šá šá a-ri-i* IN.NU-*šu al-si-ki-na-ši al-ka-ni*
	(AX) i' 8f.'	[...] ⸢^{giš}PÈŠ⸣ *ni-iq-qa-šá* / [.............]-⸢*šú al*⸣*-si-ki-na-ši al-ka-ni*
115'	NA iii 13	*ul a*[*l-si-ki-na-ši ul ta-la*]*-k*[*a-ni* ....]
	NB iii 18	⸢*ul al-si*⸣*-*[*ki-na-ši* .... *it-b*]*a-*⸢*ki-na-ši* IM.1 IM.2 IM.3⸣ [...... ....]
	NC iii 18'	*ul al-si-ki-na-ši ul ta-la-ka-ni la-am it-ba-ki-na-ši* IM.1 IM.2 IM.3 IM.4 ⸢ÉN⸣
	(AX) i' 10f.'	[...........]-⸢*na-ši*⸣ *ul tal-la-ka-ni* / [............]-⸢*na-ši*⸣ IM.1 IM.2 IM.3 IM.4 ÉN
116'	NA iii 14	KA.[INIM.MA ...] [.........]
	NB iii 19	KA.INIM.MA IGI GIG.GA.[.......]
	NC iii 19'	KA.INIM.MA IGI GIG.GA.⸢KÁM⸣

Overview of IGI 1 Manuscripts and Parallels: **AA**=BAM 20; **AB**=BAM 159; **AC**=BAM 19; **AD**=BAM 22; **AE**=BAM 18; **AmA**=BAM 165; **AX**=KAL 7/12; **bA**=BM 41293+; **EA**=EMAR 6/4; **HA**=STT 279; **NA**=BAM 510; **NB**=BAM 513; **NC**=BAM 514; **ND**=BAM 515; **NE**=BAM 516; **NJ**=AMT 12/5; **NQ**=BAM 521; **NU**=AMT 14/3; **sA**=IRAQ 65; **UA**=AuOrS 23/27; **uA**=SpTU 50; **UB**=Ugaritica 5; **UC**=AuOrS 23/14; **xA**=CM 37

(AX) i’ 12.’ [................] ⌜IGI⌝ GIG.GA.A.KÁM

117’ *dudubi šīpāti sāmāti šīpāti peṣâti ahennâ taṭammi sebet u sebet kiṣrī takaṣṣar ēma takaṣṣaru šipta tamannu*	117’Its medical application: you spin separately red (and) white wool. You shall tie seven and seven knots (on each wool). Whenever you make a knot, you shall recite the (above) incantation.
118’ *ṭurri šīpāti sāmāti ina īnīšu marušti tarakkas ṭurri šīpāti peṣâti ina īnīšu balitti tarakkasma ina’eš*	118’You tie the cord from the red wool on his sick eye. You tie the cord from the white wool on his healthy eye and then it (the eye) he should get better.

117’ NA iii 15 DÙ.DÙ.B[I SÍG S]A$_5$ SÍG BABBAR *a-he-en-n[a* ....]

NB iii 20 DÙ.DÙ.BI SÍG SA$_5$ ⌜SÍG⌝ B[ABBAR ....] ⌜7⌝ *u* 7 KA.KEŠDA KEŠDA *e-ma* KEŠDA ÉN Š[ID-*nu*]

NC iii 20’ DÙ.DÙ.BI SÍG SA$_5$ SÍG BABBAR *a-he-en-na-a* NU.NU 7 *u* 7 KA.KEŠDA KEŠDA *e-ma* ⌜KEŠDA ÉN ŠID⌝-*n*[*u*]

(AX) i’ 13f.’ [................................ SÍ]G BABBAR ⌜*a-he*⌝-*na-a* NU.NU 7 *u* 7 KA.KEŠDA KEŠDA / [.........................] ⌜ŠID-*nu*⌝ →

118’ NA iii 16 DUR S[ÍG] ⌜ SA$_5$⌝ *ina* IGI-*šú* GIG-*tì* [................................ ....]

NB iii 21 DUR SÍG SA$_5$ *ina* IGI-⌜*šú*⌝ G[IG .... D]UR SÍG BABBAR *ina* IGI-*šú* TI.LA KEŠDA-*ma* *i*[*na-eš*]

NC iii 21’ ⌜DUR SÍG SA$_5$⌝ *ina* IGI-*šú* GIG-*tì* KEŠDA DUR SÍG BABBAR *ina* $^{\text{OVER ERASURE}}$ IGI $^{\text{OVER ERASURE}}$-*šú* TI.LA KEŠDA-*ma* *ina-e*[*š*]

(AX) i’ 14f.’ DUR SÍG SA$_5$ ⌜*ina* IGI-*šú*⌝ GIG KEŠDA-⌜*ás*⌝ / [.................................. *ina* IG]I-⌜*šú ba*⌝-*lit-ti* KEŠDA-*ma* T[I.LA]

119’ *šiptu* igi bar igi bar-bar igi bar-ra bar-bar igi hul igi hul-hul igi bar-ra hul-hul	119’Incantation: The open eye is a staring eye, the opened eye stares, the evil eye is malevolent, the opened eye is malevolent!
120’ *šittāšina mārat Ani ina berūšina pitiqtu patqat*	120’The two of them are daughter(s) of Anu, between whom (the eyes) a mud-brick wall is constructed

Overview of IGI 1 Manuscripts and Parallels: **AA**=BAM 20; **AB**=BAM 159; **AC**=BAM 19; **AD**=BAM 22; **AE**=BAM 18; **AmA**=BAM 165; **AX**=KAL 7/12; **bA**=BM 41293+; **EA**=EMAR 6/4; **HA**=STT 279; **NA**=BAM 510; **NB**=BAM 513; **NC**=BAM 514; **ND**=BAM 515; **NE**=BAM 516; **NJ**=AMT 12/5; **NQ**=BAM 521; **NU**=AMT 14/3; **sA**=IRAQ 65; **UA**=AuOrS 23/27; **uA**=SpTU 50; **UB**=Ugaritica 5; **UC**=AuOrS 23/14; **xA**=CM 37

121’ *ul illak ahātu ana lēt ahātīša manna lušpur ana mārat Ani ša šamê*	(= nose). 121’A sister cannot go to the side (lit. cheek) of her sister! Whom shall I send to the heavenly daughter(s) of
122’ *liššâni kannīšina hulāli karpātīšina zaginduri ebbi*	Anu? 122’May they bring their *kannu*-jars from banded agate (onyx), their vessels of pure *zagindurû*-lapis lazuli! 123’May
123’ *lissapānimma libellâ īnī abâti īnī ašâti u dalhāti tê šipti*	they keep on drawing water and put an end to cloudy, blurred and troubled eyes. Incantation spell. 124’It is an
124’ *ka’inimma īni marušti dudubi* ŠU.BI.GIN$_7$.NAM	invocation for a sick eye. Its medical application is like the (previous) one.

119’ NA iii 17 ÉN ig[i bar] ⸢igi⸣ bar-bar igi bar-ra ⸢bar⸣-ba[r .... h]ul-⸢hul igi⸣ ba[r-ra ....]
NB iii 22 ÉN igi bar igi bar-bar igi bar-r[a bar-bar igi h]ul igi hul-hul igi bar-ra hul-h[ul]
NC iii 22’ ⸢ÉN igi bar igi⸣ bar-bar igi bar-ra bar-bar igi hul igi ⸢hul$^?$⸣-hul igi bar-ra ⸢hul⸣-h[ul]
(AX) i’ 16f.’[............................ ba]r igi bar-ra bar-[bar ...] / [.............. hu]l ⸢igi$^?$ bar$^?$-ra$^?$ hul$^?$⸣-[hul]

120’ NA iii 18 *š[i-it-t]a-⸢ši⸣-na* DUMU.MUNUS ⸢^{d}⸣ [...... *b*]*e-ru-ši-na p*[*i-tiq-tu*$_4$ ....]
NB iii 23 *ši-it-ta-ši-na* DUMU.MUNUS ⸢^{d}⸣ [... *in*]*a* ⸢*be*⸣*-ru-ši-na pi-tiq-tu*$_4$ *pat-qa*[*t*]
NC iii 23’ [*ši-it*]*-⸢ta-ši-na⸣* DUMU.MUNUS ^{d}*a-ni ina be-ru-ši-na pi-tiq-tu*$_4$ *pat-*[*qat*]

121’ NA iii 19 *u*[*l*$^?$ .... *a-ha-ti-š*]*á*$^?$ *man-na lu-uš-pur* ⸢*a*⸣-[*na* (or *a*[*na*) ....]
NB iii 24 *ul il-lak a-ha-tu a-n*[*a le-e*]*t* ⸢*a*⸣*-ha-ti-šá man-na lu-uš-pur a-na* DUMU.MUNUS ^{d}*a-nì šá* ⸢AN-*e*⸣
NC iii 24’ *ul i*[*l-la*]*k* ⸢*a-ha-tu*$_9$$^?$⸣ *ana le-et a-ha-ti-šá man-na lu-uš-pur ana* ⸢DUMU⸣.MUNUS ^{d}*a-nì šá* AN-[*e*]
(AX) ii’ 2’ *man-na* [*lušpur* ....]

122’ NA iii 20 [... D]UG.MEŠ-*ši-na* ^{na4}[...............................]
NB iii 25 *liš-šá-ni kan-ni-ši-na* ^{na4}N[ÍR] DUG.MEŠ-*ši-na* ^{na4}ZA.GÌN.DURU$_5$ *eb-bu*
NC iii 25’ *liš-šá-a-n*[*i kan-n*]*i-ši-na* ^{na4}NÍR DUG.MEŠ-*ši-na* DUG ZA.GÌN.DURU$_5$ *eb-b*[*u*]

Overview of IGI 1 Manuscripts and Parallels: **AA**=BAM 20; **AB**=BAM 159; **AC**=BAM 19; **AD**=BAM 22; **AE**=BAM 18; **AmA**=BAM 165; **AX**=KAL 7/12; **bA**=BM 41293+; **EA**=EMAR 6/4; **HA**=STT 279; **NA**=BAM 510; **NB**=BAM 513; **NC**=BAM 514; **ND**=BAM 515; **NE**=BAM 516; **NJ**=AMT 12/5; **NQ**=BAM 521; **NU**=AMT 14/3; **sA**=IRAQ 65; **UA**=AuOrS 23/27; **uA**=SpTU 50; **UB**=Ugaritica 5; **UC**=AuOrS 23/14; **xA**=CM 37

(AX) ii' 3f.' *liš-šá-⸢a⸣-[ni ....] / kar-pa-[ti-ši-na ....]*

123' NA iii 21 [... *a-b]a-tú* IGI.MIN *a-šá-ti* ⸢*ù*⸣ [..............................]

NB iii 26f. *li-is-sa-pa-ni-im-m[a] li-be-la-a* IGI.MIN *a-ba-ti* / IGI.MIN *a-šá-*⸢*ti ù*⸣ *dal-ha-a-ti* ⸢TU$_6$⸣.ÉN

NC iii 26' *li-is-sa-*⸢*pa*⸣*-ni-im-ma li-be-la-a* IGI.MIN *a-ba-tú* IGI.MIN *a-šá-ti ù dal-ha-a-ti* T[U$_6$.ÉN]

(AX) ii' 5f.' *li-s[a$^?$-pa-a-ni ....] / i-n[u ....]*

124' NA iii 22f. [....................] IGI GIG.[GA ....] / [...........] ŠU.BI.[GIN$_7$.NAM]

NB iii 28 ⸢KA.INIM.MA⸣ IGI GIG.⸢GA.A⸣.KÁM : DÙ.DÙ.BI ŠU.BI.GIN$_7$.⸢NAM⸣

NC iii 27' KA.INIM.MA ⸢IGI⸣ GIG.GA.KÁM : DÙ.DÙ.BI ŠU.⸢BI⸣.GI[N$_7$.NAM]

125' *šiptu* igi bar igi bar-bar igi bar-ra bar-bar igi sùh igi sùh-sùh igi bar-ra sùh-sùh **126'** *šitta īnū ahhātu šinama ina berūšina šadû parik[ma]* **127'** *elēnūšina kiṣirtu kaṣrat šaplānūšina pitiqtu patqat* **128'** *ayyu šāršinama ayyu lā šāršinama* **129'** *ayyu šār tībīšina ayyu lā šār tībīšina(ma$^?$)* **130'** *šār pāni ikil pāni ṣulum pāni attā puṭur Marduk [tê šipti]* **131'** *ka'inimma īni marušti dudubi* ŠU.BI.GIN$_7$.NAM	125'Incantation: The open eye is a staring eye, the opened eye stares, the blurred eye blurs vision, the opened eye is blurred! 126'Two eyes, both are sisters, between whom a mountain is parked! 127'Above whom the 'brow' is furrowed, below whom a mud-brick wall (= nose) is constructed! 128'Which one is their (toxic) wind, which one is not their (toxic) wind? 129'Which is the wind rising against them, which is not a wind, rising against them? 130'You, Marduk, disperse the resistance, gloom, and anger! [Incantation spell.] 131'It is an invocation for a sick eye. Its medical application is like the (previous) one.

125' NA iii 24 [... s]ùh igi sùh-sùh igi b[ar-ra ....]

NB iii 29 ÉN igi bar igi bar-bar igi bar-ra bar-⸢bar⸣ igi sùh igi sùh-sùh igi bar-ra sùh-sù[h]

Overview of IGI 1 Manuscripts and Parallels: **AA**=BAM 20; **AB**=BAM 159; **AC**=BAM 19; **AD**=BAM 22; **AE**=BAM 18; **AmA**=BAM 165; **AX**=KAL 7/12; **bA**=BM 41293+; **EA**=EMAR 6/4; **HA**=STT 279; **NA**=BAM 510; **NB**=BAM 513; **NC**=BAM 514; **ND**=BAM 515; **NE**=BAM 516; **NJ**=AMT 12/5; **NQ**=BAM 521; **NU**=AMT 14/3; **sA**=IRAQ 65; **UA**=AuOrS 23/27; **uA**=SpTU 50; **UB**=Ugaritica 5; **UC**=AuOrS 23/14; **xA**=CM 37

	NC iii 28’	ÉN igi bar igi bar-⸢bar igi bar⸣-ra bar-bar igi sùh igi sùh-sùh i[gi ba]r$^{?}$-⸢ra sùh⸣ s[ùh]
126’	NA iii 25	[.. *in]a be-ru-ši-na* KUR-⸢*ú*⸣ [..........]
	NB iii 30	*ši-it-ta i-nu a-ha-tu ši-[na]-ma ina be-ru-ši-na* KUR-*ú pa-ri[k-ma]*
	NC iii 29’	*ši-it-ta i-nu a-*⸢*ha-tu*⸣ *ši-na-ma ina be-r[u-š]i-na* KUR-*ú pa-r[ik-ma]*
127’	NA iii 26	[.. K]I.⸢TA⸣-*nu-ši-na pi-ti[q-tú* ....]
	NB iii 31	UGU-*nu-ši-na ki-ṣir-tu* ⸢*kàṣ-rat*⸣ KI.TA-*nu-ši-na pi-tiq-tú pat-[qat]*
	NC iii 30’	UGU-*nu-ši-na ki-*⸢*ṣir-tu kàṣ-rat* KI.TA⸣-*nu-ši-na pi-tiq-tu*$_{4}$ [...........]
128’	NA iii 27	[.......................... *a-a]-*⸢*ú*⸣ NU I[M-*ši-na-ma*]
	NB iii 32	*a-a-ú* IM-*ši-na-a-ma a-a-ú* NU IM-⸢*ši*⸣-*n[a-ma]*
	NC iii 31’	*a-a-ú* IM-*ši-na-*⸢*ma a-a*⸣*-ú* NU IM-*ši-n[a*$^{?}$*-ma]*
129’	NA iii 28	[................................ *la]-*⸢*a*⸣ I[M *ti-bi-ši-na* (*-ma*$^{?}$)]
	NB iii 33	*a-a-ú* IM *ti-bi-ši-na a-a-ú la-a* IM *ti-b[i-ši-na* (*-ma*$^{?}$)]
	NC iii 32’	*a-a-ú* IM *ti-bi-ši-*⸢*na*⸣ *a-a-ú* NU IM *ti-bi-ši-n[a*$^{?}$ (*-ma*$^{?}$)]
130’	NA iii 29	**break of K 11847**
	NB iii 34	⸢*ša*⸣*-ar pa-ni i-kíl pa-ni ṣu-lu-u[m*$^{?}$ *p]a*$^{?}$*-n[i*$^{?}$*] a[t*$^{?}$*-ta p]u-ṭu[r* ....]
	NC iii 33’	⸢*ša-ar pa-ni i-kíl pa-ni*⸣ *ṣ[u-lu-um*$^{?}$ *pa-n]i*$^{?}$ ⸢*at*⸣*-ta pu-*⸢*ṭur* ^{d}AMAR$^{?}$⸣.[UTU TU$_{6}$.ÉN]
131’	NB iii 35	[KA.INIM.M]A IGI GIG.GA.A.K[ÁM ....]
	NC iii 34’	[KA.IN]IM.[MA IGI GIG.GA.KÁM : DÙ].DÙ.B[I] ŠU.⸢BI⸣.GI[N$_{7}$.NAM]

132’ *šiptu* [igi bar] igi bar-bar [...] igi bar huš-huš **133’** [...] igi bar-ra nu gi-na **134’** ... [... *sāniq*] *qabû ša Anu tê šipti* **135’** *ka’inimma īni marušti* : *dudubi* ŠU.BI.GIN$_{7}$.NAM	132’Incantation: the open eye is a staring eye [...] the open eye is crimson. 133’[...] the opened eye is not in order. 134’... [... the one who executes] the command of Anu. Incantation spell. 135’It is an invocation for a sick eye. Its medical application is like the (previous) one.

Overview of IGI 1 Manuscripts and Parallels: **AA**=BAM 20; **AB**=BAM 159; **AC**=BAM 19; **AD**=BAM 22; **AE**=BAM 18; **AmA**=BAM 165; **AX**=KAL 7/12; **bA**=BM 41293+; **EA**=EMAR 6/4; **HA**=STT 279; **NA**=BAM 510; **NB**=BAM 513; **NC**=BAM 514; **ND**=BAM 515; **NE**=BAM 516; **NJ**=AMT 12/5; **NQ**=BAM 521; **NU**=AMT 14/3; **sA**=IRAQ 65; **UA**=AuOrS 23/27; **uA**=SpTU 50; **UB**=Ugaritica 5; **UC**=AuOrS 23/14; **xA**=CM 37

132’	NB iii 36	[............... ig]i ⸢bar-bar⸣ x [...]
	NC iii 35’	É[N igi bar i]g[i bar-bar .... i]gi bar huš-huš
133’	NC iii 36’	[...] igi bar-ra nu gi-na
134’	NC iii 37’	x [.. *sa-niq q*]*á-bu-u šá* ^{d}*a-nì* TU$_6$.ÉN
135’	NC iii 38’	[KA.INIM.MA IGI GIG.GA.KÁM : DÙ.DÙ.B]I ŠU.⸢BI⸣.GIN$_7$.NAM

136’ *šiptu* [... *īnā/ū*] *pursīt dāmi šuharratu* **137’** ... [... *īnā/ū*] *ašâtu ša dimti* **138’** ... [... *īnā/ū*] *apâtu eper sūqi u tarbaṣi* **139’** ... [...] ... *sumuktu* **140’** ... [...] ... [...] **141’** ... [...] ... [...]	136’Incantation: [... O eyes,] porous blood vessels, 137’... [... eyes] blurred (because) of tear(s). 138’... [...] cloudy (eyes) (because of) street and the stall dust. 139’... [...] ... *sumuktu*-dirt?. 140’... [...] ... [...] 141’... [...] ... [...]

136’	NC iii 39’	⸢ÉN⸣ [.................................... IGI.MIN *pur-s*]*i-*⸢*it* MÚD *šu-har-ra-tu*⸣
	(NA) ii 28’	[.................. *šu-h*]*ar-ra-tú* IGI.MIN ^{ERASURE} GIN$_7$ *nik-si* UDU.NÍTA MÚD [............]
	(NB) ii 43’	[.......................... *šu-h*]*ar-ra-te* IGI.MIN GIN$_7$ *nik-si* UDU.⸢NÍTA MÚD *še-en-a*⸣
	(NC) ii 39’	[........] ⸢MÚD? *šu*?-*har*?⸣-[*ra-t*]*e* ⸢IGI.MIN⸣ GIN$_7$ *nik-si* UDU.NÍTA ⸢MÚD⸣ *š*[*e-en-a*]
	(UB) 4f.	IGI.MEŠ *pur-sí-it* ⸢MÚD⸣.ME[Š] / *šu-har-re-tu*$_4$
	(EA) 3	*pur-si-it da-mi i-na-š*[*u*]
137’	NC iii 40’	x [... IGI.MIN *a-ša*]-⸢*a*⸣-*tu*$_4$ *ša* ÉR
138’	NC iii 41’	x [.. *a-p*]*a-a-tu* SAHAR$^{(sic!)}$ SILA *u* TÙR
139’	NC iii 42’	x [...] x x *su-muk-t*[*ú*]
140’	NC iii 43’	x [.. l]ú?-⸢tur?-a?-ke$_4$? KUM?⸣ x [....]
141’	NC iii 44’	x [...] x ⸢^{ú}HAR.HAR?⸣ x [.......]

GAP!

Overview of IGI 1 Manuscripts and Parallels: **AA**=BAM 20; **AB**=BAM 159; **AC**=BAM 19; **AD**=BAM 22; **AE**=BAM 18; **AmA**=BAM 165; **AX**=KAL 7/12; **bA**=BM 41293+; **EA**=EMAR 6/4; **HA**=STT 279; **NA**=BAM 510; **NB**=BAM 513; **NC**=BAM 514; **ND**=BAM 515; **NE**=BAM 516; **NJ**=AMT 12/5; **NQ**=BAM 521; **NU**=AMT 14/3; **sA**=IRAQ 65; **UA**=AuOrS 23/27; **uA**=SpTU 50; **UB**=Ugaritica 5; **UC**=AuOrS 23/14; **xA**=CM 37

The space on NB, between 79-7-8, 156 [AMT 8/3] and K 7105, is unclear. But there are at least ca. 11 lines missing on NB.

142’ NB iii 47a’ [...] x

143’ [*dudubi ... šīpāti sāmāti šīpāti peṣâti*] *ahennâ taṭammi* **144’** [*sebet kiṣrī takaṣṣar ēma takaṣṣaru šipta tamannu*] *ina nakkaptīšu tarakkassu*	143’[Its *medical application*:] you spin separately [red (and) white wool$^?$ ...] 144’[You shall tie seven knots. Whenever you make a knot you shall recite the incantation.] You bind it on his temple.

143’ NB iii 47b’ [DÙ.DÙ.BI ....] ⸢*a-he-en-na-a*⸣ [N]U.NU

144’ NB iii 47c’ [...] *ina* SAG.KI-*šú* KEŠDA-⸢*su*⸣

145’ [*šiptu ...*] *īni lā iraššâ tê šipti*	145’[Incantation: ... malady of] the eye must not develop. Incantation spell.

145’ NB iii 47d’ [ÉN ....] x$^?$ IGI NU TUK-*a* TU$_6$.ÉN

146’ [*dudubi ... ina nakkaptīšu*] *ša imitti*	146’[Its medical application: ... you bind it on his$^?$] right [temple$^?$]

146’ NB iii 47e’ [*dudubi* .... *ina* SAG.KI-*šú*$^?$] *šá* ZAG

147’ [*šiptu* ... ta-ma-ad-r]a-áš ta-ma-ad-ra-áš tu$_6$-én	147’[Incantation: ...] tamadraš tamadraš. Incantation spell.

147’ NB iii 47f’ [ÉN .... ta-ma-ad-r]a-áš ta-ma-ad-ra-áš tu$_6$-én

148’ [*dudubi ... ina nakkaptīšu*] *ša šumēli*	148’[Its medical application: ... you bind it on his$^?$] left [temple$^?$].

148’ NB iii 47g’ [DÙ.DÙ.BI .... *ina* SAG.KI-*šú*$^?$] *šá* GÙB

Overview of IGI 1 Manuscripts and Parallels: **AA**=BAM 20; **AB**=BAM 159; **AC**=BAM 19; **AD**=BAM 22; **AE**=BAM 18; **AmA**=BAM 165; **AX**=KAL 7/12; **bA**=BM 41293+; **EA**=EMAR 6/4; **HA**=STT 279; **NA**=BAM 510; **NB**=BAM 513; **NC**=BAM 514; **ND**=BAM 515; **NE**=BAM 516; **NJ**=AMT 12/5; **NQ**=BAM 521; **NU**=AMT 14/3; **sA**=IRAQ 65; **UA**=AuOrS 23/27; **uA**=SpTU 50; **UB**=Ugaritica 5; **UC**=AuOrS 23/14; **xA**=CM 37

Begin of K 13465 on ms. NA

149' [*ka'inimma īni marušti*] *dudubi* ŠU.BI.GIN$_7$.NAM	149'[It is an invocation for a sick eye.] Its medical application is like the (previous) one.

149' NA iii 29a' [KA.INIM.MA IGI GIG.GA.K]Á$^?$[M ....]

NB iii 47h' [.. DÙ.D]Ù.BI ŠU.BI.GIN$_7$.NA[M]

150' [*šiptu* ... gi]n$_7^?$ a a-lal-la ér gub-ba-a gub-ba-a **151'** [*Marduk ippalissuma ana*] *Ea abīšu išassi* **152'** [*minâ ēpuš ul idi ša anāku*] *īdû attā tīdi tê* [*šipti*] **153'** *ka'inimma īni marušti*	150'[Incantation: ... (pouring out)] like the water of the shaduf, o tear(s) be present, be present! 151'[Marduk noticed it (the harm) and then] cried out [to] his father Ea: 152'[what I must do I do not know: what I] know, you (already) know. Incantation spell. 153'[It is an invocation] for a sick eye.

150' NA iii 29b' [ÉN .... gi]n$_7^?$ a a-lal-la ér gub-ba[-a...............]
NB iii 47i' [ÉN .... g]ub-ba-a gub-b[a-a]

151' NA iii 29c' [*Marduk ip-pa-lis-su-ma ana*] ⸢^{d}⸣*é-a* ⸢AD⸣-*šú i-šá-a*[*s-si*]
NB iii 47j' [.. AD-š]*ú*$^?$ *i-šá-*⸢*as*⸣-[*si*]

152' NA iii 29d' [*mi-na-a e-pu-uš ul i-di ša ana-ku i-du*]-⸢*u*$^?$⸣ *at-ta ti-di* T[U$_6$.ÉN]

NB iii 47k' [..] ⸢*ti-di*⸣ T[U$_6$.ÉN]

153' NA iii 29e' [*ka'inimma* IG]I GIG.GA.[KÁM]

154' *dudubi šīpāti sāmāti šīpāti peṣâti ištēniš taṭammi sebet u sebet kiṣrī takaṣṣar ēma takaṣṣaru šipta tamannu ina nakkapātīšu tarakkasma ina'eš*	154'Its medical application: you spin together red (and) white wool. Seven and seven knots you shall tie. Whenever you make a knot you shall recite the incantation. You bind it on his temples and he will get better.

Overview of IGI 1 Manuscripts and Parallels: **AA**=BAM 20; **AB**=BAM 159; **AC**=BAM 19; **AD**=BAM 22; **AE**=BAM 18; **AmA**=BAM 165; **AX**=KAL 7/12; **bA**=BM 41293+; **EA**=EMAR 6/4; **HA**=STT 279; **NA**=BAM 510; **NB**=BAM 513; **NC**=BAM 514; **ND**=BAM 515; **NE**=BAM 516; **NJ**=AMT 12/5; **NQ**=BAM 521; **NU**=AMT 14/3; **sA**=IRAQ 65; **UA**=AuOrS 23/27; **uA**=SpTU 50; **UB**=Ugaritica 5; **UC**=AuOrS 23/14; **xA**=CM 37

154’ NA iii 29f’ [.. *e-m*]*a*$^?$ ⌜KEŠDA⌝ ÉN ŠID-*nu ina* SAG.K[I ....]

NB iv 1f. [.................. SÍ]G SA$_5$ ⌜SÍG BABBAR 1⌝-[*niš* .... / ....] KEŠDA ÉN ⌜ŠID-*nu*⌝ *i*[*na* ....]

NC iv 1 ⌜DÙ⌝.D[Ù.BI ....] ⌜1-*niš* NU.NU 7 *u* 7 KA.KEŠDA KEŠDA *e-ma* KEŠDA$^?$ ÉN ŠID-*nu ina* SAG.KI.MEŠ-*šú* KEŠDA-*ma ina-eš*⌝

155’ [*šiptu* i-gi t]i-la a-ga ti-la i-gi kún-na a-ga kún-na : ur-sag gi-na-zu gi bàn-da-zu tu$_6$-én **156’** *ka’inimma īni marušti* : *dudubi* ŠU.BI.GIN$_7$.NAM	155’[Incantation: The eye] is healthy, the back is healthy, the eye is shining, the back is shining! Your tiny reed is your faithful hero. Incantation spell. 156’It is an invocation for a sick eye. Its medical application is like the (previous) one.

155’ NA iii 29g–h’ [... n]a a-ga k[ún$^?$-na .... /............. z]u$^?$ tu$_6$-[én]

NB iv 3 [ÉN i-gi t]i-la a-ga ti-la i-gi kún-na ⌜a⌝-[ga] ⌜kún⌝-n[a.......................... ....]

NC iv 2 [............................ ti-l]a ⌜i-gi⌝ kún-na a-ga kún-⌜na : ur-sag gi⌝-na-zu gi ⌜bàn-da-zu tu$_6$-én⌝

156’ NA iii 29i’ [...Š]U.BI.GI[N$_7$.NAM]

NB iv 4 [KA.IN]IM.MA IGI GIG.GA.A.KÁ[M (:)] DÙ.DÙ.⌜BI⌝ [...........................]

NC iv 3 K[A.INIM.MA IGI] GIG.GA.A.KÁM : DÙ.DÙ.BI ŠU.BI.GIN$_7$.NAM

157’ *šiptu* pa-la huš pa-la huš pa-la huš-bi níg-gi-na-bi i-gi pa-la huš-bi tu$_6$-én **158’** *ka’inimma īni marušti dudubi* ŠU.BI.AŠ.ÀM	157’Incantation: reddish ‘robe’, reddish ‘robe’, its ‘robe’ is reddish! In truth: the eye’s ‘robe’ is reddish. Incantation spell. 158’It is an invocation for a sick eye. Its medical application is the same (as the previous one).

157’ NA iii 29j’ **Presumably two lines until the beginning of col. iv.**

Overview of IGI 1 Manuscripts and Parallels: **AA**=BAM 20; **AB**=BAM 159; **AC**=BAM 19; **AD**=BAM 22; **AE**=BAM 18; **AmA**=BAM 165; **AX**=KAL 7/12; **bA**=BM 41293+; **EA**=EMAR 6/4; **HA**=STT 279; **NA**=BAM 510; **NB**=BAM 513; **NC**=BAM 514; **ND**=BAM 515; **NE**=BAM 516; **NJ**=AMT 12/5; **NQ**=BAM 521; **NU**=AMT 14/3; **sA**=IRAQ 65; **UA**=AuOrS 23/27; **uA**=SpTU 50; **UB**=Ugaritica 5; **UC**=AuOrS 23/14; **xA**=CM 37

	NB iv 5	[ÉN pa-l]a ⌜huš⌝ pa-la huš pa-la huš-⌜bi⌝ ní[g-gi-n]a-bi i-gi pa-la ⌜huš⌝-b[i tu$_6$-én]
	NC iv 4	⌜ÉN pa-la huš pa-la huš pa-la huš-bi níg-gi-na-bi i-gi-i pa-la huš-bi tu$_6$-én⌝
158'	NB iv 6	[KA.INIM.MA] ⌜IGI GIG⌝.GA.A.⌜KÁM DÙ⌝.DÙ.BI ⌜ŠU⌝.BI.A[Š.ÀM]
	NC iv 5	⌜KA.INIM.MA IGI GIG.GA.A.KÁM⌝ : DÙ.DÙ.BI ŠU.BI.AŠ.ÀM

159' *šiptu īni eṭli marṣat īni ardati marṣat īni eṭli u ardati mannu uballiṭ*	[159']Incantation: The eye of the lad is sick; the eye of the maiden is sick! Who will heal the eye of the lad and the maiden?
160' *tašappar ileqqûnikku libbi elleti gišimmari ina pîka teheppi ina qātīka tepettil*	[160']You will send for (and) they will bring you a clean date-palm offshoot! You break (it) up with your mouth (teeth) and twist (it to thread) with your hand.
161' *eṭla u ardata ina nakkapātīšunu tukaṣṣar īn eṭli u ardati iballuṭ tê šipti*	[161']You bind (it) up on the lad's or maiden's temples and the eye of the lad and the maiden should recover. Incantation spell.
162' *ka'inimma īni marušti dudubi* ŠU.BI.AŠ.ÀM	[162']It is an invocation for a sick eye. Its medical application is the same (as the previous one).

159'	NA iv 1	⌜ÉN⌝ *i-ni* GURUŠ ⌜GIG-*at i-ni* ^{munus}KI.SIKIL⌝ GIG-*at i-ni* GURUŠ *u* ^{munus}KI.SIKIL *man-nu ú-bal-liṭ*
	NB iv 7	[ÉN *i*]-*ni eṭ-li* GIG-⌜*at i*⌝-*n*[*i* ^{munus}K]I.SIKIL GIG-*at i-ni* GURUŠ *u* ^{munus}KI.SIKIL *man-nu* ⌜*ú*⌝-[*bal-liṭ*]
	NC iv 6	⌜ÉN *i-ni* GURUŠ GIG-*at i-ni* ^{munus}KI.SIKIL GIG-*at i-ni* GURUŠ *u* ^{munus}KI.SIKIL *man-nu ú-bal*$^{?}$-*liṭ*⌝
	(HA) 17f.	ÉN IGI GURUŠ GIG-*ma* IGI KI.SIKIL GIG-*ât* / IGI GURUŠ *u* KI.SIKIL *man-nu ú-bal-laṭ*
160'	NA iv 2	*ta-šap-pár i-*⌜*le*⌝-*qu-ni-ku* ŠÀ KÙ-*ti* ^{giš}GIŠIMMAR *ina pi-i-ka te-he-pi ina* ŠU-*ka te-pe-til*
	NB iv 8	[*ta-š*]*ap-pár i-le-qu-ni-ku* ⌜ŠÀ KÙ-*ti* ^{giš}GIŠIMMAR *ina pi-i-ka te-he-pi ina* ŠU-*ka te-pe*⌝-*ti*[*l*]

Overview of IGI 1 Manuscripts and Parallels: **AA**=BAM 20; **AB**=BAM 159; **AC**=BAM 19; **AD**=BAM 22; **AE**=BAM 18; **AmA**=BAM 165; **AX**=KAL 7/12; **bA**=BM 41293+; **EA**=EMAR 6/4; **HA**=STT 279; **NA**=BAM 510; **NB**=BAM 513; **NC**=BAM 514; **ND**=BAM 515; **NE**=BAM 516; **NJ**=AMT 12/5; **NQ**=BAM 521; **NU**=AMT 14/3; **sA**=IRAQ 65; **UA**=AuOrS 23/27; **uA**=SpTU 50; **UB**=Ugaritica 5; **UC**=AuOrS 23/14; **xA**=CM 37

	NC iv 7	⸢*ta-šap-pár i-le-qu-ni-ku* ŠÀ KÙ-*ti* ^{giš}GIŠIMMAR *ina pi-i-ka te-he-pi ina* ŠU-*ka te-pe-til*⸣
	(HA) 18f.	*a-šap-par i-liq-qu-nik-ki* / ŠÀ KÙ-*ti* ^{giš}GIŠIMMAR : *ina pi-i-ka te-he-pi ina* ŠU-*ka* SÚD
161'	NA iv 3	GURUŠ *u* KI.SIKIL ⸢*ina* SAG.KI.MEŠ⸣-*šú-nu tu-ka-ṣar* IGI GURUŠ *u* KI.SIKIL *i-bal-lu-uṭ* TU$_6$.ÉN
	NB iv 9	[GURUŠ *u* K]I.SIKIL *ina* SAG.KI.MEŠ-*šú-nu tu-ka-ṣar* IGI GURUŠ *u* KI.SIKIL *i-bal-lu-uṭ* TU$_6$.⸢ÉN⸣
	NC iv 8	⸢GURUŠ *u* KI.SIKIL *ina* SAG.KI.MEŠ-*šú-nu tu-ka-ṣar* IGI GURUŠ *u* KI.SIKIL *i-bal-lu-uṭ* TU$_6$.ÉN⸣
	(HA) 20f.	IGI$^{?}$(text BAD) GURUŠ *u* KI.SIKIL *ina* SAG.KI-*šú tu*$^{?}$(text ⸢LI⸣)-*ka-ṣar* / IGI GURUŠ *u* KI.SIKIL *i-bal-luṭ* ⸢ÉN⸣
162'	NA iv 4	KA.INIM.⸢MA⸣ IGI GIG.GA.A.KÁM DÙ.DÙ.BI ERASURE ŠU.BI.AŠ.ÀM
	NB iv 10	[KA.I]NIM.MA IGI GIG.GA.A.KÁM DÙ.DÙ.BI ŠU.BI.AŠ.ÀM
	NC iv 9	⸢KA.INIM.MA IGI GIG.GA.A.KÁM DÙ.DÙ.BI ŠU.BI.AŠ.ÀM⸣
	(HA) 22	KA.INIM IGI GI[G..........]
	(HA) 23ff.	DÙ.DÙ.BI SÍG S[A$_5$ SÍG BABBAR 1-*niš* NU.NU] / ⸢7 [*u*] 7 ⸢KA.KEŠDA⸣ KE[ŠDA *e-ma* KEŠDA] / ⸢ÉN$^{?}$⸣ [Š]ID-*n*[*u* .....] / $^{\text{r.1}}$ *ana* SAG.KI.MIN-*šú* KEŠDA-*m*[*a ina-eš*/TIN]

NB.: Billingual incantation, for the Sumerian see the score text (partiture) below!

163' *šiptu ina šamê šāru izīqamma ina īn amēli simmē ištakan* **164'** *ištu šamê rūqūti* **165'** *ana īnī marṣāti simme ištakan* **166'** *ša amēlu šuātu īnāšu dalhā* **167'** *īnāšu ašâ* **168'** *amēlu šū ina ramānīšu marṣiš ibakki* **169'** *ša amēlu šuātu murussu Nammu īmurma*	163'Incantation: The wind blew in the sky and thus caused lesions in a man's eye. 164'From the distant sky, the wind blew in the sky and thus caused lesions in a man's eye. 165'It caused lesions within the sick eyes! 166'Regarding that man, his eyes are troubled, 167'his eyes are blurred! 168'This man weeps bitterly by himself. 169'It was that man's illness

Overview of IGI 1 Manuscripts and Parallels: **AA**=BAM 20; **AB**=BAM 159; **AC**=BAM 19; **AD**=BAM 22; **AE**=BAM 18; **AmA**=BAM 165; **AX**=KAL 7/12; **bA**=BM 41293+; **EA**=EMAR 6/4; **HA**=STT 279; **NA**=BAM 510; **NB**=BAM 513; **NC**=BAM 514; **ND**=BAM 515; **NE**=BAM 516; **NJ**=AMT 12/5; **NQ**=BAM 521; **NU**=AMT 14/3; **sA**=IRAQ 65; **UA**=AuOrS 23/27; **uA**=SpTU 50; **UB**=Ugaritica 5; **UC**=AuOrS 23/14; **xA**=CM 37

170’ *kasî hašlūti leqēma* **171’** *šipat apsî idīma* **172’** *īnī amēli rukusma* **173’** *Nammu ina qātīša elleti īn amēli ina labātīša* **174’** *šāru ša īn amēli uddupu ina īnīšu littaṣi* **175’** *ka’inimma īni marušti*	which the (water goddess) Nammu noticed (and said): [170’]‘Take crushed *kasû*-plant, [171’]recite the Apsû incantation, [172’](and) bandage the eyes of the man.’ [173’]When Nammu touches the man’s eye with her clean hand, [174’]may the wind which has inflated the man’s eye depart from his eye(s)! (Incantation!) [175’]It is an invocation for a sick eye.

163’ NA iv 5f. én an-na ⸢im⸣ ri-a igi lú-ka gig-ga ba-an-gar / *ina šá-me-e šá-a-ru i-zi-qam-ma ina i-in* LÚ *si-im-me iš-ta-kan*
NB iv 11f. [é]n an-na im ri-a igi lú-ka gig-ga ba-an-gar / *ina šá-me-e šá-*⸢*a*⸣*-ru i-zi-qam-ma ina i-in* LÚ *si-im-me iš-ta-kan*
NC iv 10f. ⸢én an-na im ri-a igi lú-ka gig-ga ba-an-gar / *ina šá-me-e šá-a-ru i-zi-qam-ma ina i-in* LÚ *si-im-me iš-ta-kan*⸣
(HA) r.2ff. én an-na im ⸢ri-a⸣ igi ⸢lú⸣-k[a g]i[g-ga] / ba-an-gar : *ina* AN-*e* IM *i-zi-qam-ma* / *ina i-ni* LÚ *sim-mu iš-ta-kan*

164’ NA iv 7f. an-ta ⸢sù⸣-da-ta im ri-a$^{?}$(text MIN$^{?}$) igi lú-ka gig-ga ba-an-gar / *iš-tu* AN-*e ru-qu-ti*
NB iv 13 ⸢an⸣-ta sù-da-ta im ri-a igi lú-ka gig-ga ba-an-gar : *iš-tu* AN-*e ru-qu-ti*
NC iv 12f. ⸢an-ta sù-da-ta im ri-a igi lú-ka gig-ga ba-an-gar⸣ / ⸢*iš-tu* AN-*e*⸣ *r*[*u*]-⸢*qu*⸣*-ti*
(HA) r.5ff. an-ta sù-ud-da im ri-a / igi lú gig ba-an-gar / *ul-tú* AN-*e ru-qu-ti šá-a-ru* / *i-zi-qam-ma*$^{?}$ *ina i-ni* LÚ *sim-mu* / *iš-ta-kan*

165’ NA iv 9 igi gig-⸢ga⸣ gig-ga ba-an-gar : *ana i-ni mar-ṣa-a-ti si-im-me iš-ta-kan*
NB iv 14f. ⸢igi gig⸣-ga gig-ga ba-an-gar / [...] ⸢*i*⸣*-ni mar-ṣa-a-ti si-im-ma iš-ta-kan*
NC iv 14 ⸢igi gig-ga gig-ga⸣ [...................... *i-n*]*i m*[*ar-ṣa-a-ti si-i*]*m-me iš-ta-kan*
(HA) r.10 igi gig gig ba-an-gar
(HA) r.11 *ina i-ni mar-ṣa-ti sim-mu iš-ta-kan*

166’ NA iv 10 lú-bi igi-bi lù-lù-a : *šá* LÚ *šu-a-tú i-na-šú da-al-ha*
NB iv 16f. [lú-b]i igi-bi lù-lù-a / [*šá* LÚ *šu*]-⸢*a-tú*⸣ *i-da-šú da-*⸢*al*⸣*-h*[*a*]
NC iv 15 [.. *i-n*]*a-šú* ⸢*da-al*⸣*-ha*
(HA) r.12 lú-bi igi-bi lù-lù-a

Overview of IGI 1 Manuscripts and Parallels: **AA**=BAM 20; **AB**=BAM 159; **AC**=BAM 19; **AD**=BAM 22; **AE**=BAM 18; **AmA**=BAM 165; **AX**=KAL 7/12; **bA**=BM 41293+; **EA**=EMAR 6/4; **HA**=STT 279; **NA**=BAM 510; **NB**=BAM 513; **NC**=BAM 514; **ND**=BAM 515; **NE**=BAM 516; **NJ**=AMT 12/5; **NQ**=BAM 521; **NU**=AMT 14/3; **sA**=IRAQ 65; **UA**=AuOrS 23/27; **uA**=SpTU 50; **UB**=Ugaritica 5; **UC**=AuOrS 23/14; **xA**=CM 37

	(HA) r.13	*šá* LÚ *šu-u* IGI.MIN-*šú dal-ha*
167’	NA iv 11	igi-bi ⸢ba⸣-an-⸢sùh⸣-sùh : *i-na-šú a-šá-a*
	NB iv 16f.	⸢igi-bi⸣ ba-an-⸢sùh⸣-sùh / [*i-n*]*a-š*[*ú*] *a-šá-a*
	NC iv 16	[..] ⸢*a*⸣-*šá-a*
	(HA) r.14	igi-bi sùh-sùh : *i-na-šú a-šá-a*
168’	NA iv 12f.	lú-⸢u$_{18}$-lu⸣-bi ní-te-a-ni-šè ér gig ì-šéš-šéš / LÚ ⸢*šu*⸣-*ú ina ra-ma-ni-šú mar-ṣi-iš i-bak-ki*
	NB iv 18f.	⸢lú-u$_{18}$-lu-bi ní-te-a-ni-šè ér gig ì-šéš-šéš⸣ / LÚ *šu-ú ina ra-ma-ni-šú mar-ṣi-iš i-b*[*ak-ki*]
	NC iv 17f.	[lú-u$_{18}$-lu-bi ní-te-a-ni-šè ér gig ì-š]éš-šéš / [.. ....] ⸢*i*⸣-*bak-ki*
169’	NA iv 14	lú-⸢bi tu⸣-ra-a-ni ^{d}engur-ke$_{4}$ igi ⸢im⸣-ma-an-sì : *šá* LÚ *šú-a-tú mu-ru-us-su* ^{d}MIN *i-mur-ma*
	NB iv 20f.	lú-bi tu-ra-a-ni ^{d}engur-ke$_{4}$ ⸢igi im-ma⸣-a[n$^{?}$-sì] / *šá* LÚ *šú-a-tu$_{4}$* *mu-ru-us-su* ^{d}MIN ⸢*i-mur-ma*⸣
	NC iv 19	[.. *mu-ru-us-s*]*u* ⸢^{d}MIN *i-mur*⸣-*ma*
	(HA) r.15	lú-bi tu-ra-a-ni ^{d}íd-ke$_{4}$ igi im-ma-an-sì
	(HA) r.16	LÚ *šú-a-tú* GIG-*su* ^{d}ÍD *i-mur-ma*
170’	NA iv 15	gazi$^{⸢sar⸣}$ gaz-gá šu ù-me-ti : *ka-si-i haš-lu-ti le-qé-ma*
	NB iv 22f.	gazi^{sar} kum-mà ⸢šu⸣ ù-me-ti / *ka-si-i haš-lu-ti le-qé-ma*
	NC iv 20	[.. *le-q*]*é-ma*
	(HA) r.17	gazi^{sar} al-šeg$_{6}$-gá šu u-me-ti
	(HA) r.18	⸢*ka-se-e ba*⸣-*áš-lu-te le-qé-ma*
171’	NA iv 16	⸢tu$_{6}$-tu$_{6}$⸣ abzu-ta u-me-ni-sì : *ši-pat ap-si-i i-di-ma*
	NB iv 24f.	tu$_{6}$-tu$_{6}$ abzu-ta ù-me-ni-sì / *ši-pat ap-si-i i-di-ma*
	NC iv 21	[... *i-di*]-*m*[*a*]
	(HA) r.19	[......... abzu-t]a u-m[e-ni-sì]
	(HA) r.20	too broken, no dividing line visible, but expected.
172’	NA iv 17	i[gi l]ú-ka ù-me-ni-kešda : *i-ni a-me-li ru-kus-ma*

Overview of IGI 1 Manuscripts and Parallels: **AA**=BAM 20; **AB**=BAM 159; **AC**=BAM 19; **AD**=BAM 22; **AE**=BAM 18; **AmA**=BAM 165; **AX**=KAL 7/12; **bA**=BM 41293+; **EA**=EMAR 6/4; **HA**=STT 279; **NA**=BAM 510; **NB**=BAM 513; **NC**=BAM 514; **ND**=BAM 515; **NE**=BAM 516; **NJ**=AMT 12/5; **NQ**=BAM 521; **NU**=AMT 14/3; **sA**=IRAQ 65; **UA**=AuOrS 23/27; **uA**=SpTU 50; **UB**=Ugaritica 5; **UC**=AuOrS 23/14; **xA**=CM 37

	NB iv 26f.	igi lú-ka ù-me-ni-kešda / *i-ni a-me-li ru-kus-ma*
	NC iv 22	[.. *ru-kus-m*]*a*?
	(HA) r.21	[igi l]ú-⌜bi u-me-ni-kešda⌝ : ⌜*i-ni a-me*⌝-[*li* ....]
173'	NA iv 18f.	[^{d}engu]r lú šu kù-ga-na igi lú-ba-ka šu tag-ga-ni-ta / [^{d}MI]N *ina* ŠU-*šá* KÙ-*ti i-in a-me-lì ina la-ba-ti-šá*
	NB iv 28f.	^{d}engur lú šu kù-ga-⌜na igi⌝ l[ú-ba-ka šu tag-g]a-ni-ta / ^{d}MIN *ina* ŠU-*š*[*á* .... *l*]*a*-⌜*ba*⌝-*ti-šá*
	NC iv 23f.	too broken
	(HA) r.22	^{d}íd šu kù-ga-a-ni igi lú-bi-ta šu t[ag-ga-ni-ta]
	(HA) r.23	^{d}MIN *ina* ŠU.MIN-*šú* KÙ-*te i-ni* LÚ *ina la-pa-t*[*i-šú*]
174'	NA iv 20f.	[im ig]i lú-ka sù-sù igi-bi-ta ba-ra-an-è / [*ša-a*]-*ru šá i-in a-me-lì ud-du-pu ina i-ni-šú lit-ta-ṣi*
	NB iv 30f.	im igi lú-k[a .... ba-ra-a]n-è / *šá-a-rù šá* ⌜*i*⌝-[*in* .... *lit-t*]*a-ṣi*
	NC iv 25f.	[.......................................ba-ra-a]n-⌜è⌝ / [.................................... ....*ina* I]GI-⌜*šú*⌝ *lit-ta-ṣi*
	(HA) r.24	im igi lú-geš sù-sù igi-bi-šè ba-ra-⌜è⌝
	(HA) r.25	*šá-a-ru šá i-ni* LÚ *ud-du-pu ina i-ni-šú lit-ta-ṣi* ÉN
175'	NA iv 22	[KA.I]NIM.MA IGI GIG.GA.A.KÁM
	NB iv 32	⌜KA⌝.I[NIM.MA ....].⌜A⌝.KÁM
	NC iv 27	[..................... IG]I GIG.GA.A.KÁM
	(HA) r.26	KA.INIM.MA *šá* IGI.MIN.MEŠ GIG.MEŠ
	(HA) r.27f.	DÙ.DÙ.BI GAZI^{sar} ŠEG$_6$-*šal* SÚD / ÉN *an-ni-te* 7?-*šú ana* UGU ŠID-*nu*
	(HA) r.29	LAL-*ma ina-ah*

176' [*šiptu*] *īnū apâtu īnū ašâtu īnū pursindi dāmi šuharriātu* **177'** *šina ibakkâ ana pān ummīšina Mami*	176'[Incantation.] O cloudy eyes, O blurred eyes, O porous blood vessels! 177'The two (eyes) are weeping before their mother

Overview of IGI 1 Manuscripts and Parallels: **AA**=BAM 20; **AB**=BAM 159; **AC**=BAM 19; **AD**=BAM 22; **AE**=BAM 18; **AmA**=BAM 165; **AX**=KAL 7/12; **bA**=BM 41293+; **EA**=EMAR 6/4; **HA**=STT 279; **NA**=BAM 510; **NB**=BAM 513; **NC**=BAM 514; **ND**=BAM 515; **NE**=BAM 516; **NJ**=AMT 12/5; **NQ**=BAM 521; **NU**=AMT 14/3; **sA**=IRAQ 65; **UA**=AuOrS 23/27; **uA**=SpTU 50; **UB**=Ugaritica 5; **UC**=AuOrS 23/14; **xA**=CM 37

178' *ammīn nâšima ittīni tarkusī ašâ dāma u šāra tê šipti* **179'** *ka'inimma īni marušti*	Mami: [178']'Why us and (why) did you saddle us with blurred (vision), blood, and wind?' Incantation spell. [179']It is an invocation for a sick eye.

176' NA iv 23 [ÉN *i-n*]*u a-pa-tú i-nu a-šá-tú i-nu pur-si-in-di da-a*$^{?}$(text MIN$^{?}$)-*mi šu-har-ri-a-tu*$_4$
NB iv 33 [.. *šu-har-ri-a-t*]*u*$_4$
NC iv 28 [... *pur-si-in-d*]*i da-a-mi šu-har-ri-a-tu*$_4$

177' NA iv 24 [*ši-n*]*a i-bak-ka-a ana* IGI AMA-*ši-na* ⸢^{d}*ma-mi*⸣
NB iv 33 **Broken**
NC iv 29 [............................ *ana* IG]I AMA-*ši-na* ^{d}*ma-mi*

178' NA iv 25 [*a-m*]*ì-in na-ši-ma it-ti-ni tar-ku-si a-šá-a d*[*a-a-ma* ....]
NC iv 30 [...] ⸢*a*⸣-*šá-a da-a-ma u šá-a-ra* TU$_6$.ÉN

179' NA iv 26 [KA.IN]IM.MA [..................................]
NC iv 31 [........................] ⸢IGI⸣ GIG.GA.⸢A⸣.KÁM

180' [*dudubi*] *šīpāti sāmāti šīpāti peṣâti ahennâ taṭammi ina qablīšunu lippa talpap* **181'** *šīpāti sāmāti ina īnīšu marušti šīpāti peṣâti ina īnīšu balitti tarakkasma ina'eš*	[180'][Its medical application]: You spin separately red and white wool, make a wad from their middle (parts), [181']bind the [red wool] on his sick eye and the white wool on his healthy eye, and he will get better.

180' NA iv 27 [DÙ.DÙ.BI] S[ÍG S]A$_5$ ⸢SÍG BABBAR *a-he-en-na-a*⸣ N[U.NU ....]
NC iv 32 [.. *a-he-e*]*n-*⸢*na-a* NU.NU *ina* MURUB$_4$-*šú-nu*⸣ *líp-pa tál-pap*

181' NA iv 28 [SÍG SA$_5$ *ina* I]GI-*šú* GIG SÍG BABBAR *ina* IGI-⸢*šú*⸣ T[I ....]
NC iv 33 [..................................] ⸢SÍG BABBAR *ina* IGI-*šú* TI KEŠDA-*ma*⸣ *ina-eš*

Overview of IGI 1 Manuscripts and Parallels: **AA**=BAM 20; **AB**=BAM 159; **AC**=BAM 19; **AD**=BAM 22; **AE**=BAM 18; **AmA**=BAM 165; **AX**=KAL 7/12; **bA**=BM 41293+; **EA**=EMAR 6/4; **HA**=STT 279; **NA**=BAM 510; **NB**=BAM 513; **NC**=BAM 514; **ND**=BAM 515; **NE**=BAM 516; **NJ**=AMT 12/5; **NQ**=BAM 521; **NU**=AMT 14/3; **sA**=IRAQ 65; **UA**=AuOrS 23/27; **uA**=SpTU 50; **UB**=Ugaritica 5; **UC**=AuOrS 23/14; **xA**=CM 37

182' [*šiptu* še l]á še lá hu-tu-ul hu-tu-ul igi lal hu-tu-ul min igi lal-bi hu-tu-ul min **183'** [*šatti*] *pāna magir šatti pāna magir iṭâb magir šanîš tê šipti* **184'** *ka'inimma šumma amēlu īnāšu dalhā*	[182'][Incantation: the winnowed grain], the winnowed grain! It is afflicted, the diminished eye (vision) is afflicted, it is afflicted, ditto, that diminished eye is afflicted, ditto! [183']In the spring it was favourable, in the spring it was favourable! It will be good (and) favourable, secondly (it will be good and favourable)! Incantation spell. [184']Invocation: if the man's eyes are troubled.

182' NA iv 29 [ÉN še l]á še lá hu-tu-ul hu-tu-ul igi lal ⌜hu⌝-t[u-ul ....]
NC iv 34 [......... hu-tu]-⌜ul hu-tu-ul igi lal hu-tu-ul min igi lal-bi hu-tu-ul min⌝

183' NA iv 30 [*ša-at-ti p*]*a-na* ŠE.GA *ša-at-ti pa-na* Š[E.GA ....]

NC iv 35 [..................... Š]E.⌜GA *ša-at-ti pa-na* ŠE.GA *i-ṭàb* ŠE.GA MIN TU$_6$.ÉN⌝

184' NA iv 31 [KA.INI]M.MA DIŠ N[A ....] L[Ù.LÙ]

NC iv 36 [.............] ⌜DIŠ NA IGI.MIN-*šú* LÙ.LÙ⌝

(ND) iv 45' [DIŠ NA] IGI.MIN-*šú* LÙ.LÙ LÀL BABBAR *ina* Ì [..................................]
(NE) i 1 DIŠ NA IGI.MEŠ-*šú* LÙ.LÙ ⌜LÀL⌝ BABBAR *ina* ⌜Ì⌝ [...............................]

(xA) r.9 [DI]Š NA IGI.MIN-*šú* LÙ.LÙ-⌜*ha*⌝ LÀL Ì.NUN.NA Ì.⌜SAG⌝ 1-*niš* HE.HE *ina* GE$_6$ IGI.MIN-*šú* DIR[I]

(uA) r.8f. DIŠ NA IGI.MEŠ-šú LÙ.LÙ-*ha* LÀL Ì.NUN.NA Ì.SAG gloss: *hal-ṣa* 1-*niš* x ERASURE? KÚM.KÚM-*am ta-šá-hal ana* IGI.MIN-*šú* ŠUB

185' [*dudubi*] *birki immeri teleqqe* [...] *u*? *ṭurra taṭammi ana šinīšu teṣṣip* ... [...] **186'** *sebet* [*u*] *sebet kiṣrī takaṣṣar ēma takaṣṣaru šipta tamannu ina nakkaptīšu tarakkasma ina'eš*	[185'][Its medical application]: take sheep testicle (lit. 'knee') [...], and you spin (and) twine a two-ply cord ... [...], [186']you shall tie seven [and] seven [knots]. Whenever you make a knot, you shall recite the incantation (see above), you

Overview of IGI 1 Manuscripts and Parallels: **AA**=BAM 20; **AB**=BAM 159; **AC**=BAM 19; **AD**=BAM 22; **AE**=BAM 18; **AmA**=BAM 165; **AX**=KAL 7/12; **bA**=BM 41293+; **EA**=EMAR 6/4; **HA**=STT 279; **NA**=BAM 510; **NB**=BAM 513; **NC**=BAM 514; **ND**=BAM 515; **NE**=BAM 516; **NJ**=AMT 12/5; **NQ**=BAM 521; **NU**=AMT 14/3; **sA**=IRAQ 65; **UA**=AuOrS 23/27; **uA**=SpTU 50; **UB**=Ugaritica 5; **UC**=AuOrS 23/14; **xA**=CM 37

	bind it on his temple, (and) he will get better.

185' NA iv 32 D[Ù.DÙ.BI *b*]*ir*-⸢*ki* UDU TI-*qé*⸣ [x x] *u* DUR NU.NU *ana* 2-*šú te-eṣ-ṣi-ip* x [x x]

NC iv 37f. [...................................] x x x (x) ⸢*u*? DUR NU.NU *ana* 2-*šú te-eṣ-ṣi-ip*⸣ / [x x x]

186' NA iv 33 7 [*u* 7 .... É]N? ŠID-*nu ina* SAG.KI-*šú* KEŠDA-*m*[*a* ....]

NC iv 38 [.....] ⸢7 KA.KEŠDA KEŠDA *e-ma* KEŠDA ÉN ŠID-*nu ina* SAG.KI-*šú* KEŠDA-*ma ina-eš*⸣

187' *šiptu* [*attina*] *īnā pursimīt dāmi šuharratu ammīni taššâni hāma* **188'** *handabillu šuršurra alapâ ša nāri ina sūqāti kirbāna* **189'** *ina tukqinnāte huṣāba ammīni taššâni zunnāni kīma kakkabi* **190'** *mitaqqutāni kīma nabli lām ikšudūkināši ṣurru u naglabu* **191'** *ša Gula šipat lā paṭāri šipat Asalluhi Marduk šipat Ningirimma bēlet šipti* **192'** *u Gula bēlet asûti iddīma anāku ašši tê šipti* **193'** *ka'inimma hāmū huṣāba u mimma ša īnī šūlî*	[187']Incantation: O [you] eyes are porous blood vessels! Why have you picked up chaff, [188']the *handabillu*-pebbles?, *šuršurru*-fibre?, the *alapû*-algae of the river, the clods from the streets (and) [189']twigs from the refuse heaps? Why have you carried (them) along? Rain down like (a shooting) star, [190']drop down like a meteor (lit. flame), before [191']Gula's [190']flint-razor and scalpel manage to reach you (i.e. the eyes). [191']An irreversible incantation, the incantation of Asalluhi and Marduk, the incantation of Ningirimma, mistress of incantations, [192']and Gula, mistress of the medical skill; she casts (the spell) and I (the *asû*-healer) carry (it) out. Incantation spell. [193']Invocation for removing the chaff, splinter and anything (else) from the eyes.

187' NA iv 34 ÉN *a*[*t-ti-na* .... *pu*]*r*-⸢*si-mi-it*⸣ MÚD *šu-har-ra-tú am-mi-ni ta-aš-ša-ni ha*-⸢*ma*⸣

Overview of IGI 1 Manuscripts and Parallels: **AA**=BAM 20; **AB**=BAM 159; **AC**=BAM 19; **AD**=BAM 22; **AE**=BAM 18; **AmA**=BAM 165; **AX**=KAL 7/12; **bA**=BM 41293+; **EA**=EMAR 6/4; **HA**=STT 279; **NA**=BAM 510; **NB**=BAM 513; **NC**=BAM 514; **ND**=BAM 515; **NE**=BAM 516; **NJ**=AMT 12/5; **NQ**=BAM 521; **NU**=AMT 14/3; **sA**=IRAQ 65; **UA**=AuOrS 23/27; **uA**=SpTU 50; **UB**=Ugaritica 5; **UC**=AuOrS 23/14; **xA**=CM 37

	NC iv 39’	[.................] ⸢*i-na pur-si-mi-it* MÚD *šu-har-ra-tú am-mi-ni ta-aš-šá-ni ha-ma*⸣
188’	NA iv 35	*ha-an-d[a-bi-l]u*? *šu-ur-šu-ra e-lap*?*-pa-a ša* ÍD *ina* SILA.MEŠ *kir-ba-ni*
	NC iv 40’	[.............] ⸢*šu-úr-šu-ri-im a-lap-pa-na*?*-a ša* ÍD *ina* SILA.MEŠ *kir-ba-ni*⸣
189’	NA iv 36	*ina tub-kí[n-na]-*⸢*a*⸣*-te hu-ṣa-a-ba am-mi-ni taš-ša-ni zu-un-na-ni* GIN$_7$ MUL
	NC iv 41’	[........................*-t*]*e* ⸢*hu-ṣa-a-ba am-mi-ni taš-ša-ni zu-un-na-ni* GIN$_7$ MUL⸣
190’	NA iv 37	*mi-ta-q[u-ta]-ni* GIN$_7$ *nab-li la-am ik-šu-du-ki-na-ši ṣur-ru nag-la-bu*
	NC iv 42’	[*mi-t*]*a-*⸢*qu-ta-ni* GIN$_7$ *nab-li la-am ik-šu-du-ki-na-ši ṣur-ru u nag-la-bu*⸣
191’	NA iv 38	*šá* ^{d}*gu-la* É[N N]U DU$_8$ ÉN ^{d}*asal-lú-hi* ^{d}AMAR.UTU ÉN ^{d}*nin-gi-rim-ma* EN ÉN
	NC iv 43’	[*ša* ^{d}*gu-l*]*a* ⸢ÉN NU DU$_8$ ÉN ^{d}*asal-lú-hi* ^{d}AMAR.UTU ÉN ^{d}*nin-gi-rim-ma* EN ÉN⸣
192’	NA iv 39	*u* ^{d}*gu-la* ⸢EN⸣ [A.Z]U-*ti i-di-ma ana-ku áš-ši* TU$_6$.ÉN
	NC iv 44’	[............................*-t*]*i* ⸢*i-di-ma*⸣ [..............] ⸢TU$_6$.ÉN⸣
193’	NA iv 40	KA.INIM.MA ⸢*ha-a*⸣*-mu hu-ṣa-ba u mim-ma ša* IGI.MIN *šu-li-i*
	NC iv 45’	[KA.INIM.M]A ⸢*ha-a-mu hu-ṣa-ba u mim-ma* IGI.MIN *šu-li-i*⸣

194’ *šiptu ina šurrî lām bašāmu alallû urda ana māti* **195’** *ittû šer’a ūlid šerhu habburra* **196’** *habburra kanna kannu kiṣra kiṣru šubulta šubultu* **197’** *mer’a Šamaš eṣṣid Sîn upahhar Šamaš ina eṣēdīšu Sîn ina puhhurīšu*	194’Incantation. In the beginning before creation, the shaduf descended (from heaven) to earth, 195’the seeder-plough gave birth to the furrow, the furrow to the sprout, 196’the sprout to the root-stock, the root-stock to the bud, the bud to the head-of-grain, (and) the head-of-grain to 197’the *merhu*-kernel. The Sun-god was harvesting, the Moon-god was reaping. While the Sun-god was

Overview of IGI 1 Manuscripts and Parallels: **AA**=BAM 20; **AB**=BAM 159; **AC**=BAM 19; **AD**=BAM 22; **AE**=BAM 18; **AmA**=BAM 165; **AX**=KAL 7/12; **bA**=BM 41293+; **EA**=EMAR 6/4; **HA**=STT 279; **NA**=BAM 510; **NB**=BAM 513; **NC**=BAM 514; **ND**=BAM 515; **NE**=BAM 516; **NJ**=AMT 12/5; **NQ**=BAM 521; **NU**=AMT 14/3; **sA**=IRAQ 65; **UA**=AuOrS 23/27; **uA**=SpTU 50; **UB**=Ugaritica 5; **UC**=AuOrS 23/14; **xA**=CM 37

198’ *ana īn eṭli merhu īrub Šamaš u Sîn išizzānimma merhu lilâ* [*tê šipti*] **199’** *ka’inimma merhu ša libbi īnī šūlî*	harvesting (and) the Moon-god was reaping, [198’]the *merhu*-kernel entered into the eye of the lad. O Sun-god and Moon-god stand by me, and let the *merhu*-kernel take off! [Incantation spell.] [199’]Invocation for removing the *merhu* from out of the eyes.

194’ NA iv 41 ÉN *ina šur-ri-i la-*⸢*am*⸣ *ba-ša-mu a-la-lu ur-da ana ma-t*[*i*]
NC iv 46’ [........................ *ba-ša-m*]*u* [*a-l*]*a-l*[*u*] ⸢*ur-da ana ma*⸣*-t*[*i*]

195’ NA iv 42 *it-tu-ú še-er-a* Ù.TU *še-er-hu hab-bur-r*[*a*]
NC iv 47’ [.................] ⸢Ù.TU *še*⸣*-er-hu* [..............]

196’ NA iv 43 *hab-bur-ra ka-an-na* ⸢*ka*⸣*-an-nu ki-iṣ-ra ki-iṣ-ru šu-bu-ul-ta šu-bu*[*l-tu*]
NC iv 48’ [............................. *ka-an*]*-*⸢*nu ki-iṣ-ra ki-iṣ-ru šu-bu*⸣*-*[*ul-ta* ....]

197’ NA iv 44 *mé-er-a* ^{d}UTU *e-ṣi-*⸢*id*⸣ ^{d}30 *ú-pa-har* ^{d}UTU *ina e-ṣe-di-šú* ^{d}30 *ina pu-h*[*u-ri-šú*]
NC iv 49’ [.................................. *ú-pa-ha*]*r* ^{d}UTU *ina e-*⸢*ṣe-di*⸣*-*[*šú* ....
.......]

198’ NA iv 45 *ana* IGI GURUŠ *me-er-hu* KU$_4$-⸢*ub*⸣ ^{d}UTU *u* ^{d}30 *i-ši-za-nim-ma mé-er-hu li-la-*⸢*a*⸣ [TU$_6$.ÉN]
NC iv 50’ [..] ⸢*i-ši*⸣*-*[*za-ni*]*m-*⸢*ma*⸣ *mé-e*[*r-hu*
..........................]

199’ NA iv 46 KA.INIM.MA *mé-er-hu* ⸢*ša*⸣ ŠÀ IGI.MIN *š*[*u-li-i*]
NC iv 51’ [KA.INIM.MA *me-er-hu ša*] ⸢ŠÀ IGI.MIN *šu*⸣*-*[*li-i*]

Catchline of Tablet Two **200’** *šumma amēlu īnāšu murdinnī malâ sahlê qēm labti ina šikari tarabbak taṣammid* UD.3.KAM *īnīšu* [*lā tapaṭṭar*]	**Catchline of Tablet Two** [200’]If a man’s eyes are full of *murdinnu*-brambles: you shall make an infusion from *sahlû*-plant (and) flour of roasted grain in beer, (and) bandage (his eyes).

Overview of IGI 1 Manuscripts and Parallels: **AA**=BAM 20; **AB**=BAM 159; **AC**=BAM 19; **AD**=BAM 22; **AE**=BAM 18; **AmA**=BAM 165; **AX**=KAL 7/12; **bA**=BM 41293+; **EA**=EMAR 6/4; **HA**=STT 279; **NA**=BAM 510; **NB**=BAM 513; **NC**=BAM 514; **ND**=BAM 515; **NE**=BAM 516; **NJ**=AMT 12/5; **NQ**=BAM 521; **NU**=AMT 14/3; **sA**=IRAQ 65; **UA**=AuOrS 23/27; **uA**=SpTU 50; **UB**=Ugaritica 5; **UC**=AuOrS 23/14; **xA**=CM 37

	For three days [you do not loosen (the bandage from)] his eyes.

200’ NA iv 47 DIŠ NA IGI.MIN-*šú mur-din-n*[*i* DIRI] *sah-lé-e* ZÌ [................] KA[Š ....]

(ND) i 1 [........................... *mur-di*]*n-ni* DIRI *sah-lé-e* ZÌ ŠE.SA.A *ina* KAŠ *tara-bak* LAL UD.3.KÁM IGI.MIN-*š*[*ú* NU DU₈]

Name of Tablet One	**Name of Tablet One**
201’ [*ištēn*] *tuppu šumma* [*amēlu īnāšu marṣā*]	[201’][First] Tablet [of the (Treatise)] ‘If [man’s eyes are sick’.]

201’ NA iv 48 DU[B.1$^{?}$.KÁM$^{?}$] DI[Š NA$^{?}$ IGI$^{?}$.MIN$^{?}$-*šú*$^{?}$ GIG$^{?}$]

Overview of IGI 1 Manuscripts and Parallels: **AA**=BAM 20; **AB**=BAM 159; **AC**=BAM 19; **AD**=BAM 22; **AE**=BAM 18; **AmA**=BAM 165; **AX**=KAL 7/12; **bA**=BM 41293+; **EA**=EMAR 6/4; **HA**=STT 279; **NA**=BAM 510; **NB**=BAM 513; **NC**=BAM 514; **ND**=BAM 515; **NE**=BAM 516; **NJ**=AMT 12/5; **NQ**=BAM 521; **NU**=AMT 14/3; **sA**=IRAQ 65; **UA**=AuOrS 23/27; **uA**=SpTU 50; **UB**=Ugaritica 5; **UC**=AuOrS 23/14; **xA**=CM 37

§ II The Nineveh Manuscripts of Chapter Two (IGI 2)

TITLE	If A Man's Eyes Are Full of *Murdinnu*-Brambles *šumma*(DIŠ) *amēlu*(NA) *īnāšu*(IGI.MIN-*šú*) *mur-din-ni malâ*(DIRI) = Assur Medical Catalogue l. 8.

Sigla notations:
N = Nineveh, Neo-Assyrian. A, B, C, ... designate the different manuscripts.
Translation in italics are tentative reconstructions based on parallels.

Base Manuscript:	**ND (BAM 515)**, collated.
Museum number:	British Museum, K 1845 + 2440 + K 2444 + 2500 + 2501 + 2504 + 2508 + 2762 + 3662 + 4116 + 6425 + 6652 + 6974 + 7933 + 8349 + 8832 + 9247 + 10495 + 10790 + 10892 + 11803 + 15454 + 15765 + 15769 + Sm 1308.
Origin and date:	Nineveh, 7th century BC.
Type of tablet:	Two-column, portrait-oriented tablet. The two vertical dividing rulings were made by a twisted thread. There are no round holes visible in the preserved parts.
Measurements:	ca. 31 × 18 × 3,3 (upper edge) – 3,6 (towards the middle) cm.
Copy:	BAM 515.
Photo/CDLI nr.:	Plates 19–26/P394104.
Literature:	Köcher 1980b: xif., BAM 515; Fincke 2000: 331. Scurlock and Andersen 2005: 793; Fincke 2009; Scurlock 2014: 756; Attia 2015.

§ II.1 Related Manuscripts containing IGI 1 and 3 from Nineveh

The texts included represent parallels and partial parallels from the other tablets of the IGI treatise.

Manuscript: **NA** (BAM 510), see **§ I.1**, parallels: 1, 117ff.', 215'.

Manuscript: **NB** (BAM 513), see **§ I.1**, parallels: 117ff.'.

Manuscript: **NC** (BAM 514), see **§ I.1**, parallels: 117ff.', 215'.

Manuscript: **NE** (BAM 516), see **§ III.1**, parallels: 215'.

https://doi.org/10.1515/9781501506550-005

§ II.2 Related other Manuscripts from Nineveh

The texts included represent parallels and partial parallels which are considered important for the compilation of the IGI-treatise. They come from other tablets and fragments from Nineveh containing prescriptions for sick eyes or from the UGU-treatise.

Manuscript: **NI** (BAM 480), see **§ V.1**, parallels: 62', 71', 147', 157'.

Manuscript: **NK** (BAM 518), see **§ IV.2**, parallels: 10.

§ II.3 Related Manuscripts from Different Cities

The texts included here represent parallels and partial parallels which are considered important for the compilation of the IGI-treatise. These are manuscripts coming from other periods and from cities other than Nineveh.

Sigla notations:

A = Assur, Late Assyrian. A, B, C, ... designate the different manuscripts.
b = Babylon, Late Babylonian. A, B, C, ... designate the different manuscripts.
Bo = Boğazköy, Hattuša, Hittite period. A, B, C, ... designate the different manuscripts.
K = Kalhu, Late Assyrian. A, B, C, ... designate the different manuscripts.
s = Sippar, Late Babylonian. A, B, C, ... designate the different manuscripts.
u = Uruk, Late Babylonian. A, B, C, ... designate the different manuscripts.
x = unknown provenance, Late Babylonian. A, B, C, ... designate the different manuscripts.
Initial capital letters designate tablets in Assyrian script or northern scripts, and small letters tablets in Babylonian script.
Parenthesis [()] on a siglum designate a parallel text and not a duplicate.

Hattuša

Manuscript: **BoA (KUB 4/50)**, photo collated, parallels: 145'.
Museum number: Istanbul, Bo 3928.
Origin and date: Boğazköy, Hattuša. Hittite period.
Type of tablet: Too fragmentary to judge.
Copy: KUB 4/50.
Photo: Mainzer Photoarchiv, http://www.hethport.uni-wuerzburg.de/HPM/index.html, CTH 809.
Literature: Fincke 2010; Schwemer 2013: 156.

Assyrian

Manuscript:	**AA (BAM 20)**, see **§ I.4**, parallels: 10f., 117ff.'.

Manuscript:	**AB (BAM 159)**, see **§ I.4**, parallels: 58', 117ff.'.

Manuscript:	**AD (BAM 22)**, see **§ I.4**, parallels: 22ff., 65f.', 98f.'.

Manuscript:	**AF (BAM 23),** collated, parallels: 71', 121', 137ff.'.
Museum number:	Vorderasiatisches Museum, Berlin, VAT 13782 + 13904.
Origin and date:	Assur, Late Assyrian.
Type of tablet:	One-column, landscape-oriented tablet.
Measurements:	13,3 × 6,7 × 2,2 cm.
Copy:	BAM 23.
CDLI nr.:	P285125.
Literature:	Köcher 1963: xv; Fincke 2000: 329; Scurlock and Andersen 2005: 784; Attia 2015: 47.

Manuscript:	**AG (BAM 15)**, collated, parallels: 207f.'.
Museum number:	Vorderasiatisches Museum, Berlin, VAT 13892.
Origin and date:	Assur, Late Assyrian.
Type of tablet:	Too fragmentary to judge. It was not fired, but pressure exercised over the tablet while in a wet state, thus it turned convex. It shows large script.
Measurements:	ca. 7,4 × 5,4 × 2,4 cm.
Copy:	BAM 15.
CDLI nr.:	P285118.
Literature:	Köcher 1963: xv; Fincke 2000: 329; Scurlock and Andersen 2005: 784; Attia 2015: 52.

Manuscript:	**KA (CTN 4/123),** collated, parallels: 53'.
Museum number:	British Museum, London, ND 04405/16
Origin and date:	Kalhu, Late Assyrian.
Type of tablet:	Too fragmentary for certainty.
Measurements:	ca. 5,1 × 6,7 × 2,5 cm
Copy:	CTN 4/123.
CDLI nr.:	P363537.
Literature:	Wiseman and Black 1996: no. 123; Worthington 2005: 7ff.; Scurlock 2014: 758.

Babylonian

Manuscript:	**bB (BAM 382)**, collated, parallels: 25f.
Museum number:	Vorderasiatisches Museum, Berlin, VAT 17406.
Origin and date:	Babylon, Late Babylonian.
Type of tablet:	One-column, landscape-oriented tablet.
Measurements:	7 × 4,2 × 2,1 cm.
Copy:	BAM 382.
CDLI nr.:	P285453.
Literature:	Köcher 1971: xxvii; Fincke 2000: 329; Scurlock and Andersen 2005: 790; Attia 2015: 39.

Manuscript:	**sA (IRAQ 65)**, see **§ I.4**, parallels: 10, 65f.', 98f.'.

Manuscript:	**uA (SpTU 50)**, see **§ I.4**, parallels: 58', 215'.

Manuscript:	**uB (NBC 4211)**, photo collated, parallels: 25.
Museum number:	Yale Babylonian Collection, New Haven, NBC 4211.
Origin and date:	Uruk, Late Babylonian.
Type of tablet:	One-column, portrait oriented tablet.
Measurements:	ca. 13,4 × 9,6 × 2,6 cm.
CDLI nr.:	P290281.
Literature:	Beaulieu 1994: 25.

Manuscript:	**xA (CM 37)**, see **§ I.4**, parallels: 23f., 58', 215'.

§ II.4 Synopsis of the Prescriptions of Chapter Two (IGI 2)

1ff. Prescriptions and medical applications for eyes full of *murdinnu*-brambles (a disease): bandage for three days with a plant and roasted grain in beer, three times re-bandaging the eyes and smearing the eyes with gazelle knuckle-fat. Pounding the substances into a lead salve, spattering a dried plant over the eyes, and re-bandaging. Again, three times a day re-bandaging, spattering dried plants over the head, keeping the bandage for three days. On the fourth day releasing the bandage, shaving the head, daubing the eyes: prognosis for recovery.

8f. No diagnosis in the beginning, but this time at the end; this prescription for eyes suffering from 'sun-heat' and *murdinnu*-brambles: eight drugs including a bat guano, plants, minerals, and river silt, applied as eye drops.

10 No diagnosis (but presumably the same as the previous one): a plant, a mineral, a saline solution applied as eye drops.

11	No diagnosis (but presumably the same as the previous one): a plant, a mineral, a saline solution applied as eye drops.
12ff.	Ritual/medical application for *giddagiddû*-fibers, ritual/medical application acts at the door of man's house.
16	Prescription for 'spoiled' blood; plant ingredients.
17f.	Prescription for blurred vision due to abnormal hair growth in the eyes; mixture of plants, animal fats, honey and ghee, applied by daubing.
19ff.	Prescription for eyes full of loose tissue; pounded plants in honey applied by daubing; alternative mineral treatment in ghee, applied by daubing?.
22ff.	Prescription for eyes full of loose tissue: making a 'clod' from plants, fat, and bat guano mixed in cedar 'blood' (i.e. resin) and oil; mixture is applied by daubing.
25f.	Prescription for eyes full of tissue and blood: salve with plants, bat guano; applied by daubing.
27ff.	Prescription and medical application for eyes full of *qūqānu*-'worms': ritual/medical application acts of burying materia medica and magica under a threshold.
50f.'	Prescription for ...: daubing the eys with bone marrow and; salve from bone marrow and, pounded in honey, ghee, plant oil and copper patina; applied by daubing.
52f.'	No diagnosis (but presumably as the previous one): pounded flour, grains poured directly into the eyes.
53'	Fragmentary prescription: salve from animal fats and wax, pounded in bone marrow; applied by daubing.
54f.'	Prescription for foreign objects in the eye, and dimmed eyes with chronic suffering and cloudy eyes; recipe demaged.
56'	Prescription for inflamed eyes: bandage of crushed and sifted plants with grain flour in beer.
57'	No diagnosis (but presumably as the previous one): eye drops made from a plant, a mineral, and a saline solution.
58f.'	Prescription and medical application for dim eyes: ritual/medical application acts of burying materia medica and magica under a threshold.
60'	Fragmentary prescription: daubing the eyes.
61f.'	Prescription for darkened eyes: salves from oils, copper patina, and fungus-ridden potsherd, mixed in mountain honey; applied by daubing?.
63f.'	Prescription for 'pressed' eyes: sap of a fresh plant applied over the face/eye, salve with copper patina and sesame oil; applied by daubing.
65f.'	Prescription for the same case: grated plant into milk, baked, and pounded (with) plants and a mineral; applied by daubing.
67'	Prescription for the same case: parched crumbled bread applied on the eyes as eye drops.
68'	Prescription for the same case: [bandage] with plant based powder.

69' Prescription for the same case: salve of plants in milk; applied by daubing.

70' Prescription for the same case: salve of mineral in ghee; applied by daubing; salve of mineral in bone marrow; applied by daubing.

71' Prescription for the same case: pickling of a turtle gall bladder in salt, to be dried out and pounded in oil, and a copper patina; applied by daubing.

72' Prescription for the same case: pounded substance using a bronze knife in ghee; applied daubing.

73' Prescription for the same case: plants in sesame oil, a daubing applied with the finger.

74' Two prescription for the same case: salve from lizard's head and oil; applied by daubing; salve with pounded wall lizard and charcoal; applied by daubing.

75' No diagnosis (but presumably as the previous one): salve from a sheep's ribcage; applied by daubing.

76' Prescription for closed eyes: dripping into the eyes of substance(s) mixed in ghee.

77f.' No diagnosis (but presumably as the previous one): wild cow brain mixed in sesame oil and male pigeon brain, prepared over three days [on a cosmetic palette]; applied regularly as a salve into the eyes.

79ff.' No diagnosis (but presumably as the previous one): raven egg smeared on a bronze knife, ...; applied by daubing

82' Fragmentary prescription: daubing.

83' Fragmentary prescription: daubing.

84' Fragmentary prescription: salve of substance(s) in sesame oil, pounded in red paste; applied by daubing

85' Fragmentary prescription: salve of substance(s) in sesame oil, pounded with frit and cedar oil; applied by daubing

86' Fragmentary prescription: salve of substance(s) in oil in a copper kettle; applied by daubing

87' Fragmentary prescription: salve of plants; applied by daubing

88' Fragmentary prescription: salve of substance(s) in oil; applied by daubing

89' Fragmentary prescription: medication dripped into the eyes.

90f.' Fragmentary medical application prescription: medical application acts with a lamp and its smoke, rinsing the eyes.

92f.' Fragmentary prescription: salve with bat guano, pounded with a lead spoon in oil and copper patina; applied by daubing.

94f.' Fragmentary prescription: preparation of a salve with patina in a copper kettle, daubing the eyes for seven days.

96f.' Fragmentary prescription: salve from ingredients in fat; applied by daubing.

98f.' Prescription for *kiṣâtu* 'skinned' *and closed eye lids*: salve of a skinned plant in *pūru*-oil; applied by daubing; salve of old copper in ghee; applied by repeated daubing; prognosis for recovery.

100f.' Fragmentary prescription: salve of plants pounded in patina; applied by daubing.

102' Fragmentary prescription: salve of parched and crushed ingredients, pounded in patina; applied by daubing.

103' Fragmentary medical application prescription: burying of substances under a threshold for seven days, pounded in patina into a salve; applied by daubing.

104' Fragmentary prescription: ingredients pounded in patina into a salve; applied by daubing.

105ff.' Fragmentary medical application prescription: pricking (birds') eyes with a needle, producing a salve; applied by daubing.

108ff.' Fragmentary prescription for *kurāru*-pustle on the eyelids: bandage from plants, seeds, ewe hoof, goat kidney kept fifteen days; daubing the eyes for three more days with a plant ingredient.

115' Prescription for eyes full of yellowness (jaundice): blowing pounded pomegranate peel via a reed-straw into the eyes.

116' Prescription for eyes full of yellowness (jaundice): two salves of pomegranate peel, first in oil, then in saline solution; applied by daubing.

117ff.' Prescription for sick closed eyes, with fever and filmy vision: shaving the head, cooling it with dough, salve of plants and ghee; applied by daubing and rinsing the eyes.

120' No diagnosis (but presumably as the previous one): salve of plant in mountain honey and ghee; applied by daubing.

121ff.' Prescription for membrane-covered eyes with tears and dark spots: salve from plants, bat guano mixed in cedar oil; applied by daubing: prognosis for recovery.

124f.' Prescription for membrane-covered eyes with opaque vision and white spot on the pupil: salve of plants mixed in cedar oil; applied by daubing.

126f.' Fragmentary prescription for opaque vision: salve; applied by daubing.

128ff. Fragmentary prescriptions: blowing medication into the eyes, fumigation, and daubing: prognosis for recovery.

137f. Fragmentary prescription: application with different resins for eight months.

139' Prescription for eyes full of film: salve of pounded potsherd, white plant and ghee; applied by daubing.

140' Prescription for the same case: medication containing bat guano, and spattered into the eyes.

141' Fragmentary prescription for the same case: two salves from bat guano in ghee, and pounded potsherd; applied by daubing.

142f.' No diagnosis (but presumably as the previous one): salve of a plant in ghee, applied three times, another ghee salve, daubing.

144f.' Fragmentary prescription: salve of a bat guano in ghee, daubing three times a month; bandage of plant leaf in vinegar; squeezing plant sap into the eyes.

146' Fragmentary prescription: salve of grain powder and saline solution; applied by daubing.
147' Fragmentary prescription: salve of copper patina in fat of gazelle's thigh; applied by daubing.
148' Fragmentary prescription: salve, and dripping honey and fat into the eyes.
149'–193' Fragmentary and unclear.
194' No diagnosis (but presumably as the previous one): salve of (pounded) potsherd, salt cedar oil, daubing.
195' No diagnosis (but presumably as the previous one): salve of a plant and a saline solution in honey; applied by daubing.
196' Fragmentary and unclear.
197f.' Fragmentary and unclear.
199' Prescription for eyes full of film, fragmentary and unclear.
200ff.' Surgical prescription for left and right eyes full of film: treatment with a scalpel, fragmentary and unclear.
204' Prescription for sick eyes with milk, fragmentary and unclear.
205' No diagnosis (but presumably as the previous one): eagle's brain in mothers' milk, fragmentary and unclear.
206' No diagnosis (but presumably as the previous one): plant seeds and powder, rest fragmentary.
207f.' Two prescriptions for eyes full of film: a salve applied by daubing.
209ff.' Fragmentary prescriptions, eyes full of film.
215ff.' Catchline of tablet three, designation of tablet two, and preserved Ashurbanipal colophon.

Edition of IGI 2

1 *šumma amēlu īnāšu murdinnī malâ sahlê qēm labti ina šikari tarabbak taṣammid* UD.3.KAM *īnīšu* [*lā tapaṭṭar*] **2** [*kala*] *ūme šalāšīšu tarakkas ina rebî ūmi ina suādi erri īnīšu takaddad mê ina*$^?$ [*libbi*$^?$ *īnīšu tanaddi*] **3** [*īnīšu*] *tušakkal qerša emma ištiššu šinīšu šalāšīšu īnīšu tarakkas lipi kursinni ṣabīti īnīšu* [...] ... **4** [*ina*] *arkīti ina irri abāri tasâk īnīšu teqqi hūrata tasâk ana muhhi īnīšu tābīla tazarru taṣammid* **5** *kala ūme šalāšīšu riksa ukâlma inassah kalbāna* (gloss: *ū bīna*) *zēr qudri burāša* **6** *labta sahlê taballal tābīla ana muhhi qaqqadīšu tazarru qaqqassu taṣammidma* UD.3.KAM [*lā*] *tapaṭṭar* **7** *ina rebî ūme tapaṭṭaršuma qaqqassu tugallab šamma ribka īnīšu tēteneqqi ina'eš*	[1]If a man's eyes are full of *murdinnu*-brambles: you shall make an infusion from *sahlû*-plant (and) flour of roasted grain in beer, (and) bandage (his eyes). For three days [you do not loosen (the bandage from)] his eyes. [2][Every] day you bandage (his eyes) three times. On the fourth day, you rub his eyes with parched *suādu*-aromatic, [(and) you put] water into$^?$ [his eyes.] [3]You wipe [his eyes], (and) bandage his eyes once, twice, (and) three times with a hot strip of meat, (and) you ... [his] eyes with fat from a gazelle's knuckle. [4]Afterwards you pound (the previous substances) in a lead salve and daub his eyes. You pound a dyeing sumac, spatter it in a dry state over his eyes, (and) bandage (the eyes). [5]Three times during the whole day he keeps the binding on (his eyes) and then he removes (it). [6]You mix [5]*kalbānu*-plant (gloss: or tamarisk), seed(s) of *qudru*-plant, juniper, [6]roasted grain (and) *sahlû*-plant. In dry state, you spatter (the ingredients) over his head, you bandage his head and then for three days you do [not] loosen (the bandage). [7]On the fourth day you release (the bandage) and you shave his head. You keep daubing his eyes with the drug infusion (and) he will get better.

1 ND i 1 [.......................... *mur-di*]*n-ni* DIRI *sah-lé-e* ZÌ ŠE.SA.A *ina* KAŠ *tara-bak* LAL UD.3.KÁM IGI.MIN-*š*[*ú* NU DU$_8$]

Overview of IGI 2 Manuscripts and Parallels: **AA**=BAM 20; **AB**=BAM 159; **AD**=BAM 22; **AF**=BAM 23; **AG**=BAM 15; **bB**=BAM 382; **BoA**=KUB 4/50; **KA**=CTN 4/123; **NA**=BAM 510; **NB**=BAM 513; **NC**=BAM 514; **ND**=BAM 515; **NE**=BAM 516; **NI**=BAM 480; **NK**=BAM 518; **sA**=IRAQ 65; **uA**=SpTU 50; **uB**=NBC 4211; **xA**=CM 37

https://doi.org/10.1515/9781501506550-006

(NA) iv 47 DIŠ NA IGI.MIN-*šú mur-din-n*[*i* DIRI] *sah-lé-e* ZÌ [................] KA[Š ....]

2 ND i 2 [*ka-la*] ⌜UD-*me* 3-*šú*⌝ KEŠDA *ina* 4 UD-*mi ina* ^{šim}MAN.DU *er-ri* IGI.MIN-*šú ta-kad-da-ad* A *ina* Š[À IGI.MIN-*šú* ŠUB]

3 ND i 3 [IGI.MIN-*šú t*]*u-šak-kal qer-šá em-ma* 1-*šú* 2-*šú* 3-*šú* IGI.MIN-*šú* KEŠDA Ì.UDU *kur-sin-ni* MAŠ.DÀ IG[I.MIN-*šú* (x)] x-*pap*$^{?}$

4 ND i 4 [*ina* EG]IR-*tì ina ir-ri* A.GAR$_5$ SÚD IGI.MIN-*šú* MAR ^{giš}HAB SÚD *ana* UGU IGI.MIN-*šú ta-bi-la*$_{12}$ ⌜MAR⌝ LAL

5 ND i 5 [*k*]*a-la* UD-*me* 3-*šú* KEŠDA *ú-kal-ma* ZI ^{giš}MAŠ.HUŠ $^{\text{(gloss: u giš.šinig)}}$ NUMUN ^{ú}KI.^{d}IŠKUR $^{\text{[ši]m?}}$LI

6 ND i 6 ŠE.SA.A *sah-lé-e* HE.HE *ta-bi-la*$_{12}$ *ana* UGU SAG.DU-*šú* MAR SAG.DU-*su* LAL-*ma* U[D.3.KÁM NU D]U$_8$

7 ND i 7 *ina* 4 UD-*me* DU$_8$-*šú-ma* SAG.DU-*su tu-gal-lab* Ú *rib-ka* IGI.MIN-*šú* MAR.MEŠ [*ina-e*]*š*

---

8 *šammu peṣû rikibti arkabi emesalli aban gabî uhūlu qarnānû murru qadūt* [*šikāni*] **9** *kasû naphar samānat šammī ṭīpu šumma amēlu īnāšu ṣēta hanṭā u murdinnī* [*malâ*]	[8]White plant, bat guano, *emesallu*-saline solution, alum, horned *uhūlu*-alkali, bitter-plant, river [silt], [9]*kasû*-plant: total of eight drugs, which are (used as) drops, if a man's eyes are inflamed (lit. burn) with sun-heat and [full] of a *murdinnu*- brambles.

8 ND i 8 Ú.BABBAR U$_5$.ARGAB^{mušen} ^{mun}*eme-sal-lì* NA$_4$ *ga-bi-i* NAGA.SI ^{šim}SES IM.G[Ú$^{?}$.EN$^{?}$.NA$^{?}$]

9 ND i 9 GAZI^{sar} PAP 8 Ú.MEŠ *ṭi*$_5$*-pu šum-ma* NA IGI.MIN-*šú* UD.DA *ha-an-ṭa u mur-d*[*in-ni* DIRI]

Overview of IGI 2 Manuscripts and Parallels: **AA**=BAM 20; **AB**=BAM 159; **AD**=BAM 22; **AF**=BAM 23; **AG**=BAM 15; **bB**=BAM 382; **BoA**=KUB 4/50; **KA**=CTN 4/123; **NA**=BAM 510; **NB**=BAM 513; **NC**=BAM 514; **ND**=BAM 515; **NE**=BAM 516; **NI**=BAM 480; **NK**=BAM 518; **sA**=IRAQ 65; **uA**=SpTU 50; **uB**=NBC 4211; **xA**=CM 37

10 *šammu peṣû aban gabî emesalli annû ṭīpu* [*ša īnī*]	[10]White plant, alum, *emesallu*-saline solution; these (drugs) are (used as) drops [for the eyes].
Alternative prescription 1	**Alternative prescription 1**
11 *kukru qēm labti kasû annû* [*ṭīpu ša īnī*]	[11]*Kukru*-aromatic, flour of roasted grain, *kasû*-plant; these (drugs) are (used as) [drops for the eyes.]

10	ND i 10	Ú.BABBAR NA$_4$ *ga-bi-i* ^{mun}*eme-sal-lì an-nu-ú ṭi-*[*pu šá* IGI.MIN]
	(NK) 8'	[................ NA$_4$ *g*]*a-bi-i* ^{mun}*eme-sal-lì ṭi$_5$-pu šá* ⸢IGI.MIN.MEŠ⸣
	(AA) 9'	Ú.BABBAR NA$_4$ *ga-bi-i* ^{mun}[*eme-sal-lì*]
	(AA) 10'	*an-nu-u ṭi-pu šá* I[GI(.MIN)]
	(sA) ii 20	Ú.BABBAR NA$_4$ *ga-bi-i* $^{\text{mun?}}$*eme-sal-lì* (AN ATTEMPT TO WRITE THE NUMBER 3?)
	(sA) ii 21	3 Ú.MEŠ *ṭi-pi šá* IGI.MIN
11	ND i 11	⸢^{šim}⸣GÚR.GÚR ZÌ ŠE.SA.A GAZI^{sar} *an-nu-ú* [*ṭi-pu šá* IGI.MIN]
	(AA) 7'	^{šim}GÚR.GÚR ZÌ ŠE.SA.A GA[ZI^{sar}]
	(AA) 8'	*ina* KAŠ *tara-bak an-nu-u* LAL *š*[*á*$^?$ IGI.MIN]

12 [*šumma*] *amēlu īnāšu giddagiddâ ukallā ana bīti ahî illakma bābu išassi kīma* x [...] **13** [...] *giddagiddû ašar šanîmma giddagiddûkunuma tablā šanîš* [...]	[12]If a man's eyes contain *giddagiddû*-fibers, he goes to a stranger's house and calls at the entrance door': 'like x [...] [13][...] *giddagiddû*-fibers, ditto, take away your *giddagiddû*-fibers, ditto ...!'
Alternative prescription 1	**Alternative prescription 1**
14 *ana* [*bīt* (*lā*$^?$)] *edê illakma bāba išassi kīma* x x x [...] **15** ... *giddagiddû ašar šanîmma giddagiddûkunuma tablā* ... [...]	[14]He goes [to] an (un)known [house] and calls at the entrance door: 'like ... [...]. [15]... *giddagiddû*-fibers, ditto, remove your (pl.) *giddagiddû*-fibers, ... [...]!'

12	ND i 12	[DIŠ N]A ⸢IGI.MIN-*šú* GÍD.DA.GÍD.DA *ú*⸣*-kal-la ana* É *a-hi-i* DU-*ma* KÁ$^?$ GÙ-*si ki-ma* x [...]
13	ND i 13	[... GÍD.D]A.GÍD-*du* ⸢KIMIN GÍD.DA.GÍD-*du*⸣*-ku-nu-ma tab-la* MIN [...]

Overview of IGI 2 Manuscripts and Parallels: **AA**=BAM 20; **AB**=BAM 159; **AD**=BAM 22; **AF**=BAM 23; **AG**=BAM 15; **bB**=BAM 382; **BoA**=KUB 4/50; **KA**=CTN 4/123; **NA**=BAM 510; **NB**=BAM 513; **NC**=BAM 514; **ND**=BAM 515; **NE**=BAM 516; **NI**=BAM 480; **NK**=BAM 518; **sA**=IRAQ 65; **uA**=SpTU 50; **uB**=NBC 4211; **xA**=CM 37

14 ND i 14 *a*-[*na* É (NU$^{?}$)] ⌜*e*⌝-*de-e* DU-*ma* KÁ GÙ-*si ki*-⌜*ma* x x x⌝ [...]

15 ND i 15 HI x [(x x) GÍ]D.DA.GÍD-*du* KIMIN GÍD.GÍD-*ku-nu-ma tab-la* x [...]

---

16 *šumma amēlu* [*ina*] *īnīšu lipištu kukra burāša ṭūra zēr bīni* [... *tasâk* ...]	[16]If there is a fleshy substance [in] a man's eyes; [you pound] *kukru*-aromatic, juniper, *ṭūru*-plant, seeds of tamarisk...

16 ND i 16 DIŠ N[A *ina* IGI.MI]N-*šú li-piš-tu*$_4$ ^{šim}GÚR.GÚR ^{šim}LI ^{šim}HAB NUMUN ŠI[NIG ... SÚD ...]

---

17 *šumma amēlu ina īnīšu šārtu aṣât u īnāšu ašâ ṭābta kamma lipi* [*kalīti*$^{?}$ ...] **18** *ša immeri dišip šadê malmališ tasâk ina himēti taballal īnīšu teqqi tamaš*[*šaš*$^{?}$ ...]	[17]If a hair protrudes from a man's eyes, and his eyes are blurred: [[18]you pound in equal amounts] [17]salt, *kammu*-tanning-fungus, [kidney$^{?}$] fat [...] [18]of a sheep (and) mountain honey (and) you mix (them) in ghee. You daub his eyes, (and) wipe (them) [...]

17 ND i 17 DIŠ NA *in*[*a* IG]I.MIN-*šú* SÍG *a-ṣa-at u* IGI.MIN-*šú a-šá-a* MUN *kám-ma* ⌜Ì.UDU⌝ [ÉLLAG$^{?}$ ...]

18 ND i 18 *šá* UDU.NÍ[TA LÀ]L.KUR.RA *mál-ma-liš* SÚD *ina* Ì.NUN HE.HE IGI.MIN-*šú* MAR *ta-ma*[*š-aš*$^{?}$ ...]

---

19 *šumma amēlu īnāšu šēra ālika malâ ana* [*bulluṭīšu* ...] **20** [... *zēr*] GI.ZÚ.LUM.MA *ina dišpi tasâk teqqi* : ... [...] **21** [...] *ashar ina himēti tasâk teqqi* : ... [...]	[19]If a man's eyes are full of loose tissue: in order to [heal him ...] [20]You pound ... [seed] of 'date reed' in honey and daub (his eyes) : ... [...] [21]You pound ... *ashar*-stone in ghee, you daub (his eyes) : ... [...]

19 ND i 19 DIŠ N[A IGI.MIN]-*šú* UZU *a-li-ka*$_{13}$ DIRI-*a ana* [TI-*šú* ...]

20 ND i 20 x [x NUMUN] GI.ZÚ.LUM.MA *ina* LÀL SÚD MAR : x [...]

21 ND i 21 [x x ^{n}]^{a4}*as-har ina* Ì.NUN SÚD MAR : x [...]

Overview of IGI 2 Manuscripts and Parallels: **AA**=BAM 20; **AB**=BAM 159; **AD**=BAM 22; **AF**=BAM 23; **AG**=BAM 15; **bB**=BAM 382; **BoA**=KUB 4/50; **KA**=CTN 4/123; **NA**=BAM 510; **NB**=BAM 513; **NC**=BAM 514; **ND**=BAM 515; **NE**=BAM 516; **NI**=BAM 480; **NK**=BAM 518; **sA**=IRAQ 65; **uA**=SpTU 50; **uB**=NBC 4211; **xA**=CM 37

22 [*šumma amēlu*] *īnāšu šēra ālika malâma u illak ana bulluṭīšu* [*sahlê nīnâ murra lipâ* ...] **23** *kanakta šamma peṣâ rikibti arkabi* [*emesalli ištēniš tasâk* ...] **24** *ina dām erēni lu ina šaman erēni taballal passa teppuš* [*ina mê tasâk īnāšu teqqi*]	[22][If a man's] eyes are full of loose tissue and it moves, in order to heal it: [[23]you pound together [22]*sahlû*-plant, *nīnû*-mint, bitter-plant, fat,] [23]*kanaktu*-aromatic, white plant, bat guano, [*emesallu*-saline solution, ...]. [24]You mix (them) in cedar 'blood' (i.e. resin) or in cedar oil (and) [you make] a collyrium stick [(out of it), you pound (it) in water and daub his eyes].

22	ND i 22	[DIŠ NA IGI.M]IN-*šú* UZU DU-*ka*$_{16}$ DIRI-*ma u* DU-*ak ana* TI-⸢*šú*⸣ x [...]
	(AD) 4f.'	DIŠ NA IGI.MIN-*šú* UZU DU-*ka* DI[RI-*ma* DU-*k*]*a ana* TI-*šú* / *sah-lé-e* ^{ú}KUR.RA ^{ši}[^{m}SE]S Ì.UDU →
23	ND i 23	$^{\text{[ši]m}}$GIG Ú.BABBAR U$_5$.ARGAB^{mušen} ^{mu}[^{n}*eme-sal-lì* 1-*niš* SÚD ...]
	(AD) 5f.'	^{šim}GIG / Ú.BABBAR U$_5$.ARGAB^{mušen} ^{m}[^{un}*em*]*e*-⸢*sal-lì* 1-*niš* SÚD⸣
	(xA) 2'	[...............................] ⸢U$_5$.ARGAB^{mušen}⸣
24	ND i 24	[*ina* MÚD ^{gi}]^{š}EREN *lu ina* Ì+GIŠ ⸢^{giš}⸣EREN HE.HE Z[A.NA DÙ-*uš ina* A.MEŠ SÚD IGI.MIN-*šú* MAR]
	(AD) 7'	*ina* MÚD EREN *lu ina* Ì ER[EN H]E.HE ZA.NA DÙ-*uš*
	(AD) 8'	*ina* A.MEŠ SÚD MAR
	(xA) 2'	*ina* MÚD ^{giš}ERE[N HE.H]E ⸢ZA.NA DÙ-*uš*⸣ *in*[*a* A.MEŠ SÚD MAR ....]

25 [*šumma amēlu*] *īnāšu šēra u dāma malâ murru* [*nīnû šammu peṣû lipi kanakti*] **26** *rikibti arkabi sahlû šammū annûti* [*tēqītu ša šēri āliki*]	[25]If his eyes are full of tissue and blood: bitter-plant, [*nīnû*-mint, white plant, *kanaktu*-aromatic pith,] [26]bat guano (and) *sahlû*-plant. These plants [are for an ointment (for the case when there is) a loose tissue (in the eyes).]

25	ND i 25	[DIŠ NA IG]I.MIN-*šú* UZU *u* MÚD DIRI.MEŠ ^{šim}S[ES$^{?}$ ....]
	(AD) 9f.'	DIŠ NA IGI.MIN-*šú* UZU *u* MÚD DIRI ^{š}[^{im}S]ES ^{ú}KUR.RA / Ú.BABBAR Ì.UDU ^{šim}GIG →
	(bB) 3	[...] x Ú.BABBAR ^{šim}GIG →

Overview of IGI 2 Manuscripts and Parallels: **AA**=BAM 20; **AB**=BAM 159; **AD**=BAM 22; **AF**=BAM 23; **AG**=BAM 15; **bB**=BAM 382; **BoA**=KUB 4/50; **KA**=CTN 4/123; **NA**=BAM 510; **NB**=BAM 513; **NC**=BAM 514; **ND**=BAM 515; **NE**=BAM 516; **NI**=BAM 480; **NK**=BAM 518; **sA**=IRAQ 65; **uA**=SpTU 50; **uB**=NBC 4211; **xA**=CM 37

	(uB) 16	[DIŠ LÚ] IGI.MIN.MEŠ-*šú* UZU *u* MÚD ⸢DIRI.MEŠ⸣ *ana* ⸢TI⸣-*šú*
26	ND i 26	[U_5.A]RGAB^{mušen} *sah-lu-u* Ú.MEŠ *an-nu-t*[*i* ....]
	(AD) 10'	U[$_5$].ARGAB^{mušen}
	(AD) 11'	*sah-lé-e ina* Ì S[Ú]D MAR
	(bB) 3	U_5.ARGAB^{mušen}
	(bB) 4	[...] x [... Ì].GIŠ HE.HE *te-qit šá* UZU DU

27 [*šumma amēlu*] *īnāšu qūqānī malâ gurušgaraš* [*ša šahî* ...] **28** [*ina*] *ṣubāti tessip sebet ūmē ina askuppi tetemmer* [*tušellâmma* ...] **29** [...] *malmališ* [*tasâk* ...]	[27]If a man's eyes are full *qūqānu*-'worms': [28]you collect [27]a 'vulva' of [a pig ... [28]in a] cloth. You bury (it) under the threshold for seven days, [you remove (it) and ...] [29][... you pound (it)] in equal measure [...]

27	ND i 27	[DIŠ NA IGI.MI]N-*šú qù-qa-ni* DIRI.MEŠ *gu-ru-uš-ga-r*[*a-aš ša šahî* ...]
28	ND i 28	[*ina* TÚ]G *te-sip* 7 UD-*me ina* KUN_4 *te-te-m*[*er* E_{11}-*ma* ....]
29	ND i 29	[x x *ma*]*l-má-l*[*iš* SÚD x x x x] x ⸢x⸣ [..]

GAP!

Presumably more then 20 lines are missing!

50' [... *ina lipî*] *eṣemti kurîti immeri* ... [... *tasâk teqqi*] **51'** [...] *malmališ tasâk ina dišpi himēti šaman erēni šuhti tasâk* [*teqqi*]	[50'][... you pound (them) in marrow of] a sheep's short [bone (and)] ... [... (and) daub (his) eyes.] [51']You pound [...] in equal measures. You pound (them) in honey, ghee, cedar oil, copper patina. [You daub (his eyes with it)].
Alternative prescription 1 **52'** *ana ašri šanîmma qēm* [*ašnan*] *itti labti tasâk ana muhhi īnīšu tašappak*	**Alternative prescription 1** [52']Alternatively; you pound [cereal] flour with roasted grain, (and) you pour it onto his eyes.

Overview of IGI 2 Manuscripts and Parallels: **AA**=BAM 20; **AB**=BAM 159; **AD**=BAM 22; **AF**=BAM 23; **AG**=BAM 15; **bB**=BAM 382; **BoA**=KUB 4/50; **KA**=CTN 4/123; **NA**=BAM 510; **NB**=BAM 513; **NC**=BAM 514; **ND**=BAM 515; **NE**=BAM 516; **NI**=BAM 480; **NK**=BAM 518; **sA**=IRAQ 65; **uA**=SpTU 50; **uB**=NBC 4211; **xA**=CM 37

50’ ND i 50’ [........... *ina* Ì.UDU GÌR.PAD].⌜DU LÚGUD⌝.DA UD[U$^{?}$ ...] x x x [SÚD MAR]

51’ ND i 51’ [x x] x [... *má*]*l-ma-liš* SÚD *ina* LÀL Ì.NUN Ì.GIŠ ^{giš}EREN SAHAR.URUDU S[ÚD$^{?}$ MAR]

52’ ND i 52’ ⌜DIŠ KIMIN⌝ ZÌ ^{d}[ŠE.TIR] KI ŠE.SA.A SÚD *ana* UGU IGI.MIN-*šú* DUB

53’ *šumma amēlu īnāšu [... ina lipî kalīti] immeri iškūri ištēniš taballal ina lipî eṣemti arikti tasâk teqqi*	53’If a man’s eyes are [...]: you mix together [... in kidney fat] of a [sheep] and wax. You pound (it) in marrow of a long bone (and) daub (his eyes).

53’ ND i 53’ DIŠ NA IGI.MIN-*šú* [... *ina* Ì.UDU ÉLLAG UDU.NÍ]TA$^{?}$ GAB.LÀL 1-*niš* HE.HE *ina* Ì.UDU GÌR.PAD.DU GÍD.DA SÚD *te-eq-qí*

(KA) 5’ [... *ina* A GAZI^{sa}]⌝ SILA$_{11}$ *ina* Ì.UDU GÌR.PAD.⌜DU⌝ GÍD.DA SÚD M[AR]

54’ *šumma ina īni [...] īteneṭṭâ amēlu šū (šuātu) šipiršu ilabbirma īnāšu ippâ* **55’** *ana bulluṭīšu ištēn šiqil [...] ina himēti tasâk īnīšu tēteneqqi*	54’If in the eye [...], (and both eyes) become progressively dark: the effect on this man will be long lasting and his eyes will be cloudy. 55’In order to heal it: you pound one shekel of [...] in ghee (and) keep daubing his eyes.

54’ ND i 54’ DIŠ *i-na* IGI x [x x x] x *i-te-né-ṭa-a* NA BI KIN-*šú* SUMUN-*ma* IGI.MIN-*šú ip-pa-a*

55’ ND i 55’ *ana* TI-*šú* 1 GÍ[N x x x x] x *ina* Ì.NUN SÚD IGI.MIN-*šú* MAR.MEŠ

56’ *šumma amēlu īnāšū nuppuhā [... qēm] kukri qēm labti tahaššal tanappi ina šikari tarabbak īnīšu taṣammid*	56’If a man’s eyes are inflamed [...]: you crush and sift [... powder of] *kukru*-aromatic (and) flour of roasted grain, you make an infusion from (them) in beer (and) bandage his eyes.

Overview of IGI 2 Manuscripts and Parallels: **AA**=BAM 20; **AB**=BAM 159; **AD**=BAM 22; **AF**=BAM 23; **AG**=BAM 15; **bB**=BAM 382; **BoA**=KUB 4/50; **KA**=CTN 4/123; **NA**=BAM 510; **NB**=BAM 513; **NC**=BAM 514; **ND**=BAM 515; **NE**=BAM 516; **NI**=BAM 480; **NK**=BAM 518; **sA**=IRAQ 65; **uA**=SpTU 50; **uB**=NBC 4211; **xA**=CM 37

Alternative prescription 1 **57'** *šammu peṣû aban* [*gabî emesalli*] *šammū ṭīpu ša īnī*	**Alternative prescription 1** 57'White plant, *gabû*-[alum, *emesallu*-saline solution]; drugs are (used as) eye-drops.

56' ND i 56' DIŠ NA IGI.MIN-*šú nu-u*[*p-pu-ha* ... Z]Ì ⸢^{šim}⸣GÚR.GÚR ZÌ ŠE.SA.A GAZ SIM *ina* KAŠ *tara-bak* IGI.MIN-*šú* LAL

57' ND i 57' Ú.BABBAR NA$_4$ [*ga-bi-i* ^{mun}*eme-sal-lì*] ⸢Ú.HI⸣.A *ṭi-pu šá* IGI.MIN

58' *šumma amēlu īnāšu barrā* [*dimta ukallā šamma peṣâ*] *iškūra*? [*ina himēti tasâk*] **59'** *sebet ūmē ina askuppi* [*tetemmer tušellâmma* ...]	58'If a man's eyes are flickering [and contain tear(s) you pound white plant (and)] wax? [in ghee 59'You bury (the ingredients)] under the threshold for seven days, [you remove it and ...].

58' ND i 58' DIŠ NA IGI.MIN-*šú ba*[*r-ra u* ÉR *ú-kal-la* ....] ⸢GAB??⸣.L[ÀL?] x x x (x)

(AB) iv 29f.' DIŠ NA IGI.MIN-*šú bar-ra u* ÉR *ú-kal-la* / Ú.BABBAR ⸢LÀL⸣ *ina* Ì.NUN SÚD IGI.MIN-*šú* MAR

(uA) r.2f. [DIŠ NA] IGI.MIN-*šú i-bar-ru-ra u* ÉR *ú-kal-la* Ú.BABBAR LÀL / [(x)] KUR.RA *ina* Ì SÚD MAR

(xA) r.4 [DIŠ NA I]GI.⸢MIN⸣-*šú i-bar-ru-r*[*a u* É]R ⸢*ú-kal*⸣-*la* Ú.BABBAR LÀL.KUR.RA *ina* Ì.⸢GIŠ⸣ S[ÚD MAR]

59' ND i 59' 7 UD-*me ina* KU[N$_4$ *te-te-mer* E$_{11}$-*ma* ...] x [...]

60' *šumma amēlu īnāšu* [...] *tasâk īnīšu teqqi* ... [...]	60'If a man's eyes are [...] you pound [...] and daub his eyes ... [...]

60' ND i 60' ⸢DIŠ NA IGI.MIN-*šú*⸣ [........... S]ÚD ⸢IGI.MIN-*šú* MAR⸣ x [..................]

61' *šumma amēlu īnāšu* [*arpā* ...] *ina šamni u šuhti* [*ša tangussi tasâk īnīšu teqqi*]	61'If a man's eyes [grew dark: you pound ...] in oil and patina [of a copper *tangussu*-kettle and daub his eyes.]

Overview of IGI 2 Manuscripts and Parallels: **AA**=BAM 20; **AB**=BAM 159; **AD**=BAM 22; **AF**=BAM 23; **AG**=BAM 15; **bB**=BAM 382; **BoA**=KUB 4/50; **KA**=CTN 4/123; **NA**=BAM 510; **NB**=BAM 513; **NC**=BAM 514; **ND**=BAM 515; **NE**=BAM 516; **NI**=BAM 480; **NK**=BAM 518; **sA**=IRAQ 65; **uA**=SpTU 50; **uB**=NBC 4211; **xA**=CM 37

62' *haṣba labīra ša kibša* [*išû*] *ina šamni šuhti tasâk teqqi dišip šadê* [...]	[62']You pound an old fungus-[ridden] potsherd in oil (and) copper patina (and daub his eyes). You [mix] mountain honey [in ... and you daub his eyes].

61' ND i 61' DIŠ NA IGI.MIN-*šú a*[*r-pa* ....] *ina* Ì *u* SAHAR.UR[UDU *ša* ŠEN.TUR SÚD IGI.MIN-*šú* MAR]

62' ND i 62' ŠIKA LIBIR.RA *šá ki*-˹*ib*˺-*š*[*a*$^{?}$ TUK-*ú*] ˹*ina*˺ Ì SAHAR.URUDU SÚD MAR LÀL.K[UR.RA ...]

(NI) i 56 ˹ŠIKA˺ Ì.GU.LA *ša kib*-˹*ša*$_{25}$˺ TUK-*ú ina* Ì SAHA[R.URUDU] SÚD *te-qí*

63' *šumma amēlu īnāšu ṣuhhutā karān šēlebi arqūssu tuhassa mêšu ina* [*diqāri tarabbak*] **64'** *pāna takattamma ša elēni išallu*$^{?}$ *ina šuhti u šamni* [*tasâk teqqi*]	[63']If a man's eyes are under pressure; you squeeze fox-grape while still fresh, [you make an infusion from] its sap into a [*diqāru*-pot]. [64']You cover the top, and whatever emerges$^{?}$ above, [you pound] in a copper patina and sesame oil [and daub (his eyes)].
Alternative prescription 1 **65'** *ana ašri šanîmma sahlê ina šizbi takâṣ ina tinūri teppi ma'da lā* ...[...] **66'** *lipi kanakti atā'iša aban gabî šammu peṣâ kasâ ina himēti tasâk* [*īnīšu teqqi*]	**Alternative prescription 1** [65']Alternatively: you grate a *sahlû*-plant into milk, you bake (it) in a tannour-oven. It shall not dry out very much [...]. [66']You pound *kanaktu*-aromatic pith, *atā'išu*-plant, alum, white plant (and) *kasû*-plant in ghee. [You daub his eyes with it].
Alternative prescription 2 **67'** *ana ašri šanîmma akal šibri turrar tasâk kīma ṭīpi teṭeppi*	**Alternative prescription 2** [67']Alternatively: you parch crumbled bread, you pound it (and) apply it as drops (on his eyes).
Alternative prescription 3 **68'** *ana ašri šanîmma qēm hallūri qēm kakkî qēm kasî sahlê qalâti balṭāti ina diqāri tarabbak* [*taṣammid*]	**Alternative prescription 3** [68']Alternatively: you make an infusion from powder of chickpea, powder of lentil, powder of *kasû*-plant, freshly

Overview of IGI 2 Manuscripts and Parallels: **AA**=BAM 20; **AB**=BAM 159; **AD**=BAM 22; **AF**=BAM 23; **AG**=BAM 15; **bB**=BAM 382; **BoA**=KUB 4/50; **KA**=CTN 4/123; **NA**=BAM 510; **NB**=BAM 513; **NC**=BAM 514; **ND**=BAM 515; **NE**=BAM 516; **NI**=BAM 480; **NK**=BAM 518; **sA**=IRAQ 65; **uA**=SpTU 50; **uB**=NBC 4211; **xA**=CM 37

	roasted *sahlû*-plant in a *diqāru*-pot. [You bandage (his eyes)].
Alternative prescription 4	**Alternative prescription 4**
69' *ana ašri šanîmma ballukka kasâ ina šizbi tasâk īnīšu teqqi*	69' Alternatively: you pound *ballukku*-aromatic (and) *kasû*-plant in milk (and) you daub his eyes.
Alternative prescription 5	**Alternative prescription 5**
70' *ana ašri šanîmma šamma peṣâ kutpâ turrar ina himēti tasâk teqqi* :	70' Alternatively: you parch white plant (and) black frit, you pound (them) in ghee (and) daub.
Alternative prescription 6	**Alternative prescription 6**
70' *ana ašri šanîmma lulâ ina lipî eṣemti immeri tasâk teqqi*	70' Alternatively: you pound *lulû*-antimony in the marrow of a sheep's bone (and) daub (his eyes).
Alternative prescription 7	**Alternative prescription 7**
71' *ana ašri šanîmma marat raqqi ina ṭābti tušnâl/tuštāl adi ablat tašakkan enūma ītablu ina šamni šuhti tasâk teqqi*	71' Alternatively: you cure the gall bladder of *raqqu*-turtle in salt, you leave (it) until it has dried out, when it has dried out you pound it in oil (and) copper patina (and) daub (his eyes).
Alternative prescription 8	**Alternative prescription 8**
72' *ana ašri šanîmma [marat? ...] eli patar siparri ina himēti tasâk teqqi*	72' Alternatively: you pound [gall bladder of ...] over a bronze knife in ghee, (and) you daub (his eyes with it).
Alternative prescription 9	**Alternative prescription 9**
73' *ana ašri šanîmma šamma peṣâ karān šēlebi [ina] šamni tanaddi ina ubānīka teqqi*	73' Alternatively: you put white plant (and) fox-grape in sesame oil, you daub (his eyes) with your finger.

Overview of IGI 2 Manuscripts and Parallels: **AA**=BAM 20; **AB**=BAM 159; **AD**=BAM 22; **AF**=BAM 23; **AG**=BAM 15; **bB**=BAM 382; **BoA**=KUB 4/50; **KA**=CTN 4/123; **NA**=BAM 510; **NB**=BAM 513; **NC**=BAM 514; **ND**=BAM 515; **NE**=BAM 516; **NI**=BAM 480; **NK**=BAM 518; **sA**=IRAQ 65; **uA**=SpTU 50; **uB**=NBC 4211; **xA**=CM 37

Alternative prescription 10 **74'** *ana ašri šanîmma qaqqad ṣurāri tubbal tasâk* [*ina šamni tanaddi teqqi*]	**Alternative prescription 10** 74' Alternatively: you dry a lizard's head (and) pound (it), [place it in oil (and) daub (his eyes)].
Alternative prescription 11 **74'** [*ana ašri*] *šanîmma ṣurār igāri tubbal tasâk ina mušāli*$^{?}$ *ina pēmti tašakkan teqqi*	**Alternative prescription 11** 74' Alternatively: you dry a wall-lizard (and) pound (it). You put (it) on a palette$^{?}$ over charcoal, (and) daub (his eyes).
Alternative prescription 12 **75'** *sikkat ṣēli immeri turrar tasâk* (...) UD.3.KAM *ina mušāli tašakkan kayyamānu teqqi*	**Alternative prescription 12** 75' You parch a lamb chop (and) pound it. (...) Over three days you place (it) on a palette (and) you regularly daub (his eyes).

63' ND i 63' DIŠ NA IGI.MIN-*šú ṣu-uh-hu-ta* [GEŠTI]N.KA$_5$.A SIG$_7$-*su tu-ha-sa* A.MEŠ-*šú ina* ^{d}[^{ug}ÚTUL *tara-bak*]

64' ND i 64' IGI DUL-*ma šá* AN.TA *i-*[*ša*]*l*$^{?}$*-lu ina* SAHAR.URUDU *u* Ì.GI[Š SÚD MAR]

65' ND i 65' DIŠ KIMIN ZÀ.HI.LI *ina* GA ⌜*ta-ka*⌝*-aṣ ina* NININDU *te-ep-pi ma-ʾ-da la i-ba*-x [...]

(AD) r.14f.' *sah-lé-e ina* G[A *t*]*a-ka-a-aṣ* / *in*[*a* $^{(im)}$]ŠU.RIN.NA *te-ep-pi ma-*⌜*ʾ*⌝*-da*⌝ *la ir-ri-ra*

(sA) ii 23ff. *sah-lé-e* / *ki-ṣa-a-ti ina* NININDU$^{?}$(SUG) *te-ṭe-eh-hi ma-ʾ-du* / *la ir-ri-ra*

66' ND i 66' Ì.UDU ^{šim}GIG ^{ú}KUR.KU[R N]A$_4$ *ga-bi-i* Ú.BABBAR GAZI^{sar} *ina* Ì.NUN SÚ[D IGI.MIN-*šú* MAR]

(AD) r.16' *in*[*a*] Ì *hal-ṣi* S[Ú]D MAR

(sA) ii 25f. *ina* Ì.GIŠ.BUR *tara-bak* / IGI.MIN-*šú* MAR URUDU SUMUN *ina* Ì.NUN.NA SÚD

(sA) ii 26 GIN$_7$ *rib-ki* IGI.MIN-*šú* MAR-*ma* TI-*uṭ*

Overview of IGI 2 Manuscripts and Parallels: **AA**=BAM 20; **AB**=BAM 159; **AD**=BAM 22; **AF**=BAM 23; **AG**=BAM 15; **bB**=BAM 382; **BoA**=KUB 4/50; **KA**=CTN 4/123; **NA**=BAM 510; **NB**=BAM 513; **NC**=BAM 514; **ND**=BAM 515; **NE**=BAM 516; **NI**=BAM 480; **NK**=BAM 518; **sA**=IRAQ 65; **uA**=SpTU 50; **uB**=NBC 4211; **xA**=CM 37

67’	ND i 67’	[DIŠ K]IMIN NINDA *ši-ib-ri t*[*ur-á*]*r* SÚD *ki-ma ṭi-pi te-ṭe-e*[*p-pi*]
68’	ND i 68’	[DIŠ KIMI]N ZÌ GÚ.GAL ZÌ G[Ú.TUR] ⸢ZÌ⸣ GAZI^{sar} *sah-le-e qa-la-a-ti bal-ṭa-ti ina* ^{dug}ÚTUL *tara-ba*[*k* LAL]
69’	ND i 69’	⸢DIŠ KIMIN⸣ ^{šim}BA[L G]AZI^{sar} *ina* GA SÚD IGI.MIN-*šú* [MA]R$^{?}$
70’	ND i 70’	DIŠ KIMIN ⸢Ú⸣.BA[BBAR A]N.ZAH.GE$_6$ *tur-ár ina* Ì.NUN SÚD MAR : DIŠ KIMIN KÙ.GAN *ina* Ì.UDU GÌR.PAD.DU UDU SÚD ⸢MAR⸣
71’	ND i 71’	DIŠ KIMIN ZÍ BAL.[G]I$^{⸢ku6⸣}$ *ina* MUN NÁ-*al* EN HÁD.DU GAR-*an* UD-*ma* HÁD.DU *ina* Ì SAHAR.URUDU SÚD ⸢MAR⸣
	(ND) iii 23’	[... EN HÁD.DU GAR-*an* U]D-*ma* HÁD.DU *ina* SAHAR.URUDU Ì.NUN ⸢SÚD MAR⸣
	(NI) ii 2f.	NUMUN [^{ú}E]ME.UR.GI$_7$ SIG$_7$-*su tu-hás-sà* A-*šú ana* ^{dug}BUR.ZI SUR-*at* EN HÁD.DU GAR-*an* / U[D-*m*]*a i-tab-lu ina* Ì SAHAR.URUDU SÚD MAR
	(AF) 9’	⸢ZÍ GÚ.BÍ$^{ku6⸣}$ *ina* MUN NÁ-*al* BAR ^{giš}NU.ÚR.MA ⸢^{giš}GIG *tur-ár*⸣
72’	ND i 72’	DIŠ KIMIN Z[Í x (x x)] UGU GÍR.ZABAR *ina* Ì.NUN SÚD ⸢MAR⸣ $^{gloss:(?)\ x(?)}$ [...]
73’	ND ii 1	DIŠ KIMIN Ú.BABBAR ^{ú}GEŠTIN.K[A$_5$.A *ina*] Ì$^{?}$+GIŠ$^{?}$ ŠUB *ina* ŠU.SI-*ka* MAR
74’	ND ii 2	DIŠ KIMIN SAG.DU EME.ŠID HÁD.DU S[ÚD *ina* Ì ŠUB MAR : DIŠ K]IMIN EME.ŠID É.GAR$_8$ HÁD.DU SÚD *ina* ŠU.LÚ.ZABAR$^{?}$ *ina* NE GAR-*an* MAR
75’	ND ii 3	GAG.TI.TI UDU *tur-ár* SÚ[D (...) U]D.3.KÁM *ina mu-šá-lì* GAR SAG.UŠ MAR

Overview of IGI 2 Manuscripts and Parallels: **AA**=BAM 20; **AB**=BAM 159; **AD**=BAM 22; **AF**=BAM 23; **AG**=BAM 15; **bB**=BAM 382; **BoA**=KUB 4/50; **KA**=CTN 4/123; **NA**=BAM 510; **NB**=BAM 513; **NC**=BAM 514; **ND**=BAM 515; **NE**=BAM 516; **NI**=BAM 480; **NK**=BAM 518; **sA**=IRAQ 65; **uA**=SpTU 50; **uB**=NBC 4211; **xA**=CM 37

76' *šumma amēlu īnāšu katmā* x [... *tasâk*] *ina himēti taballal ana libbi īnīšu tunattak*	76'If the man's eyes are closed: [you pound ...], mix (it) in ghee (and) you drip it into his eyes.
Alternative prescription 1 **77'** *muhha ša rīmti* [*tasâk*? (...) *ina*] *šamni u muhhi ša summati zikari* **78'** *malmališ taballal* UD.3.KAM [*ina mušāli tašakkan*] *kayyamānu ana libbi īnīšu tattanaddi*	**Alternative prescription 1** 77'You [pound?] wild cow's brain and [(...)] 78'you mix (it) in equal measure 77'in sesame oil and (in) the brain of a male pigeon. 78'Over three days [you place (it) on a cosmetic palette (and)] you keep on applying it regularly into his eyes.
Alternative prescription 2 **79'** *pel āribi* [*tasâk* (...) *arki*] *tušellâmma patar siparri himēta tapaššaš* **80'** [...] *qātēka ina mê temessi* **81'** [... *ina*] *himēti tulabbak teqqi*	**Alternative prescription 2** 79'[You pound] a raven's egg, [(...) afterwards] you remove (it), and smear ghee on a bronze knife. 80'[...] You wash your hands in water, 81'[...] You soften up ... [in] ghee and daub (his eyes with it).

The following prescriptions are fragmentary and mitght not be alternatives.

Alternative prescription 3 **82'** [... *ina mušāli tašakkan*] *kayyānam tēteneqqi*	**Alternative prescription 3** 82'[If, ... you place (it) on a cosmetic palette (and)] you keep on daubing (his eyes) regularly.
Alternative prescription 4 **83'** [...] *tasâk teqqi*	**Alternative prescription 4** 83'[...] you pound, and daub (his eyes).
Alternative prescription 5 **84'** [...] *ana šamni tarabbak rebiat kalgukki tasâk teqqi*	**Alternative prescription 5** 84'[...] you make an infusion from (it) in sesame oil, you pound one fourth measure of *kalgukku*-red paste (and) daub (his eyes).
Alternative prescription 6 **85'** [...] x SILA$_x$(KISAL) *kutpâ ina šaman erēni tasâk teqqi*	**Alternative prescription 6** 85'You pound [...] (*and*) x SILA-measures of black frit in cedar oil (and) daub (his eyes).

Overview of IGI 2 Manuscripts and Parallels: **AA**=BAM 20; **AB**=BAM 159; **AD**=BAM 22; **AF**=BAM 23; **AG**=BAM 15; **bB**=BAM 382; **BoA**=KUB 4/50; **KA**=CTN 4/123; **NA**=BAM 510; **NB**=BAM 513; **NC**=BAM 514; **ND**=BAM 515; **NE**=BAM 516; **NI**=BAM 480; **NK**=BAM 518; **sA**=IRAQ 65; **uA**=SpTU 50; **uB**=NBC 4211; **xA**=CM 37

Alternative prescription 7 **86’** [...] x :?	**Alternative prescription 7** 86’[...] x :?
Alternative prescription 8 **86’** *karān šēlebi tasâk ina šamni ina tangussi tabbalakkat teqqi*	**Alternative prescription 8** 86’You pound fox-grape, (and) transfer (it) in oil into a copper *tangussu*-kettle, you daub (his eyes).
Alternative prescription 9 **87’** [... *zēr*] *egemgīri urnê ištēniš tasâk teqqi*	**Alternative prescription 9** 87’[...] you pound together [... seeds of] *egemgīru*-plant, and *urnû*-plant (and) you daub (his eyes).
Alternative prescription 10 **88’** [...] *ina šamni tasâk teqqi*	**Alternative prescription 10** 88’[...] you pound in oil, you daub (his eyes).
Alternative prescription 11 **89’** [...] ... *ana libbi īnīšu tunattak*	**Alternative prescription 11** 89’[...] ... (and) you drip (it) into his eyes.

76’	ND ii 4	DIŠ NA IGI.MIN-*šú* DUL?-*ma* x [x SÚ]D? *ina* Ì.NUN HE.HE *ana* ŠÀ IGI.MIN-*šú tu-na-tak*
77’	ND ii 5	UGU *ša* SÚN-*tì* S[ÚD? (...) *ina*] Ì+GIŠ *u* UGU *ša* TUmušen NITA
78’	ND ii 6	*mal-ma-liš* HE.HE U[D.3.KÁM *ina mu-šá-lì* GAR S]AG.UŠ *ana* ŠÀ IGI.MIN-*šú* ŠUB.ŠUB-*di*
79’	ND ii 7	NUNUZ UG[Amušen SÚD x x x (x) EG]IR? E11-*ma* GÍR.ZABAR Ì.NUN ŠÉŠ
80’	ND ii 8	x [.. Š]U.MEŠ-*ka ina* A LUH-*si*
81’	ND ii 9	[.. *ina*] ⌜Ì⌝.NUN *tu-la-bak* MAR
82’	ND ii 10	[................................... *ina mu-šá-lì* GAR-*a*]*n ka-a-a-nam te-te-né-*⌜*qí*⌝
83’	ND ii 11	[..] ⌜SÚD⌝ MAR

Overview of IGI 2 Manuscripts and Parallels: **AA**=BAM 20; **AB**=BAM 159; **AD**=BAM 22; **AF**=BAM 23; **AG**=BAM 15; **bB**=BAM 382; **BoA**=KUB 4/50; **KA**=CTN 4/123; **NA**=BAM 510; **NB**=BAM 513; **NC**=BAM 514; **ND**=BAM 515; **NE**=BAM 516; **NI**=BAM 480; **NK**=BAM 518; **sA**=IRAQ 65; **uA**=SpTU 50; **uB**=NBC 4211; **xA**=CM 37

84' ND ii 12 [................ *a*]*na* ⌜Ì+GIŠ *tara-bak* IGI.4.GÁL⌝.LA ^{im}KAL.GUG SÚD MAR

85' ND ii 13 [.......................] x SILA$_{x}$(KISAL) *ku-ut-pa-a ina* Ì+GIŠ EREN SÚD *te-qí*

86' ND ii 14 [...........] x ⌜:$^{?}$⌝ GEŠTIN.KA$_{5}$.A SÚD *ina* Ì *ina* ^{urudu}ŠEN.TUR BAL-*at te-qí*

87' ND ii 15 [.................. (NUMUN) ^{giš}NÍG.GÁ]N.⌜GÁN⌝ *úr-né-e*$^{?}$ UR.BI *ta-sàk te-qí*

88' ND ii 16 [..] *ina* Ì SÚD *te-qí*

89' ND ii 17 [..] x-*ta ana* ŠÀ IGI.MIN-*šú tu-na-tak*

90' [... *buṣinni*$^{?}$] *ša nūri tasarrim qutra ša nūri* **91'** [...] ... *itti mê uhūli qarnānî īnīšu temessi*	$^{90'}$[...] you cut [the wick$^{?}$] of a lamp. $^{91'}$You [...] $^{90'}$the smoke of the lamp, $^{91'}$[...]... (and) you wash his eyes with the sap of horned *uhūlu*-alkali.

90' ND ii 18 [............................ *bu-ṣi-n*]*i*$^{?}$ *šá nu-rì ta-sa-rim qut-ra*$_{x}$(ÁG) *ša nu-rì*

91' ND ii 19 [..] x KI A NAGA.SI IGI.MIN-*šú* LUH-*si*

92' [... *šamma peṣâ*] *hamšat šiqil rikibti arkabi malmališ taballal* **93'** [...] *itqūr abāri ina šamni u šuhti tasâk teqqi*	$^{92'}$[...] you mix in equal measures [... white plant], (and) five shekels of bat guano. $^{93'}$[...] you pound (it with) a lead spoon in oil and copper patina, daub (his eyes with it).

92' ND ii 20 [.................. Ú.BABBA]R$^{?}$ ⌜5$^{?}$⌝ GÍN U$_{5}$.ARGAB^{mušen} ⌜*mal-ma-liš*⌝ HE.HE

93' ND ii 21 [........................ DÍL]IM ⌜A.BÁR⌝ *ina* Ì *u* ⌜SAHAR.URUDU⌝ SÚD MAR

94' [... *ina*] *tangussi tukaṣṣa ina tangussi taballal*	$^{94'}$[...] you cool (it) off in a copper *tangussu*-kettle (and) you mix (it) in a copper *tangussu*-kettle. $^{95'}$[...] you strip

Overview of IGI 2 Manuscripts and Parallels: **AA**=BAM 20; **AB**=BAM 159; **AD**=BAM 22; **AF**=BAM 23; **AG**=BAM 15; **bB**=BAM 382; **BoA**=KUB 4/50; **KA**=CTN 4/123; **NA**=BAM 510; **NB**=BAM 513; **NC**=BAM 514; **ND**=BAM 515; **NE**=BAM 516; **NI**=BAM 480; **NK**=BAM 518; **sA**=IRAQ 65; **uA**=SpTU 50; **uB**=NBC 4211; **xA**=CM 37

95' [... *šuhta*] *ša tangussi tašammaṭ sebet ūmī teqqi*	away the patina of a copper *tangussu*-kettle (and) daub (his eyes) for seven days.

94' ND ii 22 [...................... *ina* ^{urudu}ŠE]N$^{?}$.TUR *tu-kàṣ-*⸢*ṣa ina* ^{urudu}ŠEN⸣.TUR HE.HE

95' ND ii 23 [.......... SAHAR.URUD]U ⸢*ša*⸣ ^{urudu}ŠEN.TUR *ta-šam-ma-aṭ* 7 UD-*mi* MAR

96' [...] *pa'ṣūte lipâ* **97'** [... *ina irri*] *abāri tasâk teqqīma kappi īnīšu ikši*	$^{96'}$[...] crushed [(ingredients)] and fat, $^{97'}$you pound [... into a] lead [salve], daub (his eyes), then the eyelid has benefitted.

96' ND ii 24 [...] x *pa-'a-ṣú-te* Ì.UDU

97' ND ii 25 [...................... *ina ir-ri*] ⸢A⸣.GAR$_5$ SÚD *te-qí-ma* PA IGI.MIN-*šú ik-ši*

98' [*ana īnī kiṣâti bulluṭi u kappi īnīšu*] *šūṣi sahlê kiṣâti ina tinūri teṭehhīma* **99'** [*ma'da lā irrirā ina šaman pūri tarabbak īnīšu*] *teqqi erâ labīra ina himēti tasâk kīma ribki īnīšu tēteneqqīma iballuṭ*	$^{98'}$[In order to heal the irritated area around the eyes and] remove [his eyelash]: you introduce grated *sahlû*-plant into a tannour-oven, but $^{99'}$[it (= grated *sahlû*) shall not dry out much. You make an infusion from it in *pūru*-oil (and)] daub [his eyes]. You pound old copper in ghee as an infusion for the eyes, you daub his eyes again and again, then he should recover.

98' ND ii 26 [.. *š*]*u-ṣi-i sah-lé-e ki-ṣa-a-ti ina* NININDU$^{!}$(SUG) TE-*ma*

(AD) r.13ff. DIŠ ⸢*a-na* IGI.MIN⸣.MEŠ ⸢*ki*⸣-*ṣa-a-ti b*[*ul-l*]*u-ṭi u kap-pi* IGI.MIN-*šú* / ⸢*šu-ṣi*⸣-*i sah-lé-e ina* G[A *t*]*a-ka-a-aṣ* / *in*[*a* $^{(im)}$]ŠU.RIN.NA *te-ep-pi* →

(sA) ii 22ff. *a-na* IGI.MIN *ki-ṣa-a-ti bul-lu-ṭu* / *ù kap-pi* IGI.MIN *šu-ṣi-i sah-lé-e* / *ki-ṣa-a-ti ina* NININDU$^{?}$(text SUG) *te-ṭe-eh-hi*

99' ND ii 27 [.. MA]R URUDU SUMUN *ina* Ì.NUN SÚD GIN$_7$ *rib-ki* IGI.MIN-*šú* MAR.MEŠ-*ma* TI

Overview of IGI 2 Manuscripts and Parallels: **AA**=BAM 20; **AB**=BAM 159; **AD**=BAM 22; **AF**=BAM 23; **AG**=BAM 15; **bB**=BAM 382; **BoA**=KUB 4/50; **KA**=CTN 4/123; **NA**=BAM 510; **NB**=BAM 513; **NC**=BAM 514; **ND**=BAM 515; **NE**=BAM 516; **NI**=BAM 480; **NK**=BAM 518; **sA**=IRAQ 65; **uA**=SpTU 50; **uB**=NBC 4211; **xA**=CM 37

(AD) r.15f. *ma-*⌜ʾ⌝*-da*⌝ *la ir-ri-ra* / *in*[*a*] Ì *hal-ṣi* S[Ú]D MAR

(sA) ii 24ff. *ma-ʾa-du* / *la ir-ri-ra ina* Ì.GIŠ.BUR *tara-bak* / IGI.MIN-*šú* MAR URUDU SUMUN *ina* Ì.NUN.NA SÚD
(sA) ii 27 GIN$_7$ *rib-ki* IGI.MIN-*šú* MAR-*ma* TI-*uṭ*

The following prescriptions might be alternatives to the one in lines 98f.' This is, however, unclear since the diagnostic part is broken off.

100' [... *mê*] *maštakal mê lišān kalbi mê karān šēlebi* **101'** [...] *teleqqe ina šuhti tasâk īnīšu teqqi*	[100'][... sap] of *maštakal*-plant, sap of dog's tongue-plant, fox-grape sap, [101']You take [...]. You pound (them) in copper patina (gloss: in the sap of a *sahlû*-plant), (and) you daub his eyes (with it).

100' ND ii 28 [.................................. A$^?$] ⌜^{ú}⌝IN$_6$.ÚŠ A ^{ú}EME.UR.GI$_7$ A ^{ú}GEŠTIN.KA$_5$.A
101' ND ii 29 [.......................]-⌜*ti* TI⌝-*qé ina* SAHAR.URUDU SÚD ⌜IGI.MIN-*šú* MAR⌝
gloss: A *sah-lé-e* (over the dividing line)

102' [...] *turrar tapâṣ ina šuhti tasâk teqqi*	[102']You parch (and) crush [...], you pound (it) in copper patina, (and) daub (his eyes).

102' ND ii 30 [.......................... *tu*]*r-*⌜*ár ta-pa-a-aṣ ina*⌝ SAHAR.URUDU SÚD ⌜MAR⌝

103' [... *sebet ūmē ina*] *askuppi tetemmer tušellâmma ina šuhti tasâk teqqi* **104'** [...] *ina šuhti tasâk teqqi*	[103'][...] You bury (the ingredients) under the threshold [for seven days]. You remove (them) up and then you pound it in copper patina, daub (his eyes with it). [104']You pound [...] in copper patina, daub (his eyes with it).

103' ND ii 31 [... 7 UD-*me ina* KU]N$_4$ *te-tem-mer* E$_{11}$-*ma ina* SAHAR.URUDU SÚD MAR

104' ND ii 32 [...] *ina* SAHAR.URUDU SÚD MAR

Overview of IGI 2 Manuscripts and Parallels: **AA**=BAM 20; **AB**=BAM 159; **AD**=BAM 22; **AF**=BAM 23; **AG**=BAM 15; **bB**=BAM 382; **BoA**=KUB 4/50; **KA**=CTN 4/123; **NA**=BAM 510; **NB**=BAM 513; **NC**=BAM 514; **ND**=BAM 515; **NE**=BAM 516; **NI**=BAM 480; **NK**=BAM 518; **sA**=IRAQ 65; **uA**=SpTU 50; **uB**=NBC 4211; **xA**=CM 37

105' [...] *īnīšunu ina ṣillî tutakkap* **106'** [...] *šammī ša āribu ana ṣehrīšu ilqâ* **107'** [...] *šâšu tasâk teqqi*	[105'][...] you prick their eyes (of raven chicks) with a needle. [106'][... (you take)] the plants which the raven took to its chicks (in order to heal them). [107']You pound [... (these plants brought?)] by it (and) daub (his eyes).

105' ND ii 33 [..] x IGI.MEŠ-*šú-nu ina* ^giš^DÁLA *tu-ták-kap*

106' ND ii 34 [....................................] ⌜Ú.MEŠ *ša*⌝ UGA^mušen^ *ana* TUR.MEŠ-*šú il-qa-a*

107' ND ii 35 [..] *šá-šu ta-sàk te-qí*

108' [...] *kamkadi tasâk muhhi kurāri ša kappi īnīšu* **109'** [*tugallab* (...)] *ballukka zēr šammi daqqiqi? zê upputte gūra ša qanî zēr talupadi* **110'** *larsīni ša halli lahri ša šumēli ša māšī ūlidu* **111'** [*kalīt*] *lalî lakî ša šamma lā našku uṭṭata lā ṣabitu ina nemsēte taqallu* **112'** *balta ša ṭābti šarmada karān šēlebi zēr haṭṭi rē'î taqallu zēr lišān* [*kalbi*] **113'** *kurkānâ egemgīra šamma peṣâ* [*qanâ*] *ṭāba ištēniš tasâk taballal ina mê kasî sekrūti* **114'** *kaṣûti talâš* UD.15.KAM *taṣṣanammid* UD.15.KAM *šamma peṣâ* UD.3.KAM *teqqi*	[108'][...] you pound *kamkadu*-plant. [109']You [shave off] [108']the surface of the *kurāru*-pustle of his eyelids. [111']You roast in a tub [109'][...], *ballukku*-aromatic, tiny? plant seeds, excrement of *upputte*-insect, reed leaf, seeds of *talupadu*-plant, [110']a hoof of the left hind leg of an ewe which bore twins, [111'][kidney] of young suckling goat which has not (yet) bitten a plant nor grasped a grain kernel. [112']You roast salted *baltu*-(thorn) plant, *šarmadu*-plant, fox-vine (and) seeds of shepherd's-staff plant. [113']You pound (and) mix together [112']seeds of dog's-tongue plant, [113']*kurkānû*-plant, *egemgīru*-plant, white plant, sweet [reed]. [114']You knead (all the above-mentioned ingredients, first) [113']in warmed-up (and then) [114']cold [113']sap of the *kasû*-plant. [114']You continusly bandage (the eyes) for fifteen days. On the fifteenth day, you daub (his eyes) with white plant for three days.

108' ND ii 36 [......................... *k*]*am-ka-di* SÚD UGU GIG.GIR *ša kap-pi* IGI.MIN-*šú*

Overview of IGI 2 Manuscripts and Parallels: **AA**=BAM 20; **AB**=BAM 159; **AD**=BAM 22; **AF**=BAM 23; **AG**=BAM 15; **bB**=BAM 382; **BoA**=KUB 4/50; **KA**=CTN 4/123; **NA**=BAM 510; **NB**=BAM 513; **NC**=BAM 514; **ND**=BAM 515; **NE**=BAM 516; **NI**=BAM 480; **NK**=BAM 518; **sA**=IRAQ 65; **uA**=SpTU 50; **uB**=NBC 4211; **xA**=CM 37

109' ND ii 37 [*tu*$^{?}$-*gal*$^{?}$-*lab*$^{?}$] ⌜^{ú}BAL NUMUN Ú⌝ [*da-a*]*q-qí-qí* ŠE$_{10}$ *up-pu-te gu-ra šá* GI NUMUN ^{ú}*ta-lu-pa-di*

110' ND ii 38 [*la-a*]*r-sì-ni ša hal-li* ⌜U$_{8}$⌝ *ša* GÙB *ša* MAŠ.TAB.BA Ù.TU

111' ND ii 39 [ÉLLAG] MÁŠ.TUR *la-ki-i ša* Ú *la na-*⌜*aš-ku*⌝ ŠE.BAR *la ṣa-bi-tú ina nem-se-te ta-*⌜*qàl-lu*⌝

112' ND ii 40 [$^{\text{(giš)}}$*b*]*al-ta*$_{5}$ *ša* MUN ^{ú}GÚR.UŠ ^{giš}GEŠTIN.⌜KA$_{5}$.A⌝ NUMUN ^{ú}NÍG.GIDRU *ta-qal-lu* NUMUN ^{ú}EM[E.UR.GI$_{7}$]

113' ND ii 41 ⌜^{ú}⌝KUR$_{4}$.GI.RIN.NA ^{ú}*gim-gi-ra* Ú.⌜BABBAR⌝ [GI.DÙ]G.GA 1-*niš* SÚD HE.HE *ina* A GAZI^{sar} *sek-ru-t*[*i*]

114' ND ii 42 [S]ED *ta-là-aš* UD.15.KÁM LAL.M[EŠ$^{?}$] UD.15.KÁM Ú.BABBAR UD.3.KÁM *te-eq-q*[*í*]

115' [*šumma*] *amēlu īnāšu amurriqāna malâ qilip nurmî tasâk ina takkussi ana libbi īnīšu tanappah*$^{?}$	115'If a man's eyes are full of yellowness (jaundice): you pound pomegranate peel (and) [you blow$^{?}$] it into his eyes through a reed-straw.

115' ND ii 43 [DIŠ N]A IGI.MIN-*šú* IGI.SIG$_{7}$.SIG$_{7}$ DIRI BAR ^{giš}NU.Ú[R.M]A SÚD *ina* ^{gi}SAG.KUD *ana* ŠÀ IGI.MIN-*šú* B[ÚN$^{?}$]

116' [*šumma amēlu*] *īnāšu amurriqāna malâ haṣab nurmî ina šamni tasâk teqqi* : *emesalli* [*tasâk teqqi*$^{?}$]	116'If a man's eyes are full of yellowness (jaundice): you pound pomegranate peel in oil and daub (his eyes) : [(or alternative) you pound] (it in) *emesallu*-saline solution (and) [daub his eyes].

116' ND ii 44 [DIŠ NA I]GI.⌜MIN⌝-*šú* IGI.SIG$_{7}$.SIG$_{7}$ DIRI ŠIKA ^{giš}NU.ÚR.[M]A *ina* Ì SÚD MAR : ^{mun}*eme-sal-lì* S[ÚD$^{?}$ MAR$^{?}$]

Overview of IGI 2 Manuscripts and Parallels: **AA**=BAM 20; **AB**=BAM 159; **AD**=BAM 22; **AF**=BAM 23; **AG**=BAM 15; **bB**=BAM 382; **BoA**=KUB 4/50; **KA**=CTN 4/123; **NA**=BAM 510; **NB**=BAM 513; **NC**=BAM 514; **ND**=BAM 515; **NE**=BAM 516; **NI**=BAM 480; **NK**=BAM 518; **sA**=IRAQ 65; **uA**=SpTU 50; **uB**=NBC 4211; **xA**=CM 37

117' [*šumma amēlu īnāšu*] *marṣāma ūmē ma'dūti lā ipetti ina ummi qaqqadīšu īnāšu ṣilla* [*malâ*]	117'[If a man's eyes] are sick and he cannot open (them) for many days, with his head being feverish (*ummu*), (and) his eyes are a film-[filled]. 118'[...] ... You shave his head. You cool off (the head) with dough three times a day. You parch seeds of *maštakal*-plant, 119'you pound [in ghee] on a lead [spoon] (and) daub his eyes. You wash (the eyes) with water, (and) you put *kasû*-plant over his eyes, until they become clear (of film) you keep on repeating (it).
118' [...] x *qaqqassu tugallab ina ūme šalāšīšu līša tukaṣṣa zēr maštakal turrar*	
119' [*ina himēti itqūr*] *abāri tasâk teqqi mê temessi kasâ eli īnīšu tašakkan adi uzakkû tuttanār*	
Alternative prescription 1	**Alternative prescription 1**
120' [*karān*] *šēlebi dišip šadê ina himēti taballal tēteneqqi*	120'You mix fox-grape (and) mountain honey in ghee (and) keep daubing (his eyes).

117' ND ii 45 [DIŠ NA IGI.MIN-*šú* G]IG-⸢*ma* UD *ma*⸣-ʾ-*du-ti* NU ⸢BAD⸣ *ina* KÚM SAG-*šú* IGI.MIN-*šú* GIS[SU DIRI$^{?}$]

(NA) i 18' [......... IGI.M]IN-*šú* GI[G .... *ma*-ʾ-*d*]*u-ti* NU BAD *ina* KÚM [....... ....]

(NB) i 8' DIŠ NA IGI.MIN-*šú* GIG-*ma* UD.MEŠ *ma*-ʾ-*du-ti* NU BA[D ....]

(NC) i 23' [... *š*]*ú*$^{?}$

(AA) 11f.' ⸢DIŠ$^{?}$⸣ NA IGI.MIN-*šú* GIG-*ma* UD-*me* ME[Š] / NU BAD-*te ina* KÚM SAG.DU-*šú* ⸢IGI⸣.MI[N-*šú*] / ⸢GISSU DIRI⸣ →

(AB) iv 3f.' DIŠ NA IGI.MIN-*šú* GIG-*ma* UD.MEŠ *ma*-ʾ-*du-te* NU BAD-⸢*te*⸣ / *ina* KÚM SAG.DU-*šú* IGI.MIN-*šú* GISSU DIRI

118' ND ii 46 [... M]I$^{?}$ SAG.DU-*su tu-gal-*⸢*lab ina* UD-*me* 3-*šú* NÍG⸣.SILA$_{11}$.GÁ *tu-kàṣ*-⸢*ṣa* NUMUN ^{ú}IN$_{6}$.ÚŠ⸣ *t*[*ur-ár*]

(NA) i 19' [SAG.D]U-*su* SAR-*a*[*b* .... N]ÍG.SILA$_{11}$.GÁ *tu-kàṣ-ṣ*[*a* ....]

(NB) i 8f.' [....................] / SAR-*ab ina* UD-*me* 3-*šú* NÍG.SILA$_{11}$.GÁ *tu-kàṣ-ṣa* NU[MUN ....]

(NC) i 24f.' [... *tu*]-⸢*kàṣ*$^{?}$-*ṣa*$^{?}$⸣ / [......................] x ⸢*tur*$^{?}$-*ár*$^{?}$⸣

Overview of IGI 2 Manuscripts and Parallels: **AA**=BAM 20; **AB**=BAM 159; **AD**=BAM 22; **AF**=BAM 23; **AG**=BAM 15; **bB**=BAM 382; **BoA**=KUB 4/50; **KA**=CTN 4/123; **NA**=BAM 510; **NB**=BAM 513; **NC**=BAM 514; **ND**=BAM 515; **NE**=BAM 516; **NI**=BAM 480; **NK**=BAM 518; **sA**=IRAQ 65; **uA**=SpTU 50; **uB**=NBC 4211; **xA**=CM 37

(AA) 13f.' SAG.⌜DU-*su*⌝ SA[R] / *ina* UD-*me* 3-*šú* NÍG$^{?}$⌝.SILA$_{11}$.GÁ *tu-kà*[*ṣ-ṣa*] / [NU]MUN ^{ú}IN$_{6}$.ÚŠ *tur-ár* →

(AB) iv 5f.' SAG.DU-*su* SAR.SAR *ina* UD-*me* 3-*šú ša* NÍG.⌜SILA$_{11}$.GÁ⌝ / *tu-kàṣ-ṣa* NUMUN ^{ú}IN.NU.UŠ *tur-*⌜*ár*⌝

119' ND ii 47 [*ina* Ì.NUN DÍLIM] ⌜A⌝.BÁR SÚD MAR A LUH-*si* GAZI^{sar} UGU ⌜IGI.MIN-*šú* GAR$^{?}$ EN$^{?}$ *ú-za-ku*⌝-*ú* GUR.G[UR]

(NA) i 20' [*ina*] ⌜Ì⌝.NUN DÍLIM A.⌜BÁR⌝ *t*[*a-sà*]*k* IGI.MIN-*šú t*[*e*$^{?}$-*qí*$^{?}$-*ma*$^{?}$ *ina*$^{?}$-*eš*$^{?}$]

(NB) i 9f.' [.................] / DÍLIM A.BÁR *ta-sàk* IGI.MIN-*šú* [.............................]

(NC) i 26' [... *in*]*a*$^{?}$-⌜*eš*$^{?}$⌝
THE DIVIDING LINE IS NOT VISIBLE!

(AA) 15ff.' *ina* Ì.⌜NUN$^{?}$⌝ / [DÍLIM] ⌜A$^{?}$⌝.BÁR SÚD IGI.MIN-*šú* MAR.M[E(Š)] / [*bul-ṭ*]*u*$^{?}$ *lat-k*[*u*$^{?}$]

(AB) iv 7f.' *ina* Ì.NUN DÍLIM A.BÁR SÚD IGI.MIN-*šú* / [M]AR.MEŠ-*ma* *bul-ṭu lat-ku*

120' ND ii 48 ⌜^{ú}⌝[GEŠTIN$^{?}$.K]A$_{5}$.A LÀL.KUR.RA *ina* Ì.NUN HE.⌜HE⌝ *te-te-neq*(NIG)-*q*[*í*]

121' *šumma amēlu īnāšu marṣāma šišītu muhha lamassat īnīšu armat dimta illak īnāšu ṣilla malâma*	[121']If a man's eyes are sick, and a membrane covers the surface of the pupil of his eyes, tear(s) flow, (and) his eyes are film-filled:
122' *errâ sahlāna zēr lišān* [*kalbi* ...] *šamma peṣâ rikibti arkabi*	[122']*errû*-colocynth, *sahlânu*-plant, seeds of [dog's] tongue plant [...], white plant, bat guano.
123' *ištēššeret šammī šâšunu* [*ištēniš tasâk ina šaman*] *erēni taballal īnīšu teqqīma iballuṭ*	[123']Those eleven$^{sic!}$ drugs you pound [together], mix [in] cedar [oil], daub his eyes, then he should recover.

121' ND ii 49 DIŠ ⌜NA IGI.MIN⌝-*šú* GIG-*ma ši-ši-tu* UGU ^{d}LAMA IGI.⌜MIN-*šú*⌝ *á*[*r-ma*]*t* [É]R.HI.A DU-*ak* IGI.MIN-*šú* GISSU DIRI-[*ma*]

(ND) ii 65 [DIŠ N]A I[GI.M]IN-[*šú* ....] x-*ma* DUGUD *ana* TI-*šú* ILLU NU.LUH

(AF) 1 ⌜DIŠ NA IGI.MIN-*šú* GIG⌝-*ma ši-*⌜*ši*⌝-*t*[*ú*] ⌜UGU⌝ ^{d}L[AMA IGI.MIN-*šú ár-mat*]

Overview of IGI 2 Manuscripts and Parallels: **AA**=BAM 20; **AB**=BAM 159; **AD**=BAM 22; **AF**=BAM 23; **AG**=BAM 15; **bB**=BAM 382; **BoA**=KUB 4/50; **KA**=CTN 4/123; **NA**=BAM 510; **NB**=BAM 513; **NC**=BAM 514; **ND**=BAM 515; **NE**=BAM 516; **NI**=BAM 480; **NK**=BAM 518; **sA**=IRAQ 65; **uA**=SpTU 50; **uB**=NBC 4211; **xA**=CM 37

122' ND ii 50 ^{ú}⸢ÚKUŠ⸣.LAGAB *sah-la-na* NUMUN ^{ú}EM[E.UR.GI$_7$ ...] ⸢Ú⸣.BABBAR U$_5$.ARGAB$^{m[ušen]}$

123' ND ii 51 11$^{(sic!)}$ Ú.⸢HI.A⸣ *ša-šu-*⸢*nu* 1$^{?}$⸣-[*niš* SÚD *ina* Ì.GIŠ ^{giš}ER]EN HE.HE IGI.MIN-*šú* MAR-*ma* ⸢TI⸣

124' *šumma amēlu īnāšu marṣāma [šišītu muhha lamassat īnīšu armat] digalšu kabit ana pūṣi ša muhhi lamassat īnīšu nasāhi* **125'** *aktam [... tasâk ... ina šaman] erēni taballal īnīšu tēteneqqīma iballuṭ*	124'If a man's eyes are sick, and [a membrane covers the surface of the pupil of his eyes], (and) his vision is 'heavy', in order to remove the white spot from the surface of the pupil of his eyes. 125'[You pound] *aktam*-plant, [... in] cedar [oil] you mix it, you keep daubing his eyes, and then he should recover.

124' ND ii 52 DIŠ NA IGI.MIN-⸢*šú* GIG⸣-*m*[*a ši-ši-tu* UGU ^{d}LAMA IGI.MIN-*šú ár-mat di-ga*]*l*-⸢*šu* DUGUD⸣ *ana* BABBAR *ša* UGU ^{d}LAMA IGI.MIN-*šú* ⸢ZI⸣

125' ND ii 53 ^{ú}*at-ká*[*m* ... SÚD ... *ina* Ì] ⸢^{giš}⸣EREN HE.HE IGI.MIN-*šú* MAR.MES-*ma* TI

126' *šumma amēlu īnāšu [marṣāma ...] digalšu kabit* **127'** ... *[tasâk] īnīšu teqqi*	126'If a man's eyes [are sick, and ...] his vision is 'heavy', 127'[You pound ...] (and) daub his eyes.

126' ND ii 54 DIŠ NA IGI.MIN-⸢*šú*⸣ [GIG-*ma* ....] x *di-gal-šu* ⸢DUGUD⸣

127' ND ii 55 x x [.. SÚ]D IGI.MIN-*šú* MAR

128' ... **129'** [...] *tasâk teqqi*	128'... 129'[...] you pound [...] and daub (his eyes).

128' ND ii 56 [...] x UM IM DU KU BA[D/N[U ...]

129' ND ii 57 [.. S]ÚD MAR

Overview of IGI 2 Manuscripts and Parallels: **AA**=BAM 20; **AB**=BAM 159; **AD**=BAM 22; **AF**=BAM 23; **AG**=BAM 15; **bB**=BAM 382; **BoA**=KUB 4/50; **KA**=CTN 4/123; **NA**=BAM 510; **NB**=BAM 513; **NC**=BAM 514; **ND**=BAM 515; **NE**=BAM 516; **NI**=BAM 480; **NK**=BAM 518; **sA**=IRAQ 65; **uA**=SpTU 50; **uB**=NBC 4211; **xA**=CM 37

130' [...] *pillâ zikara* **131'** [...] *ikkalma* ... [...] **132'** [... *tasâk ina takkussi ana*] *libbi īnīšu tanappah* **133'** [...] *tasâk šanîš*	130'[...] male *pillû*-plant. 131'[...] he shall eat (it) and then ... [...]132'[... you pound it (and) through a reed-straw] you blow it [in]to his eyes. 133'[...] you pound] and ditto (= you daub his eyes.)
Alternative prescription 1 **134'** [...] *tanaddi ana muhhi haṣab igulê* **135'** [...] *tašarrap qutra ša šitti* **136'** [...] *ahennâ īnīšu tēteneqqīma iballuṭ*	**Alternative prescription 1** 134'[You] put [...]. You [(smear)...] on the surface of potsherd of fine salve, 135'[...] you burn it. The smoke of the remainder 136'[..]. You keep daubing his eyes separately, then he should recover.

130' ND ii 58 [.......... g]išNAM.TAR NÍT[A]

131' ND ii 59 [..........] x GU₇-*ma* x [(x)]

132' ND ii 60 [.......... SÚD *ina* gišSAG.KUD *ana* Š]À ⌜IGI.MIN-*šú* MÚ⌝-*ah*

133' ND ii 61 [.......... SÚ]D? MIN

134' ND ii 62 [.......... ŠUB-*d*]*i ana* UGU ŠIKA *ì-gu-le-e*

135' ND ii 63 [..........] x *ta-šár-rap qut-ra šá šit-ti*

136' ND ii 64 [.......... *a-he-e*]*n-na* IGI.MIN-*šú* MAR.MEŠ-*ma* TI

137' [*šumma*] *amēlu* [*īnāšu marṣāma*] ...-*ma kabit ana bulluṭīšu hīl nuhurti* **138'** *hīl baluhhi* [... *sebet*] *arhī u samānat arhī inassaha iballuṭ*	137'[If] man's eyes [sick and ...] ... and (the condition) is grave. In order to heal it: resin of *nuhurtu*-plant, 138'resin of *baluhhu*-aromatic [... seven] or eight months will elapse, (then) he should recover.

137' ND ii 65 [DIŠ N]A I[GI.M]IN-[*šú* ....] x-*ma* DUGUD *ana* TI-*šú* ILLU NU.LUH

Overview of IGI 2 Manuscripts and Parallels: **AA**=BAM 20; **AB**=BAM 159; **AD**=BAM 22; **AF**=BAM 23; **AG**=BAM 15; **bB**=BAM 382; **BoA**=KUB 4/50; **KA**=CTN 4/123; **NA**=BAM 510; **NB**=BAM 513; **NC**=BAM 514; **ND**=BAM 515; **NE**=BAM 516; **NI**=BAM 480; **NK**=BAM 518; **sA**=IRAQ 65; **uA**=SpTU 50; **uB**=NBC 4211; **xA**=CM 37

(ND) ii 49 DIŠ ⸢NA IGI.MIN⸣-*šú* GIG-*ma ši-ši-tu* UGU ^{d}LAMA IGI.⸢MIN-*šú á*[*r-ma*]*t* [É]R.HI.A DU-*ak* IGI.MIN-*šú* GISSU DIRI-[*ma*]

(AF) 1f. ⸢DIŠ NA IGI.MIN-*šú* GIG⸣-*ma ši*-⸢*ši*⸣-*t*[*ú*] ⸢UGU⸣ ^{d}L[AMA IGI.MIN-*šú ár-mat*] / ⸢*ana* TI-*šú* ILLU NU.LUH⸣

138’ ND ii 66 ILLU $^{⸢šim}$BULUH $^{ú⸣}$ [... 7 I]TI *u* 8 ITI ZI-*ha* TI

(AF) 2 ILLU ^{šim}BULUH $^{⸢ú⸣}$ [..]

(AF) 3 ⸢DIŠ NA⸣ IGI.MIN-*šú* ⸢MÚ-*ah* GISSU *ša* 7 ITI [......................................]

139’ *šumma amēlu īnāšu šišītu* [*malâ ... hamiššer*] *uṭṭat haṣbi šammi peṣî ina himēti tasâk teqqi*	139’If a man’s eyes [are full of] a film, [...] you pound [15] grains of potsherd, (and) white plant in ghee, (and) daub (his eyes).
Alternative prescription 1 **140’** *šumma amēlu šanîš ištēn šiqil rikibti* [*arkabi ina ... tasâk ...*] *tābīla tazarru*	**Alternative prescription 1** 140’If a man ditto: [you pound] one shekel of bat [guano in ...] (and) you spatter it in dry state (into his eyes).
Alternative prescription 2 **141’** *šumma amēlu šanîš ištēn šiqil rikibti arkabi ina himēti tasâk teqqi* : *hamiššer uṭṭat haṣbi* [*... ina ...*] *tasâk teqqi*	**Alternative prescription 2** 141’If a man ditto: you pound one shekel of bat guano in ghee and daub (his eyes) : you pound a 15 grain measure of potsherd [... (and) daub (his eyes).
Alternative prescription 3 **142’** *imhur-līm ina himēti* [*tasâk* (*īnīšu*) *teqqi*]	**Alternative prescription 3** 142’[You pound] *imhur-līm*-plant in ghee [(and) daub (his eyes).]
Alternative prescription 4 **143’** [*... ištiššu*] *šinīšu šalāšīšu himēta tasâk teqqi*	**Alternative prescription 4** 143’[... once], twice, three times, you pound ghee (and) daub (his eyes).

139’ ND ii 67 DIŠ NA IGI.MIN-*šú ši-š*[*i-tú* DIRI .... 1]5$^{?}$ ŠE ŠIKA Ú.BABBAR *ina* Ì.NUN SÚD MAR

(AF) 4 DIŠ NA IGI.⸢MIN-*šú*⸣ *ši*-⸢*ši-tú*⸣ DIRI LAG MUN GAZI^{s}[^{ar} ....]

Overview of IGI 2 Manuscripts and Parallels: **AA**=BAM 20; **AB**=BAM 159; **AD**=BAM 22; **AF**=BAM 23; **AG**=BAM 15; **bB**=BAM 382; **BoA**=KUB 4/50; **KA**=CTN 4/123; **NA**=BAM 510; **NB**=BAM 513; **NC**=BAM 514; **ND**=BAM 515; **NE**=BAM 516; **NI**=BAM 480; **NK**=BAM 518; **sA**=IRAQ 65; **uA**=SpTU 50; **uB**=NBC 4211; **xA**=CM 37

140'	ND ii 68	DIŠ NA MIN 1 GÍN U[5.ARGAB^mušen^ .... SÚD ....] x [x *t*]*a-bi-la*12 MAR
	(AF) 5	DIŠ ⌜NA IGI⌝.MIN-*šú* ⌜*ši*⌝-*š*[*i-t*]*ú* DIRI 1/2 GÍN U5.⌜ARGAB^mušen^⌝ x x x [...]
141'	ND ii 69	DIŠ NA MIN 1 GÍN U5⌜.ARGAB^mušen^ *ina* Ì.NUN SÚD MAR :⌝ 15 ŠE Š[IKA ... *ina* ... S]ÚD ⌜MAR⌝
	(AF) 6	⌜DIŠ NA⌝ IGI.⌜MIN-*šú ši-ši-tú*⌝ *ú*-⌜*kal-la* U5.AGRAB⌝^mu^[^šen^ ... M]AR?
	(AF) 7	⌜15 ŠE LÀL⌝.KUR-*e* ⌜SÚD⌝ *te-qé*
142'	ND ii 70	^ú^*im-hur-lim ina* Ì.NUN [SÚD (IGI.MIN-*šú*) MAR]
	(AF) 8	⌜^ú^⌝*im-hur*-⌜*lim*⌝ *ina* Ì.NUN SÚD ⌜*te-qí*⌝

GAP!

143'	ND iii 9'	[... 1-*šú*] ⌜2-*šú* 3-*šú* Ì.NUN SÚD MAR⌝

NB.

The following prescriptions might be alternatives to the one on lines 139f.' This is, however, unclear since the diagnostic part is broken off.

144' [... *ina*] *himēti tasâk ina arhi šalāšīšu teqqi rikibti arkabi ina himēti tasâk teqqi* [*arti*] *bīni arti ēri* **145'** [*ina*] *ṭābāti talâš īnīšu taṣammid šamma peṣâ uhūla qarnānâ uzun lalî lā patān ana libbi īnīšu tamazza'*	[144'] [...:] you pound in ghee (and) you daub (his eyes) three times in a month. You pound bat guano in ghee (and) daub (his eyes). [145']You knead [144'][leaf] of tamarisk, leaf of *ēru*-tree [145'][in] vinegar?, (and) you bandage his eyes. Without (him) eating, you squeeze out into his eyes white plant, horned *uhūlu*-alkali, (and) kid's-ear plant.

144'	ND iii 10'	[............ *ina*] ⌜Ì.NUN SÚD *ina* ITI 3-*šú* MAR U5.ARGAB^mušen^ *ina* Ì.NUN SÚD MAR⌝ P[A ^giš^]*bi-ni* PA ^giš^MA.NU
145'	ND iii 11'	[*ina* A.GEŠTI]N.NA *ta-la-aš* IGI.MIN-*šú* LAL Ú.BABBAR NAGA.SI UR.TÁL.TÁL NU ⌜*pa-tan*⌝ [*ana*] ⌜ŠÀ⌝ IGI.MIN-*šú ta-ma-za-a'*

Overview of IGI 2 Manuscripts and Parallels: **AA**=BAM 20; **AB**=BAM 159; **AD**=BAM 22; **AF**=BAM 23; **AG**=BAM 15; **bB**=BAM 382; **BoA**=KUB 4/50; **KA**=CTN 4/123; **NA**=BAM 510; **NB**=BAM 513; **NC**=BAM 514; **ND**=BAM 515; **NE**=BAM 516; **NI**=BAM 480; **NK**=BAM 518; **sA**=IRAQ 65; **uA**=SpTU 50; **uB**=NBC 4211; **xA**=CM 37

(BoA) 3ff.' [BE KIMIN *m*]*ar-ṣa-ma* ^{ú}ÚR.TÁ[L.TÁL ...] / *ta-na-za-a' ta-pa-*[*aš* ...] / *a-na* ŠÀ IGI.MEŠ-*šú i-z*[*a* ...]

146' [...] ... *emesalli sīkti labti taballal turrar tasâk teqqi*	146'[...] ...: you mix *emesallu*-saline solution (and) roasted grain powder, you parch (the mixture), pound it (and) daub his eyes.

146' ND iii 12' [...] x $^{\text{⸢mun⸣}}$*eme-sal-lì si-ik-ti* ŠE.SA.⸢A HE.HE⸣ *tur-ár* SÚD MAR

147' [*šumma* ...] *šuhta ina libbi lipi sāqi ṣabīti tasâk teqqi*	147'[If ...:] you pound copper patina into fat of a gazelle's thigh and daub (his eyes).

147' ND iii 13' [DIŠ .... SAH]AR.URUDU *ina* ŠÀ Ì.UDU *sa-a-qí* M[AŠ.D]À SÚD MAR

(NI) i 44 [.. *sa*]*-a-qí* MAŠ.⸢DÀ SÚD⸣ *te-qí*

148' [*šumma* ... *murru ina šizbi musukkati ša zikara*] *ūlidu tasâk teqqi dišpa himēta ana libbi īnīšu tunattak*	148'[If ...:] you pound [bitter-plant in milk from a woman in maternity, who] gave birth [to a male] (and) daub (his eyes), you drip into his eyes honey (and) ghee.

148' ND iii 14' [DIŠ ... ^{šim}SES GA ^{munus}Ú.ZÚG *šá* NI]TA$^{?}$ Ù.TU SÚD ⸢MAR LÀL⸣ Ì.NUN.NA *ana* ŠÀ IGI.MIN-*šú tu-na-ták*

149' [*šumma* ...] x x [...] *šāru ul uṣṣâ* **150'** [...] ... *ina himēti taballal teqqi*	149' [If ...] x x [...] wind does not come out. 150'[...] ... you mix [...] in ghee (and) daub (his eyes).

149' ND iii 15' [DIŠ ....] x x [...] IM NU È-*a*

150' ND iii 16' [...] x *ina* Ì.NUN HE.HE MAR

151' [...] *tašaqqal teqqi*	151'[...] you weigh (it and) daub (his eyes).

151' ND iii 17' [..] *ta-ša-qàl* MAR

Overview of IGI 2 Manuscripts and Parallels: **AA**=BAM 20; **AB**=BAM 159; **AD**=BAM 22; **AF**=BAM 23; **AG**=BAM 15; **bB**=BAM 382; **BoA**=KUB 4/50; **KA**=CTN 4/123; **NA**=BAM 510; **NB**=BAM 513; **NC**=BAM 514; **ND**=BAM 515; **NE**=BAM 516; **NI**=BAM 480; **NK**=BAM 518; **sA**=IRAQ 65; **uA**=SpTU 50; **uB**=NBC 4211; **xA**=CM 37

152' [... *rikibti arkabi*] *tābīla ina himēti taballal ašar šanîmma*	[152'][...], you mix [bat guano] in dry state in ghee (and) ditto.

152' ND iii 18' [........................... U$_5$.ARGAB^{m}]^{ušen} ⸢*ta-bi-la*$_{12}$ *ina*⸣ Ì.NUN HE.HE KIMIN

153' [...] *ubāni-aṣi arqūssu ina mê temessi tahaššal mêšunu* **154'** [...] *tubbal šihiltu šuhta malmališ taballal* [*ina mê*] *temessi dišip šadê tasâk teqqi*	[153'][...] you wash *ubāni-aṣi*-plant in water while still fresh, crush it (and) you ... (filter out) their saps, [154']dry (it) out, ... (and) mix in equal measure the filtrate (with) the copper patina. You wash (it) [in water], pound mountain honey (and) you daub (his eyes).

153' ND iii 19' [.....................] ⸢*ú-ba-ni*⸣-*a-ṣi* SIG$_7$-*su ina* ⸢A LUH⸣-*si* GAZ A.MEŠ-*šú-nu*

154' ND iii 20' [.....................] ⸢HÁD.DU⸣ *ši-hi-il-tú* SAHAR.URUDU *mal-ma-liš* HE.HE [*ina* A LU]H LÀL.KUR-*e* SÚD MAR

155' [... *ina*] *šizbi musukkati malmališ taballal tasâk teqqi*	[155'][...] you mix in equal measure [... *in the*] milk from a woman in maternity, pound it (and) daub (his eyes with it).

155' ND iii 21' [............................ *ina* G]A ^{munus}Ú.ZÚG *mal-ma-liš* HE.HE ⸢SÚD⸣ MAR

156' [...] *mêšunu ana pursīti taṣahhat* **157'** [... *adi ablat tašakkan*] *enūma ītablu ina šuhti himēta tasâk teqqi*	[156'][...] you press out their sap into a *pursītu*-bowl. [157'][... you leave it until it has dried], when it has dried out you pound it in copper patina (and) ghee, (and) daub (his eyes).

156' ND iii 22' [... A.M]EŠ-*šú-nu ana* ^{dug}BUR.ZI [SU]R-⸢*at*⸣

157' ND iii 23' [... EN HÁD.DU GAR-*an* U]D-*ma* HÁD.DU *ina* SAHAR.URUDU Ì.NUN ⸢SÚD MAR⸣

Overview of IGI 2 Manuscripts and Parallels: **AA**=BAM 20; **AB**=BAM 159; **AD**=BAM 22; **AF**=BAM 23; **AG**=BAM 15; **bB**=BAM 382; **BoA**=KUB 4/50; **KA**=CTN 4/123; **NA**=BAM 510; **NB**=BAM 513; **NC**=BAM 514; **ND**=BAM 515; **NE**=BAM 516; **NI**=BAM 480; **NK**=BAM 518; **sA**=IRAQ 65; **uA**=SpTU 50; **uB**=NBC 4211; **xA**=CM 37

(ND) i 71' DIŠ KIMIN ZÍ BAL.[G]I⌜^{ku_6}⌝ *ina* MUN NÁ-*al* EN HÁD.DU GAR-*an* UD-*ma* HÁD.DU *ina* Ì SAHAR.URUDU SÚD ⌜MAR⌝

(NI) ii 2f. NUMUN [^{ú}E]ME.UR.GI$_7$ SIG$_7$-*su tu-hás-sà* A-*šú ana* ^{dug}BUR.ZI SUR-*at* EN HÁD.DU GAR-*an* / U[D-*m*]*a i-tab-lu ina* Ì SAHAR.URUDU SÚD MAR

158' [... *ana*] *libbi īnīšu tunattak lipâ ina šuhti tasâk teqqi*	158'[... into] his eyes you drip (it). You pound fat in copper patina (and) daub (his eyes).

158' ND iii 24' [...................... *ana* Š]À IGI.MIN-*šú tu-na-ták* Ì.UDU *ina* SAHAR.URUDU SÚD ⌜MAR⌝

159' [*šumma* ...] *īnāšu katmā kurṣipti eqli ina mešēlti tasâk libbi īnīšu* **160'** [...] ... *šadâna ṣābita šuruš gišimmari zikari* **161'** [...] *gabâ ahê tasâk teqqi*	159'[If ..., (and)] his eyes are closed: you pound a field-butterfly on *mešēltu*-whetstone. The inner part of his eyes 160'[...] magnetite, root of male date palm, 161'[...] you pound [...], (and) alum separately, (and) daub (his eyes).

159' ND iii 25' [DIŠ .... IGI.M]IN-*šú kát-ma kur-ṣip-ti* A.ŠÀ *ina* ^{na_4}BAR.DÙ.E SÚD ŠÀ IGI.MIN-*šú*

160' ND iii 26' [............................] x ^{na_4}KA.GI.NA.DAB.BA SUHUŠ ^{giš}GIŠIMMAR NÍTA

161' ND iii 27' [... IM.SAHAR.N]A$_4$.KUR.RA *a-he-e* SÚD MAR

162' [...] ... *inib errî tahaššal ina šamni tasâk teqqi*	162'[...:] you crush [...], (and) fruit of *errû*-colocynth, pound it in oil (and) daub (his eyes).

162' ND iii 28' [..................................] x GURUN ^{ú}ÚKUŠ.LAGAB GAZ *ina* Ì SÚD MAR

163' [... *ina dišip*] *šadê himēta šanîš*	163'[... in] mountain [honey] (and) ghee, ditto.

Overview of IGI 2 Manuscripts and Parallels: **AA**=BAM 20; **AB**=BAM 159; **AD**=BAM 22; **AF**=BAM 23; **AG**=BAM 15; **bB**=BAM 382; **BoA**=KUB 4/50; **KA**=CTN 4/123; **NA**=BAM 510; **NB**=BAM 513; **NC**=BAM 514; **ND**=BAM 515; **NE**=BAM 516; **NI**=BAM 480; **NK**=BAM 518; **sA**=IRAQ 65; **uA**=SpTU 50; **uB**=NBC 4211; **xA**=CM 37

163’ ND iii 29’ [.. *ina* LÀ]L.⸢KUR⸣.RA Ì.NUN MIN

164’ [...] *tasâk teqqi*	164’[...] you pound (and) daub (his eyes).

164’ ND iii 30’ [.. S]ÚD ⸢MAR⸣

GAP!

Break of approximately four lines!

165’ [...] *tasâk ina himēti* [*taballal* ...]	165’You pound [...], [mix] in ghee (and) [...]

165’ ND iii 34’ [..........................] ⸢SÚD *ina* Ì⸣.N[UN HE.HE ....]

166’ [...] *īnīšunu ina ṣillî tutakkap** **167’** [...] *ina itqūr abāri* [*tasâk teqqi*]	166’[...] you prick their eyes with a needle. 167’[... you pound ...] into a lead spoon-salve, [(and daub his eyes)]

166’ ND iii 35’ [... IGI.MEŠ]-*šú-nu ina* ^{giš}DÁLA *t*[*u-ták-kap*]

167’ ND iii 36’ [..] *ina* DÍLIM A.BÁR [SÚD MAR]

168’ [...] *billata tubbal tahaššal ina himēti* [*tasâk teqqi*]	168’[...] you dry out beer mash (and) crush (it) [...], (and) [pound] in ghee, [(and daub his eyes)]

168’ ND iii 37’ [..................................... *b*]*i-la-ta* HÁD.DU GAZ *ina* Ì.NU[N SÚD MAR]

169’ [...] *tasâk ana libbi īnīšu tunattak*	169’[...] you pound [...], you drip (it) into his eyes.

169’ ND iii 38’ [... SÚ]D$^{?}$ *ana* ŠÀ IGI.MIN-*šú t*[*u-na-ták*]

170’ [...] *teqqi*	170’[...], (and) you daub (his eyes).

170’ ND iii 39’ [.. M]AR

171’ [...] ... **172’** [...] ...	171’[...] ... 172’[...] ...

171’ ND iii 40’ [...] x-*ti-i* BAD

Overview of IGI 2 Manuscripts and Parallels: **AA**=BAM 20; **AB**=BAM 159; **AD**=BAM 22; **AF**=BAM 23; **AG**=BAM 15; **bB**=BAM 382; **BoA**=KUB 4/50; **KA**=CTN 4/123; **NA**=BAM 510; **NB**=BAM 513; **NC**=BAM 514; **ND**=BAM 515; **NE**=BAM 516; **NI**=BAM 480; **NK**=BAM 518; **sA**=IRAQ 65; **uA**=SpTU 50; **uB**=NBC 4211; **xA**=CM 37

172' ND iii 41' [..] x-*hap-pi*

173' [...] *tasâk teqqi*	173'[...] you pound (and) daub (his eyes).

173' ND iii 42' [..] SÚD MAR

174' [... *ina*] *ṣubāti*? *tessip* **175'** [... *ana libbi īnīšu*] *tunattak*	174'[...] you collect [... in a] cloth. 175'[...] you drip (it) [into his eyes].

174' ND iii 43' [.. *ina* TÚ]G? *te-sip*

175' ND iii 44' [.. *ana* ŠÀ IGI.MIN-*šú tu*]-*na-ták*

176' [...] ... *inassah*	176'[...] ... he uproots.

176' ND iii 45' [...] GIŠ *i-na-sah*

177' [...] *piqan ṣabīti* **178'** [...] *tasâk teqqi*	177'[...], (and) gazelle droppings, 178'[...] you pound [...], (and) daub (his eyes).

177' ND iii 46' [...] x A.GAR.GAR MAŠ.DÀ

178' ND iii 47' [...] ⌜*ta*⌝-*sàk* MAR

179' [...]	179'[...] ...

179' ND iii 48' [..] x

180' [...] *ina mê tasâk teqqi*	180'[...] you pound [...] in water, (and) daub (his eyes).

180' ND iii 49' [..] x *ina* A SÚD *te-qí*

181' [...] *ina šikari talâš īnīšu taṣammid*	181'[...] you knead [...] in beer, (and) bandage (his eyes).

181' ND iii 50' [.. *in*]*a* ⌜KAŠ⌝ *ta-là-aš* IGI.MIN-*šú* LAL

Overview of IGI 2 Manuscripts and Parallels: **AA**=BAM 20; **AB**=BAM 159; **AD**=BAM 22; **AF**=BAM 23; **AG**=BAM 15; **bB**=BAM 382; **BoA**=KUB 4/50; **KA**=CTN 4/123; **NA**=BAM 510; **NB**=BAM 513; **NC**=BAM 514; **ND**=BAM 515; **NE**=BAM 516; **NI**=BAM 480; **NK**=BAM 518; **sA**=IRAQ 65; **uA**=SpTU 50; **uB**=NBC 4211; **xA**=CM 37

182’ [...] *teqqi* **183’** [...] *tasâk teqqi*	182’[...], you daub (his eyes). 183’[...], you pound [...], (and) you daub (his eyes).

182’ ND iii 51’ [...] *te-qí*

183’ ND iii 52’ [...] x SÚD *te-qí*

184’ [...] *ina šamni tasâk teqqi*	184’[...] you pound [...] in oil, (and) you daub (his eyes).

184’ ND iii 53’ [.. *in*]*a* Ì SÚD *te-qí*

185’ [... *ina īnīšu*] *marušti tummad*	185’[...] you apply (it) on [his] sick [eye].

185’ ND iii 54’ [... *ina* IGI-*šú* G]IG *tu-mad*

186’ [...] *tasâk teqqi*	186’[...] you pound [...], (and) daub (his eyes).

186’ ND iii 55’ [... *t*]*a-sàk te-qí*

187’ [...] *tasâk teqqi* **188’** ... [...] *tarakkas* **Alternative prescription 1** **189’** *šīnāta* [...] *atāʾiša* **190’** *libbi īnīšu* [...] *teṭên*	187’[...] you pound [...], (and) daub (his eyes). 188’... [...] you bind on. **Alternative prescription 1** 189’[You ...] urine, [..] *atāʾišu*-plant, 190’the inner part of his eyes [...] you grind up [...]

187’ ND iii 56’ [.. S]ÚD MAR
188’ ND iii 57’ x x [...] KEŠDA

NB.

The following prescription 189f.’ starts as an alternative one, but it is unclear if it refers to l. 187f.’ or earlier.

189’ ND iii 58’ ⸢KÀŠ⸣ [..] ⸢ú⸣KUR.KUR

190’ ND iii 59’ ŠÀ IGI.MI[N-*šú* .... ÀR]A-⸢*en*⸣

Overview of IGI 2 Manuscripts and Parallels: **AA**=BAM 20; **AB**=BAM 159; **AD**=BAM 22; **AF**=BAM 23; **AG**=BAM 15; **bB**=BAM 382; **BoA**=KUB 4/50; **KA**=CTN 4/123; **NA**=BAM 510; **NB**=BAM 513; **NC**=BAM 514; **ND**=BAM 515; **NE**=BAM 516; **NI**=BAM 480; **NK**=BAM 518; **sA**=IRAQ 65; **uA**=SpTU 50; **uB**=NBC 4211; **xA**=CM 37

191' *šumma īnāšu* [...] *sahlê* **192'** *šammi ašî* [... *ina*] *šizbi taballal teqqi*	[191']If his eyes are [... [192']you ...] [191']*sahlû*-plant, [192']*ašû*-disease-plant, [...] you mix (the ingredients) [in] milk, (and) daub (his eyes).

191' ND iii 60' DIŠ IGI.MIN-*š*[*ú* ....] ZÀ.HI.LI

192' ND iii 61' Ú *a-ši-i* [... *ina* G]A HE.HE MAR

193' *ana nuhhi* [...] *ina šamni taballal teqqi* **Alternative prescription 1** **194'** *lipâ haṣab ṭābti ana libbi īnīšu* [...] *ina šaman erēni taballal teqqi* **Alternative prescription 2** **195'** *emesalli aktam tasâk ina dišpi* [...] *ina dišpi peṣî patar siparri šanîš*	[193']In order to soothe [...], you mix [...] in oil (and) daub (his eyes). **Alternative prescription 1** [194'][You apply] fat and flake of salt into [his] eyes, (and) you mix [...] in cedar oil, (and) daub (his eyes). **Alternative prescription 2** [195']You pound *emesallu*-saline solution (and) *aktam*-plant in honey, [you ...] in honey. [...] in white honey with a bronze knife, ditto (i.e. you mix and daub his eyes).

193' ND iii 62' *a-na nu-úh-hi* x [..] x *ina* Ì HE.HE MAR

194' ND iii 63' Ì.UDU ŠIKA MUN *ana* ŠÀ IGI.MI[N-*šú* ...] *ina* Ì.GIŠ ^{giš}EREN HE.HE MAR

195' ND iii 64' ^{mun}*me*$_5$-SILIM ^{ú}*ak-tam* SÚD *ina* LÀ[L ...] ⸢*ina*⸣ LÀL BABBAR GÍR.ZABAR MIN

196' *šumma amēlu īnāšu madirā* [...] *šamma peṣâ zēr* GI.ZÚ.LUM.MA **Alternative prescription 1** **197'** *rikibti arkabi* [...]	[196']If a man's eyes are rotten: [...] white plant, seeds of 'date reed' **Alternative prescription 1** [197'][...] bat guano, [...]

Overview of IGI 2 Manuscripts and Parallels: **AA**=BAM 20; **AB**=BAM 159; **AD**=BAM 22; **AF**=BAM 23; **AG**=BAM 15; **bB**=BAM 382; **BoA**=KUB 4/50; **KA**=CTN 4/123; **NA**=BAM 510; **NB**=BAM 513; **NC**=BAM 514; **ND**=BAM 515; **NE**=BAM 516; **NI**=BAM 480; **NK**=BAM 518; **sA**=IRAQ 65; **uA**=SpTU 50; **uB**=NBC 4211; **xA**=CM 37

Alternative prescription 2	Alternative prescription 2
198' *abāra ina himēti taqallu* [...]	[198']You refine lead in ghee [...]

196' ND iii 65' DIŠ NA IGI.MIN-*šú ma-di-ra* x [...] x-*ra* Ú.BABBAR NUMUN GI.ZÚ.LUM.MA

197' ND iv 1 U$_5$.ARGAB^{muš}[^{en} ....]

198' ND iv 2 A.GAR$_5$ *ina* Ì.NUN BÍL x [..]

199' *šumma amēlu īnāšu ṣilluma šamhā* [...]	[199']If a man's eyes have grown bulky with a film ... [...]

199' ND iv 3 DIŠ NA IGI.MIN-*šú* GISSU-*ma* ⸢*šam-ha*⸣ [..]

200' *šumma amēlu īn imittīšu ṣillu*[*ma šamhat* ...] **201'** *ina naglabi* [*šēli* ...]	[200']If a man's right eye has [grown bulky] with a film [...] [201']with a [sharp] scalpel [...]

200' ND iv 4 DIŠ NA IGI ZAG-*šú* ⸢GISSU⸣-[*ma* ....]

201' ND iv 5 *ina* GÍR.ŠU.I *š*[*e-e-li*? ....]

202' *šumma amēlu īn šumēlīšu ṣillu*[*ma šamhat* ...] **203'** *ina naglabi* [...]	[202']If a man's left eye has [grown bulky] with a film [...] [203']with a scalpel [...]

202' ND iv 6 DIŠ NA IGI GÙB-*šú* GISS[U-*ma* ....]
203' ND iv 7 *ina* GÍR.ŠU.I [..]

204' *šumma amēlu īnāšu marṣā namrā* [...]	[204']If a man's eyes are sick and shiny [you ...]
Alternative prescription 1	**Alternative prescription 1**
205' *muhha ša erî ina šizbi musukkati* [*tasâk* ...]	[205'][You pound] the brains of an *erû*-eagle in the milk from a woman in maternity [...]

Overview of IGI 2 Manuscripts and Parallels: **AA**=BAM 20; **AB**=BAM 159; **AD**=BAM 22; **AF**=BAM 23; **AG**=BAM 15; **bB**=BAM 382; **BoA**=KUB 4/50; **KA**=CTN 4/123; **NA**=BAM 510; **NB**=BAM 513; **NC**=BAM 514; **ND**=BAM 515; **NE**=BAM 516; **NI**=BAM 480; **NK**=BAM 518; **sA**=IRAQ 65; **uA**=SpTU 50; **uB**=NBC 4211; **xA**=CM 37

Alternative prescription 2 **206'** *zēr* GI.ZÚ.LUM.MA *sīkti* [*labti taballal* ...]	**Alternative prescription 2** $^{206'}$[You mix] seeds of 'date reed' (and) powder [of roasted grain ...]

204'	ND iv 8	DIŠ NA IGI.MIN-*šú* GIG.GA ⸢ZALAG.GA⸣ x [.......................................]
205'	ND iv 9	UGU *ša* TI$_8$^{mušen} *ina* GA ⸢^{munus}Ú$^{?}$⸣.[ZÚG$^{?}$ SÚD$^{?}$.......................................]
206'	ND iv 10	NUMUN GI.ZÚ.LUM.MA *si-ik-t*[*i* ŠE.SA.A HE.HE ....]

207' *šumma amēlu lamassāt īnīšu ṣilla* [*malâ* ...] **208'** *īnīšu teqqi ana ašri šanîmma hīl abukkati* [...]	$^{207'}$If the man's pupils [are full] of a film, [you ...] $^{208'}$you daub his eyes. Alternatively: resin of *abukkatu*-plant [...]

207'	ND iv 11	DIŠ NA ^{d}LAMA.MEŠ IGI.MIN-*šú* GI[SSU DIRI$^{?}$ ....]
	(AG) r.5f.'	[DIŠ N]A$^{?}$ ⸢^{d}LAMA.MEŠ IGI⸣.M[IN-*šú* ...] / [... NA]GA.SI MÚD ER[EN$^{?}$...]
208'	ND iv 12	[I]GI.MIN-*šú* MAR DIŠ KIMIN ILLU L[I.TAR/DUR ....]
	(AG) r.7'	[DI]Š ⸢KIMIN⸣ ILLU LI.DUR [..]

209' *šumma īn amēli ṣillu* [*ṣirihta mali* ...] **210'** [...] ... [...]	$^{209'}$If a man's eye [is full of] a film (and) [has inflammation ...] $^{210'}$[...] ... [...]

209'	ND iv 13	[DIŠ IG]I ⸢LÚ⸣ GISSU ⸢*ṣi*⸣-[*ri-ih-ta*$_5$ DIRI ....]
210'	ND iv 14	[........] x x [...]

GAP!

Ca. 25 lines are missing!

211' [...] **212'** [...] ... *ana ašri šanîmma* [...]	$^{211'}$[...] ... [...] $^{212'}$[...] ... Alternatively: [...]

211'	ND iv 41'	[.....................]-⸢*ri-i*⸣ [...]
212'	ND iv 42'	[................] x DIŠ K[IMIN$^{?}$ ....]

Overview of IGI 2 Manuscripts and Parallels: **AA**=BAM 20; **AB**=BAM 159; **AD**=BAM 22; **AF**=BAM 23; **AG**=BAM 15; **bB**=BAM 382; **BoA**=KUB 4/50; **KA**=CTN 4/123; **NA**=BAM 510; **NB**=BAM 513; **NC**=BAM 514; **ND**=BAM 515; **NE**=BAM 516; **NI**=BAM 480; **NK**=BAM 518; **sA**=IRAQ 65; **uA**=SpTU 50; **uB**=NBC 4211; **xA**=CM 37

213' [*šumma amēlu īnāšu*] ... *malâ* ... [...] **214'** [...] *dām kurṣipti alpi ṣalmi u* [...]	[213']If a man's eyes] are full of ... [...] [214'][You ...] ..., blood of a black ox-fly and [...]

213' ND iv 43' [DIŠ NA IGI.MIN-*šú*] x ⸢x⸣ DIRI x [...]

214' ND iv 44' [........................] x MÚD *kur-ṣib-ti* GU$_4$ GE$_6$ *u* x [..................................]

Catchline of Tablet Three **215'** *šumma amēlu īnāšu dalhā dišpa peṣâ ina himēti* [*ištēniš taballal* ...]	**Catchline of Tablet Three** [215']If a man's eyes are troubled: [you mix together] white honey in ghee (and) [...]

215' ND iv 45' [DIŠ NA] IGI.MIN-*šú* LÙ.LÙ LÀL BABBAR *ina* Ì.[NUN 1-*niš* HE.HE ......]

(NE) i 1 DIŠ NA IGI.MEŠ-*šú* LÙ.LÙ ⸢LÀL⸣ BABBAR *ina* ⸢Ì⸣ [...............................]

(NA) iv 31 [KA.INI]M.MA DIŠ N[A ....] L[Ù.LÙ]

(NC) iv 36 [.............] ⸢DIŠ NA IGI.MIN-*šú* LÙ.LÙ⸣

(xA) r.9 [DI]Š NA IGI.MIN-*šú* LÙ.LÙ-⸢*ha*⸣ LÀL Ì.NUN.NA Ì.⸢SAG⸣ 1-*niš* HE.HE *ina* GE$_6$ IGI.MIN-*šú* DIR[I]

(uA) r.8f. DIŠ NA IGI.MEŠ-šú LÙ.LÙ-*ha* LÀL Ì.NUN.NA Ì.SAG [gloss: *hal-ṣa*] 1-*niš* x [ERASURE?] KÚM.KÚM-*am ta-šá-hal ana* IGI.MIN-*šú* ŠUB

Name of Tablet Two **216'** *šanû tuppu šumma amēlu* [*īnāšu marṣā*]	**Name of Tablet Two** [216'] Second [tablet] of the (treatise) 'If a man's [eyes are sick'.]

216' ND iv 46' [DUB].⸢2⸣.KÁM DIŠ NA [IGI.MIN-*šú* GIG]

Ashurbanipal's Colophon, BAK no. 329

217' [*ēkal Aššur-bāni-apli šar kiššati šar māt Aššur ša Nabû u Tašmētu uznu rapaštu išrukūšu* **218'** *ēhuzzu īnu namirtu nisiq tupšarrūti*	[217'][Palace of Ashurbanipal king of the world, king of the Land Assyria, to whom Nabû and Tašmētu granted understanding,] [218'][(who) acquired] clear insight [(and) a high level of scribal proficiency,] [219']that skill which among the kings, my predecessor(s)

Overview of IGI 2 Manuscripts and Parallels: **AA**=BAM 20; **AB**=BAM 159; **AD**=BAM 22; **AF**=BAM 23; **AG**=BAM 15; **bB**=BAM 382; **BoA**=KUB 4/50; **KA**=CTN 4/123; **NA**=BAM 510; **NB**=BAM 513; **NC**=BAM 514; **ND**=BAM 515; **NE**=BAM 516; **NI**=BAM 480; **NK**=BAM 518; **sA**=IRAQ 65; **uA**=SpTU 50; **uB**=NBC 4211; **xA**=CM 37

219' *ša ina šarrāni ālik mahrīya mamma šipru* [*šuātu lā ēhuzzu*] **220'** *bulṭī ištu muhhi adi ṣupri liqtī ahûti tāhīzu nakla* **221'** *azugallūt Ninurta u Gula mala bašmu ina tuppāni ašṭur asniq abrēma* **222'** *ana tāmarti šitassīya qereb ēkallīya ukīn*	no one [acquired]. [221'][I wrote,] checked, and collated tablets with [220']medical prescriptions from cranium to the (toe-) nail, non-canonical material, elaborate teaching(s), (and) [221']the advanced healing art(s) of Ninurta and Gula, as much as created, (and) [222']I placed (them) within of my palace for consultation (and) my reading.

217' ND iv 47' [É.GAL ^{m}*Aš-šur*-DÙ.A LUGAL ŠÚ 20 KUR AN.ŠÁR^{ki} *ša* ^{d}AG *u* ^{d}*taš-me-tu*$_{4}$ GEŠTU.MIN *ra-pa-áš-tu*$_{4}$ *iš-ru-ku-šú*]

218' ND iv 48' [*e-hu-uz-z*]*u* [IGI.MIN *n*]*a-*⸢*mir*⸣*-t*[*u*$_{4}$ *ni-siq tup-šar-ru-ti*]

219' ND iv 49' *ša ina* LUGAL.MEŠ-*ni a-lik mah-*⸢*ri*⸣*-ia* ⸢*mám-ma šip-ru*⸣ [*šu-a-tú* NU *e-hu-uz-zu*]

220' ND iv 50' ⸢*bul*⸣*-ṭi* TA *muh-hi* EN UMBIN ⸢*liq-ti* BAR.MEŠ *ta*⸣*-h*[*i-zu nak-l*]*a*

221' ND iv 51' *a-zu-gal-lu-ut* ^{d}*Nin-urta u* ^{d}*Gu-la ma-la ba-áš-mu* ⸢*ina*⸣ *ṭ*[*up-pa-a-ni áš-ṭùr as-n*]*iq* IGI.KÁR-*ma*

222' ND iv 51' ⸢*a*⸣*-na ta-mar-ti* ^{ERASURE} *ši-ta-si-ia qé-reb* É.GAL-⸢*ia ú*⸣*-kin*

Overview of IGI 2 Manuscripts and Parallels: **AA**=BAM 20; **AB**=BAM 159; **AD**=BAM 22; **AF**=BAM 23; **AG**=BAM 15; **bB**=BAM 382; **BoA**=KUB 4/50; **KA**=CTN 4/123; **NA**=BAM 510; **NB**=BAM 513; **NC**=BAM 514; **ND**=BAM 515; **NE**=BAM 516; **NI**=BAM 480; **NK**=BAM 518; **sA**=IRAQ 65; **uA**=SpTU 50; **uB**=NBC 4211; **xA**=CM 37

§ III The Nineveh Manuscripts of Chapter Three (IGI 3)

TITLE	IF A MAN'S EYES ARE TROUBLED *šumma*(DIŠ) *amēlu*(NA) *īnāšu*(IGI.MEŠ-*šú*) *dalhā*(LÙ.LÙ) = Assur Medical Catalogue l. 9.

Sigla notations:
N = Nineveh, Neo-Assyrian. A, B, C, ... designate the different manuscripts.
Translation in italics are tentative reconstructions based on parallels.

Base Manuscript:	**NE (BAM 516)**, collated.
Museum number:	British Museum, K 2533 + 2545 + 2575 + 3320 + 5906 + 8110 + 13439 + 13719 + 14786 + 16424 + Sm 970A (+) K 4120 [top left col. i].
Origin and date:	Nineveh, 7th century BC.
Type of tablet:	Two-column, portrait-oriented tablet. The two vertical dividing rulings of the tablet were done with an instrument, presumably with the stylus. There are round holes visible at empty spaces.
Measurements:	ca. 25 × 16,4 × 2,6 cm (lower edge).
Copy:	BAM 516.
Photo/CDLI nr.:	Plates 27–31/P432416.
Literature:	Köcher 1980b: xii-xiii, BAM 516; Fincke 2000: 331; Scurlock and Andersen 2005: 793; Scurlock 2006: nos. 121–125, 128; Fincke 2009; Geller 2010a: 193; Scurlock 2014: 756; Attia 2015.

§ III.1 Related Manuscripts containing IGI 1 and 2 from Nineveh

The texts included represent parallels and partial parallels from the other tablets of the IGI treatise.

Manuscript: **NA** (BAM 510), see **§ I.1**, parallels: 1.

Manuscript: **NC** (BAM 514), see **§ I.1**, parallels: 1.

Manuscript: **ND** (BAM 515), see **§ II.1**, parallels: 1.

§ III.2 Related other Manuscripts from Nineveh

The texts included represent parallels and partial parallels which are considered important for the compilation of the IGI-treatise. They come from other tablets and fragments from Nineveh containing prescriptions for sick eyes or from the UGU-treatise.

https://doi.org/10.1515/9781501506550-007

Manuscript: **NI** (BAM 480), see **§ V.1**, parallels: 54'.

Manuscript: **NF** (BAM 520), see **§ IV.1**, parallels: 2ff.

Manuscript: **NS** (AMT 18/4), see **§ IV.6**, parallels: 49f.'.

§ III.3 Related Manuscripts from Different Cities

The texts included here represent parallels and partial parallels which are considered important for the compilation of the IGI-treatise. These are manuscripts coming from other periods and from cities other than Nineveh.

Sigla notations:

A = Assur, Late Assyrian. A, B, C, ... designate the different manuscripts.
Am = Assur, Middle Assyrian. A, B, C, ... designate the different manuscripts.
Bo = Boğazköy, Hattuša, Hittite period. A, B, C, ... designate the different manuscripts.
x = unknown provenance, Late Babylonian. A, B, C, ... designate the different manuscripts.
Initial capital letters designate tablets in Assyrian script or northern scripts, and small letters tablets in Babylonian script.
Parenthesis [()] on a siglum designate a parallel text and not a duplicate.

Hattuša

Manuscript: **BoB (KUB 37/2)**, photo collated, parallels: 81f.', 89'.
Origin and date: Boğazköy, Hattuša. Hittite period.
Type of tablet: Too fragmentary to judge.
Copy: KUB 37/2.
Photo: Mainzer Photoarchiv, http://www.hethport.uni-wuerzburg.de/HPM/index.html, CTH 890.
Literature: Stol 1986: 297; Schwemer 1998: 17 fn. 56 (Paläeographie); Fincke 2000: 333; Arnott 2002: 43; Schwemer 2005/6: 224 fn. 43; Schwemer 2013: 156. Abusch et al. 2016: 10.

Manuscript: **BoC (KUB 4/55)**, ph. collated, parallels: 81f.', 89'.
Museum number: Istanbul, Bo 5726.
Origin and date: Boğazköy, Hattuša. Hittite period.
Type of tablet: Too fragmentary to judge.
Copy: KUB 4/55.
Photo: Mainzer Photoarchiv, http://www.hethport.uni-wuerzburg.de/HPM/index.html, CTH 890.

Literature: Schwemer 2013: 156; Abusch et al. 2016: 10.

Assyrian

Manuscript: **AmB (BAM 25)**, collated, parallels: 75ff.', 81f.'
Museum number: Vorderasiatisches Museum, Berlin, VAT 16464.
Origin and date: Assur, Middle Assyrian.
Type of tablet: Fragment of a presumably multi-column tablet. BAM 25 seems to be an indirect join to BAM 13 and 17. The paleography of all fragments suggest Middle- or Early Neo-Assyrian dating rather than Late Assyrian.
Measurements: 3,6 × 3 × 1,2 cm.
Copy: BAM 25.
CDLI nr.: P285127.
Literatur: Köcher 1963a: xvi, BAM 25; Stol 1986: 297; Scurlock and Andersen 2005: 784; Attia 2015: 76f.

Manuscript: **AH (BAM 209)**, collated, parallels: 9ff.
Museum number: Vorderasiatisches Museum, Berlin, VAT 13756 + 13771 (+) 14162
Origin and date: Assur, Late Assyrian.
Type of tablet: One-column, portrait oriented tablet.
Measurements: ca. 16 × 8,5 × 2,3 (towards the middle) cm.
Copy: BAM 209.
CDLI nr.: P285298.
Literature: Köcher 1964: xii, BAM 209; Fincke 2000: 329; Scurlock and Andersen 2005: 188, 788; Scurlock 2006: 95 fn. 171, no. 126, Attia 2015: 72, 80.

Babylonian

Manuscript: **uA (SpTU 50)**, see **§ I.4**, parallels: 1,

Manuscript: **xA (CM 37)**, see **§ I.4**, parallels: 1.

Manuscript: **xB (BM 40737)**, collated, parallels: 37ff.'.
Museum number: British Museum, BM 40737.
Origin and date: According to Fincke 2009: 84, 93, the tablet's provenance is unknown. But, according to the British Museum Collection online, the tablet comes from Jimjima (Babylon). Late Babylonian.
Type of tablet: Too fragmentary to judge.

Measurements:	6,4 × 3,7 × 0,23 cm.
Copy:	Fincke 2009: 94.
Photo:	Fincke 2009: 104.
Literature:	Fincke 2009.

§ III.4 Synopsis of the Prescriptions of Chapter Three (IGI 3)

1	Prescription for troubled eyes: preparation of medication with honey in oil.
2ff.	Prescription against flash of light and ghost afflictions: magnetite, minerals, stones, copper, and plants crushed and spattered into the eyes; salve from kidney of black ox in fat, daubing: prognosis for recovery.
7f.	Prescription, presumably for the same case as the previous: seeds of plants and trees used for fumigation of the eyes and temples.
9ff.	Prescription against ghost affliction and light phenomena, behavior like a goat: plants, resin ...
14ff.	Too broken.
24ff.'	Broken incantations: the second one concerns cloudy and blurred eyes.
27ff.'	Medical application with plants and activities on the roof during the night; collecting drugs in the morning; application onto the eyes; rinsing the eyes with the sap of a *kasû*-plant.
32f.'	Eye salve against ghost affliction: stones, minerals and plants in water; maceration overnight; mixed in sesame oil and smeared onto the eyes; also, dissolved in beer and consumed; additionally, the drugs were put in a leather bag around the neck of the patient: prognosis for recovery.
36'	The previous prescription has to be applied on the 21st day.
37'	Prescription for the same case: smearing the eyes with minerals.
38'	Prescription for the same case: pounded black frit in ghee smearing the eyes; pounded lapis lazuli in ghee smearing the eyes.
39'	Prescription for the same case: pounded sardonyx in ghee and smearing the eyes; pounded *šimbizidû*-galena in the milk from a woman in maternity, smearing the eyes.
40'	Prescription for the same case: pounded obsidian in ghoose fat and smearing the eyes: prognosis for recovery.
41ff.'	Prescription against ghost affliction: plants, magnetite, stones, old partridge fat, wax; these 11 drugs are mixture against 'Hand of the Ghost' applied by daubing onto the eyes: prognosis for recovery.
44f.'	Too fragmentary.
46ff.'	No diagnosis (but presumably same as the previous): mixture of marrow from a sheep's bone, black cumin, pomegranate; ingredients pounded in honey, ghee and cedar oil, probably with daubing.

49f.' Prescription for a man who cannot see and has heat stroke: bat guano, white plant, saline solution in mountain honey and ghee, daubing the eyes.

51ff.' Prescriptions for diminished eyesight: pounded black snake fat, plants, resins, saline solution, black cumin in copper patina and mountain honey; daubing; washing the eyes with a *plant sap*; daubing and application with a lead spoon (or salve).

55f.' Fragmentary prescription: bandaging with plants.

57ff.' Fragmentary prescription: bandaging and daubing: prognosis for recovery.

62ff.' Fragmentary prescription: Hands of Šulpaea and Ištar, presumably fumigation over charcoal, daubing: prognosis for recovery.

66f.' Fragmentary prescription, vision problems caused by Hand of Ištar, pounded ingredient(s) in honey and ghee, daubing: prognosis for recovery.

68f.' Prescription for eye 'perforation' (*šīlu*), sleepless state and abnormal condition: mixture of fat from black snake in ghee and mountain honey, daubing.

70ff.' Prescriptions for lengthened eye 'perforation' (*šīlu*), the patient cannot get out of bed: heated up leaves of different trees in water and in a tannour-oven; crushing and sifting gazelle droppings, ox dung, flour of roasted grain, and knead (everything) in the sap of a *kasû*-plant; bandaging. In addition, drinking of *aktam*-plant in beer: prognosis for recovery.

73 Definition of *Sîn-lurmâ* as day blindness.

74 Definition of *Sîn-lurmâ* as night blindness.

75ff.' Prescription for day/night blindness: parts of donkey liver and neck tendons twisted into a string and placed on the neck of the person. Ritual/medical application in the morning with holy water vessel and cloth, fumigation with juniper in an incense burner. Colloborative ritual/medical application action by the physician (*asû*), the exorcist (*mašmašu*) and the patient. The *mašmašu* and the patient utter short spells.

81ff.' Prescription for day/night blindness: incisions in the 'pole' of a liver: The physician (*asû*) gathers apprentice exorcists (*mašmašu*) giving them instruction; mixture of ghee and first class sesame oil, daubing.

84' There was presumably a medical application with the above prescription.

85f.' Incantation addressing Ea.

87f.' Medical application accompanying the previous incantation involving eating of the lobe of the lung.

89ff.' Prescription presumably for day/night blindness: incision of the 'pole' of a liver, involvement of the lips: prognosis for recovery. Rest too fragmentary.

93ff.' Instruction for making a salve with a lead spoon: pounded plants, different sulphurs, bitumen, ox kidney fat (mixed) into lead, daubing with finger. The prescription is labelled as a tested and a checked healing ointment from the *ummânu*.

The following lines contain no prescriptions but enumerations of drugs and memos for remedies.

97f.' Enumeration of nine plant drugs and wax as a mixture for the eyes.

99ff.' Enumeration of nine plant-based drugs and instruction for making a softening ointment: boiling of drugs over charcoal, pounding and mixing them in oil and white wax.

102f.' Enumeration of seven plant-based drugs and instruction for making a mixture for the eyes: roasting the drugs, pounding them in fat, wax and ghee, daubing.

104f.' Enumeration of minerals, stones, plants, sulphur, ox fat, lead, 'lead spoon' (salve), designated as belonging to the physician (*asû*).

106ff.' Further fragmentary enumeration of drugs.

Edition of IGI 3

1 *šumma amēlu īnāšu dalhā dišpa peṣâ ina himēti [ištēniš taballal ...]*	[1]If a man's eyes are troubled: [you mix together] white honey in ghee (and) [...]

1 NE i 1 DIŠ NA IGI.MEŠ-*šú* LÙ.LÙ ⌜LÀL⌝ BABBAR *ina* ⌜Ì⌝ [...............................]

(ND) iv 45' [DIŠ NA] IGI.MIN-*šú* LÙ.LÙ LÀL BABBAR *ina* Ì.[NUN 1-*niš* HE.HE ......]
(NA) iv 31 [KA.INI]M.MA DIŠ N[A ....] L[Ù.LÙ]

(NC) iv 36 [.............] ⌜DIŠ NA IGI.MIN-*šú* LÙ.LÙ⌝

(xA) r.9 [DI]Š NA IGI.MIN-*šú* LÙ.LÙ-⌜*ha*⌝ LÀL Ì.NUN.NA Ì.⌜SAG⌝ 1-*niš* HE.HE *ina* GE$_6$ IGI.MIN-*šú* DIR[I]

(uA) r.8f. DIŠ NA IGI.MEŠ-šú LÙ.LÙ-*ha* LÀL Ì.NUN.NA Ì.SAG [gloss: *hal-ṣa*] 1-*niš* x [ERASURE?] KÚM.KÚM-*am ta-šá-hal ana* IGI.MIN-*šú* ŠUB

2 *enūma īnāšu burṣa iddanaggalā šugidimmakku* [...]	[2]When his eyes repeatedly see a flash of light: (it is) a 'Hand of the Ghost' [...] [3]In order to heal this condition (lit. it): magnetite, tin, [black] frit [...] [4]*mūṣu*-stone, *zalāqu*-stone, lapis lazuli, *šubû*-stone, *tašrītu*-stone, male copper (bead), [...]-stone [...] [5][seed] of tamarisk, seed of *ēru*-tree, seed of male rush, *ashar*-stone [... you crush these drugs together], [6]sprinkle, and pound (them) in kidney fat of a black ox – like (you pound) *kammu*-tanning-fungus over copper – and [you regularly daub his eyes, and he will get better.]
3 *ana bulluṭīšu šadânu ṣābitu annakku kutpû* [...]	
4 *mūṣu zalāqu uqnû šubû aban tašrīti erû zikaru* [...]	
5 [*zēr*] *bīni zēr ēri zēr ašli zikari ashar* [... *šammī annûti ištēniš tahaššal*]	
6 *tašappah ina lipî kalīt alpi ṣalmi kīma kamma ina muhhi erî tasâkma* [*īnīšu kayyamānamma teqqīma ina'eš*]	
Alternative prescription 1	**Alternative prescription 1**
7 [*ana ašri šanîmma*] *zēr bīni zēr ēri zēr ašli* [*zēr* ...]	[7][Alternatively: (when his eyes repeatedly see a flash of light)]: seed of tamarisk, seed of *ēru*-tree, seed of *ašlu*-rush [*seed of ..., and*] [8][*seed*] of
8 [*zēr*] *burāšī kīma qutāri īnīšu u pūti* [...]	

Overview of IGI 3 Manuscripts and Parallels: **AH**=BAM **209**; **AmB**=BAM 25; **BoB**=KUB 37/2; **BoC**=KUB 4/55; **NA**=BAM 510; **NC**=BAM 514; **ND**=BAM 515; **NE**=BAM 516; **NF**= BAM 520; **NI**=BAM 480; **NS**=AMT 18/4; **uA**=SpTU 50; **xA**=CM 37; **xB**=BM **40737**

https://doi.org/10.1515/9781501506550-008

	juniper like fumigation for the eyes and forehead [...]

2 NE i 2 ⸢*e*⸣-*nu-ma* IGI.MIN-*šú bu-ur-ṣa id-da-nag-ga-la* ŠU.GI[DIM.MA ....]
(NF) i' 8' [..] x ⸢KU$^?$⸣ [.................. T]I$^?$[............] x

3 NE i 3 ⸢*ana* TI⸣-*šú* ^{na4}KA.GI.NA.DAB.BA ^{na4}AN.NA ^{na4}AN.Z[AH.GE$_6$ ....]
(NF) i' 9' [........................^{na4}AN.ZA]H$^?$.GE$_6$ →

4 NE i 4 ⸢^{na4}*mu-ṣa*⸣ ^{na4}ZÁLAG ^{na4}ZA.GÌN ^{na4}ŠUBA NA$_4$ BAL URUDU.NITA N[A$_4$ ...]
(NF) i' 9' ^{na4}*mu-ṣa* ⸢^{na4}ZÁLAG⸣ ^{na4}GUG ^{n}[^{a4} x (x)]

5 NE i 5 [NUMUN ^{giš}Š]INIG NUMUN ^{giš}MA.NU NUMUN *áš-li* NITA ^{na4}*ás-ha*[*r* ....]
(NF) i' 10f.'[... ^{na4}A]N$^?$.NA ^{na4}MUŠ.GÍR ⸢NUMUN⸣ ^{giš}*bi-ni* NUMUN ^{giš}⸢MA.NU⸣ /
[......... Ú.M]EŠ ŠEŠ 1-*niš* GAZ →

6 NE i 6 [*ta-š*]*a-pah ina* Ì.UDU ÉLLAG GU$_4$ GE$_6$ GIN$_7$ *kám-ma ina* UGU URUDU SÚD-*m*[*a* ...]

(NF) i' 11' *ta-ša-pah ina* Ì.UDU ÉLLAG GU$_4$ GE$_6$
(NF) i' 12' [........................ IG]I.MEŠ-*šú ka-a-a-man-nam-ma* MAR-*ma ina-eš*

7 NE i 7 [DIŠ KIMIN] NUMUN ^{giš}ŠINIG NUMUN ^{giš}MA.NU NUMUN *áš*-⸢*li*⸣ [NUMUN ...]

8 NE i 8 [NUMUN ^{šim}L]I GIN$_7$ *qu-ta-ri* IGI.MIN-*šú u* SAG.KI [.............................]

9 [*šumma amēla*] *šugidimmakku iṣbassuma ina pāni īnīšu kīma nūri* [*lū kīma berqi rūqi* (...)]	[9][If 'Hand of] the Ghost' afflicts a man and (the ghost) [10]shows itself [9]in front of a man's eyes like a lamp-light [or like distant lightning] [10][or like a (...)]
10 [*lū kīma* (...)] ... *lū kīma enzi ištanakkan amēlu šū* [*šugidimmakku iṣbassu* ...]	..., or like a goat; this man [has been seized by a 'Hand of the Ghost' ...] [11][In order to uproot it (the 'Hand of the Ghost') ...] [12]you pound together [11][...]
11 [*ana nasāhīšu* ...] *burāšu kukru* [...] 12 [...] *ištēniš tasâk* [...]	juniper, *kukru*-aromatic, [...]

9 NE i 9 [DIŠ NA ŠU.G]IDIM.MA DAB-*su-ma i-na* IGI IGI.MIN-*šú* GIN$_7$ *nu-ri* x [.......................]

Overview of IGI 3 Manuscripts and Parallels: **AH**=BAM **209**; **AmB**=BAM 25; **BoB**=KUB 37/2; **BoC**=KUB 4/55; **NA**=BAM 510; **NC**=BAM 514; **ND**=BAM 515; **NE**=BAM 516; **NF**= BAM 520; **NI**=BAM 480; **NS**=AMT 18/4; **uA**=SpTU 50; **xA**=CM 37; **xB**=BM **40737**

(AH) r.19f.’⸢DIŠ NA⸣ ŠU.GIDIM$_4$.MA DAB-⸢*su-ma ina* IGI.MIN.MEŠ-*šú* GIN$_7$⸣ [*nu-ri* (...)] / ⸢*lu*⸣-*u* GIN$_7$ NIM.GÍR ⸢SÙ⸣.[UD$^?$.DA$^?$] →

10 NE i 10 [*lu-u* GIN$_7$ (...)] x ⸢x *lu*⸣-*u* GIN$_7$ UD$_5$ GAR.GAR-*an* NA BI Š[U$^?$.GIDIM.MA DAB-*su* ....]

(AH) r.20f.’[*l*]*u-u* GIN$_7$ x [...] / ⸢*lu-u* GIN$_7$ UD$_5$ GAR-*an*$^?$ NA BI ŠU⸣.GI[DIM.MA DAB-*su* (...)]

(AH) r.22’ *i-kal* x [...] x ⸢IGI.MIN.MEŠ-*šú*⸣ [............................]

11 NE i 11 [............. ^{ši}]^{m}⸢LI⸣ ^{šim}GÚR.GÚR x [..]

(AH) r.23’ *ana* ZI-*šú* ⸢^{šim}⸣L[I..]

12 NE i 12 [...] 1-*niš* SÚD x [....................................]

(AH) r.24’ Ì$^?$(text DÙ$^!$).A.⸢BÁR⸣ SUR-⸢*at*⸣ [..]

(AH) r.25’ ⸢*te-qí*⸣-*tu šá* ŠU.GI[DIM.MA ....]

(AH) r.26’ *ana* IGI ^{d}⸢*Gu*⸣-*la* [..]

13 [...] *hīl abukkati* [...]	13[...] resin of *abukkatu*-plant [...]

13 NE i 13 [..................................] ⸢ILLU⸣ LI.[DUR ....]

14 [...] ... [...] **15** [...] ... [...]	14[...]-*sulphur* [...] 15[...] ... [...]

14 NE i 14 [... -^{d}]ÍD [...]

15 NE i 15 [..] x [...]

GAP!

A gap of unknown length, but there are more then 15 lines to be expected. According to Köcher in BAM VI, no. 516, Taf. 36 there are ca. 19 lines missing.

16’ [...] *teqqi*	16’[...] you daub (his eyes).

16’ NE i 35’ [.. M]AR$^?$

17’ [...] *teqqi*	17’[...] you daub (his eyes).

Overview of IGI 3 Manuscripts and Parallels: **AH**=BAM **209**; **AmB**=BAM 25; **BoB**=KUB 37/2; **BoC**=KUB 4/55; **NA**=BAM 510; **NC**=BAM 514; **ND**=BAM 515; **NE**=BAM 516; **NF**= BAM 520; **NI**=BAM 480; **NS**=AMT 18/4; **uA**=SpTU 50; **xA**=CM 37; **xB**=BM **40737**

17’ NE i 36’ [.. M]AR

18’ [...] *sāma/malâ* **19’** [...] *teqqi*	18’[...] reddish/full of 19’[...] you daub (his eyes).

18’ NE i 37’ [.. S]A$_5$/D]IRI

19’ NE i 38’ [.. M]AR

20’ NE i 39’ [..] x

GAP!

A gap of ca. 10 lines.

21’ ... [...]	21’... [...]
Alternative prescription 1’ **22’** *suluppa* [...]	**Alternative prescription 1’** 22’[...] date [...]
Alternative prescription 2’ **23’** *ana ašri šanîmma bīna* [...]	**Alternative prescription 2’** 23’Alternatively: [...] tamarisk, [...]

21’ NE i 50’ [x (x)] x [...]

22’ NE i 51’ ZÚ.LU[M].M[A..]

23’ NE i 52’ DIŠ KIMIN ^{giš}ŠINIG [...]

24’ *šiptu* ... [...] **25’** *adappātu*$^?$ x [...] **26’** *ka’inimma īnī apâti īnī* [*ašâti* ...]	24’Incantation: ... [...] 25’canals$^?$ x [...] 26’Invocation for cloudy (and) [blurred] eyes [...]

24’ NE i 53’ ÉN KI SA DI x [..]

25’ NE i 54’ *a-da-pa-tu$_4$ in-*⸢x⸣ [..]

26’ NE i 55’ KA.INIM.MA IGI.MIN *a-pa-ti* IGI.MEŠ ⸢*a*⸣-[*ša-ti* ....]

Overview of IGI 3 Manuscripts and Parallels: **AH**=BAM **209**; **AmB**=BAM 25; **BoB**=KUB 37/2; **BoC**=KUB 4/55; **NA**=BAM 510; **NC**=BAM 514; **ND**=BAM 515; **NE**=BAM 516; **NF**= BAM 520; **NI**=BAM 480; **NS**=AMT 18/4; **uA**=SpTU 50; **xA**=CM 37; **xB**=BM **40737**

27’ *dudubi sebe uṭṭat hīl abukkati* [...]	[27’]Its medical application: seven grain measures of resin of *abukkatu*-[plant ...]
28’ *ina mūši ina ūri ana pān* [...]	[28’]During the night on the roof (you place the drugs) in front of [a star ...]
29’ *ina šēri lām ṣīt šamši šammī annûti* [...]	[29’]In the morning, before sunrise [you ... (process)] these drugs. [30’]You apply
30’ ... *ana libbi tanaddi īnīšu teqqi arkīšu* [*itqūr abāri ul tapaṭṭar*]	... in the inner part, (and) daub his eyes. Afterwards, [you do not remove the lead spoon ointment]. [31’]You treat
31’ *īnīšu tušamhar ina mê kasî īnīšu tuhappap* [...]	his eyes in the same way, and rinse his eyes in the sap of a *kasû*-plant [...]

27’ NE i 56’ DÙ.DÙ.BI 7 ŠE ILLU ⸢LI⸣.[DUR ....]

28’ NE i 57’ *ina* GE₆ *ina* ÙR *ana* IGI ⸢MUL⸣ x [...] x [..]

29’ NE i 58’ *ina še-rì la-am* ⸢dUTU.È Ú⸣.HI.A *an-*⸢*nu*⸣*-*[*ti* ....]

30’ NE i 59’ ⸢x x⸣ *ana* ŠÀ ŠUB-*di* IGI.MIN-*šú* MAR EGI[R-*šú* DÍLIM A.BÁR *ul* DU₈-*ár*]

31’ NE i 60’ IGI.MIN-*šú tu-šam-har ina* A GAZI^sar^ IGI.MIN-*šú tu-ha-pa*[*p* ....]

32’ *tēqīt īnī ša šugidimmakki mūṣa* [...]	[32’]Ointment for the eyes against ‘Hand of the Ghost’: [you ...] *mūṣu*-stone, [...]-stone [...] [33’]*huluhhu*-stone, black frit,
33’ *huluhha kutpâ lulû arti pillî zikari arti* [...]	*lulû*-antimony, leaf of male *pillû*-mandragora, leaf [...].[34’]You put all
34’ *naphar ištēššeret abnī u šammī annûti ana mê tanaddi ina kakkabi tušbât* [...]	these 11 stones and drugs into water, (and) let (them) stay under a star (= stay overnight) [...].[35’]You put (them)
35’ *ana šamni tanaddi īnīšu tapaššaš ana šikari tanaddīma išatti ina kišādīšu* [*ina maški*] *tašakkanma išallim*	in sesame oil, you smear his eyes (with it), you put (them) into beer and he drinks (it). You place (them) on his neck [in a leather bag] and then he will be safe. [36’]From now on, you do (this) in (any) one month on the
36’ *annânam ina* ITI.1.KAM UD.21.KAM *teppušma išallim*	twenty first day, and then he will be safe.

Overview of IGI 3 Manuscripts and Parallels: **AH**=BAM **209**; **AmB**=BAM 25; **BoB**=KUB 37/2; **BoC**=KUB 4/55; **NA**=BAM 510; **NC**=BAM 514; **ND**=BAM 515; **NE**=BAM 516; **NF**= BAM 520; **NI**=BAM 480; **NS**=AMT 18/4; **uA**=SpTU 50; **xA**=CM 37; **xB**=BM **40737**

Alternative prescription 1 **37'** *ana ašri šanîmma abnu sāmu kīma bulāli īnīšu tapaššaš*	**Alternative prescription 1** [37']Alternatively: with a stone red like the *bulālu*-plant you smear his eyes.
Alternative prescription 2 **37'** *šumma ašar* [*šanîmma*] *mūṣam ašar šanîmma*	**Alternative prescription 2** [37']If ditto, *mūṣu*-stone, ditto (=you smear his eyes).
Alternative prescription 3 **38'** *šumma ašar šanîmma kutpâ ina himēti tasâk ašar šanîmma*	**Alternative prescription 3** [38']If ditto; you pound black frit in ghee, ditto (smear his eyes).
Alternative prescription 4 **38'** *šumma ašar šanîmma uqni šadê* [*ina*] *hīmeti tasâk ašar šanîmma*	**Alternative prescription 4** [38']If ditto: you pound mountain lapis lazuli in ghee, ditto.
Alternative prescription 5 **39'** *šumma ašar šanîmma muššara ašar šanîmma*	**Alternative prescription 5** [39']If ditto; sardonyx, ditto (you pound in ghee).
Alternative prescription 6 **39'** *šumma ašar šanîmma šimbizida ina šizbi musukkati tasâk īnīšu tapaššaš*	**Alternative prescription 6** [39']If ditto; you pound *šimbizidû*-galena in the milk from a woman in maternity, you smear his eyes (with it).
Alternative prescription 7 **40'** *šumma ašar šanîmma ṣurri ṣalmi ina šaman kurkî tasâk ašar šanîmma*	**Alternative prescription 7** [40']If ditto; you pound obsidian in goose fat, ditto (you smear his eyes with it and he will be safe).

32' NE i 61' *te-qí-it* IGI.MIN *ša* ŠU.GIDIM.MA ^{na4}*mu-ṣa* NA$_4$ [..................................]

33' NE i 62' ^{na4}AN.ZAH.BABBAR ^{na4}AN.ZAH.GE$_6$ KÙ.GAN PA ^{giš}NAM.TAR NÍTA P[A ...]

34' NE i 63' PAP 11 NA$_4$.MEŠ *u* Ú.HI.A ŠEŠ *ana* A ŠUB-*di ina* UL *tuš-bat* [...............]

Overview of IGI 3 Manuscripts and Parallels: **AH**=BAM **209**; **AmB**=BAM 25; **BoB**=KUB 37/2; **BoC**=KUB 4/55; **NA**=BAM 510; **NC**=BAM 514; **ND**=BAM 515; **NE**=BAM 516; **NF**= BAM 520; **NI**=BAM 480; **NS**=AMT 18/4; **uA**=SpTU 50; **xA**=CM 37; **xB**=BM **40737**

35'	NE i 64'	*ana* Ì+GIŠ ŠUB-*di* IGI.MIN-*šú* ŠÉŠ-*aš ana* KAŠ ŠUB-*di-ma* ⸢NAG *ina*⸣ G[Ú-*šú ina*$^{?}$ KUŠ$^{?}$ GA]R-*an-ma* ⸢SILIM⸣-*im*
36'	NE i 65'	*an-na-nam ina* ITI.1.KÁM UD.21.KÁM D[Ù-*ma*] ⸢*i*⸣-*šal*-⸢*lim*⸣
37'	NE i 66'	DIŠ KIMIN NA$_{4}$ SA$_{5}$ *ki-ma bu-la-li* IGI.MIN-*šú* ŠÉŠ-*aš* : DIŠ K[IMIN ^{na4}*m*]*u-ṣa-am* KIMIN
	(xB) 2'	[DIŠ KIMI]N ⸢^{na4}*mu-ṣa* KIMIN :⸣ [DIŠ KIMIN ... : DIŠ KIMIN]
38'	NE i 67'	DIŠ KIMIN ^{na4}*kut-pa-a ina* Ì.NUN SÚD KIMIN : DIŠ KIMIN ^{na4}ZA.GÌN KUR.R[A *ina*] ⸢Ì⸣.NUN SÚD KIMIN
39'	NE i 68'	DIŠ KIMIN ^{na4}MUŠ.GÍR KIMIN : DIŠ KIMIN *šim-bi-zi-da*$_{4}$ *ina* G[A ^{munus}] ⸢Ú⸣.ZÚG SÚD IGI.MIN-*šú* ŠÉŠ-*aš*
	(xB) 3'	1 ^{na4}MUŠ.⸢GÍR KIMIN : DIŠ KIMIN⸣ [...]
40'	NE i 69'	DIŠ KIMIN ^{na4}ZÚ GE$_{6}$ *ina* Ì KUR.G[I SÚ]D KIMIN
	(xB) 4'	*ina* Ì KUR.GI^{mušen} KIMIN ⸢: DIŠ KIMIN⸣ x [...]

41' *kukru miriq šammi ašî nīnû kasû lipi qanî* **42'** *šadânu ṣābitu mūṣa šaman iṣṣūr hurri*$^{?}$ *labīri iškūru* **43'** *ištēššeret šammī annûti ribku ša šugidimmakki īnīšu tēteneqqīma iballuṭ*	41'*Kukru*-aromatic, *mirqu*-powder$^{?}$ of *ašû*-disease-plant, *nīnû*-'mint', *kasû*-plant, pith of reeds, 42'magnetite, *mūṣu*-stone, fat from an old partridge$^{?}$, (and) wax. 43'These eleven drugs are an infusion against 'Hand of the Ghost' (affliction): you keep daubing his eyes (with the mixture), then he should recover.

41'	NE i 70'	^{šim}GÚR.GÚR *mi-ríq* Ú *a-ši-i* ^{ú}K[UR.RA GA]ZI^{sar} Ì.UDU GI.MEŠ
42'	NE i 71'	^{na4}KA.GI.NA.DAB.BA ^{na4}*mu-ṣa* Ì.GIŠ ⸢MUŠEN.HABRUD$^{?}$⸣ LIBIR.RA GAB.LÀL
43'	NE i 72'	11 Ú.HI.A ŠEŠ *rib-ku ša* ŠU.⸢GIDIM.MA⸣ IGI.MIN-*šú* MAR.MEŠ-*ma* TI

Overview of IGI 3 Manuscripts and Parallels: **AH**=BAM **209**; **AmB**=BAM 25; **BoB**=KUB 37/2; **BoC**=KUB 4/55; **NA**=BAM 510; **NC**=BAM 514; **ND**=BAM 515; **NE**=BAM 516; **NF**= BAM 520; **NI**=BAM 480; **NS**=AMT 18/4; **uA**=SpTU 50; **xA**=CM 37; **xB**=BM **40737**

44' [...] ... *ina tišît ūme* [...] **45'** *niqâ teppušma šēršunu* [...]	44'[...] on the 9th day [...] 45'you make an offering *and* [...] their flesh [...]

44' NE ii 1' [...............] x ⸢*ina*⸣ 9 UD.K[AM? ....]

45' NE ii 2' ⸢UDU.SISKUR DÙ⸣-*ma* UZU-*šu-nu* [..]

46' *muhha ša eṣemti kurīti immeri* [...] **47'** *zība mê nurmî* ... [...] **48'** *ištēniš taballal ina dišpi himēti šaman erēni* [*tasâk* ...] x [...]	48'You mix together 46'marrow of a short sheep-bone, [...] 47'black cumin, sap of pomegranate, ... [...] 48'You pound (them) in honey, ghee and cedar oil, [(and) ...]

46' NE ii 3' UGU *ša* GÌR.PAD.DU LÚGUD.DA ⸢UDU⸣ x [..]

47' NE ii 4' GAMUN.GE₆ A ^giš^NU.ÚR.MA ^giš^x [..]

48' NE ii 5' 1-*niš* HE.HE *ina* LÀL Ì.NUN Ì.GIŠ EREN S[ÚD? ....] x [................]

49' *šumma amēlu īnāšu lā inaṭṭalā amēlu šū ṣēta hamiṭ ištēn šiqil rikibti arkabi* **50'** *mišil šiqil šamma peṣâ rebiat emesalli ina dišip šadê u himēti* [*tasâk*] *īnīšu teqqi*	49'If a man's eyes cannot see: that man is inflamed with sun heat: 50'[you pound] 49'one shekel of bat guano, 50'half shekel of white plant, (and) one fourth shekel of *emesallu*-saline solution in mountain honey and ghee, (and) you daub his eyes (with it).

49' NE ii 6' DIŠ NA IGI.MIN-*šú la ina-ṭa-la* NA BI UD.DA TAB.⸢BA 1 GÍN U₅.ARGAB⸣^mušen^

(NS) 6' DIŠ NA IGI.MIN-*šú la ina-ṭa-la* N[A BI ....]

50' NE ii 7' 1/2 GÍN Ú.BABBAR IGI.4.GÁL.LA ^mun^*eme-sal-lì ina* ⸢LÀL⸣.KUR *u* Ì.N[UN SÚD I]GI.MIN-*šú* MAR

(NS) 7' 1/2 GÍN Ú.⸢BABBAR⸣ IGI.4.GÁL.[LA ....]

(NS) 8' *u* Ì.NUN S[ÚD] x [..]

NO DIVIDING LINE TO BE SEEN!

51' *šumma amēlu digil īnīšu maṭi lipi ṣallāmti maštakal suluppa? bīna*	51'If a man's eyesight is diminished: 53'you mix and pound in equal

Overview of IGI 3 Manuscripts and Parallels: **AH**=BAM **209**; **AmB**=BAM 25; **BoB**=KUB 37/2; **BoC**=KUB 4/55; **NA**=BAM 510; **NC**=BAM 514; **ND**=BAM 515; **NE**=BAM 516; **NF**= BAM 520; **NI**=BAM 480; **NS**=AMT 18/4; **uA**=SpTU 50; **xA**=CM 37; **xB**=BM **40737**

52’ *lipi nēši hīl tīyati errâ*$^{(\text{gloss: } \textit{ṭūra})}$ *uhūla qarnānâ šamma peṣâ emesalli zība* **53’** *malmališ ina šuhti ina dišip šadê taballal tasâk teqqi* [*passa*$^?$] *teppuš ušû uhūla qarnānâ īnīšu temessi* **54’** [*arkīšu*] *īnīšu teqqīma* UD$^?$.X$^?$.KAM$^?$ ... *tanaddi adi sebîšu teqqi arkīšu itqūr abāri ul tapaṭṭar*	measures $^{51'}$fat from a black snake, *maštakal*-plant, date$^?$, tamarisk, $^{52'}$fat from a lion, resin of *tīyatu*-plant, *errû*-colocynth$^{(\text{or } \textit{ṭūru}\text{-plant})}$, horned *uhūlu*-alkali, white plant, *emesallu*-saline solution, (and) black cumin $^{53'}$in copper patina (and) in mountain honey. You daub (his eyes). You make a [collyrium stick] (out of it). You wash his eyes (with it in the sap of) *ušû*-plant and horned *uhūlu*-alkali. $^{54'}$[Afterwards] you daub his eyes. On day x, you apply ..., up to seven times you daub (his eyes). Afterwards you do not stop using the lead spoon (salve).

51’ NE ii 8’ ⌜DIŠ NA⌝ *di-gi-il* IGI.MIN-*šú ma-a-ṭi* Ì.UDU MUŠ.⌜GE$_6$ ^{ú}IN⌝.NU.UŠ Z[Ú.LUM.M]A$^?$ ^{giš}ŠINIG

52’ NE ii 9’ ⌜Ì⌝.UDU UR.MAH ILLU ^{ú}*ti-iá-tu* ⌜ÚKUŠ.LAGAB $^{(\text{gloss: ŠIM.HAB})}$ NAGA.SI⌝ [Ú].BABBAR ^{mun}*eme-sal-lì* ⌜^{ú}GAMUN⌝.GE$_6$

53’ NE ii 10’ [*mal-m*]*a-liš ina* SAHAR.URUDU *ana* LÀL.KUR.RA HE.HE SÚD MAR Z[A.NA *te-p*]*u-uš* ^{ú}ESI NAGA.⌜SI⌝ IGI.MIN-*šú* LUH-*si*

54’ NE ii 11’ [EGIR-*šú* I]GI.⌜MIN⌝-*šú* MAR-*ma* UD$^?$.x$^?$.KÁM$^?$ x [...] x ŠUB EN 7-*šú* ⌜MAR EGIR-*šú* DÍLIM A.BÁR *ul* DU$_8$-*ár*⌝

(NI) ii 6f. *te-qí* EGIR-*šú* / [DÍLIM A.B]ÁR NU DU$_8$-*šú*

It is unclear of the next prescription is not an alternative one to 51ff.’

55’ [...] *burāša uhūla qarnānâ nuhurta sahlê* **56’** [... *ina* ...] *talâš taṣammid*	$^{55'}$[..: $^{56'}$you pound] horned *uhūlu*-alkali, *nuhurtu*-plant, *sahlû*-plant $^{56'}$[...] you knead [(it) in ...], (and) you bandage (his eyes).

55’ NE ii 12’ [.. ^{ši}]^{m}LI NAGA.⌜SI⌝ NU.LUH.HA *sah-lé-e*

56’ NE ii 13’ [... *ina* ...] SILA$_{11}$-*aš* LAL

Overview of IGI 3 Manuscripts and Parallels: **AH**=BAM **209**; **AmB**=BAM 25; **BoB**=KUB 37/2; **BoC**=KUB 4/55; **NA**=BAM 510; **NC**=BAM 514; **ND**=BAM 515; **NE**=BAM 516; **NF**= BAM 520; **NI**=BAM 480; **NS**=AMT 18/4; **uA**=SpTU 50; **xA**=CM 37; **xB**=BM **40737**

57’ [*šumma* ...] ...-*ma īnīšu* **58’** [...] ... *emesalli* **59’** [...] *tasâk* **60’** [... *kala ūme* ...] *riksa ukâl* **61’** [...] *īnīšu tēteneqqīma iballuṭ*	57’[If ...] and his eyes, 58’[...] *emesallu*-saline solution, 59’[...] you pound, 60’[... x times during the whole day] he keeps the bandage on. 61’[...] you keep daubing his eyes, and then he should recover.

57’ NE ii 14’ [..] x-⸢*ma*⸣ IGI-*šú*

58’ NE ii 15’ [..] x x ⸢^{mun}*eme-sal-lì*⸣

59’ NE ii 16’ [...] x SÚD

60’ NE ii 17’ [.. *ka-la* UD-*me* X-*šú* KE]ŠDA *ú-kal*

61’ NE ii 18’ [.. IG]I.⸢MIN⸣-*šú* MAR.MEŠ-*ma* TI

62’ [... *qāt*] *Šulpaea* (gloss: *Adad rāhiṣ*) **63’** [...] *qāt Ištar* **64’** [...] *ina pēmti tašakkan* **65’** [...] *tasâk tēteneqqīma iballuṭ*	62’[... hand of the] god Šulpaea(gloss: Adad, the rain-maker), 63’[...] hand of Ištar, 64’[...] you put [...] over charcoal. 65’You pound [...], daub (his eyes) again and again, then he should recover.

62’ NE ii 19’ [.. ŠU] ⸢^{d}⸣*Šul-pa-è-a* (gloss: ⸢^{d}IŠKUR *ra-hi-iṣ*⸣)

63’ NE ii 20’ [..] ŠU ^{d}15

64’ NE ii 21’ [.. *i*]*na* NE GAR-*an*

65’ NE ii 22’ [.. SÚ]D$^{?}$ MAR.MEŠ-*ma* TI

66’ [...] *šumma lā inaṭṭalā qāt Ištar* **67’** [... *ina*] *dišpi u himēti tasâk īnīšu tēteneqqīma iballuṭ*	66’[...], if (his eyes) do not see, (it is the) hand of Ištar. 67’You pound [... in] honey and ghee, you daub his eyes, then he should recover.

66’ NE ii 23’ [..] x MI *šum*$_4$-*ma la i-na-aṭ-ṭa-la* ŠU ^{d}*Iš*$_8$-*tár*

Overview of IGI 3 Manuscripts and Parallels: **AH**=BAM **209**; **AmB**=BAM 25; **BoB**=KUB 37/2; **BoC**=KUB 4/55; **NA**=BAM 510; **NC**=BAM 514; **ND**=BAM 515; **NE**=BAM 516; **NF**= BAM 520; **NI**=BAM 480; **NS**=AMT 18/4; **uA**=SpTU 50; **xA**=CM 37; **xB**=BM **40737**

67’ NE ii 24’ [........................ *ina* LÀ]L *u* Ì.NUN SÚD IGI.MIN-*šú* MAR.MEŠ-*ma* TI

68’ *šumma amēlu šīlī* [*īnīšu* ...] ...-*ma lā iṣallal eli minâtēšina ikabbitā* **69’** *lipi ṣallamti ina himēti dišip šadê taballal teqqi*	68’If the perforations of a man’s [eyelids ...] ... and he cannot sleep, the ‘condition’ (of the eyes) is heavy: 69’You mix ‘fat from a black snake’ in ghee and mountain honey, (and) you daub (his eyes).

68’ NE ii 25’ DIŠ NA *ši*-[*li*? IGI.MIN-*šú* ...] x x x x x NU NÁ ⸢UGU⸣ *mi-na-te-ši-na* DUGUD

69’ NE ii 26’ Ì.UDU ⸢MUŠ⸣.GE$_6$ *ina* Ì.NUN ⸢LÀL⸣.KUR-*e* ⸢HE⸣.HE *te-qí*

70’ *šumma amēlu šīlī īnīšu šaddūma mayyāla lā inašši arti šunê arti titti* **71’** *arti lipāri arti* GI.ZÚ.LUM.MA *ina mê ina tinūri tesekker ana libbi tattanaddīšu* **72’** *piqan ṣabīti kabūt alpi ištēniš tahaššal tanappi itti qēm labti taballal ina mê kasî talâš taṣammid aktam ina šikari išattīma iballuṭ*	70’If perforations of a man’s eye(lids) are lengthened, and he cannot ‘lift his bed’ (get out of bed): 71’you heat up 70’leaf of *šunû*-tree, fig leaf, 71’leaf of *lipāru*-tree, (and) leaf of ‘date reed’in water in a tannour-oven, you keep on putting (the mixture) into it. 72’You crush and sift together gazelle droppings (and) ox dung, you mix (them) with flour of roasted grain. You knead (it) in the sap of a *kasû*-plant (and) bandage (his eys). (In addition,) he shall drink *aktam*-plant in beer, then he should recover.

70’ NE ii 27’ DIŠ NA *ši*-⸢*li* IGI⸣.MIN-*šú šad-du-ma* KI.⸢NÁ NU ÍL⸣ PA ^{giš}ŠE.NÚ.A PA ^{giš}PÈŠ

71’ NE ii 28’ PA ^{giš}MI.⸢PÀR⸣ PA GI.ZÚ.LUM.MA *ina* A *ina* ⸢NININDU ÚŠ⸣-*ker ana* ŠÀ ŠUB.ŠUB-*šú*

72’ NE ii 29’ A.GAR.GAR MAŠ.⸢DÀ ŠURUN⸣ GU$_4$ 1-*niš* GAZ SIM KI ZÌ ŠE.SA.A HE.HE *ina* ⸢A GAZI⸣^{sar} SILA$_{11}$-*aš* LAL ^{ú}*ak-tam ina* KAŠ NAG-*ma* TI

Overview of IGI 3 Manuscripts and Parallels: **AH**=BAM **209**; **AmB**=BAM 25; **BoB**=KUB 37/2; **BoC**=KUB 4/55; **NA**=BAM 510; **NC**=BAM 514; **ND**=BAM 515; **NE**=BAM 516; **NF**= BAM 520; **NI**=BAM 480; **NS**=AMT 18/4; **uA**=SpTU 50; **xA**=CM 37; **xB**=BM **40737**

73’ *šumma amēlu ūma kala lā immar mūša kala immar Sîn-lurmâ*	[73’]If a man cannot see during the whole day, (but) sees during the whole night: (it is) a day blindness.

73’ NE ii 30’ DIŠ ⸢NA UD DÙ⸣.A.BI NU IGI.DU$_8$ GE$_6$ DÙ.A.BI IGI.⸢DU$_8$ ^{d}30⸣-*lu-ur-ma-a*

74’ *šumma amēlu ūma kala immar mūša kala lā immar Sîn-lurmâ*	[74’]If a man sees during the whole day, (but) cannot see during the whole night: (it is) a night blindness.

74’ NE ii 31’ DIŠ ⸢NA UD⸣ DÙ.A.BI IGI.DU$_8$ GE$_6$ DÙ.A.BI NU IGI.⸢DU$_8$⸣ ^{d}30-⸢*lu-ur*⸣-*ma-a*

75’ *šumma amēlu īnāšu sillurmâ makūt gabīdi ša imēri šēr labânīšu* **76’** *ina pitilti tašakkak ina kišādīšu tašakkan agubbâ tukān ina šēri šahhâ* **77’** *ana pān šamši tatarraṣ nignak burāši tašakkan amēla šuātu ina kutal šahhî ana pān šamši* **78’** *tušzassu mašmašu sebet akalī inašši ša īnāšu marṣā sebet akalī inaššīma* **79’** [*mašmašu*?] *ana marṣi muhra namra īni iqabbi* **80’** *marṣu ana mašmaši muhra balṣa īni iqabbi*	[75’]If a man’s eyes (have) a day/night blindness: [76’]you twist (lit. thread) into a string [75’]the ‘pole’ of a donkey liver (and) its neck tendons, [76’](and) place (it) on his neck. You set up a holy water vessel (and) in the morning [77’]you spread out [76’]a *šahhû*-cloth [77’]facing the sun, you install an incense burner with juniper. [78’]You have [77’]that man [78’]stand [77’]behind the *šahhû*-cloth facing the sun. [78’]The *mašmašu*-healer lifts up seven loafs of bread. The one whose eyes are sick (also) lifts up seven loafs of bread. [79’][A *mašmašu*-healer?] shall say to the patient: ‘accept (the bread), O shining of eye(s)’. [80’]The patient shall say to the *mašmašu*-healer: ‘accept (the bread), O staring of eye(s)’.

75’ NE ii 32’ DIŠ NA ⸢IGI⸣.MIN-*šú si-lu-ur-ma-a ma-ku-ut ga-bi-di ša* ANŠE UZU *la-ba-ni-šú*

(AmB) 4 [... *ga-b*]*i-di ša* ANŠE UZU ⸢GÚ⸣

76’ NE ii 33’ *ina* ⸢ŠU.SAR⸣ *ta-šak-kak ina* GÚ-*šú* GAR-*an* A.GÚB.BA.A GIN-*an ina še-rì* ^{túg}ŠÀ.HA

Overview of IGI 3 Manuscripts and Parallels: **AH**=BAM **209**; **AmB**=BAM 25; **BoB**=KUB 37/2; **BoC**=KUB 4/55; **NA**=BAM 510; **NC**=BAM 514; **ND**=BAM 515; **NE**=BAM 516; **NF**= BAM 520; **NI**=BAM 480; **NS**=AMT 18/4; **uA**=SpTU 50; **xA**=CM 37; **xB**=BM **40737**

(AmB) 5 [...] ⸢A⸣.GUB.BA.A *ana* IGI ^{d}UTU GI[N-*an*]

77’ NE ii 34’ *ana* ⸢IGI ^{d}⸣UTU LAL-*aṣ* NÍG.NA ^{šim}LI GAR-*an* LÚ *šú-a-tú ina ku-tal* ^{túg}ŠÀ.HA *ana* IGI ^{d}UTU
(AmB) 6 [... *ta-t*]*a-ra-aṣ*

78’ NE ii 35’ *tuš-*⸢*za-as*⸣*-su* MAŠ.MAŠ 7 NINDA ÍL-*ši šá* IGI.MIN-*šú* GIG 7 NINDA ÍL-*ši-ma*
(AmB) 6ff. [...] TA 7 NINDA.MEŠ TI-*qé* / [... T]A *ana* NA *ša* IGI.MEŠ-*šú* GIG [...] / [...] x A.GUB.BA.A-*e*

79’ NE ii 36’ M[AŠ.MAŠ$^{?}$ *a*]*na* ^{lú}TU.RA *mu-uh-ra nam-ra i-ni i-qab-bi*

80’ NE ii 37’ [^{lú}TU.R]A *ana* MAŠ.MAŠ *mu-*⸢*uh-ra*⸣ *bal-ṣa i-ni i-qab-bi*

81’ [*šumma amēlu īnāšu sillurmâ*] *makūt gabīdi taharraṣ* **82’** [... *ikkal* ...] ... *ṣehrī tupahharma kīam iqabbû* **83’** [... *šá*] *iqabbû himēta u šaman rūšti ištēniš taballal īnīšu tēteneqqi*	81’[If a man’s eyes (have) a day/night blindness:] you cut into the ‘pole’ of a liver, 82’[... he shall eat it ...] ... You assemble children, and they shall say thus: 83’[...] is [what] they shall say. You mix together ghee and first class sesame oil (and) daub his eyes again and again.

81’ NE iii 1 [DIŠ NA IGI.MIN-*šú si-lu-ur-ma-a m*]*a-ku-ut ga-bi-di ta-har-ra-aṣ*
(AmB) 9 [... *ta-har-r*]*a-aṣ* →
(BoB) 26f.’ [.................. *s*]*í-nu-ri* DAB-*su* UZU ŠU.SI NÍTA / [... *ga*]*-bi-id-dì a-na šu-me-e*
(BoC) 5f.’ [... IGI.MEŠ-*š*]*u sí-nu-*⸢*ri*⸣ DAB-*su* UZU [......] / [... *g*]*a-bi-id-*⸢*dì*$^{?}$⸣ *a-na šu-me-e*
(BoB) 28’ [...] ⸢14⸣ *ki-ir-ṣí ta-kar-ra-aṣ*
(BoC) 7’ [........ *ki-i*]*r-*⸢*ṣí ta*⸣*-kar-ra-aṣ*

82’ NE iii 2 [............................. M]AŠ$^{?}$ ^{lú}TUR.MEŠ *tu-pa-har-ma ki-a-am i-qab-bu-u*
(AmB) 9f. GU$_{7}$ / [.......... *tu-pa-h*]*ar ki-am* DUG$_{4}$.GA-*u*
(BoB) 29ff.’ [...] ⸢*ta*⸣*-na-di-in-ma* ^{lú}GIG *ina* ⸢NIGIN-x⸣ / [... *i*$^{?}$*-n*]*a*$^{?}$ ZAG-*ka a-na* IGI-*šu tu-*⸢*up*$^{?}$⸣*-x* [x] / [...] x *ù ki-a-am* [...............]

Overview of IGI 3 Manuscripts and Parallels: **AH**=BAM **209**; **AmB**=BAM 25; **BoB**=KUB 37/2; **BoC**=KUB 4/55; **NA**=BAM 510; **NC**=BAM 514; **ND**=BAM 515; **NE**=BAM 516; **NF**= BAM 520; **NI**=BAM 480; **NS**=AMT 18/4; **uA**=SpTU 50; **xA**=CM 37; **xB**=BM **40737**

(BoC) 8ff.' [............................ ^{lú}GI]G *ina* NIGIN-*šu i-ma*[*h* ...] / [...] x *ina* ZAG-*ka a-n*[*a* ...] / [...] x *ù k*[*i-* ...]

83' NE iii 3 [....] ⸢*i*⸣-*qab-bu-u* Ì.NUN *u* Ì.GIŠ.SAG 1-*niš* HE.HE IGI.MIN-*šú* MAR.MEŠ

84' [*dudubi* (...)] *šuātu* ŠU.BI.GIN$_7$.NAM	[84']'[This *medical application* (...)] is like the (previous) one.

84' NE iii 4 [DÙ.DÙ.BI (............................)] *šu-a-tu* ŠU.BI.GIN$_7$.NAM

85' [*šiptu* ... *šemēma*$^?$] *muhra Ea lišmâ Ea limhura* **86'** [...] *amur namra īni amur balṣa īni tê šipti*	[85']'[Incantation: ... hear and] accept! May Ea hear, may Ea accept (it)! [86']'[...] see O, shining of eye, see O, staring of eye. Incantation spell.

85' NE iii 5 [ÉN .... *še*$^?$-*me-ma*$^?$ *mu*]-*úh-ra* ^{d}*É-a liš-ma-a* ^{d}*É-a lim-hu-ra*

86' NE iii 6 [....................................... *a-m*]*ur nam-ra i-ni a-mur bal-ṣa i-ni* TU$_6$.ÉN

87' [*dudubi* ...] *sebet*$^?$ *ubān hašê teleqqēma šipta annītu* **88'** [*tamannu* ... *ina*] *dalti ina qātīšu tašakkanma ikkal*	[87']'[Its medical application: ...] you take seven$^?$ 'lobes' of the lung and [[88']' recite] [87']'this incantation. [88']'You place [... at] the door in his hand and he shall eat (it).

87' NE iii 7 [DÙ.DÙ.BI ....] ⸢7$^?$⸣ ŠU.SI *ha-še-e* TI-*ma* ÉN *an-ni-tú*

88' NE iii 8 [ŠID-*nu* .... *ina*] ^{giš}IG *ina* ŠU-*šú* GAR-*ma* GU$_7$

89' [...] ... *makūt gabīdi ēma herṣi* **90'** [*taharraṣ*$^?$...] *šaptāšu u* [...]-*ma ina'eš*	[89']'[...] ... 'pole' of a liver, wherever [[90]' you cut] a piece. [90']'[...] his lips and [...] and then he should get better.

89' NE iii 9 [..............................] x PA *ma-ku-ut* ⸢*ga-bi-di e-ma*⸣ *her-ṣi*
(BoB) 27f.' [... *ga*]-*bi-id-dì a-na šu-me-e* / [...] ⸢14⸣ *ki-ir-ṣí ta-kar-ra-aṣ*
(BoC) 6f.' [... *g*]*a-bi-id*-⸢*dì*$^?$⸣ *a-na šu-me-e* / [.... *ki-i*]*r*-⸢*ṣí ta*⸣-*kar-ra-aṣ*

90' NE iii 10 [*ta-har-ra-aṣ* ....] ⸢NUNDUM⸣-*šú* ⸢*ù*⸣ [..............]-⸢*ma ina-eš*⸣

Overview of IGI 3 Manuscripts and Parallels: **AH**=BAM **209**; **AmB**=BAM 25; **BoB**=KUB 37/2; **BoC**=KUB 4/55; **NA**=BAM 510; **NC**=BAM 514; **ND**=BAM 515; **NE**=BAM 516; **NF**= BAM 520; **NI**=BAM 480; **NS**=AMT 18/4; **uA**=SpTU 50; **xA**=CM 37; **xB**=BM **40737**

91’ [...] ... *minâta*$^?$ [...] ... **92’** [...] *labta* [...]	91’[...] ... ‘limbs/condition’$^?$ [...] ... 92’[...] roasted grain [...]

91’ NE iii 11 [.......................] x GI *mi-na-t*[*a*$^?$ ....] x x [x]

92’ NE iii 12 [.........................] PA ⌜ŠE.SA$^?$.A$^?$⌝ [..]

GAP!

Ca. 60 lines are lost!

93’ *itqūr abāri kīma līši*$^?$ *tašakkanu burāša kukra* [...] **94’** *kasâ uhūla qarnānâ sahlê šammi aši kibrīta ru’tīta iṭṭâ* [...] **95’** *lipi kalīti alpi ištēniš tasâk ana libbi abāri tanaddīma ubāna* [*teqqi*$^?$] **96’** *tēqītu šalimtu ša qāt ummâni latek bari*	93’A ‘lead spoon’-salve, which you have to place (on the eyes) like dough$^?$: 95’you pound together 93’juniper, *kukru*-aromatic, [...]-plant, 94’*kasû*-plant, horned *uhūlu*-alkali, *sahlû*-plant, *ašû*-disease-plant, *kibrītu*-sulphur, *ru’tītu*-sulphur, liquid bitumen, [...], 95’and ox kidney fat, and put it into the lead. [(Then) you daub$^?$] (the eyes with your) finger. 96’A healing ointment from the hand of the *ummânu*-wise man, tested and checked.

93’ NE iv 1 DÍLIM A.BÁR GIN$_7$ ⌜NÍG⌝.[SILA$_{11}$.GÁ$^?$] ⌜GAR⌝-*nu* ^{šim}LI ^{šim}GÚR.GÚR ⌜Ú⌝ [...]

94’ NE iv 2 GAZI^{sar} NAG[A.SI Z]À.⌜HI⌝.LI Ú *a-ši-i* PIŠ$_{10}$-^{d}ÍD ÚH-^{d}ÍD ES[IR ...]

95’ NE iv 3 Ì.UDU ÉLLAG ⌜GU$_4$ 1-*niš ta*⌝-*sàk ana* ŠÀ A.BÁR ŠUB-*ma* ŠU.SI [MAR$^?$]

96’ NE iv 4 *te-qí-tu ša-lim-tu ša* ŠU UM.ME.A *la-te-ek ba-r*[*i*]

97’ *kasû sahlê atā’išu māš(t)u kukru iškūru nīnû lipi kanakti zēr burāši* **98’** *tišît šammū ribku ša īnī*	97’*Kasû*-plant, *sahlû*-plant, *atā’išu*-plant, *māš(t)u*-twin plant, *kukru*-aromatic, wax, *nīnû*-mint, *kanaktu*-aromatic pith, seed of juniper. 98’Nine drugs which (are used as) an infusion for the eyes.

Overview of IGI 3 Manuscripts and Parallels: **AH**=BAM **209**; **AmB**=BAM 25; **BoB**=KUB 37/2; **BoC**=KUB 4/55; **NA**=BAM 510; **NC**=BAM 514; **ND**=BAM 515; **NE**=BAM 516; **NF**= BAM 520; **NI**=BAM 480; **NS**=AMT 18/4; **uA**=SpTU 50; **xA**=CM 37; **xB**=BM **40737**

97’ NE iv 5 GAZI⌜sar ZÀ⌝.HI.LI úKUR.KUR úMAŠ.TAB.BA šimGÚR.GÚR GAB.LÀL úKUR.RA Ì.UDU šimGIG NUMUN ⌜šimLI⌝

98’ NE iv 6 ⌜9⌝ Ú.HI.A *rib-ku ša* IGI.MIN

99’ *nīnâ sahlê kasâ nuhurta atā’iša māš(t)a* **100’** *kammu kukra hašâ ina pēmti tušabšal ina šamni u iškūri peṣî tasâk* **101’** *tišīt šammū ša napšalti lubki*	[100]’You boil over charcoal [99]’*nīnû*-mint, *sahlû*-plant, *kasû*-plant, *nuhurtu*-plant, *atā’išu*-plant, *māš(t)u*-twin plant, [100]’*kammu*-tanning-fungus, *kukru*-aromatic, *hašû*-thyme, (and) pound (them into a salve) in sesame oil and white wax. [101]’Nine drugs which (are used as) a softening salve.

99’ NE iv 7 úKUR.RA *sah-lé-e* GAZIsar úNU.LUH.HA úKUR.KUR úMAŠ.TAB.BA

100’ NE iv 8 *kam-mu* šimGÚR.GÚR úHAR.HAR *ina* NE ŠEG₆-*šal ina* Ì.GIŠ *u* GAB.LÀL BABBAR SÚD

101’ NE iv 9 9 Ú.HI.A *ša nap-šal-ti lu-ub-ki*

102’ *nīnâ atā’iša kasâ māš(t)a murra zēr burāši kammu ša aškāpi sebet šammī* **103’** *ribku ša īnī ina pēmti taqallu ina lipî iškūri u himēti tasâk īnīšu teqqi*	[103]’You roast over charcoal [102]’*nīnû*-mint, *atā’išu*-plant, *kasû*-plant, *māš(t)u*-twin plant, bitter-plant, seeds of juniper, *kammu*-tanning-fungus of a leather worker – seven drugs – [103]’(used as) an infusion for the eyes: you pound (them into salve) in fat, wax and ghee. You daub his eyes.

102’ NE iv 10 úKUR.RA úKUR.KUR GAZIsar úMAŠ.TAB.BA šimSES NUMUN šimLI *kam-mu šá* AŠGAB 7 Ú.HI.A

103’ NE iv 11 *rib-ku ša* IGI.MIN *ina* NE *ta-qal-lu ina* Ì.UDU GAB.LÀL *u* Ì.NUN SÚD IGI.MIN-*šú* MAR

For parallels see IGI 1: 32f.

Overview of IGI 3 Manuscripts and Parallels: **AH**=BAM **209**; **AmB**=BAM 25; **BoB**=KUB 37/2; **BoC**=KUB 4/55; **NA**=BAM 510; **NC**=BAM 514; **ND**=BAM 515; **NE**=BAM 516; **NF**= BAM 520; **NI**=BAM 480; **NS**=AMT 18/4; **uA**=SpTU 50; **xA**=CM 37; **xB**=BM **40737**

104’ *kutpû tuškû ashar mūṣa uhūlu qarnānû kukru šammu peṣû sahlû* **105’** *kammu kibrītu lipi alpi abāra itqūr abāri qāt asî*	104’Black frit, *tuškû*-mineral, *ashar*-stone, *mūṣu*-stone, horned *uhūlu*-alkali, *kukru*-aromatic, white plant, *sahlû*-plant, 105’*kammu*-tanning-fungus, *kibrītu*-sulphur, ox fat, lead: lead spoon-salve – handiwork of an *asû*-physician.

104’ NE iv 12 ^{na4}AN.ZAH.GE$_6$ *tuš-ku* ^{na4}*as-har* ^{na4}*mu-ṣa* NAGA.SI ^{šim}GÚR.GÚR Ú.BABBAR ZÀ.HI.LI

105’ NE iv 13 *kam-mu* PIŠ$_{10}$-^{d}ÍD Ì.UDU GU$_4$ A.GAR$_5$ DÍLIM A.BÁR ŠU ⸢^{lú}A.ZU⸣

106’ *kutpû kibrītu kupru* [...] **107’** *zību kasû sahlû* [...] **108’** *lipi alpi lipi eṣemti* [...] **109’** *itqurti* [...]	106’Black frit, *kibrītu*-sulphur, *kupru*-dry bitumen [...] 107’black cumin, *kasû*-plant, *sahlû*-plant, [...] 108’Ox fat, bone marrow, [...]109’a spoon/salve of$^?$ [...]

106’ NE iv 14 AN.ZAH.GE$_6$ PIŠ$_{10}$-^{d}ÍD *ku*-⸢*up*⸣-*r*[*a* ....]

107’ NE iv 15 ^{ú}GAMUN.GE$_6$ GAZI^{sar} Z[À.HI.LI ....]

108’ NE iv 16 Ì.UDU GU$_4$ Ì.UDU GÌR.PAD.D[U ....]

109’ NE iv 17 *it-qur-ti* ⸢IR$^?$⸣ [..........]

110’ *kukru*$^?$ [...]	110’*Kukru*-aromatic$^?$, [...]

110’ NE iv 18 ⸢$^{šim?}$GÚR$^?$⸣.[GÚR$^?$ ....]

BREAK!

Ca. 55 lines are missing until the end of the tablet.

Overview of IGI 3 Manuscripts and Parallels: **AH**=BAM **209**; **AmB**=BAM 25; **BoB**=KUB 37/2; **BoC**=KUB 4/55; **NA**=BAM 510; **NC**=BAM 514; **ND**=BAM 515; **NE**=BAM 516; **NF**= BAM 520; **NI**=BAM 480; **NS**=AMT 18/4; **uA**=SpTU 50; **xA**=CM 37; **xB**=BM **40737**

§ IV Additional texts from Nineveh

Some fragments might belong to the Nineveh UGU or IGI, but they cannot as yet be properly placed. Other texts, not belonging to the IGI or the UGU Treatises, comprise loose collections of material that have not been edited into a standardized treatise. Such texts might be *ahû* 'extraneous / non-canonical' collections or oral collections, recorded by scribes in the Royal Library of Ashurbanipal (Panayotov 2018: 112 and elsewhere in BAM 9).

The two-column fragmentary tablet **NF (BAM 520)** probably represents the fourth tablet of the Nineveh IGI treatise. The main clue that a fourth tablet existed in Nineveh comes from the Assur Medical Catalogue (Panayotov 2018: 97, edition in BAM 9: 210):

II EYES

8) B3'(+)A8 — DIŠ NA IGI.MIN-*šú* ⸢GIG :⸣ D[IŠ NA IGI.MIN-*šú mur-din-n*]*i* ⸢DIRI$^{?}$⸣ 'If a man's eyes are sick. [If a man's eyes] are full of [(*a*)*murdin*]*nu* ('bramble').'

9) B4'(+)A9 — DIŠ NA IGI.MIN-*šú* LÙ.LÙ [: DIŠ NA? x x x x] ⸢x x x-*šú*$^{?!}$⸣ ⸢DIRI⸣ 'If a man's eyes are constantly troubled. [If a man's] ... are full of [...]. '

10) B5'(+)A10 — NÍGIN 4 DUB.MEŠ DIŠ NA IGI.MIN-*šú* G[IG EN (...) *šum*$_4$$^{?}$-*m*]*a*$^{?}$ ⸢IGI.SIG$_7$.SIG$_7$⸣ *u sin-*⸢*lu-ur-ma-a*⸣ 'Total of four tablets (of the section) 'If a man's eyes are si[ck.' Including (prescriptions) for the case] that (he has) jaundice or night-blindness.'

Another argument in favour of **NF (BAM 520)** as the fourth tablet of IGI is the fact that it shares recipes with IGI 3, since a common feature of the Nineveh Medical Encyclopaedia is that the same prescription could be used in different contexts, as happens in the first three tablets of the IGI-Treatise.

§ IV.1 NF (BAM 520)

Base Manuscript: **NF (BAM 520 (+) AMT 14/2)**, collated.
Museum number: British Museum, K 8784 + K 9503 + 81-7-27, 85 (+) K 11723. Join K 8784 + is courtesy of Eric Schmidtchen.
Origin and date: Nineveh, 7th century BC.
Type of tablet: Middle fragment of a two column, portrait-oriented tablet. The vertical dividing rulings were made by a twisted thread. There are no holes.

https://doi.org/10.1515/9781501506550-009

Measurements: ca. 10 × 14 × 3,5 cm.
Copy: BAM 520, AMT 14/2.
Photo/CDLI nr.: Plates 31–32a/P398154/P397754.
Literature: Caplice 1967: text 33; Finkel 1976: 254; Köcher 1980b: xiv (BAM 520); Maul 1994: 461ff.; Fincke 2000: 331; Scurlock and Andersen 2005: 793; Scurlock 2006: 782; Scurlock 2014: 756; Attia 2015: 71 and 79; Scurlock 2017: 286; Zomer 2018.

§ IV.1.1 Related Manuscripts containing IGI 3 from Nineveh

The text included represent parallels and partial parallels from the other tablets of the IGI treatise.

Manuscript: **NE** (BAM 516), see **§ III.1**, parallels: 8ff.'.

§ IV.1.2 Related other Manuscripts from Nineveh

These texts represent parallels and partial parallels which are considered important for the compilation of the IGI-treatise. They come from other tablets and fragments from Nineveh containing prescriptions for sick eyes or from the UGU-treatise.

Manuscript: **NL (AMT 49/4)** collated, parallels: 26'.
Museum number: British Museum, K 2462 + K 7824.
Origin and date: Nineveh, 7th century BC.
Type of tablet: Fragment from the top left of a two-column, portrait-oriented tablet. The vertical orienting rulings (see edge of col. iv) were made by a twisted thread. There are no round holes. This fragment is part of the 3rd tablet of the Nineveh Treatise 'BRONCHIA', DIŠ NA KIR_4-*šu* DUGUD.
Measurements: ca. 6,2 × 6,5 × 2,2 cm.
Copy: AMT 49/4.
CDLI nr.: P394449.
Literature: Scurlock and Andersen 2005: 781; Scurlock 2014: 298f., 752; Panayotov 2018: 101; Bácskay 2018a: 93f. and 234ff.

Manuscript: **NM (BAM 489 + 508),** collated, parallels: 29ff.'.
Museum number: British Museum, K 239 + K 2509 + K 3261 + K 9080.
Origin and date: Nineveh, 7th century BC.

Type of tablet: Fragmentary two-column, portrait-oriented tablet. The vertical orienting rulings were done by an instrument or stylus. There are no round holes.
Measurements: ca. 19,3 × 12,4 × 2,7 cm.
Copy: Finkel 1976: pl. 20; BAM 489 + 508.
Photo/CDLI nr.: Plates 44/P393804.
Literature: Finkel 1976: nr. 25, ms. L, pl. 20; Köcher 1980a: xxviii (BAM 489), xxxv–xxxvi (BAM 508); Scurlock and Andersen 2005: 793; Scurlock 2006: 782; Attia and Buisson 2007: 48; Scurlock 2014: 756; Scurlock 2017: 286, 288; Zomer 2018.

Manuscript: **NN (K 6329)**, collated, parallels: 29ff.'.
Museum number: British Museum, K 6329.
Origin and date: Nineveh, 7th century BC.
Type of tablet: Middle fragment of three[?]-column, portrait-oriented tablet. The vertical orienting rulings were done by an instrument or stylus. There are no round holes.
Measurements: ca. 8,1 × 5,3 × ... cm.
Photo/CDLI nr.: Plate 45; P396459.
Literature: Köcher 1964: xv (BAM 216); Finkel 1976: 57, 253f., 279; Köcher 1980a: xxxvi (BAM 508); Köcher 1980b: xiv (BAM 520); Scurlock 2006: 351, 727. Scurlock 2017: 286 (K 6239[sic!]); Zomer 2018.

Manuscript: **NO (K 8211+... (+) BM 98589+ ...)**, collated, parallels: 29ff.'.
Museum number: British Museum, K 8211 + K 4609a (+) BM 98589 + 98584 (K 5416a).
Origin and date: Nineveh, 7th century BC.
Type of tablet: Fragments of three-column, portrait-oriented tablet. The vertical orienting rulings were done by an instrument or stylus. There are no round holes.
Measurements: BM 98584 + BM 98589: ca. 10,6 × 13,1 × 2,6 - 3,5 (towards the middle) cm.; ca. K 8211 + K 4609a: 13,4 × 13,8 × 2,6 - 3,6 (towards the middle) cm.; K 8211 + K 4609a (+) BM 98584 + BM 98589: ca. 13,4 × 23,6+ × 2,6 - 3,6 (towards the middle) cm.
Copy: ABRT 2/11; AMT 45/5; Finkel 1976: pl. 27.
Photo/CDLI nr.: Plate 45–46/P397537+P395655+P396019.
Literature: Köcher 1964: xv (BAM 216); Finkel 1976: 77, 146, 252, no. 30, ms. S, pl. 27; Köcher 1980a: xxxvi (BAM 508); Köcher 1980b: xiv (BAM 520); Scurlock 2006: 351, 727; Böck 2007: 328 (diverse); Scurlock 2017: 286; Zomer 2018.

Manuscript: **NT (AMT 85/2)**, see **§ IV.7**, parallels: 13', 15'.

Manuscript: **NX (BAM 482)**, see **§ V.2**, parallels: 29'.

Manuscript: **NXa (AMT 19/1, AMT 20/1)**, collated, parallels: 29'.
Museum number: British Museum, K 6066 + Sm 1063
Origin and date: Nineveh, 7th century BC.
Type of tablet: Middle fragment of a two-column, portrait-oriented tablet. The vertical dividing rulings were made by a twisted thread. There are numerous round holes pierced in patterns at empty spaces. Serialized tablet belonging to UGU 2 duplicating NX (BAM 482).
Measurements: ca. 11,2 × 17,1 × 2,3–3,1 (towards the middle) cm.
Copy: AMT 19/1, AMT 20/1.
CDLI nr.: P396343.
Literature: Edition and secondary literature in Attia and Buisson 2003.

§ IV.1.3 Related Manuscripts from Different Cities

The texts included here represent parallels and partial parallels which are considered important for the compilation of the IGI-treatise. These are manuscripts coming from other periods and from cities other than Nineveh.

Sigla notations:

A = Assur, Late Assyrian. A, B, C, … designate the different manuscripts.
dk = Dūr Kurigalzu, Middle Babylonian.
X = unknown provenance, Late Assyrian. A, B, C, … designate the different manuscripts.
s = Sippar, Late Babylonian. A, B, C, … designate the different manuscripts.
u = Uruk, Late Babylonian. A, B, C, … designate the different manuscripts.
Initial capital letters designate tablets in Assyrian script or northern scripts, and small letters tablets in Babylonian script.
Parenthesis [()] on a siglum designate a parallel text and not a duplicate.

Assyrian

Manuscript: **AI (LKA 145)**, not collated, parallels: 29ff.'.
Museum number: Istanbul?
Origin and date: Assur, 8th or 7th century BC.
Type of tablet: Landscape-oriented tablet.
Copy: LKA 145.
CDLI nr.: CDLI P414054.
Literature: Scurlock 2017: 286; Zomer 2018.

Manuscript:	**AJ (BAM 216)**, collated, parallels: 29'.
Museum number:	Vorderasiatisches Museum, Berlin, VAT 8911.
Origin and date:	Assur, 8th or 7th century BC.
Type of tablet:	One-column tablet with round holes at empty spaces.
Measurements:	ca. 17,9 × 9,3 × 2,3 (towards the middle) cm.
Copy:	BAM 216.
CDLI nr.:	CDLI P285303.
Literature:	Köcher 1964: viv-xv (BAM 216); Scurlock 2006: nos. 87, 113, 114b, 117, 137c, 182, 184, 205, 206, 208, 211, 212, 214, 248, 249, 295. Scurlock 2017: 286.

Manuscript:	**AK (AO 11447)**, collated, parallels: 29'.
Museum number:	Louvre, AO 11447.
Origin and date:	Assur, 8th or 7th century BC.
Type of tablet:	One-column tablet with round holes at empty spaces.
Measurements:	ca. 23 × 10,7 × 2 cm.
Copy:	JMC 10: 5f.
CDLI nr.:	P493334.
Literature:	Edition and secondary literature in Geller 2007b; Scurlock 2017: 285ff.

Manuscript:	**XA (BM 123362)**, collated, parallels:29ff.'.
Museum number:	British Museum, BM 123362.
Origin and date:	Unclear, 7th century BC.
Type of tablet:	Rests of the lower right hand corner of a two-column tablet. The tablet is unearthed in Niniveh but it is unclear from where the tablet originates. The script might suggest Assur as well. There are round holes in empty spaces.
Measurements:	ca. 8,4 × 8,7 × 2,5 - 3,0 (towards the middle) cm.
Copy:	Plate 47.
Photo/CDLI nr.:	Plate 47–48/P422463.
Literature:	Lambert and Millard 1968: 19; Scurlock 2006: 351, 727; Scurlock 2017: 286; Zomer 2018.

Babylonian

Manuscript:	**dk (Sumer 9/29)**, not collated, parallels: 29ff.'.
Museum number:	National Museum of Iraq, Baghdad, IM 49981
Origin and date:	Dūr Kurigalzu, Middle Babylonian.
Type of tablet:	Fragment of a one-column, portrait oriented tablet?
Copy:	Sumer 9: no. 29.

Literature:	Gurney 1953: no. 29. Finkel 1976: 254, ms. i; Zomer 2018.

Manuscript:	**sA (IRAQ 65)**, see **§ III.4**, parallels: 29’.

Manuscript:	**uC (SpTU 22+85)**, not collated, parallels: 13f.’.
Museum number:	National Museum of Iraq, Baghdad, Excavation no. W 22664.
Origin and date:	Uruk, Late Babylonian.
Type of tablet:	One-column, portrait oriented tablet.
Measurements:	6,5 × 5,1 cm.
Copy:	SpTU 22+85.
CDLI nr.:	P348627+ P348689.
Literature:	von Weiher 1983: no. 22; von Weiher 1988: no. 85; Fincke 1998; Fincke 2000: 241 fn. 1792; Scurlock and Andersen 2005: 187.

Edition of NF (BAM 520)

1’ [...] **2’** [...] *teqqi* **3’** [...] ... *teqqi*	1’[...]. 2’[...] you daub (his eyes). 3’[...] ... you daub (his eyes).

1’	NF i’ 1’	[...] *x-ti*
2’	NF i’ 2’	[... *t*]*e-qí*
3’	NF i’ 3’	[...] x *te-qí*

4’ [...] ... **5’** [...] *ina šamni tasâk ašar šanîmma* **6’** [...] *ašar šanîmma* **7’** [...] *īnīšu teqqi*	4’[...].5’[...] you pound [in] oil, ditto. 6’[...], ditto (=you daub his eyes). 7’[...] you daub his eyes.

4’	NF i’ 4’	[...] TE GI
5’	NF i’ 5’	[... *in*]*a* ⌜Ì⌝ SÚD ⌜KIMIN⌝
6’	NF i’ 6’	[...] KIMIN
7’	NF i’ 7’	[...] x ⌜IGI.MEŠ-*šú* MAR⌝

Overview of Manuscripts and Parallels concerning NF (BAM 520): **AI**=LKA 145; **AJ**=BAM 216; **AK**=AO 11447; **dk**=Sumer 9/29; **NE**=BAM 516; **NF**=BAM 520 (+); **NL**=AMT 49/4; **NM**=BAM 489+508; **NN**=K 6329; **NO**=K 8211+... (+) BM 98589...; **NT**=AMT 85/2; **NX**=BAM 482; **NXa**=AMT 19/1; **sA**=IRAQ 65; **uC**=SpTU22+; **XA**=BM 123362

8’ [...] ... [...] ... [...] x	[8’][...] ... [...] ... [...] x [9’][...] black [frit]
9’ [...] *kutpâ*$^?$ *mūṣa zalāqa sāmta* [...]	*mūṣu*-stone, *zalāqu*-stone, carnelian, ...-stone, [10’][...] tin, sardonyx, seeds of
10’ [...] *annakka muššara zēr bīni zēr ēri*	tamarisk, seeds of *ēru*-tree. [11’][...] you crush these [drugs]
11’ [... *šammī*] *annûti ištēniš tahaššal tašappah ina lipî kalīt alpi ṣalmi*	together.[11’]Sprinkle, and pound (them) in kidney fat of a black ox [– [12’]like (you pound) *kammu*-tanning-fungus
12’ [*kīma kamma ina muhhi erî tasâkma*] *īnīšu kayyamānamma teqqīma ina’eš*	over copper – and] you regularly daub his eyes, and he will get better.

8’ NF i’ 8’ [...] x ⌜KU$^?$⌝ [.................. T]I$^?$[..........] x
(NE) i 3 ⌜*ana* TI⌝-*šú* ^{na4}KA.GI.NA.DAB.BA →

9’ NF i’ 9’ [................ ^{na4}AN.ZA]H$^?$.GE$_6$ ^{na4}*mu-ṣa* ⌜^{na4}ZÁLAG⌝ ^{na4}GUG ^{n}[^{a4} x (x)]
(NE) i 3f. ^{na4}AN.NA ^{na4}AN.Z[AH.GE$_6$ ...] / ⌜^{na4}*mu-ṣa*⌝ ^{na4}ZÁLAG ^{na4}ZA.GÌN ^{na4}ŠUBA →

10’ NF i’ 10’ [............. ^{na4}A]N$^?$.NA ^{na4}MUŠ.GÍR ⌜NUMUN⌝ ^{giš}*bi-ni* NUMUN ^{giš}⌜MA.NU⌝
(NE) i 4f. NA$_4$ BAL URUDU.NITA N[A$_4$ ...] / [NUMUN ^{giš}Š]INIG NUMUN ^{giš}MA.NU →

11’ NF i’ 11’ [......... Ú.M]EŠ ŠEŠ 1-*niš* GAZ *ta-ša-pah ina* Ì.UDU ÉLLAG GU$_4$ GE$_6$
(NE) i 5 NUMUN *áš-li* NITA ^{na4}*ás-ha*[*r* ...]
(NE) i 6 [*ta-š*]*a-pah ina* Ì.UDU ÉLLAG GU$_4$ GE$_6$ →

12’ NF i’ 12’ [............................... IG]I.MEŠ-*šú ka-a-a-man-nam-ma* MAR-*ma ina-eš*
(NE) i 6 GIN$_7$ *kám-ma ina* UGU URUDU SÚD-*m*[*a* ...]

13’ [*šumma amēlu enūma birṣa*] *ītanammaru šalāšīšu kīam liqbi ša Enlil u Ninlil*	[13’][If a man] constantly [sees a flash of light:] he should say three times as follows: ‘[14’]I belong to [13’]Enlil and Ninlil,
14’ [*anāku ša Ištar u Nanāya*$^?$] *anāku iqabbīma iballuṭ*	[14’][I belong to Ištar and Nanaya$^?$].’ He says this, then he should recover.

Overview of Manuscripts and Parallels concerning NF (BAM 520): **AI**=LKA 145; **AJ**=BAM 216; **AK**=AO 11447; **dk**=Sumer 9/29; **NE**=BAM 516; **NF**=BAM 520 (+); **NL**=AMT 49/4; **NM**=BAM 489+508; **NN**=K 6329; **NO**=K 8211+... (+) BM 98589...; **NT**=AMT 85/2; **NX**=BAM 482; **NXa**=AMT 19/1; **sA**=IRAQ 65; **uC**=SpTU22+; **XA**=BM 123362

13' NF i' 13' [DIŠ NA *e-nu-ma bir-ṣ*]*a* ⌜IGI-*ru*⌝ 3-*šú ki-a-am liq-bi šá* $^{d+}$*En-líl u* ^{d}*Nin-líl*
(uC) i 18f. DIŠ NA *e-nu-ma bir-ṣi i-ta-nam-ma-ru ki-a-am* DUG$_4$.GA / *šá* $^{d+}$*En-líl u* ^{d}*Nin-líl*
(NT) 4' DIŠ NA *ina* IGI.MEŠ-*šú bir-ṣi* I[GI(.IGI)-*mar* ....]

14' NF i' 14' [*ana-ku šá* ^{d}*Iš-tar u* ^{d}*Na-na-a*] *ana-ku i-qab-bi-ma* TI-*uṭ*
(uC) i 19f. *ana-ku šá* ^{d}*Iš-tar u* ^{d}*Na-na-a ana-ku / šá* ^{d}*Uraš u* ^{d}*Nin-é-gal ana-ku* 3-*šú* DUG$_4$.GA-*ma* DIN

15' [*šumma* ... *ana imitti*] *izzizzu teleqqe ina išāti tukabbab* **16'** [... *ina*] *dišpi himēti tasâk īnīšu teqqīma ina'eš*	$^{15'}$[If ...] you take [...] which stands [on the right] and you burn (it) in the fire. $^{16'}$[...] You pound (it) [in] honey and ghee. You daub his eyes and then he should get better.

15' NF i' 15' [DIŠ .... *ana* ZA]G$^{?}$ GUB-*zu* TI-*qé ina* IZI *tu-kab-ba-ab*
(NT) 6' GUB-*zu* TI-*qé ina* IZI *t*[*u-kab-ba-ab* ....]

16' NF i' 16' [.......................... *ina* L]ÀL Ì.NUN SÚD IGI.MIN-*šú te-eq-qí-ma ina-eš*

17' [... *lumun birṣi*] *ana amēli lā ṭehê agubbâ tukān ana libbi bīna maštakal* **18'** [(...) *sikilla gišimmara*] *ēra ašūha hašhūra titta šunâ nikipta zikar u sinniš* **19'** [(...) *ina kakkabi tušbât ina*] *šēri pān Šamaš ina bīti ṭābi tarammukšu kalâ kalgukka imbu' tâmti* **20'** [(...) *ina šaman asi taballal*] *tapaššassuma kaspa hurāṣa īmarma lumun birṣi ana amēli lā iṭehhe*	$^{17'}$[...] in order that [the evil of a flash of light] does not approach a man. You set up a holy water vessel (and you put) in (it) tamarisk, *maštakal*-plant, [(...) $^{18'}$*sikillu*-plant, date palm], *ēru*-tree, *ašūhu*-pine, apple, a fig, *šunû*-tree, male and female *nikiptu*-plant $^{19'}$[... and let (them) stay under a star (= stay overnight). In] the morning, in front of the Sun-god, in a friendly house you wash him. ^{20}[In oil of *asu*-aromatic you mix] $^{19'}$*kalû*-paste, *kalgukku*-red paste, algae, ^{20}you anoint him and he shall look upon silver and gold, and then the evil of a flash of light will not approach a man.

Overview of Manuscripts and Parallels concerning NF (BAM 520): **AI**=LKA 145; **AJ**=BAM 216; **AK**=AO 11447; **dk**=Sumer 9/29; **NE**=BAM 516; **NF**=BAM 520 (+); **NL**=AMT 49/4; **NM**=BAM 489+508; **NN**=K 6329; **NO**=K 8211+... (+) BM 98589...; **NT**=AMT 85/2; **NX**=BAM 482; **NXa**=AMT 19/1; **sA**=IRAQ 65; **uC**=SpTU22+; **XA**=BM 123362

17’ NF i’ 17’ [... HUL *bir-ṣ*]*i*$^{?}$ ⸢*a-na* LÚ NU TE-*e* A.GÚB.BA GIN-*an ana* ŠÀ-*bi* ^{giš}ŠINIG⸣ ^{ú}IN$_{6}$.ÚŠ

18’ NF i’ 18’ [(...) ^{ú}SIKIL ^{giš}GIŠIMMAR $^{gi]š}$MA.NU ^{giš}Ù.SUH$_{5}$ ^{giš}HAŠHUR ^{giš}PÈŠ ^{giš}ŠE.NÚ.A $^{šim\ d}$MAŠ NÍTA *u* MUNUS

19’ NF i’ 19’ [(...) *ina* UL *tuš-bat ina* Á.G]Ú.ZI.GA IGI ^{d}UTU *ina* É *ṭa-bi* TU$_{5}$-*šú* ^{im}KAL ^{im}KAL.GUG KA.A.AB.BA

20’ NF i’ 20’ [(...) *ina* Ì ^{šim}GÍR HE.HE Š]É[Š$^{?}$-*s*]*u*$^{?}$-⸢*ma*$^{?}$ KÙ.BABBAR KUG⸣.GI *i-mar-ma* HUL *bir-ṣi ana* LÚ NU TE

21’ [*šumma* ...] ... [*bīna maštakal gišimmara*] *hašhūra titta ašūha ana libbi mê būrti tanaddīma* **22’** [(...) *ina kakkabi tušbât ina*] *šēri* [...] *kalâ kalgukka imbuʾ tâmti ina šaman ballukki* **23’** [*taballal tapaššassuma*] *ṣubāta ebba* [...] *lumun birṣi ana amēli lā iṭehhe*	21’[If ...] ... you throw in well water [tamarisk, *maštakal*-plant, date palm], apple, a fig, *ašūhu*-pine. 22’[(...) and let (them) stay under a star (= stay overnight). In] the morning 23’[you mix] 22’*kalû*-paste, *kalgukku*-red paste in oil of *ballukku*-aromatic. 23’[You anoint him and you ...] pure cloth, (and then) the evil of a flash of light will not approach a man.

21’ NF i’ 21’ [DIŠ ...] x x [^{giš}ŠINIG ^{ú}IN$_{6}$.ÚŠ ^{giš}GIŠIMMA]R$^{?}$ ⸢^{giš}HAŠHUR$^{?}$⸣ ^{giš}PÈŠ ^{giš}Ù.SUH$_{5}$ *ana* ŠÀ A PÚ ŠUB-*di-ma*

22’ NF i’ 22’ [(...) *ina* UL *tuš-bat ina*] ⸢Á.GÚ.Z[I.GA .... ^{im}KA]L ⸢^{im}KAL.GUG⸣ KA.A.AB.BA *ina* Ì ^{šim}BAL

23’ NF i’ 23’ [HE.HE ŠÉŠ-*su-ma* TÚ]G DADA[G ....] ⸢HUL⸣ *bir-ṣi ana* LÚ NU TE

24’ NF i’ 24’ traces

BREAK OF UNKNOWN LENGTH!

25’ NF ii’ 1’ x x [..]

26’ *šumma amēlu mukīl rēš* [*lemutti iṣbassu* ...] **27’** *lū zikara lū sinništa ina ūri tušēlīma* [...]	26’If a supporter-of-[evil seized] a man [...] 27’You shall have either a man or a woman climb on to the roof, and [...]. 28’May (it) be left behind. In the night, as soon as the sun [sets ...]. 29’You set

Overview of Manuscripts and Parallels concerning NF (BAM 520): **AI**=LKA 145; **AJ**=BAM 216; **AK**=AO 11447; **dk**=Sumer 9/29; **NE**=BAM 516; **NF**=BAM 520 (+); **NL**=AMT 49/4; **NM**=BAM 489+508; **NN**=K 6329; **NO**=K 8211+... (+) BM 98589...; **NT**=AMT 85/2; **NX**=BAM 482; **NXa**=AMT 19/1; **sA**=IRAQ 65; **uC**=SpTU22+; **XA**=BM 123362

28’ *linnaddi ina mūši kīma Šamaš* [*erēbi* ...] **29’** *mahar apti zidubdubbâ tattanaddi* [...] **30’** *ul ipettūšu* [...] **31’** *u mūšu šâti eršu ṣallu* [...]	out constantly small heaps of flour in front of the window [...]. [30’]They shall not open it [...]. [31’]and that night, the reclining bed [...]

26’ NF ii’ 2’ DIŠ NA *mu-*⸢*kíl*⸣ S[AG HUL-*tì* DAB-*su* ....]

27’ NF ii’ 3’ *lu* NITA *lu* MUNUS ⸢*ina* ÙR *tu-še*⸣*-l*[*i-ma* ....]

28’ NF ii’ 4’ *li-in-*⸢*na-di*⸣ *ina* GE$_6$ GIN$_7$ ^{d}UTU ⸢*e*⸣*-*[*re-bi* ....]

29’ NF ii’ 5’ IGI *ap-ti* ZÌ.DUB.DUB.BU ŠUB.ŠU[B-*di* ....]

30’ NF ii’ 6’ NU *i-pet-tu-šu* [...]

31’ NF ii’ 7’ *ù mu-šu ša-*⸢*a*⸣*-ti* ^{giš}NÁ *ṣa-al-lu* x [..]

(XA) ii’ 8’ [............... ^{giš}N]Á ⸢*ṣa-al-lu la* x x MA BAL x U⸣ x [...............................]

32’ *šumma amēlu mukīl rēš lemutti iṣbassu mašqīta narmakta* [...] **33’** *ana ašri šanîmma ummu ina zumrīšu lazizma u magal ilihhib* x [...] **34’** *u zūta iraššì mê bāqili u šīnāti amēlūti erēna burāša* [...] **35’** *ina tinūri tesekker irtanahhaṣma ešeret* SILA$_x$(KISAL) *ašāga* ... [...]	[32’]If a supporter-of-evil seized a man: a potion, a bath [and ...]. [33’]Alternatively: (=if a supporter-of-evil seized a man) and *ummu*-fever persists constantly in his body, and he growls loudly [...], [34’]and he sweats. [35’]You heat up [34’]maltster-water and human urine, cedar, *burāšu*-juniper, [tree-cone ...] [35’]in a tannour-oven. It (the mixture) shall be continually drenched, and [you ...] 10 SILA-measures of *ašāgu*-acacia [...].

32’ NF ii’ 8’ DIŠ NA *mu-kíl* SAG HUL-*tì* DAB-*su maš-qí-ta nar-ma-ak-t*[*a* ....]
(XA) ii’ 9 [.. D]AB ⸢*maš-qí-ta nar*$^{?}$⸣-.................. [.........]

33’ NF ii’ 9’ DIŠ KIMIN KÚM *ina* SU-*šú la-zi-iz-ma u ma-gal i-li-hi-ib* x [.................]

Overview of Manuscripts and Parallels concerning NF (BAM 520): **AI**=LKA 145; **AJ**=BAM 216; **AK**=AO 11447; **dk**=Sumer 9/29; **NE**=BAM 516; **NF**=BAM 520 (+); **NL**=AMT 49/4; **NM**=BAM 489+508; **NN**=K 6329; **NO**=K 8211+... (+) BM 98589...; **NT**=AMT 85/2; **NX**=BAM 482; **NXa**=AMT 19/1; **sA**=IRAQ 65; **uC**=SpTU22+; **XA**=BM 123362

(XA) ii' 10f.'[.................................... *l*]*a*-⸢*zi-iz-ma u*$^{?}$ *ma*$^{?}$⸣-*g*[*al*]$^{?}$ ⸢*i*⸣-[*l*]*i*-⸢*ib*⸣ KA-*šú*⸣ x [...] / [...] x MA →
(NL) iv 2' [... DIŠ KI]MIN KÚM ⸢*ina* SU-*šú*⸣ *l*[*a*$^{?}$ ....]

34' NF ii' 10' *u* IR TUK A SAR.MUNU$_{6}$ *u* KÀŠ *a-me-lu-ti* ^{giš}EREN ^{šim}L[I$^{?}$ ....]
(XA) ii' 11f.' *u* IR ⸢TUK A SAR$^{?}$.MUNU$_{6}$⸣ [*u* KÀ]Š *a-me-l*[*u-ti* ... / ...] ⸢^{šim}LI$^{?}$ ⸢^{giš}ŠE.Ù.SUH$_{5}$ NAGA$^{?}$.SI$^{?}$⸣x [... D]Ù$^{?}$.⸢A$^{?}$⸣.BI$^{?}$ →

35' NF ii' 11' *ina* NININDU ÚŠ-*er ir-ta-na-haṣ-ma* 10$^{?}$ SILA$_{x}$(KISAL) ^{giš}KIŠI$_{16}$ x x [...]
(XA) ii' 12f.' *ina* NININD[U ÚŠ-*er* / *ir-ta-n*]*a*-⸢*haṣ-ma ina* Ì.GIŠ ^{giš}KIŠI$_{16}$ ... ŠÉŠ-*su-ma*⸣ [... TI$^{?}$]

36' én ur-sag ^{d}asal-lú-hi igi-bi hé-p[à sag-hul-ha-za hé-pà] **37'** ur-sag ^{d}šà-zu igi-bi h[é-pà sag-hul-ha-za hé-pà] /$^{(AI)}$ur-sag ^{d}en-ki-ke$_{4}$ kimin **38'** ur-sag ^{d}en-ki igi-b[i hé-pà sag-hul-ha-za hé-pà] /$^{(AI)}$ ur-sag ^{d}šà-zu kimin **39'** ur-sag ^{d}nin-urta i[gi-bi hé-pà sag-hul-ha-za hé-pà] **40'** ad-da-mu / $^{(var.)}$ ^{d}da-mu / dumu-sag ^{d}[ag-ke$_{4}$ gù mu-un-na-an-dé-e] **41'** dumu-mu nam-tar [...] / $^{(NO)}$ dumu-mu nam ba-ši-in-tal lú igi nu-un-bar-ra **42'** ^{lú}a-zu di-k[u$_{5}$ inim-bi nu-mu-un-tar-ra tu$_{6}$-én] / $^{(AI)}$ ^{lú}a-zu tag-ga [inim]-bi nu-tar-ra tu$_{6}$-én **43'** [ka-inim-ma] sag-hul-ha-za-[kám]	36'Incantation: O hero Asalluhi, may this eye be adjured, [may the supporter-of-evil be adjured!] 37'O Šazu (Marduk), may this eye be adjured, [may the supporter-of-evil be adjured!] / $^{(AI)}$ O hero of Enki, ditto! 38'O hero (of) Enki, may this eye be adjured, [may the supporter-of-evil be adjured!] / $^{(AI)}$ O hero Šazu, ditto! 39'O hero Ninurta, may this eye be adjured, [may the supporter-of-evil be adjured!] 40'My father (var. Dāmu), the first-born son [of Nabû speaks to him.]/ 41' 'My son, the decision has been made (for this case): the man can not see!' 42'The *asû*-physician (is) a judge (who) cannot [decide this case!] / $^{(AI)}$ The attending (lit. touching) *asû*-physician cannot decide this [case]. 43'Incantation spell. [It is an invocation against] the supporter-of-evil!

36' NF ii' 12' én ur-sag ^{d}asal-lú-hi igi-bi hé-p[à ....]
(NM) i' 37' én ur-sag ⸢^{d}⸣ [asal- ....]
(NN) ii' 9f.'⸢én ur⸣-sag ^{d}asal-lú-hi igi-bi hé-⸢pà⸣ / sag-hul-ha-za ⸢hé-pà⸣
(NO) ii 10f.' én ur-sag ^{d}asal-lú-hi igi-bi hé-pà / sag-hul-ha-za hé-pà

Overview of Manuscripts and Parallels concerning NF (BAM 520): **AI**=LKA 145; **AJ**=BAM 216; **AK**=AO 11447; **dk**=Sumer 9/29; **NE**=BAM 516; **NF**=BAM 520 (+); **NL**=AMT 49/4; **NM**=BAM 489+508; **NN**=K 6329; **NO**=K 8211+... (+) BM 98589...; **NT**=AMT 85/2; **NX**=BAM 482; **NXa**=AMT 19/1; **sA**=IRAQ 65; **uC**=SpTU22+; **XA**=BM 123362

(NX) iv 32' ⌜én ur⌝-sag ^{d}asal-lú-hi *š[á* ...]
(NXa) iv 13' [é]n ur-sag ^{d}as[al-lú-hi ...]
(XA) ii' 14' [é]n ur-sag ^{d}asal-lú-hi igi-bi hé-pà sag-hul-ha-za h[é-pà]
(AI) 10 ur-sag ^{d}asal-lú-hi ⌜igi⌝-bi hé-pà sag-hul-ha-za hé-pà
(AJ) 15' [én u]r-sag ^{d}asal-⌜lú⌝-hi ŠID-⌜*nu*⌝
(AK) 19 én ur-sag ^{d}asal-lú-hi *ana* UGU ŠI[D ...]
(sA) i 19 én ur-sag ^{d}asal-lú-hi *i-na* UGU ŠID LAL
(dk) 6' [................................ hé]-pà sag-⌜hul⌝-ha-za ⌜hé⌝-pà

37' NF ii' 13' ur-sag ^{d}šà-zu igi-bi h[é-pà ....]
(NM) i' 38' ur-sag ^{d}š[à ....]
(NN) ii' 11' ur-sag ^{d}šà-zu igi-bi hé-pà sag-hul-h[a- ....]
(NO) ii 12f.' ur-sag ^{d}šà-zu igi-bi hé-pà / sag-hul-ha-za hé-pà
(XA) ii' 15' [u]r-sag ^{d}šà-zu igi-bi hé-⌜pà⌝ →
(AI) 11 ur-sag ^{d}en-ki-ke$_4$ ⌜kimin⌝
(dk) 7' [................................] hé-pà sag-⌜hul⌝-ha-za hé-pà

38' NF ii' 14' ur-sag ^{d}en-ki ⌜igi⌝-b[i hé-pà ....]
(NM) i' 39' ur-sag ^{d}en-k[i ....]
(NN) ii' 12' ur-sag ^{d}en-ki-ke$_4$ igi-bi hé-pà sag-hul [......................]
(NO) ii' 14f.' ur-sag ^{d}en+ki-ke$_4$ igi-bi hé-pà / sag-hul-ha-za hé-pà
(XA) ii' 15' ur-sag ^{d}en-ki igi-bi hé-p[à]
(AI) 12 ur-sag ^{d}šà-zu ki[min]
(dk) 8' [................................ -b]i hé-pà sag-⌜hul⌝-ha-za hé-pà

39' NF ii' 15' ur-sag ^{d}nin-urta i[gi-bi hé-pà ....]
(NM) i' 40' ur-sag ^{d}ni[n-urta ....]
(NN) ii' 13f.' ur-sag ^{d}nin-urta igi-bi h[é-pà] / sag-hul-ha-za [........]
(NO) ii' 16f.' ur-sag ^{d}nin-urta igi-bi hé-pà / sag-hul-ha-za hé-pà
(XA) ii' 16' ur-sag ^{d}nin-urta ⌜igi-bi hé-pà⌝ →
(AI) 13 ur-sag ^{d}nin-urta ⌜igi⌝-bi hé-⌜pà sa[g-hul-ha-za hé-pà]
(dk) 9' [................................ -b]i hé-pà sag-hul-ha-za hé-pà
(dk) 10' [................................]-bi hé-pà sag-hu[l-h]a-za hé-pà
(dk) 11' [................................ sa]g-hul-ha-za [hé]-pà

40' NF ii' 16' ad-da-mu dumu-sag ⌜d⌝ [............... -n]a-an-d[é ....]
(NM) i' 41' ad-mu dumu-sag ⌜d⌝ [..]
(NN) ii' 15' ^{d}da-mu dumu-sag ^{d}ag-ke$_4$ ⌜gù⌝ m[u ....]

Overview of Manuscripts and Parallels concerning NF (BAM 520): **AI**=LKA 145; **AJ**=BAM 216; **AK**=AO 11447; **dk**=Sumer 9/29; **NE**=BAM 516; **NF**=BAM 520 (+); **NL**=AMT 49/4; **NM**=BAM 489+508; **NN**=K 6329; **NO**=K 8211+... (+) BM 98589...; **NT**=AMT 85/2; **NX**=BAM 482; **NXa**=AMT 19/1; **sA**=IRAQ 65; **uC**=SpTU22+; **XA**=BM 123362

(NO) ii' 18' ^{d}da-mu dumu-sag ^{d}ag-ke$_4$ gù mu-un-na-an-dé-e
(XA) ii' 16' ⸢^{d}da-mu dumu-sag ^{d}ag gù mu-un-na⸣-a[n-dé-e]
(AI) 14 ad-da-mu dumu-sag ⸢nam⸣-ma-kal gù x [.................]
(dk) 12' [...................................... g]ù mu-un-na-an-⸢dé$^{?}$⸣-e

41' NF ii' 17' dumu-mu nam-tar [........................] nu-un-b[ar ....]
(NM) i' 42' dumu-mu nam-ba-š[i- ....]
(NN) ii' 16' dumu-mu nam ba-ši-in-[..]
(NO) ii' 19' dumu-mu nam ba-ši-in-tal lú igi nu-un-bar-⸢ra⸣
(XA) ii' 17' dumu-mu nam-tar-meš [..................................] →
(AI) 15 dumu-mu nam ba-ši-in-tal lú igi ⸢bi$^{?}$⸣ [............]
(dk) 13' [..] x lú igi mi-in-bar-re

42' NF ii' 18' ⸢^{lú}a-zu⸣ di-k[u$_5$ ....] nu-tar-re tu[$_6$-én]

(NM) i' 43' ^{lú}a-zu di-ku$_5$ x [...]

(NN) ii' 17' ^{lú}a-zu di-ku$_5$ inim-bi n[u ....]

(NO) ii' 20' ^{lú}a-zu di-ku$_5$ inim-bi nu-mu-un-tar-ra tu$_6$-é[n]

(XA) ii' 17' [...-z]u ⸢di⸣-k[u$_5$ ...]
DIVIDING LINE IS PROBABLE BUT NOT TO BE SEEN!

(AI) r 1 ^{lú}a-zu tag-g[a inim]-⸢bi nu⸣-tar-ra tu[$_6$-én]

(dk) 14' [.. t]ar-⸢re⸣

43' NF ii' 19' ka-inim-⸢ma⸣ sag-hul-ha-za-[kám]

44' *dudubi sebe* [...] *ina ṭurri šīpāti sāmāti tašakkak* [...] **45'** *imhur-līm* [...] *sikillu kiškanû zēr bīni* [...] **46'** [... *talappap*] *ina pūtīšu tarakkassu* [...]	44'Its medical application: you thread seven ... on a cord of red wool [...] 46'[you wrap] 45'*imhur-līm*-plant [...] *sikillu*-plant, *kiškanû*-plant, tamarisk seed [...], 46'you bind it on his forehead [...]

44' NF ii' 20' DÙ.DÙ.BI 7 x [...... *i*]*na* DUR SÍG SA$_5$ È-*ak* Ú x [.......]

45' NF ii' 21' ^{ú}IGI-*l*[*im* ...] x ^{ú}SIKIL *giš-kan-u$_5$* NUMUN ^{giš}ŠINI[G ...]

46' NF ii' 22' x x [... *ta-la-pa*]*p*$^{?}$ *ina* SAG.KI-*šú* KEŠDA-⸢*su*⸣ x [......]

Overview of Manuscripts and Parallels concerning NF (BAM 520): **AI**=LKA 145; **AJ**=BAM 216; **AK**=AO 11447; **dk**=Sumer 9/29; **NE**=BAM 516; **NF**=BAM 520 (+); **NL**=AMT 49/4; **NM**=BAM 489+508; **NN**=K 6329; **NO**=K 8211+... (+) BM 98589...; **NT**=AMT 85/2; **NX**=BAM 482; **NXa**=AMT 19/1; **sA**=IRAQ 65; **uC**=SpTU22+; **XA**=BM 123362

47' NF ii' 23' x [.................................] x x [.................................]

§ IV.2 NK (BAM 518)

Manuscript:	**NK (BAM 518),** collated.
Museum number:	British Museum, BM 121042.
Origin and date:	Nineveh?, 8th–7th century BC.
Type of tablet:	Fragment from the right side of possibly two-column tablet, written in a large Assyrian script. Köcher 1982b: xiii considered the text as coming from Nineveh, which is why he included it in BAM 6. However, the form of the signs and the nature of the fragment might also suggest Assur as the tablet's provenance.
Measurements:	ca. 6,6 × 7,3 × 2 cm.
Copy:	BAM 518.
Photo/CDLI nr.:	Plate 33/P398602.
Literature:	Lambert and Millard 1968: 5; Köcher 1982b: xiii; Fincke 2000: 331; Scurlock and Andersen 2005: 793; Scurlock 2014: 756; Parys 2014: 20, 55ff.; Attia 2015: 38, 59.

Ll. 6ff.', 9ff.'	parallels	AB (BAM 159) iv 9f.', iv 10ff.'	§ I.4
L. 8'		IGI 2, ND (BAM 515) i 10	§ II.1

Edition

1' NK 1' [...] x x x x

2' [...] *kamūna uhūla qarnānâ* **3'** [...] *nīnâ sahlâ eṣemti amēlūti* **4'** [...] *lipi kalīti alpi ina kalli gulgul amēli* **5'** [... *ina*] *pēmti tuqattaršu*	2'[If ... You ...] cumin, horned *uhūlu*-alkali 3'[...] *nīnû*-mint, *sahlû*-plant, 'human bone'. 4'[...] fat from ox kidney in the cranium of a human skull. 5'You fumigate him [with it ... over] charcoal.

2' NK 2' [...] x ⸢úGAMUN⸣ NAGA.SI

3' NK 3' [...] x ⸢úKUR.RA ZÀ.HI.LI⸣ GÌR.PAD.DU NAM.LÚ.U19.LU

4' NK 4' [...] ⸢Ì⸣.UDU ÉLLAG GU4 *ina+kal-li gul-gul* LÚ.U19.LU

5' NK 5' [... *ina* N]E *tu-qat-tar-šu*

6’ [*šumma amēlu īnāšu*] *nuppuhāma šāra leqâ qēm kukri* **7’** [*qēm kasî*] *taqallu qēm labti ina šikari tarabbak īnīšu taṣammid*	$^{6'}$[If man’s eyes are] swollen and affected by wind (lit. taken): $^{7'}$ you roast $^{6'}$ powder of *kukru*-aromatic, $^{7'}$[powder of *kasû*-plant], (and) you make an infusion from flour of roasted grain in beer (and) bandage his eyes.
Alternative prescription 1 **8’** [*šammu peṣû aban*] *gabî emesalli ṭīpu ša īnī*	**Alternative prescription 1** $^{8'}$[White plant,] alum, *emesallu*-saline solution (used as) eye drops.

6’ NK 6’ [.................................. M]Ú.MEŠ-*ma* IM TI.MEŠ ZÌ ^{šim}GÚR.GÚR
(AB) iv 9f.’ [DIŠ N]A IGI.MIN-*šú* MÚ.MEŠ-*ma u* IM *le-qa-a* / [ZÌ ^{š}]^{im}GÚR.GÚR →

7’ NK 7’ [ZÌ GAZI^{sar} BÍ]L-*lu* ZÌ ŠE.⌜SA⌝.A *ina* KAŠ *tara-bak* IGI.MIN-*šú* LAL

(AB) iv 10f.’ ZÌ GAZI^{sar} BÍL.MEŠ ZÌ ŠE.SA.A / [*ina*$^?$ KAŠ$^?$] SAG *tara-bak* IGI.MIN-*šú* LAL

8’ NK 8’ [Ú.BABBAR NA$_4$ *g*]*a-bi-i* ^{mun}*eme-sal-lì ṭi*$_5$*-pu šá* ⌜IGI.MIN.MEŠ⌝

(ND) i 10 Ú.BABBAR NA$_4$ *ga-bi-i* ^{mun}*eme-sal-lì an-nu-ú ṭi-*[*pu šá* IGI.MIN]

More parallels in IGI 2: 10 above.

9’ [*šumma amēlu īnāšu šāra*] *uddupāma ašâ apâ* **10’** [*u dimta ittanaddâ*] *qēm hallūri qēm kakkî* **11’** [(*qēm šunê*) *qēm labti*] *qēm kukri qēm burāši* **12’** [*qēm kasî qēm suādi*] *ištēniš taballal ina mê kasî taṣammid*	$^{9'}$[If man’s eyes] are blown [by wind], and are blurred, cloudy, $^{10'}$[and constantly throwing off tear(s)] $^{12'}$you mix together $^{11'}$powder of chickpea, powder of lentil, $^{11'}$[(powder of *šunû*-tree), flour of roasted grain] powder of *kukru*-aromatic, powder of juniper, $^{12'}$[powder of *kasû*-plant$^?$, powder of *suādu*-aromatic.] (You make an infusion from them) in the sap of a *kasû*-plant (and) bandage (his eyes).

9’ NK 9’ [..................................] ⌜*ud*⌝*-du-pa-a-ma a-šá-a a-pa-a*
(AB) iv 12f.’ DIŠ N[A IGI].MIN-*šú* IM *ud-du-pa-a-ma a-pá-a* / *a-*⌜*šá-a*⌝ →

10’ NK 10’ [..................]-⌜*a*⌝ ZÌ GÚ.GAL ZÌ GÚ.TUR
(AB) iv 13’ ⌜*u*⌝ ÉR ŠUB.ŠUB-*a* ZÌ GÚ.GAL ⌜ZÌ GÚ.TUR⌝

11’ NK 11’ [(ZÌ ^{giš}ŠE.NÚ.A) ZÌ ŠE.SA].⌜A⌝ ZÌ ^{šim}GÚR.GÚR ZÌ ^{šim}LI
(AB) iv 14f.’ ZÌ ⌜^{ú}⌝ [ŠE.DÙ].⌜A ZÌ ŠE⌝.SA.A ZÌ GAZI^{sar} ZÌ ^{šim}GÚR.GÚR / ZÌ ^{šim}⌜LI⌝ →

12’ NK 12’ [ZÌ GAZI^{sar} ZÌ ^{šim}MAN.DU 1-*n*]*iš* HE.HE *ina* A GAZI^{sar} LAL
(AB) iv 15f.’ ⌜ZÌ ^{šim}⌝MAN.DU 1-*niš* HE.HE / *ina* A GAZI⌜^{sar} *tara-bak* SAG.KI.MIN-*šú* IGI.MIN-*šú* LAL-*ma* TI⌝

13’ [...] *erbēt šiqil qēm hallūri erbēt šiqil qēm kakkî* 14’ [...*erbēt*] *šiqil sahlê šumma kūṣu* 15’ [...] *uznīšu u īnīšu taṣammid* 16’ [...] *ballukku*? *kukru kasû* 17’ [...]	13’[...] four shekels powder of chickpea, four shekels powder of lentil, 14’[... four] shekels of *sahlû*-plant. When it is winter 15’[...] you bandage his ears and eyes. 16’[...] *ballukku*-aromatic, *kukru*-aromatic, *kasû*-plant. 17’ ...

13’ NK 13’ [...] ⌜4⌝ GÍN ZÌ GÚ.GAL 4 GÍN ZÌ GÚ.⌜TUR⌝

14’ NK 14’ [.. G]ÍN *sah-le-e šum*$_4$*-ma* EN.TE.⌜NA⌝

15’ NK 15’ [...] ⌜GEŠ.TÚG.MIN-*šú u* IGI.MIN⌝-*šú* LAL

16’ NK 16’ [.. ^{ši}]$^{m?}$MUG? ⌜^{šim}GÚR.GÚR GAZI^{sar}⌝

17’ NK 17’ [...] x

§ IV.3 NP (BAM 517)

Manuscript: **NP (BAM 517)**, collated.
Museum number: British Museum, K 10280.
Origin and date: Nineveh?, 7th century BC.
Type of tablet: Fragment from the right side of a two-column tablet. Written in big Assyrian script. As is the case with Ms. **NK (BAM 518)**, the origin might be Assur and not Nineveh.
Measurements: ca. 4,7 × 3,4 × 2,5 cm.
Copy: BAM 517.
Photo/CDLI nr.: Plate 33/P398602.
Literature: Köcher 1980b: xiii.

Edition

Obverse?

1' [...] x **2'** [...] *tasâk teqqi*	1'[...] x 2'[...] you pound (it and) daub (his eyes).

1' NP 1' [...] x

2' NP 2' [... SÚ]D ⌜MAR⌝

3' [...] *tasâk teqqi*	3'[...] you pound (it and) daub (his eyes).

3' NP 3' [.. SÚ]D MAR

4' [...] *tasâk teqqi*	4'[...] you pound (it and) daub (his eyes).

4' NP 4' [.. S]ÚD MAR

5' [...] *tasâk teqqi*	5'[...] you pound (it and) daub (his eyes).

5' NP 5' [.. S]ÚD MAR

6' [...] *taṣammid* **7'** [...] *īnīšu teqqi* **8'** [...] *teqqi*	6'[...] you bandage. 7'[...] and daub his eyes. 8'[...] (and) daub (his eyes).

6' NP 6' [...] x LAL

7' NP 7' [.. IGI].⌜MIN-*šú*⌝ MAR

8' NP 8' [.. R]I? ⌜MAR⌝

Reverse?

1' [*šiptu* ...] *izzazzu/ū* **2'** [...] ... **3'** [... *tê*] *šipti*	1'[Incantation ... which/they] stand/s, 2'[...] ... 3'[... (Incantation)] spell.

1' NP r.?1' [ÉN .... GU]B-*zu*

2' NP r.?2' [...] x SI

3’	NP r.[?]3’	[.. (TU_6.)] ⌜ÉN⌝
4’	NP r.[?]4’	[...] x

§ IV.4 NQ (BAM 521)

Manuscript:	**NQ (BAM 521)**, collated.
Museum number:	British Museum, K 5954.
Origin and date:	Nineveh, 7th century BC.
Type of tablet:	Flake from the middle of a neatly written tablet in large Late Assyrian script.
Measurements:	ca. 4,1 × 4 × 0,9 cm.
Copy:	BAM 521.
Photo/CDLI nr.:	Plate 34/P396287.
Literature:	Köcher 1980b: xiv; Fincke 2000: 331; Scurlock and Andersen 2005: 794; Parys 2014: 20; Scurlock 2014: 756.

Ll. 5’, 10ff.’	parallels	AB (BAM 159) iv 13’, 17ff.’	§ I.4
L. 8’		IGI 1, NA (BAM 510) i 30’	§ I.1
Ll. 10ff.’		NS (AMT 18/4) 1ff.’	§ IV.6
Ll. 11ff.		bB (BAM 382) 9ff.	§ II.4

Edition

1’ [...] x [...] **2’** [...] x [...] **3’** [...] *šammi aši* [...] **4’** [...] ... [...]	[1’][...] x [...] [2’][...] x [...] [3’][...] *ašû*-disease-plant, [4’][...] x [...]

1’	NQ 1’	[...............] x [..]
2’	NQ 2’	[...............] x R[A ....]
3’	NQ 3’	[................ Ú] ⌜*a*⌝-*ši-i* [...]
4’	NQ 4’	[.............] x PI [...]

5' [*šumma amēlu īnāšu abâ*] *ašâ*$^{?}$ *u dimta ittanaddâ* [...] **6'** [...] ... [...] **7'** [...] *īnā marṣā* [...]	5'[If a man's eyes are cloudy], blurred and are constantly giving off tear(s) [...]. 6'[...] ... [...] 7'[...] sick eyes [...]

5' NQ 5' [............................ *a-šá*]*-a u* ÉR Š[UB.ŠUB-*a* ....]
(AB) iv 13' *a-˹šá-a u˺* ÉR ŠUB.ŠUB-*a* ...
(AB) iv 17' DIŠ NA IGI.MIN-*šú a-˹ba-a a-šá-a u˺* ÉR ŠUB.ŠUB-*a* ...

6' NQ 6' [..........] x RI [..]
7' NQ 7' [........ IG]I$^{?}$.MIN GIG [...]

8' [*šumma amēlu*] *īnāšu marṣā sahlê* [*ina šizbi tušabšal* ...] **9'** [...] *šuršummī šikari rūšti* [...]	8'[If man's] eyes are sick: [you boil] *sahlû*-plant [in milk ...] 9'[...] dregs of premium beer [...].

8' NQ 8' [DIŠ NA IGI.MIN]-*šú* GIG *sah-lé-˹e˺* [....................................]
(NA) i 30' [... : DIŠ NA] ˹IGI.MIN-*šú* GIG *sah-lé˺-e ina* GA ŠEG$_6$-*šal* LAL

more parallels in IGI 1: 35' above

9' NQ 9' [........................... *šur-šu*]*m-mi* KAŠ.SAG [...]

10' [*šumma amēlu īnāšu*] *apâ ašâ u dimta ittanaddâ* [*naṭāla*] **11'** [*muṭṭu ana bulluṭīšu*] *murra šamma peṣâ rikibti arkabi* [...] **12'** [*emesalli kukra šammi ašî*] *nīnâ* [*tasâk* ...]	10'[If man's eyes are] cloudy, blurred, and constantly giving off tear(s), [(and his) seeing ability 11'is diminished. In order to heal it: 12'you pound] 11'bitter-plant, white plant, bat guano [...] 12'[*emesallu*-saline solution, *kukru*-aromatic, *ašû*-disease-plant], *nīnû*-mint' [...]

10' NQ 10' [.......................... *a-p*]*a-a a-šá-a u* ÉR Š[UB.ŠUB-*a* ....]
(AB) iv 17' DIŠ NA IGI.MIN-*šú a-˹ba-a a-šá-a u˺* ÉR ŠUB.ŠUB-*a na-ṭa-la*
(NS) 1' ˹DIŠ NA˺ [IGI.MIN-*š*]*ú ˹a-pa-a˺* [...]

11' NQ 11' [............................ ^{šim}S]ES ˹Ú˺.BABBAR U$_5$.ARGAB[^{mušen} ...]
(AB) iv 18' *mu-uṭ-ṭu ana* TI-*šú* ˹^{šim}˺SES Ú.BABBAR U$_5$.ARGAB^{mušen}
(NS) 2' ˹^{šim}˺SES Ú.BABBAR ˹U$_5^{?}$˺.[ARGAB^{mušen} ...]
(bB) r.1 ^{šim}SES Ú.BABBAR ˹U$_5$˺.ARGAB^{mušen} →

12' NQ 12' [..] ˹^{ú}KUR.RA˺ [SÚD ....]
(AB) iv 19' ^{mun}*eme-sal-lì* ^{šim}GÚR.˹GÚR˺ Ú *a-ši-i* ^{ú}KUR.RA
(NS) 3' Ú *a-ši-i* ^{ú}˹KUR.RA˺ [.............................]
(bB) r.1f. ^{mun}*eme-sal-la* / ^{ú}GÚR.GÚR Ú *a-˹ši˺-i* ^{ú}KUR.RA^{sar}

§ IV.5 NR (BAM 522) and NRa (K 19831)

Manuscript:	**NR (BAM 522)**, collated.
Museum number:	British Museum, K 11695 + K 11805.
Origin and date:	Nineveh, 7th century BC.
Type of tablet:	A flake from the middle of a neatly written tablet in medium large Late Assyrian script. The script is very similar to ms. NA, BAM 510 (IGI 1). On the other hand, according to Köcher 1980b: xiv fn. 22, **NR** might belong to ms. NE, BAM 516 (IGI 3), thus NRa (below) might be a duplicate of IGI 3.
Measurements:	ca. 5,7 × 3,5 × 0,5 cm.
Copy:	BAM 522.
Photo/CDLI nr.:	Plate 34/P396287.
Literature:	Köcher 1980b: xiv; Fincke 2000: 331; Scurlock and Andersen 2005: 794; Attia 2015: 42.

Manuscript:	**NRa (K 19831)**, photo-collated.
Museum number:	British Museum, K 19831.
Origin and date:	Nineveh, 7th century BC.
Type of tablet:	A flake duplicating NR (BAM 522).
Photo/CDLI nr.:	P404600
Literature:	Discovered via eBL, recorded as a duplicate to NR (BAM 522) by Henry Stadhouders.

Edition

1’ [...] x x [...] **2’** [...] *tasâk*? *īnīšu teqqi ashar aban gabî* [...]	1’[...] x x [...] 2’[...] you pound and daub his eyes: *ashar*-stone, alum [...]

1’	NR 1’	[...] x x [..................]
2’	NR 2’	[................ SÚ]D? ⌜IGI.MIN-*šú* MAR na4⌝*às-har* NA4 *ga-bi-*⌜*i*⌝ x [............]

3’ [*šumma amēlu īnīšu dāma*] *iṭrīma izziz marat immeri lipâ sāma ina ṭābti tušnâl*/*tuštāl* **4’** [...] *aktam ina himēti tasâk teqqi ashar ina himēti* [*tasâk teqqi*]	3’[If man’s eyes] oozed [blood] and it stays: you cure the gall-bladder of a sheep and red fat in salt [...]. 4’[...] You pound ... (and) *aktam*-plant in ghee (and) daub (his eyes); [you pound] *ashar*-stone in ghee (and) [daub (his eyes)].

3' NR 3' [DIŠ NA IGI.MIN-*šú* MÚD *iṭ-r*]*i*?-⌜*ma*⌝ GUB-*iz* ZÍ UDU.NÍTA Ì.⌜UDU⌝ SA₅ *ina* MUN NÁ-*al* x [...]

NRa 1' [..] x ⌜Ì.UDU SA₅ *ina* MUN NÁ-*al*⌝ x [...]

4' NR 4' [........................... ᵘ*a*]*k-tam ina* Ì.NUN SÚD MAR ⌜ⁿᵃ⁴⌝*às-har ina* Ì.NUN [SÚD MAR]

NRa 2' [.. S]ÚD MAR ⌜ⁿᵃ⁴*as*⌝-*har ina* Ì.NUN SÚD M[AR]

5' [*šumma amēlu īnīšu*] *dāma iṭrīma izziz murra ina šizbi musukkati ša zikara* [*ūlidu tasâk īnīšu teqqi*]	5'[If man's eyes] oozed blood and it stayed: [you pound] bitter-plant in the milk from a woman in maternity, who [gave birth] to a male [and daub his eyes]

5' NR 5' [DIŠ NA IGI.MIN-*šú* MÚ]D *iṭ-ri-ma* GUB-*iz* ˢⁱᵐSES ⌜*ina* GA⌝ ᵐᵘⁿᵘˢÚ.ZÚG ⌜*šá* NITA Ù?⌝ [.TU SÚD IGI.MIN-*šú* MAR]

NRa 3' [.. *ina* G]A ᵐᵘⁿᵘˢÚ.ZÚG *ša* NITA *ul-du ta-s*[*àk* ....]

6' [*šumma amēlu*] *īnīšu dāma ṭiri dalhā nīnâ šamma peṣâ uhūla qarnānâ atā'iša sahlâ* [...] **7'** [... *aban*] *gabî kammu ištēniš tamarraq šumma kūṣu ina šikari tasappan* ... **8'** [... *ina*] *mê temessi talâš ina tinūri teppi tušellâmma ina himēti*? [...] **9'** [...] *tābīla* [...]	6'[If] blood oozed [(from) man's] eyes (and) they are troubled: 7'you grind together 6'*nīnû*-mint, white plant, horned *uhūlu*-alkali, *atā'išu*-plant, *sahlû*-plant ... 7'[...] alum (and) *kammu*-tanning-fungus. When it is winter you [soften (it)] in beer, 8'[(and) when it is summer in ...]. You wash [(it) in] water, knead (it, and) bake (it) in a tannour-oven. You remove (it), and you [...] in ghee? [...] 9'[...] in a dry state [...]

6' NR 6' [DIŠ NA IGI.M]IN-*šú* MÚD *ṭi-ri* LÙ.MEŠ ᵘKUR.RA? ⌜Ú⌝.BABBAR NAGA.SI ⌜ᵘKUR⌝.KU[R ...]

NRa 4' [..] ⌜Ú⌝.BABBAR NAGA.⌜SI ᵘ⌝KUR.KUR ZÀ.HI.L[Iˢᵃʳ ...]

7' NR 7' [... N]A₄ *ga-bi-i kam-mu* 1-*niš ta-mar-ra*[*q š*]*um₄-ma* EN.TE.NA *ina* ⌜KAŠ⌝ [...]

NRa 5' [.. EN.T]E.⸢NA⸣ *ina* KAŠ *t*[*a-sa-pan* ...]

8' NR 8' [... *ina*] ⸢A⸣ LUH SILA$_{11}$-*aš ina* NININDU *te-*⸢*pi* E$_{11}$⸣-*ma ina* ⸢Ì⸣.N[UN$^{?}$ ...]
NRa 6' [...] x x [...]

9' NR 9' [...................... *ta-bi-l*]*a*$_{12}$$^{?}$ [...]

10' [*šumma amēlu īnīšu dāma*] *iṭrīma izziz* [...]	10'[If man's eyes] oozed [blood] and it stays [...]

10' NR 10' [DIŠ NA IGI.MIN-*šú* MÚD *i*]*ṭ-ri-ma* G[UB-*iz* ....]

11' [...] *kasû*-plant [...]	11'[...] *kasû*-plant [...]

11' NR 11' [............................... GA]ZI^{sar} [..]

§ IV.6 NS (AMT 18/4)

Manuscript:	**NS (AMT 18/4)**, collated.
Museum number:	British Museum, K 9555.
Origin and date:	Nineveh, 7th century BC.
Type of tablet:	Flake from the left side of a one or possibly two-column tablet.
Measurements:	3,2 × 4,7 × 1,5 cm.
Copy:	AMT 18/4.
Photo/CDLI nr.:	Plate 34/P398184.
Literature:	Köcher 1980b: xiii; Fincke 2000: 331; Scurlock and Andersen 2005: 779; Parys 2014: 20; Scurlock 2014: 751; Attia 2015: 75, 82.

Ll. 1ff.'	parallels	NQ (BAM 521) 10ff.'	§ IV.6
Ll. 1ff.'		AB (BAM 159) iv 17ff.'	§ I.4
Ll. 2ff.		bB (BAM 382) 9ff.	§ II. 4
Ll. 6ff.'		IGI 3, NE (BAM 516) ii 6f.'	§ III.1

Edition

1' *šumma amēlu* [*īnāšu*] *apâ* [*ašâ u dimta ittanaddâ naṭāla muṭṭu ana bulluṭīšu*]	1'If a man's [eyes] are cloudy [blurred, and constantly giving off tear(s), (and his) seeing ability is diminished. In order to heal it:] 2'bitter-plant, white

2’ *murru šammu peṣû rikibti* [*arkabi emesalli kukru*] **3’** *šammi ašî nīnû* [*sebet šammī annûti rebiat*] **4’** *ina pāni Šamaš ina gišrinni bīti tašakkan* [*ina dišpi tasâk īnīšu teqqi*] **5’** *ašar šanîmma tābīla teṭeppima* [...]	plant [bat] guano, [*emesallu*-saline solution, *kukru*-aromatic] 3’*ašû*-disease-plant, *nīnû*-mint. 4’You put [3’one fourth (shekel?) of these seven plants] on a domestic scale in front of the sun. [You pound (the drugs) in honey and daub his eyes.] 5’ditto, you administer (the medication) in a dry state and ... [...]

1’ NS 1’ ⸢DIŠ NA⸣ [IGI.MIN-*š*]*ú* ⸢*a-pa-a*⸣ [...]
(AB) iv 17f.’ DIŠ NA IGI.MIN-*šú a*-⸢*ba-a a-šá-a u*⸣ ÉR ŠUB.ŠUB-*a na-ṭa-la* / *mu-uṭ-ṭu ana* TI-*šú*
(NQ) 10f.’ [........................ *a-p*]*a-a a-šá-a u* ÉR Š[UB.ŠUB-*a* /...........................]

2’ NS 2’ ⸢^{šim}⸣SES Ú.BABBAR ⸢U$_5$$^{?}$⸣.[ARGAB^{mušen} ....]
(AB) iv 18f.’ ⸢^{šim}⸣SES Ú.BABBAR U$_5$.ARGAB^{mušen} / ^{mun}*eme-sal-lì* ^{šim}GÚR.⸢GÚR⸣
(NQ) 11f.’ [^{šim}S]ES ⸢Ú⸣.BABBAR U$_5$.ARGAB[^{mušen} ....]
(bB) r.1f. ^{šim}SES Ú.BABBAR ⸢U$_5$⸣.ARGAB^{mušen} ^{mun}*eme-sal-la* / ^{ú}GÚR.GÚR

3’ NS 3’ Ú *a-ši-i* ^{ú}⸢KUR.RA⸣ [...]
(AB) iv 19f.’ Ú *a-ši-i* ^{ú}KUR.RA / 7 Ú.HI.A ŠEŠ IGI.4.GÁL.LA.⸢TA⸣.ÀM
(NQ) 12’ [....] ⸢^{ú}KUR.RA⸣ [..]
(bB) r.2 Ú *a*-⸢*ši*⸣-*i* ^{ú}KUR.RA^{sar}

4’ NS 4’ *ina* IGI ^{d}UTU *ina* GIŠ.ERÍN É GAR [...]
(AB) iv 20f.’ *ina* IGI ^{d}UTU$^{?}$ / *ina* GIŠ.ERÍN LAL-*al ina* LÀL SÚD ⸢IGI⸣.MIN-*šú* MAR

5’ NS 5’ KIMIN *ta-bi-la te-ṭep-pi*-⸢*ma*⸣ x [...]

6’ *šumma amēlu īnāšu lā inaṭṭalā amēlu* [*šū ṣēta hamiṭ ištēn šiqil rikibti arkabi*] **7’** *mišil šiqil šamma peṣâ rebiat* [*emesalli ina dišip šadê*] **8’** *u himēti tasâk* ... [*īnīšu teqqi* ...]	6’If a man’s eyes cannot see: [that] man [is inflamed with sun heat]: 8’you pound [6’one shekel of bat guano], 7’half shekel of white plant, (and) one fourth (shekel) of [*emesallu*-saline solution in mountain honey] 8’and in ghee, ... [you daub his eyes (with it) ...]

6’ NS 6’ DIŠ NA IGI.MIN-*šú la ina-ṭa-la* N[A BI ....]
(NE) ii 6’ DIŠ NA IGI.MIN-*šú la ina-ṭa-la* NA BI UD.DA TAB.⸢BA 1 GÍN U$_5$.ARGAB⸣^{mušen}

7’ NS 7’ 1/2 GÍN Ú.⸢BABBAR⸣ IGI.4.GÁL.[LA ....]

(NE) ii 7' 1/2 GÍN Ú.BABBAR IGI.4.GÁL.LA ^mun^*eme-sal-lì ina* ⌜LÀL⌝.KUR →

8' NS 8' *u* Ì.NUN S[ÚD] x [..]

NO DIVIDING LINE TO BE SEEN!

(NE) ii 7' *u* Ì.N[UN SÚD I]GI.MIN-*šú* MAR

§ IV.7 NT (AMT 85/2)

Manuscript:	**NT (AMT 85/2)**, collated.
Museum number:	British Museum, K 2557.
Origin and date:	Nineveh, 7th century BC.
Type of tablet:	Flake from the left side of one or possibly two-column tablet.
Measurements:	ca. 5 × 3 × 2,8 cm.
Copy:	AMT 85/2.
Photo/CDLI nr.:	Plate 34/P394510.
Literature:	Stol 1993: 73 fn. 63; Fincke 2000: 328; Scurlock and Andersen 2005: 782; Scurlock 2006: nos. 122, 129, 130 and 303; Scurlock 2008b: 197.

L. 4'	parallels	NF (BAM 520) i' 13'	§ IV.1
		uC (SpTU 22+85) i 18f.	§ IV.1.3
L. 6'		NF (BAM 520) i' 15'	§ IV.1

Edition

1' *itti x* [...] **2'** *u minât šēri* [...] **3'** *ina abi u ṭebēti teppušma* ... [...]	... ^1'^with [...] ^2'^and parts of [his] flesh [...] ^3'^You perform (it) in the month Abu (5) and the month Tebet (10) and ... [...]

1' NT 1' ⌜*it-ti*⌝ x [..]

2' NT 2' *ù* ⌜*mi-na-at* UZU⌝ [..]

3' NT 3' *ina* ^iti^NE *u* ^iti^AB DÙ-*ma* x [..]

4' *šumma amēlu ina īnīšu birṣī* [*ītanammar* ...] **5'** *eṭem harbāti murtappidu* [...]	^4'^If a man [constantly sees] flashes of light in his eyes [and ...] ^5'^a roving ghost of abandoned places [afflicts him ...]. ^6'^You take ^5'^[... (a plant)]

6' *izzizzu teleqqe ina išāti* [*tukabbab* ...] **7'** *ašgikû* [...] **Alternative prescription 1** **8'** *ištēn anzahhu ištēn* [*kutpû* / *huluhhu* ...] **9'** *ištēn uṭṭat parzilli elli* [...] **10'** *ištēn aban sābi* [...] **11'** *ištēn zēr bīni* [...]	$^{6'}$which stands [$^{5'}$on a grave$^{?}$]. You [burn (it)] in fire [...] $^{7'}$*ašgikû*-stone [...] **Alternative prescription 1** $^{8'}$One *anzahhu*-glass bead, one [black frit / *huluhhu*-slag bead ...] $^{9'}$one clean iron bead (lit. grain) [...] $^{10'}$one *sābu*-stone [...] $^{11'}$one seed of tamarisk [...]

4'	NT 4'	DIŠ NA *ina* IGI.MEŠ-*šú bir-ṣi* I[GI(.IGI)-*mar* ....]
	(NF) i' 13'	[DIŠ NA *e-nu-ma bir-ṣ*]*a* ⌜IGI-*ru*⌝ 3-*šú ki-a-am liq-bi šá* $^{d+}$*En-líl u* ^{d}*Nin-líl*
	(uC) i 18f.	DIŠ NA *e-nu-ma bir-ṣi i-ta-nam-ma-ru ki-a-am* DUG$_4$.GA / *šá* $^{d+}$*En-líl u* ^{d}*Nin-líl*
5'	NT 5'	GIDIM *har-ba-ti mu-ú*[*r*$^{?}$*-tap-pi-du* ....]
6'	NT 6'	GUB-*zu* TI-*qé ina* IZI *t*[*u-kab-ba-ab*..]
	(NF) i' 15'	[.................................... *ana* ZA]G$^{?}$ GUB-*zu* TI-*qé ina* IZI *tu-kab-ba-ab*
7'	NT 7'	^{na4}ÁŠ.GI$_4$.GI$_4$ [..]
8'	NT 8'	1 ^{na4}AN.ZAH 1 ^{na4}A[N.ZAH.BABBAR/.GE$_6$ ....]
9'	NT 9'	⌜1⌝ KU.KU AN.BAR K[Ù ....]
10'	NT 10'	⌜1⌝ NA$_4$ *sa-a-b*[*i*$^{?}$ ....]
11'	NT 11'	⌜1⌝ NUMUN ^{giš}ŠINI[G ....]

12' *enūma* [...] **13'** [x] x x [...]	$^{12'}$When/If [...] $^{13'}$... [...]

12'	NT 12'	[*e*]-*nu-ma* x [..]
13'	NT 13'	[x] x x [..]

§ IV.8 NU (AMT 14/3)

Manuscript:	**NU (AMT 14/3)**, collated.
Museum number:	British Museum, K 5415a.
Origin and date:	Nineveh, 7th century BC.
Type of tablet:	Flake from the middle part of a one or possibly two-column tablet.
Measurements:	ca. 7,2 × 8 × 2 cm.
Copy:	AMT 14/3.
Photo/CDLI nr.:	Plate 35/P396018.
Literature:	Thompson 1926: 47f.; Farber 1974: 89; Kinnier Wilson 2011: 19.

Edition

1’ NU 1’ [....................] x [..]

2’ [...] *kalgukka nikiptu ina šamni* [...]	2’[...] you [...] *kalgukku*-red paste (and) *nikiptu*-plant in oil [...]

2’ NU 2’ [... ^{i}]^{m}KAL.GUG *ni-kip-*⸢*tú ina* Ì⸣ [..]

3’ [...] *burāša kukra imbuʾ tâmti šamma ēda tasâk ina tangussi* [...]	3’[...] you pound [...], juniper, *kukru*-aromatic, algae, (and) single plant. [You ...] in copper *tangussu*-kettle [...]

3’ NU 3’ [... ^{ši}]^{m}LI ^{šim}GÚR.GÚR KA.A.AB.BA Ú.DILI SÚD *ina* ⸢^{urudu}⸣Š[EN.TUR .....]

4’ [...] *hašû imhur-līm imhur-ešrā tarmuš ina kišādīšu tašakkan* [...]	4’[...]: you place [(...)], *hašû*-thyme, *imhur-līm*-plant, *imhur-ešrā*-plant, *tarmuš*-lupine on his neck, [...]

4’ NU 4’ [...] ⸢^{ú}⸣HAR.HAR ^{ú}IGI-*lim* ^{ú}IGI-NIŠ ^{ú}*tar-muš*$_8$ *ina* ⸢GÚ-*šú* GAR⸣-*a*[*n* ....]

5’ [...] *zalāqu tasâk ina libbi šamni tanaddi libbi īnīšu tapaššašma* [*iballuṭ*?]	5’[...] you pound [...], (and) *zalāqu*-stone, you put (them) into sesame oil, and you smear the inner part of his eyes with it, then [he should recover?.]

5’ NU 5’ [... ^{n}]$^{\text{a4}}$ZÁLAG SÚD *ina* ŠÀ Ì+GIŠ ŠUB-*di* ŠÀ IGI.MIN-*šú* ŠÉŠ-*m*[*a*? TI?]

6’ [...] *teqqi mê bīni* UD.20.KAM *īnīšu temessīma mê bīni šalāšīšu irammukma iballuṭ*	6’[...] you daub (his eyes). For twenty days, you wash his eyes with tamarisk sap, then he bathes three times with

	the tamarisk sap, then he should recover.

6’ NU 6’ […] x MAR A ^{giš}ŠINIG UD.20.KAM* IGI.MIN-*šú* LUH-*ma* A ^{giš}ŠINIG 3-*šú* TU$_5$-*ma* T[I]

7’ […] *arqūssu tasâk mêšu taṣahhat ina kakkabi tušbât ašar šanîmma*	7’[…] you pound […] while still green, you press its sap out, let it stay under a star (= stay overnight), ditto (= he should recover).

7’ NU 7’ [… S]IG$_7$-*su* SÚD A.MEŠ-*šú* SUR-*at ina* UL *tuš-bat* KIMI[N]

8’ […] *ana bulluṭi aban mūṣi mê bīni ša ina pēmti tašakkanuma* **9’** [… *ina*] *libbi tušeṣṣi šamna lipi eṣemti ṣabīti ištēniš tasâk teqqi*	8’[…] in order to heal (it): *mūṣu*-stone (and) tamarisk sap, which you put over charcoal and then 9’[…] you remove (it) [from the] middle (of a vessel). You pound together oil and gazelle bone marrow (and) daub (his eyes).

8’ NU 8’ [… *a*]*na* TI $^{\text{na4}}$*mu-ṣi* A.MEŠ ^{giš}ŠINIG *šá ina* NE GAR-*nu-m*[*a*]

9’ NU 9’ [… *ina*] ⌜*lìb*⌝-*bi* È Ì Ì.UDU GÌR.PAD.DU MAŠ.DÀ 1-*niš* SÚD MA[R]

10’ […] *kabūt Šeriš hašâ atā’iša ina itqi talammi ina kišādīšu tašakkan* (…)]	10’[…]. You wrap up ox dung, *hašû*-thyme (and) *atā’išu*-plant in a woollen tuft, (and) you place (it) on his neck (…).

10’ NU 10’ [… ŠU]RUN ^{d}GU$_4$ ^{ú}HAR.HAR ^{ú}KUR.KUR *ina* ^{síg}ÀKA NIGIN *ina* GÚ-*šú* GAR-*a*[*n*$^?$ (…)]

11’ […] *lū mukīl rēš lemutti lū* **12’** […*lū eṭemmu*] *lemnu iṣbassuma ana bulluṭīšu*] **13’** […] … *teleqqe ina ṭurri šīpāti peṣâti tašakkak šuruš ēri* […] **14’** […] *maštakal qilip šūmī šammu ēdu kibrītu uhūlu qarnānû sebet šammī* [*annûti*] **15’** […] *ina itqi talappap ēma lippi* [*talpap*]	11’[If, …] either the supporter-of-evil, or [(…)] 12’[…, or] evil [ghost] afflicts him: in order to heal (him): 13’[…] you take […], (and) thread white wool on a cord. Root of *ēru*-tree […] 14’[…] *maštakal*-plant, peel of garlic, single plant, sulphur, horned *uhūlu*-alkali, [*these*$^?$] seven drugs 15’[…] You wrap […] in a woollen tuft, wherever you [wrap] a wrapping, 16’[…] You shall recite [the

16’ [... *šipta Ea*] *linīhka tamannu kišādu* [...]	incantation]: ‘May [Ea] appease you’, [*place it on*] the neck [...]

11’	NU 11’	[... *l*]*u-ú* SAG.HUL.HA.ZA *lu-*[*ú* (...)]
12’	NU 12’	[... *lu-ú*$^{?}$ ... H]UL DAB-*su-ma ana* T[I-*šú*]
13’	NU 13’	[...........] x TI-*qé ina* DUR SÍG BABBAR È-*ak* SUHUŠ ^{giš}MA.[NU ....]
14’	NU 14’	[... ^{ú}IN$_{6}$.Ú]Š BAR SUM^{sar} Ú.DILI PIŠ$_{10}$-^{d}ÍD NAGA.SI 7 Ú.HI.A Š[EŠ.$^{?}$ MEŠ]
15’	NU 15’	[.. *in*]*a* ⌜^{síg}⌝ÀKA *ta-la-pap e-ma líp-p*[*i tal-pap*]
16’	NU 16’	[................................. *šiptu* ^{d}*É-*] ⌜*a*⌝ *li-ni-ih-ka* ŠID-*nu* GÚ x [..............]
17’	NU 17’	[..................] x x [..]

§ IV.9 NV (AMT 18/3)

Manuscript:	**NV (AMT 18/3)**, collated.
Museum number:	British Museum, K 10535.
Origin and date:	Nineveh, 7th century BC.
Type of tablet:	Flake from the right part of a tablet/column inscribed in Babylonian Hand.
Measurements:	ca. 4,3 × 3,4 × 0,1 - 1,1 (towards the middle) cm.
Copy:	AMT 18/3.
Photo/CDLI nr.:	Plate 35/P238920.
Literature:	Thompson 1926: 52; Scurlock and Andersen 2005: 779.

Ll. 6f.’	parallels	NX (BAM 482) ii 62f.’	§ V.2.

Edition

1’ [*šumma amēlu īnāšu/qaqqassu*$^{?}$] *kiṣṣata iraššâ aktam uhūlu qarnānû* [...] **2’** [...] *urâna ina šamni šammi peṣî tasâk ina šamni*$^{?}$ [...] **3’** [... *tasâk*] *napṭa tapaššassuma* [*iballuṭ*]	1’[If man’s eyes/head$^{?}$] have *kiṣṣatu*-skin disease, *aktam*-plant, horned *uhūlu*-alkali, [...] 2’[...], you pound [...] *urânu*-plant in oil of white plant, you [...] in oil [...]. 3’[You pound ... and] you smear him with naphtha and [then he should recover.]

1'	NV 1'	[DIŠ NA IGI.MIN-*šú*/SAG.DU-*su ki-i*]*ṣ-ṣa-ta*5 TUK ú*ak-tam* NAGA.S[I ...]
2'	NV 2'	[.......................................] ⌜ú⌝HA *ina* Ì.GIŠ Ú.BABBAR SÚD *ina* ⌜Ì?⌝ [...]
3'	NV 3'	[.. SÚ]D Ì.KUR.RA ŠÉŠ-*su-ma* [TI]

4' [...] *murra burāša tasâk ina* [...] **5'** [...]... UD.14.KAM *taṣammid* [...]	4'[...], you pound [...], bitter-plant (and) juniper, [*you* ...] in [...] 5'[...]... You bandage (his eyes) for fourteen days [...]

4'	NV 4'	[..ši]mSES šimLI SÚD *ina* [...]
5'	NV 5'	[..] x UD.14.KAM* LAL [...]

6' [*šumma amēlu nakkapti imittīšu ikkalšu*]*ma īn imittīšu naphat u dimta* [*inaqqi*] **7'** [*šugidimmak šani*] *Ištar ana bulluṭīšu sīhu* [...]	6'[If man's right temple hurt him] and his right eye is inflamed and [pours out] tear(s). 7'[It is the 'Hand of the Ghost' as a deputy of Ištar.] In order to heal it: [you mix] *sīhu*-plant [...]

6'	NV 6'	[.. *m*]*a* IGI.MIN 15-*šú nap-hat u* É[R BAL-*qí*]
	(NX) ii 62'	DIŠ NA SAG.KI ZAG-*šú* GU7-*šú-ma* IGI ZAG-*šú nap-hat ù* ÉR BAL-*qí* →
7'	NV 7'	[.............................. d*Iš*8-*t*]*ár*? ⌜*ana* TI⌝-*šú* ú*s*[*i-hu* ...]
	(NX) ii 62f.'	ŠU.GIDIM.MA *šá-ni* d*Iš*8-*tár* / ⌜*ana* TI⌝-*šú* giš*si-hu*

§ IV.10 NW (BAM 439)

Manuscript:	**NW (BAM 439)**, collated.
Museum number:	British Museum, K 13474.
Origin and date:	Nineveh, 7th century BC.
Type of tablet:	Flake from the middle part of a tablet.
Measurements:	ca. 3,1 × 2,6 × 1 cm.
Copy:	BAM 439.
Photo/CDLI nr.:	Plate 35/P400318.
Literature:	Köcher 1980a: no. 439.

Edition

1'	NW 1'	[.........................] x x [..]

2’ [...] ... *mê kasî bašlūti* [...]	²’[...] ... (and) the boiled sap of a *kasû*-plant [...]

2’ NW 2’ [.......................] x ⸢*ti*⸣ A GAZI^{sar} ŠEG$_{6}$.G[Á ....]

3’ [...] *emesalli* [...]	³’[...] *emesallu*-saline solution [...]

3’ NW 3’ [...................... ^{mu}]⸢*eme-sal-lì* x [..]

4’ [... *dāmu*?] *lā paris dāmu ša ina niksīšu aṣû* ...[...] **5’** [...] *teleqqe*? *dām bīni ina himēti* [...]	⁴’[... the blood?] is not stopped, the blood which comes out from its incision [...] ⁵’you take [...] [(and) you ...] tamarisk ‘blood’ (i.e. resin) in ghee [...]

4’ NW 4’ [............ MÚ]D? NU KUD-*is* MÚD *ša ina* KUD-*šú* È x [............................]

5’ NW 5’ [..................... T]I?-*qé* MÚD ^{giš}*bi-ni ina* Ì.N[UN ....]

6’ [...] ... *ina šamni u šuhti* [*tasâk* ...]	⁶’[...] ... [you pound ...] in oil and copper patina [...]

6’ NW 6’ [.............] x *ina* Ì *u* ⸢SAHAR⸣.URUDU [SÚD ....]

§ IV.11 NZb (AMT 17/2)

Manuscript: **NZb**, collated.
Museum Number: Rm 402.
Origin and date: Nineveh, 7th century BC.
Type of tablet: This small fragment represents the left side of a tablet (one or two column).
Measurements: ca. 2,3 × 4,6 × 3 cm.
Copy: AMT 17/2.
Photo/CDLI nr.: Plate 36/P424742.
Literature: Borger 1975: 280.

Edition

1’ *Gula bulliṭīma* [...]	¹’Gula keep (me) healthy [...]

1’ NZb 1’ ⸢^{d}*Gu-la bul*⸣-*l*[*i-ṭi-ma* ....]

2' *šalāšat ka'inimma* [...]	[2']Three invocations [for ...]

2' NZb 2' 3 KA.INIM.MA [.......................................]

3' *dudubi šīpāti sāmāti šīpāti* [*peṣâti* ...] **4'** *aban hurāṣi aban sābi* [...] **5'** *kurkānû talpap* [...]	[3']Its medical application: [you spin separately/together] red (and) [white] wool [...]. [5']You wrap up [4']a golden bead, *sābu*-stone [...] [5'](and) *kurkānû*-plant [...].

3' NZb 3' DÙ.DÙ.BI SÍG SA$_5$ SÍG [BABBAR ....]

4' NZb 4' NA$_4$ KUG.GI NA$_4$ *sa-a-*[*bi* ....]

5' NZb 5' ^{ú}*kur-ka-nu-u tál-p*[*ap* ....]

6' *šiptu abkū īnāšu* [...] **7'** *ēmuršuma* [...] **8'** *ana eṭemmi nāq mê* [*inaqqi*$^{?}$ ...] **9'** *ai iṭhîka* [...] **10'** *ai iṭhîka* [...] **11'** *ina šērti ina napāhi* [...] **12'** ... **13'** *šipta* [...]	[6']Incantation: reversed are his eyes [...] [7']One has seen him [...] [8']The pourer of water [makes a libation$^{?}$] for the ghost ... [...] [9']may he not come near you [...] [10']may he not come near you [...] [11']In the morning at sunrise [...] [12']... [...] [13']Incantation [...].

6' NZb 6' ÉN *ab-ku* IGI.MIN-*šú* PA [.......................................]

7' NZb 7' *e-mur-šú-ma* ^{d}x [.......................................]

8' NZb 8' *ana* GU$_4$ *naq me-e i-*[*naq*$^{?}$*-qi*$^{?}$.......................................]

9' NZb 9' *a-a iṭ-hi-k*[*a* ....]

10' NZb 10' *a-a iṭ-hi-k*[*a* ....]

11' NZb 11' *ina šèr-ti ina na-p*[*a-hi* ....]

12' NZb 12' *na-ás*-x x x [.......................................]

13' NZb 13' ÉN x [.......................................]

§ V From the Nineveh UGU treatise (BAM 480, 482)

The so-called UGU is the first treatise from the Nineveh Medical Encyclopaedia. Since, the general topic of the UGU Treatise is the human head, human eyes were also addressed.

§ V.1 UGU 1 (BAM 480)

Base Manuscript:	**NI (BAM 480)**, collated.
Museum Number:	K 2354 + K 2412 + K 2463 + K 2491 + K 3237 + K 6447 + K 7086 + K 8356 + K 8800 + K 8842 + K 9828 + K 11868 + K 13398 + K 13399 + Sm 637 + Sm 1156 + K 10428 [BAM 488] + K 16451 [AMT 3/4].
Origin and date:	Nineveh, 7th century BC.
Type of tablet:	Two-column, portrait-oriented tablet. Vertical column rulings done with a twisted thread, and horizontal dividing lines were drawn with an instrument. Round firing holes visible on the obverse but not to be seen on the reverse. Several lines on col iii (46–47; 55) have been been intentionally erased after the tablet dried out (see also Finkel in Worthington 2005: 6).
Measurements:	ca. 27,5 × 16,7 × 3,5 cm.
Copy:	BAM 480, BAM 488, AMT 3/4.
Photo/CDLI nr.:	Plates 36–39/P365742.
Literature:	Köcher 1980a: xxiii-xxv. Finkel 1998: 81 fn. 10. Foster 2005: 992; Worthington 2005; 2007; Stol 2007a: 3ff.; Heeßel 2010: 48ff.; Scurlock 2014: 306ff.; Panayotov 2016a,b; Bácskay 2018a: 47ff.

NB: It is not necessary to provide parallels here, since this text is cross-referenced many times, see especially the works of Worthington 2005; 2007.

Edition of the Relevant Prescriptions

1	*šumma amēlu muhhašu umma ukâl šer'ān tīb nakkapti iraššīma īnāšu iṣapparā*	[1]If a man's cranium/brain holds heat (i.e. 'fever'), he has throbbing of the blood vessel of the temple, (and) his eyes blink, [2]his eyes are blurred with dimness, cloudiness, blurring of the vision, *murdinnu*-'bramble', *qūqānu*-'worm', [3]and are constantly giving off tear(s): You grind up one third litre of
2	*īnāšu birrata ipīta išīta murdinna qūqāna ašâ*	
3	*u dimta ittanaddâ šuššān qa sahlê buṭutta ina erî teṭên tanappi*	

https://doi.org/10.1515/9781501506550-010

4 *rēška ukâl ina libbi šuššān qa teleqqe ina mê kasî talâš tugallab taṣammidma* UD.3.KAM *lā ipaṭṭar*	*sahlû*-plant (and) *buṭutta*-terebinth with a pestle (and) you sift (it). [4](Now) it requires your attention, you take one third litre out of it (the mixture prepared above), knead (it) in the sap of a *kasû*-plant. You shave (his head), bandage it (with it), and he shall not remove (the bandage) for three days.
Alternative prescription 1	**Alternative prescription 1**
5 *šuššān qa sahlê šuššān qa qēm labti ina mê kasî talâš tugallab taṣammidma* UD.3.KAM *lā ipaṭṭar*	[5]You knead one third litre of *sahlû*-plant (and) flour of roasted grain in the sap of a *kasû*-plant. You shave (his head), bandage it (with it), and he shall not remove (the bandage) for three days.
Alternative prescription 2	**Alternative prescription 2**
6 *sahlê ṭēnēti kukra uhūla qarnānâ ina šikari talâš ašar šanîmma*	[6]You knead ground *sahlû*-plant, *kukru*-aromatic (and) horned *uhūlu*-alkali in beer, ditto (= you shave his head, bandage it, and he shall not remove it for three days.)
Alternative prescription 3	**Alternative prescription 3**
7 *murra emesalli malmališ taballal ina himēti tasâk īnīšu teqqi*	[7]You mix in equal amounts bitter-plant (and) *emesallu*-saline solution. You pound (it) in ghee (and) daub his eyes.
Alternative prescription 4	**Alternative prescription 4**
8 *šuššān qa sahlê šuššān qa haṣab tinūri ešeret šiqil hīqāti* [...] 9 *ina mê kasî talâš tugallab taṣammidma* UD.3.KAM [*lā ipaṭṭar*]	[9]You knead [8]one third litre of *sahlû*-plant, one third litre of sherd(s) of a tannour-oven (and) ten shekels of diluted beer [...] [9]in the sap of a *kasû*-plant. You shave (his head), bandage it, and [he shall not remove (the bandage)] for three days.
Instruction for the patient and the healer	**Instruction for the patient and the healer**
10 *arki naṣmadāti annâti ešeret šiqil sahlê ša pî urṣi* [...]	[10]After these bandages (are applied): [11]he (= the patient) shall collect into a loaf of bread [10]ten shekels of *sahlû*-plant from the mouth of the mortar [which] [11]was

11 *ṭābta ṭābātu lā šulputū ina akali issipma ikkal hamšat šiqil* [...]
12 *ina šikari rūšti tamahhaṣma išattīšu* [...]

never crushed (together with) salt (or) vinegar, then he shall eat (it). [12]You shall beat (it) in premium beer [11]five shekels of [ground *sahlû*-plant ...] [12]and he drinks it, [... Bandages of sahlû-plant for the eyes.]

Instructions for the healer

13 UD.1.KAM *anzahha tasâk* [...]

Instructions for the healer

[13]On day one you pound *anzahhu*-glass [...]

Alternative prescription 1'

14 *ešeret šiqil inib kalbāni* [...]
15 *tahaššal tanappi ina mê kasî* [*talâš* ...]

Alternative prescription 1'

[15]You crush and sift [14]ten shekels fruit of *kalbānu*-plant, [...] [15][You knead (them)] in the sap of a *kasû*-plant. [...]

Alternative prescription 2'

16 *šimbizidâ* [...]

Alternative prescription 2'

[16][You pound] *šimbizidû*-galena [...]

Alternative prescription 3'

17 [x] x [...]
18 *tahaššal tanappi* [...]

Alternative prescription 3'

[18]You crush and sift [17][x] x [...] [18][...]

Alternative prescription 4'

19 *ešeret šiqil qēm kupsi tubbal* [...]

Alternative prescription 4'

[19]You dry ten shekels of sesame husks powder [...]

Alternative prescription 5'

20 *ešeret šiqil qēm kupsi tubbal* [...]
21 UD.1.KAM *irassu taṣammid qaqqassu* [...]
22 *ana qaqqadīšu tašappak ina bīti* [*ša tarāna išû tušeššebšu* ...]

Alternative prescription 5'

[20]You dry ten shekels of sesame husks powder [...] [21]You bandage his chest for one day, (and) [...] his head [22]You pour [[21]x litre of sesame oil] [22]over his head, (and) [let him sit] in a room [which has a canopy. You keep doing this for three days.]

Alternative prescription 6'

23 *ištēn šiqil rikibti arkabi mišil šiqil* [*šamma peṣâ* ...]

Alternative prescription 6'

[23][You pound] one shekel of bat guano, half shekel of [white plant and ...]

Alternative prescription 7'

24 *šuššān qa zēr papparhî šuššān qa zēr lapti*[?] [...]

Alternative prescription 7'

[24][You ...] one third litre seed(s) of *papparhû*-purslane, one third litre seed(s) of *laptu*-turnip' [...]

Alternative prescription 8' **25** *šuššān qa isqūqa ešeret šiqil arti* ... [...]	**Alternative prescription 8'** [25][You ...] one third litre of coarse flour (and) ten shekel(s) of ... leaves [...]
Alternative prescription 9' **26** *zēr sahlê* [...]	**Alternative prescription 9'** [26][You pound] seed(s) of *sahlû*-plant [...]

Although the beginning of i 27 is broken, structurally it seems that the following fragmentary lines are most probably alternative prescriptions as well.

Alternative prescription 10' **28** [...] *talâš ašar šanîmma*	**Alternative prescription 10'** [28][...] you knead (it), ditto.
Alternative prescription 11' **29** *kalgukku* [...] *tasâk teqqi*	**Alternative prescription 11'** [29]You pound *kalgukku*-red paste [...] (and) daub (his eyes).
Alternative prescription 12' **30** *šuššān qa arti titti* [... *tubbal* ...] *ina mê kasî talâš* **31** *tatârma tubbal tahaššal* [*tanappi* ... *tugallab*] *taṣammidma ašar šanîmma*	**Alternative prescription 12'** [30][You dry] one third litre of fig leave(s) [...] you knead (them) in the sap of a *kasû*-plant, [31]You dry again (and) crush [(and) sift ... you shave (his head)], you bandage (his head) and ditto (= and daub his eyes).
Alternative prescription 13' **32** *šuššān qa būšāna šuššān qa* x [...]*-ma ašar šanîmma*	**Alternative prescription 13'** [32][You ...] one third litre of *būšānu*-plant, one third litre of x [............] and ditto (= and daub his eyes).
Alternative prescription 14' **33** *uhūla qarnānâ* [...] *teqqi*	**Alternative prescription 14'** [33][You ...] horned *uhūlu*-alkali, [...] you daub (his eyes).
Alternative prescription 15' **34** *šuššān* [...] *ašar šanîmma*	**Alternative prescription 15'** [34][You ...] one third [...] and ditto.

The passage until line i 40 is broken off, but structurally it seems that the following fragmentary lines are most probably alternative prescriptions as well.

Alternative prescription 16’ **41** [... *talâš*] *tugallab taṣammidma ašar* [*šanîmma*]	**Alternative prescription 16’** [41][... you knead (it) ...], shave (his head), bandage it (with it) and ditto (daub (his eyes).
Alternative prescription 17’ **42** [... *tatârma*] *tubbal tahaššal tanappi ina mê kasî talâš tugallab taṣammidma ašar* [*šanîmma*] **43** [... *ina lipî eṣemti*] *arikti tasâk teqqi*	**Alternative prescription 17’** [42]You [dry again], crush and sift [...]. You knead (it) in the sap of a *kasû*-plant. You shave (his head), bandage it and ditto (daub (his eyes). [43][...] You pound [... in the marrow] of a long [bone] (and) daub (his eyes).
Alternative prescription 18’ **44** [... *šuhta ina libbi lipi*] *sāqi ṣabīti tasâk teqqi*	**Alternative prescription 18’** [44][...] You pound [copper patina into fat of a] gazelle’s thigh and daub (his eyes).
Alternative prescription 19’ **45** [...... *tahaššal tanappi ina mê kasî*] *talâš tugallab taṣammidma* UD.3.KAM *lā ipaṭṭar*	**Alternative prescription 19’** [[45]You crush and sift ...] You knead (it) in [the sap of a *kasû*-plant]. You shave (his head), bandage it (with it), and he shall not remove (the bandage) for three days.
Alternative prescription 20’ **46** [... *ina*] *šizbi* [*talâš*] *tugallab taṣammidma ašar šanîmma*	**Alternative prescription 20’** [46][... you knead (it) in milk]. You shave (his head), bandage it (with it), and ditto (= he shall not remove (the bandage) for three days).
Alternative prescription 21’ **47** [...] x [*ina*[?]] *dišip šadî šuhat hurāṣi tasâk teqqi*	**Alternative prescription 21’** [47]You pound ... [in[?]] mountain honey, patina of gold, you daub his eyes.
Alternative prescription 22’ **48** [.... *tahaššal*] *tanappi ina mê kasî talâš tugallab taṣammidma* UD.3.KAM *lā ipaṭṭar*	**Alternative prescription 22’** [48][You crush] and sift [...] You knead (it) in the sap of a *kasû*-plant. You shave (his head), bandage it, and he shall not remove (the bandage) for three days.
Alternative prescription 23’ **49** [.... *tahaššal*] *tanappi ina šuršummī šikari bašli talâš tugallab taṣammidma* UD.3.KAM *lā ipaṭṭar*	**Alternative prescription 23’** [49][You crush and] sift [...]. You knead (it) in boiled beer dregs. You shave (his head), bandage it, and he shall not remove (the bandage) for three days.

Alternative prescription 24' **50** [...] *arti*$^{?}$ *dumuqšina tatabbal ina dišpi tasâk teqqi*	**Alternative prescription 24'** [50][...] ... you remove the best parts of the foilage$^{?}$, pound (them) in honey, (and) daub (his eyes).
Alternative prescription 25' **51** [... *dumuqšina*] *tahaššal tanappi ina mê kasî talâš tugallab taṣammidma* UD.3.KAM *lā ipaṭṭar*	**Alternative prescription 25'** [51]You crush and sift [... their best] parts. You knead (them) in the sap of a *kasû*-plant. You shave (his head), bandage it, and he shall not remove (the bandage) for three days.
Alternative prescription 26' **52** [*qēm*] *labti*$^{?}$ *tahaššal tanappi ina mê kasî talâš tugallab taṣammidma* UD.3.KAM *lā ipaṭṭar*	**Alternative prescription 26'** [52]You crush and sift [flour] of roasted grain. You knead (them) in the sap of a *kasû*-plant. You shave (his head), bandage it, and he shall not remove (the bandage) for three days.
Alternative prescription 27' **53** *rikibti arkabi ina dišpi tasâk teqqi*	**Alternative prescription 27'** [53]You pound bat guano in honey (and) daub (his eyes).
Alternative prescription 28' **54** *šuššān qa arti marišmalê tahaššal tanappi ina mê kasî talâš tugallab taṣammidma* UD.3.KAM *lā ipaṭṭar*	**Alternative prescription 28'** [54]You crush and sift one third litre of *marišmalû*-plant leaves. You knead (them) in the sap of a *kasû*-plant. You shave (and), bandage (his head), and he shall not remove (the bandage) for three days.
Alternative prescription 29' **55** *gaṣṣa bašla ina šaman sirdi talâš tugallab taṣammidma ašar šanîmma*	**Alternative prescription 29'** [55]You knead boiled gypsum in olive oil. You shave (and) bandage (his head), and ditto (= he shall not remove the bandage for three days).
Alternative prescription 30' **56** *haṣab igulê ša kibša išû ina šamni šuhti tasâk teqqi*	**Alternative prescription 30'** [56]You pound a fungus-ridden fine-ointment potsherd in oil (and) copper patina (and) daub (his eyes).

Alternative prescription 31'	**Alternative prescription 31'**
57 *supāla sahlê tahaššal tanappi ina šuršummī šikari rūšti talâš tugallab taṣammidma* UD.3.KAM *lā ipaṭṭar*	[57]You crush and sift *supālu*-juniper (and) *sahlû*-plant. You knead (them) in the dregs of premium beer. You shave (and), bandage (his head), and he shall not remove (the bandage) for three days.
Alternative prescription 32'	**Alternative prescription 32'**
58 *haltappāna kalbāna tahaššal tanappi ina šuršummī šikari bašli talâš tugallab taṣammidma* UD.3.KAM *lā ipaṭṭar*	[58]You crush and sift *haltappānu*-plant (and) *kalbānu*-plant. You knead (them) in the dregs of boiled beer. You shave (and) bandage it (his head), and he shall not remove (the bandage) for three days.
Alternative prescription 33'	**Alternative prescription 33'**
59 *burāša kukra baluhha sahlê uhūla qarnānâ temessi ina šizbi talâš tugallab taṣammidma* UD.3.KAM *lā ipaṭṭar*	[59]You wash juniper, *kukru*-aromatic, *baluhhu*-aromatic, *sahlû*-plant (and) horned *uhūlu*-alkali, and knead (them) in milk. You shave (and) bandage it (his head), and he shall not remove (the bandage) for three days.
Alternative prescription 34'	**Alternative prescription 34'**
60 *šuhta ina dišpi tasâk teqqi*	[60]You pound copper patina in honey, (and) daub (his eys).
Alternative prescription 35'	**Alternative prescription 35'**
61 *šuššān qa sahlê šuššān qa billata* [...] *talâš tugallab taṣammidma* UD.3.KAM *lā ipaṭṭar*	[61]You knead one third litre of *sahlû*-plant, one third litre of beer mash, [... *in* ...]. You shave (and) bandage it (his head), and he shall not remove (the bandage) for three days.
Alternative prescription 36'	**Alternative prescription 36'**
62 *šuššān qa sahlê* [...] *talâš tugallab taṣammidma* UD.3.KAM *lā ipaṭṭar*	[62]You knead one third litre of *sahlû*-plant, [...] [*in* ...]. You shave (and), bandage (his head), and he shall not remove (the bandage) for three days.
Alternative prescription 37'	**Alternative prescription 37'**
63 *lulâ anzahha* [...] *tasâk teqqi*	[63]You pound *lulû*-antimony, *anzahhu*-glass, [...], (and) daub (his eyes).

Alternative prescription 38'	**Alternative prescription 38'**
64 *šuššān qa qēm hallūri [šuššān qa qēm kakkî ... talâš tugallab taṣammidma]* UD.3.KAM *lā ipaṭṭar*	[64][You knead] one third litre of chickpea powder, [one third litre of lentil powder ... You shave (and) bandage (his head)], and he shall not remove (the bandage) for three days.
Alternative prescription 39'	**Alternative prescription 39'**
65 *kasâ taqallu tahaššal tanappi ina šuršummī šikari talâš tugallab taṣammidma* UD.3.KAM *lā ipaṭṭar*	[65]You roast *kasû*-plant. You crush and sift (it). You knead (it) in beer dregs. You shave (and) bandage (his head), and he shall not remove (the bandage) for three days.
Alternative prescription 40'	**Alternative prescription 40'**
66 *zēr lišān kalbi arqūssu tuhassâ mēšu ana pursīti taṣahhat adi ablat tašakkan* 67 *enūma ītablu ina šamni šuhti tasâk teqqi*	[66]You squeeze out seed(s) of 'dog's-tongue plant', while still green. You press its liquid into a *pursītu*-bowl. You leave (it) until it is dried out. [67]When it has dried out you pound it in oil (and) copper patina (and) daub (his eyes).
Alternative prescription 41'	**Alternative prescription 41'**
68 *šamma peṣâ rikibti arkabi lipi kanakti ṣumlalâ zēr šurdunî kamūn bīni zēr maštakal* 69 *zê*[?] *kalbi*[?] *arti bīni emesalli nīnâ zibâ mala nīš īnīka teleqqe* 70 *tapâṣ ina šamni tasâk īnīšu ina uhūli qarnānî temessi adi dimtu parsu teqqi enūma taṣammidušu teqqi arkīšu* 71 [*itqūr*] *abāri ul tapaṭṭaršu mê šunê tušabšal ana urî tessip ina kakkabi tušbât ina šēri qaqqassu* 72 *tapaššaš mê šunê bašlūti ana qaqqadīšu tuqarrar qaqqassu kunša pušikki tarakkas*	[69]You take as much as you feel are required of [68]white plant, bat guano, *kanaktu*-aromatic pith, *ṣumlalû*-aromatic, seed(s) of *šurdunû*-plant, 'tamarisk cumin', seed(s) of *maštakal*-plant, [69]dog's dung[?], leaf of tamarisk, *emesallu*-saline solution, mint, (and) black cumin. [70]You crush (and) pound (the drugs) in oil. You wash his eyes in horned *uhūlu*-alkali – until the tear(s) stop – and you daub (his eyes). When you bandage his (head) you daub (his eyes). Afterwards [71]you do not stop treating him with the lead spoon-salve. You boil sap of a *šunû*-tree (and) collect (it) into an *urû*-bowl, let it stay under a star (= stay overnight). In the morning [72]you smear his head. You trickle the

73 [*šuššān*] *qa šamna ana qaqqadīšu tašappak ina bīti ša tarāna išû tušeššebšu* UD.3.KAM *annâ tēteneppuš*	boiled sap of a *šunû*-tree onto his head (and) tie his head with braid of combed wool. [73]You pour [one third] litre of sesame oil over his head, (and) let him sit in a room, which has a canopy. You keep doing this for three days.

1	NI i 1	DIŠ NA UGU-*šú* KÚM *ú-kal* SA ZI SAG.KI TUK-*ma* IGI.MIN-*šú i*-BÀR
2	NI i 2	IGI.MIN-*šú bir-ra-ta*$_{5}$ *i-pi-ta*$_{5}$ *i-ši-ta*$_{5}$ *mur-din-na qù-qa-na a-šá-a*
3	NI i 3	*ù* ÉR ŠUB.ŠUB-*a* 1/3 SÌLA ZÀ.HI.LI *bu-ṭu-ta*$_{5}$ *ina* ^{na4}UR$_{5}$ ÀRA-*en* SIM
4	NI i 4	SAG-*ka ú-kal ina* ŠÀ 1/3 SÌLA TI-*qé ina* A GAZI^{sar} SILA$_{11}$-*aš* SAR-*ab* LAL-*ma* UD.3.KAM NU DU$_{8}$
5	NI i 5	1/3 SÌLA *sah-lé-e* 1/3 SÌLA ZÌ ŠE.SA.A *ina* A GAZI^{sar} SILA$_{11}$-*aš* SAR-*ab* LAL-*ma* UD.3.KAM NU DU$_{8}$
6	NI i 6	*sah-lé-e* ÀRA-*tì* ^{šim}GÚR.GÚR NAGA.SI *ina* KAŠ SILA$_{11}$-*aš* ⸢KIMIN⸣
7	NI i 7	^{šim}SES ^{mun}*eme-sal-lì mál-ma-liš* HE.HE *ina* Ì.NUN SÚD IGI.⸢MIN-*šú*⸣ *t*[*e*$^{?}$-*qí*]
8	NI i 8	1/3 SÌLA ZÀ.HI.LI 1/3 SÌLA ŠIKA IM.ŠU.RIN.NA 10 GÍN *hi-qa-t*[*i* ....]
9	NI i 9	*ina* A GAZI^{sar} SILA$_{11}$-*aš* SAR-*ab* LAL-*ma* ⸢UD.3⸣.K[AM NU DU$_{8}$]
10	NI i 10	EGIR *na-aṣ-ma-da-ti an-na-ti* 10 GÍN ZÀ.HI.LI *ša* KA ⸢*ur*⸣-*ṣ*[*i* ....]
11	NI i 11	MUN A.GEŠTIN.NA NU TAG.TAG *ina* NINDA *is-sìp-ma* GU$_{7}$ 5 G[ÍN .....]
12	NI i 12	*ina* KAŠ.SAG SÌG-*aṣ-ma* NAG-*šú* [...]
13	NI i 13	UD.1.KÁM AN.ZAH SÚ[D ....]
14	NI i 14	10 GÍN GURUN ^{giš}MAŠ.HUŠ [..]
15	NI i 15	GAZ SIM *ina* A GAZ[I^{sar} SILA$_{11}$-*aš* ....]

16	NI i 16	*šim-bi-*⌜*zi*⌝*-*[*da* ....]
17	NI i 17	[x] x [..]
18	NI i 18	GAZ SI[M ....]
19	NI i 19	10 GÍN ZÌ ⌜DUH.ŠE.GIŠ.Ì⌝ H[ÁD.DU ....]
20	NI i 20	10 GÍN ZÌ DUH.ŠE.GIŠ.Ì HÁD.D[U ....]
21	NI i 21	UD.1.KAM GABA-*su* LAL SAG.DU-*s*[*u* ....]
22	NI i 22	*ana* SAG.DU-*šú* DUB-*ak ina* ⌜É⌝ [..]
	(NI) ii 9	*ana* SAG.DU-*šú* DUB *ina* É *šá ta-ra-na*$_{7}$ TUK-*ú* DÚR-*šú* UD.3.KAM *an-na*$_{7}$ DÙ.DÙ-*uš*
23	NI i 23	1 GÍN U$_{5}$.ARGAB^{mušen} 1/2 GÍ[N Ú.BABBAR ....]
24	NI i 24	1/3 SÌLA NUMUN BABBAR.HI^{sar} 1/3 SÌLA NUMUN LU.[ÚB$^{sar?}$ ....]
25	NI i 25	⌜1/3⌝ SÌLA ZÌ.KUM ⌜10 GÍN PA⌝ GI[Š ....]
26	NI i 26	[NUM]UN$^{?}$ *sa*[*h*$^{?}$*-lé-e* ....]
27	NI i 27	**Broken**
28	NI i 28	[..SI]LA$_{11}$-*aš* ⌜KIMIN⌝
29	NI i 29	^{im}KA[L.GUG.. SÚ]D *te-qí*
30	NI i 30	1/3 SÌLA PA ^{giš}PÈ[Š ... HÁD.A .... *in*]*a* A GAZI^{sar} SILA$_{11}$-*aš*
31	NI i 31	GUR-*ma* HÁD.A G[AZ SIM .... SAR-*a*]*b* LAL-*ma* KIMIN
32	NI i 32	1/3 SÌLA ^{ú}HAB 1/3 SÌLA x [..]-⌜*ma* KIMIN⌝
33	NI i 33	NAGA.S[I .... *t*]*e-*⌜*qí*⌝

34	NI i 34	1[/3 ....] x ⸢KIMIN⸣
35	NI i 35	[.. *te-q*]*í*
36	NI i 36	[..] x
37	NI i 37	[..] x
38	NI i 38	**Broken**
39	NI i 39	**Broken**
40	NI i 40	[...] ⸢SÚD⸣ *te-q*[*í*]
41	NI i 41	[.. SILA$_{11}$-*a*]*š* SAR-*ab* LAL-*ma* K[IMIN]
42	NI i 42	[................ GUR-*ma* HÁD.]A GAZ SIM *ina* A GAZI$^{⸢sar⸣}$ SILA$_{11}$-*aš* SAR-*ab* LAL-*ma* KI[MIN]
43	NI i 43	[...................................... *ina* Ì.UDU GÌR.PAD.D]A GÍD.DA ⸢SÚD⸣ MAR
44	NI i 44	[............... SAHAR.URUDU *ina* ŠÀ Ì.UDU *sa*]-*a-qí* MAŠ.⸢DÀ SÚD⸣ *te-qí*
45	NI i 45	[........... GAZ SIM *ina* A GAZI^{sar} SIL]A$_{11}$-⸢*aš* SAR-*ab* LAL⸣-*ma* UD.3.KÁM NU DU$_8$
46	NI i 46	[...................................... *ina*] ⸢GA⸣ [SILA$_{11}$-*aš* SA]R-*ab* LAL-*ma* KIMIN
47	NI i 47	[...................................] x [*ina*] ⸢LÀL⸣.KUR-*i šu-hat* KUG.GI SÚD MAR
48	NI i 48	[......... GAZ SI]M *ina* A GAZI^{sar} SILA$_{11}$-*aš* ⸢SAR⸣-*ab* LAL-*ma* UD.3.KÁM NU DU$_8$
49	NI i 49	[............ GAZ SI]M ⸢*ina*⸣ *šur-šum-mi* KAŠ ŠEG$_6$.GÁ ⸢SILA$_{11}$-*aš*⸣ SAR-*ab* LAL-*ma* UD.3.KÁM NU DU$_8$

50	NI i 50	[.. P]A$^{??}$ *du-muq-ši-na ta-tab-bal* ⸢*ina*⸣ LÀL SÚD *te-qí*
51	NI i 51	[.................. *du-muq-ši*]-⸢*na*⸣ GAZ SIM *ina* A GAZI^{sar} SILA$_{11}$-*aš* SAR-⸢*ab*⸣ LAL-*ma* UD.3.KÁM NU D[U$_{8}$]
52	NI i 52	[ZÌ ŠE.SA].⸢A$^{?}$⸣ GAZ SIM *ina* A GAZI^{sar} SILA$_{11}$-*aš* SAR-⸢*ab*⸣ LAL-*ma* UD.3.KÁM ⸢NU DU$_{8}$⸣
53	NI i 53	⸢U$_{5}$⸣.[ARGAB^{mu}]^{šen} *ina* LÀL ⸢SÚD *te*⸣-*qí*
54	NI i 54	1/3 SÌLA PA ^{giš} (OVER ERASURE) M[Á.ERI.I]Š.MÁ.RA GAZ SIM *ina* A GAZI^{sar} [SILA$_{11}$-*aš* S]AR-⸢*ab*⸣ LA[L-*ma*] UD.3.KÁM NU DU$_{8}$
55	NI i 55	IM.BABBAR *ba-aš-la* ⸢*ina* Ì⸣ *sír-di* SILA$_{11}$-*aš* SAR-*ab* [L]AL-*ma* KIMIN
56	NI i 56	⸢ŠIKA⸣ Ì.GU.LA *ša kib-*⸢*ša*$_{25}$⸣ TUK-*ú ina* Ì SAHA[R.URUDU] SÚD *te-qí*
57	NI i 57	^{ú}ZA.BA.LAM *sah-lé-e* ⸢GAZ SIM⸣ *ina šur-šum-mi* KAŠ.S[AG SILA$_{11}$-*aš* S]AR-*ab* LAL-*ma* UD.3.KÁM NU DU$_{8}$
58	NI i 58	^{ú}*hal-tap-pa-na*$_{7}$ ^{giš}MAŠ.HUŠ GA[Z SI]M *ina šur-šum-mi* KAŠ Š[EG$_{6}$.G]Á SILA$_{11}$-*aš* SAR-*ab* LAL-*ma* UD.3.KÁM NU DU$_{8}$
59	NI i 59	^{šim}LI ^{šim}GÚR.GÚR ^{šim}BULUH ZÀ.HI.L[I NA]GA.SI L[U]H-*si ina* GA SILA$_{11}$-*aš* SAR-*ab* LAL-*ma* UD.3.KÁM NU DU$_{8}$
60	NI i 60	SAHAR.URUDU [*ina* L]ÀL SÚD *te-qí*
61	NI i 61	⸢1/3⸣ SÌLA ZÀ.⸢HI⸣.LI 1/3 SÌLA DI[DA ... S]ILA$_{11}$-*aš* SAR-*ab* LAL-*ma* UD.3.KÁM NU DU$_{8}$
62	NI i 62	1/3 SÌLA ZÀ.HI.L[I .... SI]LA$_{11}$-*aš* SAR-*ab* LAL-*ma* UD.3.KÁM NU DU$_{8}$
63	NI i 63	KÙ.GAN AN.Z[AH$^{?}$ .... S]ÚD MAR

64 NI i 64 1/3 SÌLA ZÌ G[Ú.GAL 1/3 SÌLA ZÌ GÚ.TUR … SILA$_{11}$-*aš* SAR-*ab* LAL-*m*]*a* UD.3.KÁM NU DU$_8$

---

65 NI ii 1 GAZ[I^{sar}] ⸢BÍL⸣-*lu* ⸢GAZ SIM *ina*⸣ *šur-šum-mi* KAŠ SILA$_{11}$-*aš* ⸢SAR⸣-*ab* LAL-*ma* UD.3.KÁM NU DU$_8$

---

66 NI ii 2 NUMUN [^{ú}E]ME.UR.GI$_7$ SIG$_7$-*su tu-hás-sà* A-*šú ana* ^{dug}BUR.ZI SUR-*at* EN HÁD.DU GAR-*an*

67 NI ii 3 U[D-*m*]*a i-tab-lu ina* Ì SAHAR.URUDU SÚD MAR

---

68 NI ii 4 ⸢Ú.BABBAR⸣ U$_5$.ARGAB^{mušen} Ì.UDU ^{šim}GIG ^{šim}GAM.MA NUMUN ^{ú}SI.SÁ *ka-mun* ^{giš}ŠINIG NUMUN ⸢^{ú}IN.NU.UŠ⸣

69 NI ii 5 Š[E$_{10}$$^{?}$ U]R$^{?}$.GI$_7$ PA ^{giš}ŠINIG ^{mun}*eme-sal-lì* ^{ú}KUR.RA ^{ú}GAMUN.GE$_6$ *ma-la ni-iš* IGI.MIN-*ka* ŠU.⸢TI⸣

70 NI ii 6 [*t*]*a-pa-aṣ ina* Ì SÚD IGI.MIN-*šú ina* NAGA.SI LUH-*si* EN ÉR KUD-*su te-qí* UD-*ma* LAL-*šú te-qí* EGIR-*šú*

71 NI ii 7 [DÍLIM.A.B]ÁR NU DU$_8$-*šú* A ^{giš}ŠE.NÚ.A ŠEG$_6$-*šal ana* ^{dug}GAN.SAR *te-sip ina* UL *tuš-bat ina še-rì* SAG.DU-*su*

72 NI ii 8 [Š]ÉŠ A ^{giš}ŠE.NÚ.A ŠEG$_6$.GÁ *ana* SAG.DU-*šú tu-qar-ra-ár* SAG.DU-*su kun-ša$_{25}$* ^{síg}GA.RÍG.AG.A KEŠDA

73 NI ii 9 [1/3$^{?}$ SÌL]A$^{?}$ Ì.GIŠ *ana* SAG.DU-*šú* DUB *ina* É *šá ta-ra-na$_7$* TUK-*ú* DÚR-*šú* UD.3.KAM *an-na$_7$* DÙ.DÙ-*uš*

---

74 [*šumma amēlu*] *muhhašu*$^{?}$ *ītenemmem gaṣṣa uhūla qarnānâ barma kibrīt(a) eṣemta uhūla qarnānâ napṭa u šaman nūni* **75** [*ištēniš*] *taballal ina pēmti ašāgi qaqqassu tuqattar*	[74][If man's] cranium/brain$^{?}$ is constantly hot: [75]You mix [together] [74]gypsum, (multi-)coloured horned *uhūlu*-alkali, *kibrītu*-sulphur, bone, horned *uhūlu*-alkali, naphtha and fish oil. [75]You fumigate his head over charcoal of *ašāgu*-acacia.

74 NI ii 10 [DIŠ NA$^{?}$ UG]U$^{?}$-*šú* KÚM.KÚM-*em* IM.BABBAR NAGA.SI IN.GÙN *kib-rit* GÌR.PAD.DA NAGA.SI Ì.HUL *u* Ì.KU$_6$

75 NI ii 11 [1-*niš* H]E.HE *ina* NE ^{giš}KIŠI$_{16}$ SAG.DU-*su* *tu-qat-tar*

76 [*šumma amēlu*] *muhhašu*? *umma išûma īnāšu ibarrurā dāma ukallā šuššān qa sahlê tahaššal tanappi* **77** *ina mê kasî talâš qaqqassu tugallab taṣammidma* UD.3.KAM *lā ipaṭṭar*	[76][If man's] cranium/brain? has *ummu*-fever, his eyes flicker (and) contain blood. You crush and sift one third litre of *sahlû*-plant, [77]you knead (it) in the sap of a *kasû*-plant. You shave his head, bandage (it, and) ditto (= he shall not remove the bandage for three days).
Alternative prescription 1 **78** *šuššān qa sahlê šuššān qa isqūqa ina ṭābāti kasî talâš qaqqassu tugallab taṣammidma* UD.3.KAM *lā ipaṭṭar*	**Alternative prescription 1** [78]You knead one third litre of *sahlû*-plant (and) one third litre of coarse flour in vinegar. You shave his head, bandage (it, and) ditto (= he shall not remove the bandage for three days).
Alternative prescription 2 **79** *šuššān qa arti titti ina šizbi talâš*? [*tugallab ašar*] *šanîmma šuššān qa būšāna ina šizbi talâš tugallab ašar šanîmma*	**Alternative prescription 2** [79]You knead one third litre of fig leaf in milk, [shave his head] ditto. You knead one third litre of *būšānu*-plant in milk. You shave (his head), ditto (= bandage it and he shall not remove the bandage for three days).
Alternative prescription 3 **80** *šuššān qa urâna* [...] *ina šizbi talâš tugallab ašar šanîmma*	**Alternative prescription 3** [80]You knead one third litre of *urânu*-plant [...] in milk. You shave (his head), bandage (it, and) ditto (= he shall not remove the bandage for three days).
Alternative prescription 4 **81** *šuššān qa ṣadānu* [...] *ina šizbi talâš tugallab ašar šanîmma*	**Alternative prescription 4** [81]You knead one third litre of *ṣadānu*-plant [...] in milk. You shave (his head), bandage (it, and) ditto (= he shall not remove the bandage for three days).
Alternative prescription 5 **82** *samāna* [...] *ina šizbi talâš tugallab ašar šanîmma*	**Alternative prescription 5** [82]You knead '*samāna*-disease-plant' [...........] in milk. You shave (his head), bandage (it, and) ditto (= he shall not remove the bandage for three days).

76	NI ii 12	[DIŠ NA$^{?}$ UG]U$^{?}$-*šú* KÚM TUK-*ma* IGI.MIN-*šú i-bar-ru-ra* MÚD *ú-kal-la* 1/3 SÌLA ZÀ.HI.LI GAZ SIM
77	NI ii 13	⸢*ina* A⸣ [GAZI^{s}]^{ar} SILA$_{11}$-*aš* SAG.DU-*su* SAR-*ab* LAL-*ma* UD.3.KÁM NU DU$_{8}$
78	NI ii 14	⸢1/3⸣ SÌLA ⸢ZÀ.HI.LI 1/3 SÌLA⸣ ZÌ.KUM *ina* A.GEŠTIN.NA SILA$_{11}$-*aš* SAG.DU-*su* SAR-*ab* LAL-*ma* UD.3.KÁM NU DU$_{8}$
79	NI ii 15	1/3 SÌLA PA ^{giš}PÈŠ *ina* GA ⸢SILA$_{11}$$^{?}$-*aš*$^{?}$⸣ [SAR-*ab* KI]MIN ⸢1/3⸣ SÌLA ^{ú}HAB *ina* GA SILA$_{11}$-*aš* SAR-*ab* KIMIN
80	NI ii 16	1/3 SÌLA ^{ú}*u$_{5}$-r*[*a-na* ....] *ina* GA SILA$_{11}$-*aš* SAR-*ab* KIMIN
81	NI ii 17	1/3 SÌLA ^{ú}*ṣa-da-n*[*u* .... *in*]*a* ⸢GA⸣ SILA$_{11}$-*aš* SAR-*ab* KIMIN
82	NI ii 18	^{ú}*sa-ma-n*[*a$_{7}$* .... *ina* G]A SILA$_{11}$-*aš* SAR-*ab* KIMIN

§ V.2 UGU 2 (BAM 482)

Base Manuscript:	**NX (BAM 482)**, collated.
Museum number:	K 2392 + 2574 + 3430 + 3924 + 4091 + 10509 + 11744 + 16407 (+) K 2611
Origin and date:	Nineveh, 7th century BC.
Type of tablet:	Two-column, portrait-oriented tablet. Vertical column rulings done with an instrument, presumably a stylus. Several round firing holes visible on the reverse but not to be seen on the obverse.
Measurements:	ca. 17,5 × 18,2 × 3,6 cm. (K 2392 +); ca. 8,5 × 18,2 × 3,6 cm. (K 2611).
Copy:	BAM 482; JMC 9: 47.
Photo/CDLI nr.:	Plates 40–41/P365744.
Literatur:	Attia and Buisson 2003, additions in Attia and Buisson 2007: 47ff.; Heeßel 2010: 50ff.

NB.

It is not necessary to provide parallels here since this text is cross-referenced many times, see especially the works of Attia and Buisson 2003, 2007.

Edition of the Relevant Prescriptions

1 *šumma [amēlu nakkapti] imittīšu iṣbassuma īn imittīšu dimta ukâl sahlê qēm labti* 2 *[pappas] buqli ištēniš taballal ina mê kasî tarabbak nakkaptašu taṣammidma iballuṭ*	[1]If a man's [right temple] afflicts him and his right eye contains tear(s): [2]You mix together [1]*sahlû*-plant, flour of roasted grain, [2](and) malt [porridge]. You make an infusion from (them) in the sap of a *kasû*-plant. You bandage his (right) temple, then he should recover.

1 NX ii 20 DIŠ [NA SAG.KI ZAG-š]*ú* ⸢DAB-*su-ma*⸣ IGI ZAG-*šú* ÉR *ú-kal sah-lé-e* ZÌ ŠE.SA.A

2 NX ii 21 B[A.BA.ZA M]UNU$_{6}$ 1-*niš* HE.HE *ina* A GAZI^{sar} *tara-bak* SAG.KI-*šú* LAL-*ma* TI-*úṭ*

---

3 *šumma amēlu nakkapti šumēlīšu iṣbassuma īn šumēlīšu dimta ukâl sahlê hašâ tahaššal tanappi* 4 *ina šikari bašli tarabbak nakkaptašu taṣammidma iballuṭ*	[3]If a man's left temple afflicts him and his left eye contains tear(s): you crush and sift *sahlû*-plant and *hašû*-thyme. [4]You make an infusion from (them) in boiled beer. You bandage his (left) temple, then he should recover.

3 NX ii 22 ⸢DIŠ NA SAG.KI⸣ GÙB-*šú* DAB-*su-ma* IGI GÙB-*šú* ÉR *ú-kal sah-lé-e* ^{ú}HAR.HAR GAZ ⸢SIM⸣

4 NX ii 23 *ina* KAŠ AL.ŠEG$_{6}$.GÁ *tara-bak* SAG.KI-*šú* LAL-*ma* TI-⸢*úṭ*⸣

---

5 *šumma amēlu nakkaptāšu ṣabtāšuma īnāšu dimta ukallā sahlê hašâ kasâ* 6 *qēm labti pappas buqli ištēniš ina kanni ina mê kasî tarabbak nakkaptīšu takaṣṣarma iballuṭ*	[5]If both man's temples are afflicted and his both eyes contain tear(s): [2]you make an infusion from *sahlû*-plant, *hašû*-thyme, *kasû*-plant [6]flour of roasted grain (and) malt porridge in a *kannu*-jar, in the sap of the *kasû*-plant. You bind his temples, then he should recover.

5 NX ii 24 DIŠ NA SAG.KI.MIN-*šú ṣab-ta-šú-ma*$^{?}$ IGI.MIN-*šú* ÉR *ú-kal-la sah-lé-e* ^{ú}HAR.HAR GAZI^{sar}

6 NX ii 25 ZÌ ŠE.SA.A BA.BA.ZA MUNU$_{6}$ 1-*niš ina* ^{dug}GAN *ina* A GAZI^{sar} *tara-bak* SAG.KI.MIN-*šú* KEŠDA-*ma* TI-*uṭ*

---

7 *šumma amēlu nakkapti imittīšu iṣbassuma īn imittīšu dāma ukâl sahlê hašâ gaṣṣa* **8** *dadāna qēm labti pappas buqli ištēniš tahaššal tanappi ina ṭābāti tarabbak* ŠU.BI.AŠ.ÀM	[7]If a man's right temple afflicts him and his right eye contains blood: [8]you crush and sift together *sahlû*-plant, *hašû*-thyme, gypsum, *dadānu*-acacia, flour of roasted grain (and) malt porridge. You make an infusion from (them) in vinegar. Ditto (= you tie his temple, then he should recover.)

7 NX ii 26 DIŠ NA SAG.KI ZAG-*šú* DAB-*su-ma* IGI ZAG-*šú* MÚD *ú-kal sah-lé-e* ^{ú}HAR.HAR IM.BABBAR

8 NX ii 27 ^{giš}KIŠI$_{16}$.HAB ZÌ ŠE.SA.A BA.BA.ZA MUNU$_6$ 1-*niš* GAZ SIM *ina* A.GEŠTIN.NA *tara-bak* ŠU.BI.AŠ.ÀM

---

9 *[šumma] amēlu nakkapti šumēlīšu iṣbassuma īn šumēlīšu dāma ukâl larda* **10** *šumutta ballukka ištēniš tahaššal tanappi ina* [...] *tarabbak šanîš*	[9][If] man's left temple afflicts him and his left eye contains blood: [10]you crush and sift together [9]*lardu*-plant [10]*šumutta*-plant (and) *ballukku*-aromatic, you make an infusion in [... and] ditto (= you tie his temple, then he should recover.)

9 NX ii 28 [DIŠ N]A ⸢SAG⸣.KI GÙB-*šú* DAB-*su-ma* IGI GÙB-*šú* MÚD *ú-kal* [^{ú}K]I.⸢KAL⸣.HI.RÍ.IN

10 NX ii 29 [^{ú}S]U.⸢AN⸣.DAR ^{šim}MUG 1-*niš* GAZ SIM ⸢*ina*⸣ x [... *tar*]*a-bak* MIN

BREAK OF UNKNOWN LENGTH!

11' *šumma amēlu nakkapti imittīšu ikkalšuma īn imittīšu naphat u dimta inaqqi šugidimmak šani Ištar* **12'** *ana bulluṭīšu sīhu argānu barīrāta ištēn šiqil ru'tītu maštakal* **13'** *qan šalāli ina isqūqi taballal ina šikari tarabbak taṣammid*	[11']If man's right temple hurt him and his right eye is inflamed and gushes tear(s): (The cause is) 'Hand of the Ghost', deputy of Ištar. [12']In order to heal it: [13']you mix [12']*sīhu*-artemisia, *argānu*-plant, *barīrātu*-sagapenum', one shekel of *ru'tītu*-sulphur, *maštakal*-plant [13'](and) *šalālu*-reed in coarse flour. You make an infusion from (them) in beer (and) bandage (his head and eyes).

Alternative prescription 1	**Alternative prescription 1**
šumma ašar šanîmma šuršummī šiqqi šuršummē ṭābāti dannāti **14'** *šuršummī šikari rūšti suluppi Dilmun ištēn šiqil lipi kanakti ina himēti tasâk teqqi*	If ditto (= in order to heal it): [14']you pound [13']residue of garum (fish sauce), residue of strong vinegar, [14']dregs of premium beer, Dilmun date(s) (and) one shekel of *kanaktu*-aromatic pith in ghee, (and) daub (his eyes).

11' NX ii 62' DIŠ NA SAG.KI ZAG-*šú* GU$_7$-*šú-ma* IGI ZAG-*šú nap-hat ù* ÉR BAL-*qí* ŠU.GIDIM.MA *šá-ni* ^{d}*Iš*$_8$-*tár*

12' NX ii 63' *ana* TI-*šú* ^{giš}*si-hu* ^{giš}*ár-ga-nu* ^{giš}*ba-ri-ra-tú* 1 GÍN ÚH-^{d}ÍD ^{ú}IN$_6$.ÚŠ

13' NX ii 64' GI.ŠUL.HI *ina* ZÌ.KUM HE.HE *ina* KAŠ *tara-bak* LAL : DIŠ KIMIN *šur-šum-mi ši-iq-qí šur-šum-me* A.GEŠTIN.NA KALA.GA

14' NX ii 65' *šur-šum-mi* KAŠ.SAG ZÚ.LUM.MA *Dilmun*^{ki} 1 GÍN Ì.UDU ^{šim}GIG *ina* Ì.NUN SÚD *te-qi*

15' *šumma amēlu nakkapti šumēlīšu ikkalšuma īn šumēlīšu naphat u dimta inaqqi suluppi Dilmun* **16'** *šammi ašî dām erēni ina šamni asi tasâk ina kakkabi tušbât ina šēri lā patān teqqi*	[15']If man's left temple hurt him and his left eye is inflamed and gushes tear(s): [16']you pound [15']Dilmun date(s), [16']*ašû*-disease-plant (and) cedar 'blood' (i.e. resin) in the oil of *asu*-aromatic. You let it stay under a star (= stay overnight). In the morning, without (him) eating, you daub (his eyes).

15' NX iii 1 DIŠ NA SAG.KI GÙB-*šú* GU$_7$-*šú*-⌜*ma*⌝ IGI 150-*šú nap-hat u* ÉR BAL-*qí* ZÚ.LUM.MA *Dilmun*^{ki}

16' NX iii 2 Ú *a-ši-i* MÚD ^{giš}EREN ⌜*ina*⌝ Ì ^{šim}GÍR SÚD *ina* UL *tuš-bat ina še-rì* NU *pa-tan* MAR

17' *šumma ašar šanîmma gaṣṣi Purattu qēm buqli qēm hallūri qēm kakkî qēm kasî* **18'** *tahaššal tanappi ina mê kasî tarabbak nakkaptašu īnšu taṣammid*	[17']If ditto: you crush and sift Euphrates' gypsum, malt flour, chickpea powder, lentil powder (and) powder of a *kasû*-plant. [18']You make an infusion (from them) in the sap of a *kasû*-plant, (and) bandage his temple (and) eye.

17' NX iii 3 DIŠ KIMIN IM.BABBAR *pu-rat-tú* ZÌ MUNU$_6$$^{\text{(sic!)}}$ ZÌ GÚ.GAL ZÌ GÚ.TUR ZÌ GAZI^{sar}

18’	NX iii 4	GAZ SIM *ina* A GAZI^{sar} *tara-bak* SAG.KI-*šú* ^{ERASURE} IGI-*šú* LAL

19’ *šumma amēlu nakkapta iṣbassuma īmim ikaṣṣâ īnāšu nuppuhā šugidimmakku* **20’** *eṣemti amēlūti turrar tasâk ina šamni erēni taptanaššassuma iballuṭ*	19’If man’s temple afflicts him and becomes hot and cold, his eyes are inflamed: (the cause is) ‘Hand of the Ghost’. 20’You parch human bone (and) pound (it) in cedar oil, you constantly smear him (with it), then he should recover.

19’	NX iii 5	DIŠ NA SAG.KI DAB-*su-ma i-mim* ⌜*i*⌝-*kàṣ-ṣa* IGI.MIN-*šú nu-up-pu-ha* ŠU.GIDIM.MA
20’	NX iii 6	GÌR.PAD.DU NAM.LÚ.U$_{18}$.LU *tur-ár* SÚD *ina* Ì ^{giš}EREN EŠ.MEŠ-*su-ma* TI

§ V.3 NY (AMT 25/8)

Manuscript:	**NY (AMT 25/8)**, collated.
Museum number:	British Museum, K 16449.
Origin and date:	Nineveh, 7th century BC.
Type of tablet:	The flake comes from the middle part of a possibly two-column tablet and might duplicate BAM 494 ii 53–57 (UGU 5$^?$), but the lines do not seem to fit.
Measurements:	ca. 3,1 × 2,4 × 0,5 cm.
Copy:	AMT 25/8
Photo/CDLI nr.:	Plate 41/P402032.
Literature:	Bácskay and Simkó 2017: ms. M.

Ll. 1ff.’	parallels	BAM 494 ii 52ff.’

Edition

1’ [...] ... [...] **2’** [...] *ittamuh* [...]	1’[...] ... [...] 2’[...] it has seized [...]

1’	NY 1’	[...]-⌜a$^?$ ba-an-x$^{?}$⌝ [..................]
2’	NY 2’	[.. -*u*]*h*$^?$ [............................]
	BAM 494 ii 53	[... *i*]*t-ta-mu-uh* x [...........................]

3' [...] *ašâ* ... [...]	[3'][If man's eyes are ....(and)] blurred [(...)]: [4']you fumigate him with [3][(...)]
4' [...] *zēr ašli ina pēmti tuqattaršuma ašâ innassah*	[4'][...] (and) seed(s) of rush over charcoal, and the *ašû*-disease will be removed

3' NY 3' [..] *a-šá-a* [..]
BAM 494 ii 54 [..] *a-šá-a* KA x [..]

4' NY 4' [...] x NUMUN $^{\text{(OVER ERASURE OF Ú)}}$ ^{ú}*aš-lì ina* NE SAR-*šú-ma* M[AŠ ....]
BAM 494 ii 55 [..^{ú}*a*]*š-lì ina* NE SAR-*šú-ma* MAŠ.TAB.BA Z[I]

[5'][Invocation: ...] upak bappak[?] [6'][... upak up]ak: incantation spell.

5' NY 5' [...] ⸢ú⸣-pa-ak ba-ap-pa-a[k[?]]

6' NY 6' [.. -a]k tu$_6$-é[n]
BAM 494 ii 56 [...] x pa ú-pa-ak ú-pa-ak tu$_6$-é[n]

7' [...] *dudubi mê nurmî* [...]	[7'][...] this medical application: ([8'][...] you pour) [7']pomegranate sap [...] into his
7a' [...] *ana pîšu tašappakma ina'eš*	mouth [8']and then he should get better.

7' NY 7' [...^{gi}]^{š}NU.⸢ÚR⸣.M[A ...]
BAM 494 ii 57 [... : D]Ù.DÙ.BI A ^{giš}NU.⸢ÚR⸣.MA x [...]

7a' BAM 494 ii 58 [...] *ana* KA-*šú ta-šap-pa*[*k-ma in*]*a*-[*eš*]

§ V.4 NZ (AMT 5/3)

Manuscript:	**NZ (AMT 5/3)**, collated.
Museum Number:	K 10655 + K 10926.
Origin and date:	Nineveh, 7th century BC.
Type of tablet:	Fragment of a two-column tablet, containing typical prescriptions for the head. It is presumably to be placed somewhere in the Nineveh UGU treatise.
Measurments:	ca. 7,3 × 5,5 × 1,5 cm.
Copy:	AMT 5/3.
Photo/CDLI nr.:	Plate 41/P398808.
Literature:	Borger 1967: 529; Köcher 1980a: xxiv; Stol 1991/92: 58 note 102; Worthington 2005: 6.

Edition

1’ [...] *teleqqe* **2’** [... *ina*] *šamni tasâk* **3’** [...] *lā ipparras*	1’[...] you take 2’[...], (and) pound [in] sesame oil 3’[...] (but the disease) cannot be removed.

1’ NZ i 1’ [..] x TI-*qé*

2’ NZ i 2’ [.. *ina* Ì.G]IŠ SÚD

3’ NZ i 3’ [.. N]U KUD-*as*

4’ [... *īnāšu*] *dāma*$^{?}$ *ukallā* **5’** [...] *talâš taṣammid* **6’** [...] *talâš ašar šanîmma* **7’** [...] *talâš ašar šanîmma*	4’[... his eyes] contain blood. 5’[...] you knead [...] (and) bandage. 6’[...] you knead [...] (and) ditto. 7’[...] you knead [...] (and) ditto.

4’ NZ i 4’ [.. IGI.MIN-*šú* MÚ]D$^{?}$ *ú-kal-la*

5’ NZ i 5’ [.. SI]LA$_{11}$-*aš* LAL

6’ NZ i 6’ [..] x SILA$_{11}$-*aš* KIMIN

7’ NZ i 7’ [..] x SILA$_{11}$-*aš* KIMIN

8’ [...] *īnāšu ibarrurā* **9’** [...] *burāša ṣumlalâ baluhha* **10’** [...] *ina šizbi talâš taṣammidma iballuṭ*	8’[...] (and) his eyes flicker. [10’You pound$^{?}$ ...], 9’juniper, *ṣumlalû*-aromatic, *baluhhu*-aromatic’, 10’you knead in milk [...] bandage (his eyes), then he should recover.

8’ NZ i 8’ [.. IG]I.MIN-*šú* ⸢*i-bar*⸣-*ru-ra*

9’ NZ i 9’ [.. ^{šim}L]I ^{šim}GAM.MA ^{šim}BULUH

10’ NZ i 10’ [.. *in*]*a* GA SILA$_{11}$-*aš* LAL-*ma* TIN-*uṭ*

11’ [...] *ina* UD.1.KAM *ša Nisanni* **12’** [... *ṭurri*$^{?}$] *nabāsi taṭammi*	11’[...] on the first day of the month *Nisannu* 12’[...] you spin [a cord] of red wool

11’ NZ i 11’ [..] x *ina* UD.1.KÁM *šá* ^{iti}BÁRA

12' NZ i 12' [.............................. DUR$^{?}$ ^{s}]^{ig}⸢HÉ$^{?}$.MED$^{?}$.DA$^{?}$ NU.NU⸣

BREAK OF UNKNOWN LENGTH!

13' *idra* x [...]	$^{13'}$*idru*-saltpeter [...]

13' NZ ii 1' *id-ra* x [..............................]

14' *kukru* x [...] **15'** *qēm kibti billata* [...] **Alternative prescription 1** **16'** *kukru* x [...] **17'** *qēm kibti haṣab* [...] **18'** *ištēniš ina billati* [...]	$^{14'}$[You ...] *kukru*-aromatic, [...]-aromatic [...] $^{15'}$wheat flour (and) beer mash [...] **Alternative prescription 1** $^{16'}$[You ...] *kukru*-aromatic, [...]-aromatic [...] $^{17'}$wheat flour (and) potsherd [...] $^{18'}$[You mix] together in beer mash [...]

14' NZ ii 2' ^{šim}GÚR.GÚR ^{ši}[^{m}..............................]

15' NZ ii 3' ZÌ GIG DIDA x [..............................]

16' NZ ii 4' ^{šim}GÚR.GÚR ^{ši}[^{m}..............................]

17' NZ ii 5' ZÌ GIG ŠI[KA$^{?}$..............................]

18' NZ ii 6' 1-*niš ina* DID[A ....]

19' *šumma amēlu qaqqassu* [...] **20'** *zappi šahî ina* x$^{?}$ [...] **21'** *tugallab šamna* [...] **22'** *qēm buqli isqūqu eṣēmti* [...] **23'** *tatârma annuharu* [...] **24'** *ištēniš taqallu tazarru* [...] **25'** *ṭābāti bašlāti* [...] ...	$^{19'}$If man's head [...] $^{20'}$[*You* ...] pig's bristle in ... [and ...] $^{21'}$You shave (his head) [and ...] sesame oil [...] $^{22'}$malt flour, coarse flour, bone of [...] $^{23'}$You do ... again and $^{24'}$you roast $^{23'}$*annuharu*-mineral [...] $^{24'}$(and) spatter (his eyes/head) [...] $^{25'}$boiled vinegar [...] ...

19' NZ ii 7' ⸢DIŠ NA SAG.DU⸣-*su* x [..............................]

20' NZ ii 8' *zap-pí* ŠAH *ina* x [..............................]

21' NZ ii 9' SAR-*ab* Ì.GIŠ x [..............................]

22' NZ ii 10' ZÌ MUNU$_{6}$ ZÌ.KUM ⸢GÌR⸣.PA[D ....]

23’	NZ ii 11’	GUR-*ma an-nu-ha-*[*ru* ....]
24’	NZ ii 12’	1-*niš* BIL-*lu* MAR x [..........]
25’	NZ ii 13’	A.GEŠTIN.NA ŠEG$_6$.G[Á$^{?}$ ....]
26’	NZ ii 14’	x x x x [..........]

§ V.5 NZa (AMT 13/5 + 14/5)

Manuscript:	**NZa (AMT 13/5 + 14/5)**, collated.
Museum Number:	K 2974.
Origin and date:	Nineveh, 7th century BC.
Type of tablet:	Corner of possibly two-column tablet, which belongs to the treatise UGU 3, duplicating K 2516 (+) 2566+ i, bottom.
Measurements:	ca. 7,7 × 7 × 3 cm.
Copy:	AMT 13/5 + AMT 14/5.
Photo/CDLI nr.:	Plate 41/P394756.
Literature:	Thomspon 1937b: 29 (no. 8), 32; Borger 1976: 529 and 236, 102/1 etc.; Scurlock 2006: 165f. (nos. 98 and 108–109, 116), 224 (com. ii 2f.), 681.

Edition of the Relevant Prescription

8’ [*šumma amēlu šer’ān*] *nakkaptīšu tebīma īn imittīšu dimta ukalla īnāšu dāma malâ* **9’** [*pānūšu*] *iṣṣanundū ezzuš iṣbassuma šuruš ašāgi*$^{??}$ *ša*$^{??}$ **10’** [*ina*] *nasāhīšu Šamaš lā īmaru tubbal tupâṣ nakkaptīšu uṣammad*$^{?}$	8’[If man’s] temple veins throb and his right eye contains tear(s), his both eyes are full of blood 9’he has a vertigo (and) his anger$^{?}$ afflicts him:you dry and crush root of *ašāgu*-acacia’, which 10’has not seen the sun when it was torn out, (and) he bandages both his temples (with it).

8’	NZa 8’	[DIŠ NA SA SA]G.KI-*šú* ZI-*ma* IGI ZAG-*šú* ÉR *ú-kal-la* IGI.MIN-*šú* MÚD DIRI-*a*
9’	NZa 9’	[IGI.MEŠ-*šú*] ⌜*i*⌝-*ṣa-nun-du e-zu-uš* DAB-*su* SUHUŠ KI[ŠI$_{16}$ *š*]*á*$^{?}$
10’	NZa 10’	[*ina* Z]I-*šú* ^{d}UTU NU IGI.DU$_8$ *tu-bal tu-pa-áṣ* SAG.KI.MIN-*šú ú-ṣa-a*[*m-mad*$^{?}$]

§ VI Diagnostic Medical Omens Concerned with Sick Eyes (Diagnostic Handbook, *Sakikkû* Chapter 5)

Manuscripts transliterated with bound text by Eric Schmidtchen, translated and edited by Strahil V. Panayotov.

TITLE *šumma marṣu īn imittišu ikkalšu qāt il abīšu*[?] ... *imarraṣma*[?] *iballuṭ*
If the sick man's right eye hurts him: (the cause is) the hand-of-his-father's-god; he (the patient) will be sick (for x-days), but should recover.

Manuscripts

A	K 6629	AMT 75/2	TDP I, 44–46	1'–16'
B	BM 121063	forthcoming copy by Schmidtchen	– mentioned in Heeßel 2000: 133 fn. 20.	17'–31' 56'–65'
C	K 6737	CT 37/50	TDP I, 46–48	32'–41' 70'–78' (*BAD* 49'–60')
D	K 13985	TDP II, Pl. IX	TDP I, 46–48	42'–49', 79'–84' (*BAD* 61'–67')
E	K 10570	TDP II, Pl. IX	TDP I, 48–50	50'–56' 87'–98' (*BAD* 68'–80')
F	K 8078	–	–	57'–69'
G	W 17360g	TDP II, Pl. LXVI	TDP I, 48	79'–86' (*BAD* 61'–67')
H	K 3957 + K 6347 + K 9350	AMT 105/2	TDP I, 50–54	99'–112' (*BAD* 81'–99')
I	K 7099	CT 37/50	TDP I, 50–52	113'–135' (*BAD* 100'–126')

https://doi.org/10.1515/9781501506550-011

J	K 10691	TDP II, Pl. XVIII	– uncertain placement, but see Schmidtchen, forthcoming, *Mesopotamische Diagnostik*, Tafel 5	132'–142'(?)

Commentary

a	W 22307/16	SpTU I, Nr. 31	SpTU I, 39–40; Clancier 2009: 480;	1, 11', 14'(?), 52', 56'–57'(?), 58'–59'(?), 100'(?), 104(?), 107', 108', 120'

NB.

For an eclectic English edition of tablet 5, without variants, but with concise explanatory notes, compare Scurlock 2014: 45ff.

Edition

BREAK OF UNKNOWN LENGTH!	**BREAK OF UNKNOWN LENGTH!**
1' [*šumma*] *īn šumēlišu*[?] [...] *amēlu šū*[?] [...]	1'[If] his left eye [...] this man will[?] [...]
2' [*šumma*] *īn imittišu pa'ṣatma* [...]	2'[If] his right eye is injured and [...]
3' [*šumma*] *īn šumēlišu pa'ṣatma* [...]	3'[If] his left eye is injured and [...]
4' [*šumma*] *īnāšu pa'ṣāma* [...]	4'[If] his both eyes are injured and [...]
5' [*šumma*] *īn imittišu pa'ṣatma* [...]	5'[If] his right eye is injured and [...]
6' *šumma īn šumēlišu pa'ṣatma* [...]	6'If his left eye is injured and [...]
7' *šumma īnāšu pa'ṣāma kalâ*[?] [*nadâ* ...]	7'If his both eyes are injured and [discharge] yellowish *kalû*-secretion [...]
8' *šumma īn imittišu kalâ nadât* [...]	8'If his right eye discharges yellowish *kalû*-secretion [...]
9' *šumma īn šumēlišu kalâ nadât* [...]	9'If his left eye discharges yellowish *kalû*-secretion [...]
10' *šumma īnāšu kalâ nadâ* [...]	10'If his both eyes discharge yellowish *kalû*-secretion [...]
	11'If his right eye is dark [...]
11' *šumma īn imittišu tarkat* [...]	12'If his left eye is dark: it will be prolonged and [...]

12' *šumma īn šumēlišu tarkat irrikma* [...]	13'If his both eyes are dark: it will be prolonged and [...]
13' *šumma īnāšu tarkā irrikma* [...]	14'If his right eye is dark and he cannot open (it) ... [...]
14' *šumma īn imittišu tarkatma lā ipettē* ... [...]	15'[If his left eye[is dark and he cannot open [(it) ...]
15' [*šumma īn šumēlišu*] *tarkatma lā ipettē* [...]	16'[If his both eyes are dark and he] cannot open (them) [...]
16' [*šumma īnāšu tarkāma*] *lā ipettē* [...]	
BREAK OF UNKNOWN LENGTH!	**BREAK OF UNKNOWN LENGTH!**
17' [*šumma* ...] *ibalIuṭ*	17'[If ...] he should recover.
18' ...	18'...
19' [*šumma* ...] *iballuṭ*?	19'[If ...] he should recover.?
20' [*šumma* ...] *iballuṭ*	20'[If ...] he should recover.
21' [*šumma* ... *qāt*] *ilišu*?	21'[If ... (the cause is) the hand]-of-his god.
22' [*šumma* ...] *iballuṭ*	22'[If ...] he should recover.
23' [*šumma* ... *qāt*] *il ālišu*	23'[If ... (the cause is) the hand]-of-his city god.
24' [*šumma* ...] *iballuṭ*?	24'[If ...] he should recover.?
25' [*šumma* ... *murussu*] *ikabbit*?	25'[If ... his sickness] will be grave.?
26' [*šumma* ... *murussu*] *ikabbit*?	26'[If ... his sickness] will be grave.?
27' [*šumma* ...] *imât*	27'[If ...] he will die.
28' [*šumma* ...] *irrikma*? *iballuṭ*	28'[If ...] it will be prolonged and he should recover.
29' [*šumma* ...] *irrikma*? *iballuṭ*?	29'[If ...] it will be prolonged? and he should recover.? 30'[If ...] he will die.? 31'...
30' [*šumma* ...] *imât*?	
31' ...	
BREAK OF UNKNOWN LENGTH!	**BREAK OF UNKNOWN LENGTH!**
32' [*šumma* ...] *imât*	32'[If ...] he will die.
33' [*šumma* ...] *imât*	33'[If ...] he will die.
34' [*šumma* ... *murussu*?] *irrik*	34'[If ... his sickness?] will be prolonged.
35' [*šumma* ...] *imât*	35'[If ...] he will die.
36' [*šumma* ... *murussu*?] *ikabbitma imât*	36'[If ... his sickness?] will be grave and he will die.
37' [*šumma* ... *murussu*?] *irrikma na'id*	37'[If ... his sickness?] will be prolonged and he/it is worried/worrying.
38' [*šumma* ... *murussu*] *irrikma iballuṭ*	38'[If ... his sickness] will be prolonged but he should recover.
39' [*šumma* ...] *imât*	39'[If ...] he will die.
40' [*šumma* ...] *imât*	40'[If ...] he will die. 41'[If ...] there is no fault.
41' [*šumma* ...] *ḫīṭa ul īšū*	
BREAK OF UNKNOWN LENGTH!	**BREAK OF UNKNOWN LENGTH!**
42' [*šumma* ... *qāt*] *Ištar*	42'[If ... (the cause is) hand]-of-Ištar.

43’ [*šumma* … *qāt*] *Ištar*	43’[If … (the cause is) hand]-of-Ištar.
44’ [*šumma* … *qāt*] *Ištar*	44’[If … (the cause is) hand]-of-Ištar.
45’ [*šumma* … UD] x *imât*	45’[If … on day] x he will die.
46’ [*šumma* …] … *imât*	46’[If …] … he will die.
47’ [*šumma* …] *imât*	47’[If …] he will die.
48’ [*šumma* …] *turrā*? *imât*	48’[If … are] turned back, he will die.
49’ [*šumma* …] *murṣu izzib*? […]	49’[If …] the sickness will *leave*? […]
BREAK OF UNKNOWN LENGTH	**BREAK OF UNKNOWN LENGTH**
50’ …	50’…
51’ [… *qāt*?] *māmīti*? […]	51’[… hand]-of-the-(broken)-oath? […]
52’ [*šumma īn imittišu*] *ilawwī u issušu nūš iballuṭ*	52’[If his right eye] goes around and his jaw shakes, he should recover.
53’ [*šumma īn šumēlišu*] *ilawwī*? *u issušu nūš murussu ikabbitma iballuṭ*	53’[If his left eye] goes around and his jaw shakes, his sickness will be grave, but he should recover.
54’ [*šumma īnšu ša šumēli kapṣat u*] *issāšu nuššā qāt Sîn*	54’[If his left eye squints and] his jaws shake, (the cause is)-hand-of-Sîn.
55’ [*šumma* … *īn*] *šumēlišu kapṣat pūssu* […] *šapassu ša imitti našallulū* […] *ša imitti šāru ina ṣimrišu*? […] *našâ lā ile’’ē* […] *ru’assu ina nadê* […] *ana arkati maḫiṣ*	55’[If …] his left [eye] squints, his forehead […], his lip to the right creeps, […] his right […] is not able to take air in his bloatedness, […], his spittle […] while throwing up: he is affected at the back.
56’ *šumma īn imittišu* [*napalkatma*? …] *usukkašu* […] *lū šuru’šu* […] *ša šumēli išaggum* […] *ša imitti šāru lā irrub ša* […] *naṣāpa lā ile’’ē u ru’assu* […] *qāt mišitti*? […]	56’If his right eye [is wide open? …], his upper cheek […] or his eyebrow, [his ear] to the left buzzes?, […], no air enters [… in his nostril?] to the right, […] he is not able to suck, and his spittle [… (the cause is)] hand-of-the-stroke? […]
57’ *šumma īn šumēlišu napalkatma īn imittišu kapṣat* […] *murdinnu*? *uqqū*? *imitta u šumēla miḫra maḫiṣ*	57’If his left eye is wide open and his right eye drops […] *murdinnu*-brambles covered it?: he is struck to the right, left and front.
58’ *šumma īn imittišu marṣatma kalât* […] *uznu ša šumēli dāma ukâl u mādiš ana šaplānu imqut*? *igâš*? *imât*	58’If his right eye is sick and holds still […?], his left ear contains blood, and much drops downwards, (and) he vomits?: he will die.
59’ *šumma īn šumēlišu marṣatma kalât u lā inaššī imât*	59’If his left eye is sick, holds still and he cannot lift (it): he will die.
60’ *šumma īn imittišu maḫṣatma katmatma lā ipettē qāt Marduk ana* UD 3 *imât*	60’If his right eye is struck, thus closed and he cannot open (it, the cause is) hand-of-Marduk: he will die in three days.

61’ *šumma īn šumēlišu maḫṣatma katmatma lā ipettē qāt Adad ana* UD 4 *imât*	61’If his left eye is struck, thus closed and he cannot open (it, the cause is) hand-of-Adad: he will die in four days.
62’ *šumma īn šumēlišu maḫṣatma kalât te’ât u lā inaṭṭal imât*	62’If his left eye is struck, holds still, smothered and he cannot see: he will die.
63’ *šumma īn šumēlišu*$^{?}$ *katmat irrikma imât*$^{?}$	63’If his left eye is closed, (the sickness) will be prolonged and he will die.
64’ [*šumma īn imittišu/šumēlišu*$^{?}$] *katmatma lā ipettē* [...]	64’[If his right/left eye] is closed and he cannot open [(it) ...]
65’ ...	65’...
66’ [*šumma*...] *qāt* [...]	66’[If ... (the cause is)] hand-of-[...]
67’ [*šumma*...] *iraššī qāt* [...]	67’[If ...], he has (... the cause is) hand-of-[...]
68’ [*šumma*...] *ītenezzebšu*$^{?}$ *ikaṣṣaṣ*$^{?}$ [...] *qāt* [...]	68’[If ... it$^{?}$] always abandons him, he gnashes (his teeth) [... (the cause is)] hand-of-[...]
69’ [*šumma*...] *qāt* [...]	69’[If ... (the cause is)] hand-of-[...]
BREAK OF UNKNOWN LENGTH	**BREAK OF UNKNOWN LENGTH**
70’ ...	70’...
71’ *šumma īnāšu qadūta* [*sāmta malâ* ...]	71’If his eyes [are full of red] silt [...] 72’If his eyes [are full of red] silt [...]
72’ *šumma īnāšu qadūta* [*sāmta malâ* ...]	73’If his eyes [are full of] red silt [...] / this sick man should recover. [...]
73’ *šumma īnāšu qadūta sāmta* [*malâ* ...] / *marṣu šū iballuṭ* [...]	74’If his eyes are full of blood: [he will die$^{?}$].
74’ *šumma īnāšu dāma malâ* [*imât*$^{?}$]	75’If his eyes are full of blood: [...]
75’ *šumma īnāšu dāma malâ* [...]	76’If his eyes are full of blood: [...]
76’ *šumma īnāšu dāma malâ* [...]	77’If his eyes are full of blood: [... (the cause is)] wind-blast$^{?}$ [...]
77’ *šumma īnāšu dāma malâ* [...] *šibiṭ šāri*$^{?}$ [...] **78’** *šumma īnāšu* [...]	78’If his eyes [...]
BREAK OF UNKNOWN LENGTH	**BREAK OF UNKNOWN LENGTH**
79’ *šumma* [*īnāšu* ...]	79’ If his [eyes ...]
80’ *šumma īnāšu kīma*$^{?}$ [...]	80’If his eyes are like [...]
81’ *šumma īnāšu kīma*$^{?}$ [...]	81’If his eyes are like [...]
82’ *šumma īnāšu ibakkâ* [...]	82’If his eyes weep [...]
83’ *šumma īnāšu ibakkâ birdu*$^{?}$ [...]	83’If his eyes weep, (having) pockmark [...]
84’ *šumma īnāšu dimāti irtanaššâ* [...]	84’If his eyes have tears [...]
85’ [*šumma īnāšu*] *dimāti ittanaddâ* [...]	85’[If his eyes] are constantly giving off tears [...]
86’ ...	86’...
BREAK OF UNKNOWN LENGTH	**BREAK OF UNKNOWN LENGTH**
87’ *šumma īnāšu* [...]	87’If his eyes are [...]
88’ *šumma īnāšu* [...] *marṣu šū*$^{?}$ [...]	88’If his eyes are [...] this sick-man [...]
89’ *šumma īnāšu balṣā*$^{?}$ [...]	89’If his eyes are staring [...]

90’ *šumma īnāšu balṣā?* [...]	90’If his eyes are staring [...]
91’ *šumma īnāšu nabalkutma?* [...]	91’If his eyes are twisted and [...]
92’ *šumma īnāšu nabalkutma?* [...]	92’If his eyes are twisted and [...]
93’ *šumma īnāšu maqtā/muqqutā ina?* [...]	93’If his eyes are sunken, in? [...]
94’ *šumma īnāšu maqtāma* [...]	94’If his eyes are sunken, [...]
95’ *šumma īnāšu maqtāma* [...]	95’If his eyes are sunken and [...]
96’ *šumma īnāšu maqtāma* [...]	96’If his eyes are sunken and [...]
97’ *šumma īnāšu maqtāma* [...]	97’If his eyes are sunken and [...]
98’ *šumma īnāšu maqtāma* [...]	98’If his eyes are sunken and [...]
BREAK OF UNKNOWN LENGTH	**BREAK OF UNKNOWN LENGTH**
99’ [*šumma*] *īnāšu* [...]	99’[If] his eyes [...]
100’ *šumma īnāšu* [(*burkāšu kirrāšu ... mitḫāriš ikkalāšu?*)] *ištū* [*murussu ittabšû ana aganutillê*] *itâršumma* [*ina ūm tīk šamê imât?*]	100’If his eyes, [(his knee, his collarbone and ... hurt him altogether?)], since [his sickness appeared] and changed [into dropsy] then [he will die on a rainy day.]
101’ *šumma īnāšu* [*itteneprikkā?* ...]	101’If his eyes [constantly malfunction ...]
102’ *šumma īnāšu* [*itteneprikkā?* ...]	102’If his eyes [constantly malfunction ...]
103’ *šumma īnāšu* [*lapit/ulappat?* ...]	103’If he [touches] his eyes [...]
104’ *šumma īnāšu iṣṣanundā* [...] *u minâtūšu illakā?* [...]	104’If his eyes circle around [...] and his limbs move [...]
105’ *šumma īnāšu iṣṣanundā u* [...]	105’If his eyes circle around [...]
106’ *šumma īnāšu izzakâ/izzakkâ?* ... [...]	106’If his eyes are clear? [...]
107’ *šumma īnāšu u’ammaṣ* [... *dāmū?*] / *ina pîšu illakū* [...]	107’If he *flays* his eyes [... blood?] / flows out of his mouth [...]
108’ *šumma īnāšu bērā* [...]	108’If his eyes are barely opened [...]
109’ *šumma īnāšu kabtāma* [...]	109’If his eyes are heavy [...]
110’ *šumma īnāšu elī* [...]	110’If his eyes are over [...]
111’ *šumma īnāšu* ... [...]	111’If his eyes are ... [...]
112’ *šumma īnāšu* ... [...]	112’If his eyes are ... [...]
BREAK OF UNKNOWN LENGTH	**BREAK OF UNKNOWN LENGTH**
113’ [*šumma pūṣ? īnīšu qû?*] *arqūtu iprikū?* [...]	113’[If] yellow [filament] covers [the white of his eyes ...]
114’ [*šumma pūṣ? īnīšu*] *urqa balil* [...]	114’[If the white of his eyes] is mixed with yellow colour [...]
115’ [*šumma pūṣ? īnīšu*] *nabalkutma* [...]	115’[If the (white) of his eyes] is rolled up [...]
116’ [*šumma pūṣ? īnīšu*] *nabalkutma elēnu u* [*šaplānu* ...]	116’[If the (white) of his eyes] is rolled up from above [and below ...]
117’ *šumma pūṣ īnīšu nabalkutma šēpāšu kaṣâ* [...]	117’[If the white of his eyes] is rolled up and his feet cold [...]

118’ *šumma pūṣ īnīšu nabalkutma šēpāšu tebâ*? [...]	118’[If the white of his eyes] is rolled up and his feet throb [...]
119’ *šumma ṣulum īnīšu nabalkutma* [...]	119’If the pupil (lit. 'black') of his eyes is rolled up, then [...]
120’ *šumma ṣulum īnīšu nabalkutma šēpāšu ana libbišu* [*turrā*? ...]	120’If the pupil (lit. 'black') of his eyes is rolled up and his feet are [turned] towards his belly [...]
121’ *šumma šer’ānū īnīšu kīma unqi kappū* [...] *nakid* [...]	121’If the blood vessels of his eyes are bowed like a ring [...]: he is in a critical state [...]
122’ *šumma šer’ānū īnīšu kīma šitê* [... *lū*] *qāt ilišu lū qāt il ālišu* [...]	122’If the blood vessels of his eyes are [...] like a textile [... or ... (the cause is)] hand-of-his-god or hand-of-his-city [...]
123’ *šumma šer’ānū īnīšu illakūma ša nakkapti šaknū* [...]	123’If the blood vessels of his eyes are moving, but those on his temple are still [...]
124’ *šumma šer’ānū kakkulti īn imittišu ṣalmū* [...]	24’If the blood vessels of his right eyeball are black [...]
125’ *šumma šer’ānū kakkulti īn šumēlišu ṣalmū* [...]	125’If the blood vessels of his left eyeball are black [...]
126’ *šumma šer’ānū kakkulti īnīšu ṣalmū* [...]	126’If the blood vessels of his both his eyeballs are black [...]
127’ *šumma šer’ānū kakkulti īn imittišu tarkū* [...]	127’If the blood vessels of his right eyeball are dark [...]
128’ *šumma šer’ānū kakkulti īn šumēlišu tarkū* [...]	128’If the blood vessels of his left eyeball are dark [...]
129’ *šumma šer’ānū kakkulti īn imittišu* [*du’’umū*? ...]	129’If the blood vessels of his right eyeball are [dark-red ...]
130’ *šumma šer’ānū kakkulti īn šumēlišu* [*du’’umū*? ...]	130’If the blood vessels of his left eyeball are [(dark-red?) ...]
131’ *šumma šer’ānū kakkulti īnīšu* [*du’’umū*? ...]	131’If the blood vessels of his both eyeballs are [(dark-red?) ...]
132’ *šumma kibrāt īnīšu napḫā* [...] *napḫū* [...]	132’If the corners of his both eyes are swollen [...] swollen [...]
133’ *šumma kappū īnīšu šinnâ*? *tiṣbutū* [...]	133’If the lids of his both eyes grasp each other [...]
134’ *šumma kappū īnīšu ša imitti* [...] *tiṣbutū*? *u ummu ṣarḫu* [...] *qāt Sîn*? : *qāt Šamaš*	134’If the lids of his right eye [...] the grasp and flaring up *ummu*-fever [...] hand-of-Sîn : hand-of-Šamaš.
135’ *šumma* [...] *īnīšu* [...] *qû*? *iprikū*? *qāt Sîn* : *qāt Šamaš*	135’If [...] of his eyes [... and] filaments cover: hand-of-Sîn : hand-of-Šamaš.
136’ [*šumma... īnīšu* ...] *šer’ānu*? *arqu iprik qāt Sîn* : *qāt Šamaš*	136’[If ... his eyes ...] yellow colour covers the blood vessels: hand-of-Sîn : hand-of-Šamaš.
137’ [*šumma*...] *qāt Ninurta*	137’[If ...] hand-of-Ninurta.

138’ [*šumma*...] *Marduk*	$^{138'}$[If ... hand-of-Marduk
139’ [*šumma*...] *imât*	$^{139'}$[If ...] he will die.
140’ [*šumma*...] *imât*	$^{140'}$[If ...] he will die.
141’ [*šumma*...] *malâ*/*sāmā*$^{?}$ *imât*	$^{141'}$[If ... his eyes] are full/red$^{?}$: he will die.
142’ [*šumma*...] *turrā imât*	$^{142'}$[If ...] are turned (back): he will die.
Catchline	**Catchline**
1 [*šumma marṣu appašu sām*] *iballuṭ*	^{1}[If the nose of the sick man is red]: he should recover.
Colophon H	**Colophon H**
1 [... *gabri*$^{?}$] *akkadê*$^{?}$	^{1}[... copy$^{?}$ from] Akkad ^{2}[...] many ^{3}[...] wrote checked and collated ^{4}[...] main healer (*asû*) ^{5}[...] of Assur.
2 [...] *ma’dūti*	
3 [...] *šaṭir issaniq barī*	
4 [...] *rab asî*	
5 [...] *Aššur*	

Transliteration

1’ A 1f.’ [DIŠ] IGI ⌜150$^{?}$⌝ [...] / [(x)] LÚ ⌜BI$^{?}$⌝ [...]

2’ A 3’ [DIŠ I]GI 15-*šú p*[*a-a’-ṣa-at* ...]

3’ A 4’ [DIŠ IG]I 150-*šú pa-*[*a’-ṣa-at* ...]

4’ A 5’ [DIŠ I]GI.MIN-*šú pa-a’-*[*ṣa-ma* ...]

5’ A 6’ [DIŠ] IGI 15-*šú pa-a’-ṣa-*⌜*at*⌝-[*ma* ...]

6’ A 7’ DIŠ IGI 150-*šú pa-a’-ṣa-at-ma*⌝ [...]

7’ A 8’ DIŠ IGI.MIN-*šú pa-a’-ṣa-ma* IM.G[Á.LI$^{?}$ ŠUB.MEŠ$^{?}$ ...]

8’ A 9’ DIŠ IGI 15-*šú* IM.GÁ.LI ŠUB-*át* [...]

9’ A 10’ DIŠ IGI 150-*šú* IM.GÁ.LI ŠUB-*át* [...]

10’ A 11’ DIŠ IGI.MIN-*šú* IM.GÁ.LI ŠUB.MEŠ [...]

11’ A 12’ DIŠ IGI 15-*šú tar-kàt* [...]

12’ A 13’ DIŠ IGI 150-*šú tar-kàt* GÍD-*ma* [...]

13'	A 14'	DIŠ IGI.MIN-*šú tar-ka* GÍD-*ma*⌉ [...]
14'	A 15'	⌈DIŠ IGI 15⌉-*šú tar-kàt-ma* NU BAD *qu-b*[*u-ra*? ...]
15'	A 16'	[DIŠ IGI 150-*šú tar*]-*kàt-ma* NU BAD [...]
16'	A 17'	[DIŠ IGI.MIN-*šú tar-ka-ma* N]U⌉ ⌈BAD⌉ [...]

BREAK OF UNKNOWN LENGTH?

17'	B i 1'	[..........] ⌈TIN⌉
18'	B i 2'	[..........] ⌈x⌉
19'	B i 3'	[..........] ⌈TIN?⌉
20'	B i 4'	[..........] ⌈TIN⌉
21'	B i 5'	[.......... ŠU DING]IR?-⌈*šú*?⌉
22'	B i 6'	[..........] ⌈TIN⌉
23'	B i 7'	[.......... ŠU] ⌈DINGIR⌉ URU-*šú*
24'	B i 8'	[..........] ⌈TIN?
25'	B i 9'	[..........] ⌈DUGUD?⌉
26'	B i 10'	[..........] ⌈DUGUD?⌉
27'	B i 11'	[..........] ⌈x⌉ GAM
28'	B i 12'	[..........] ⌈GÍD?-*ma*⌉ ⌈TIN⌉
29'	B i 13'	[.......... GÍ]D?⌉-*ma*?⌉ ⌈TIN?⌉
30'	B i 14'	[..........] ⌈GAM?⌉
31'	B i 15'	[..........] ⌈x⌉ [x (x)]

BREAK OF UNKNOWN LENGTH?

32’	C 1’	[..] ⸢GAM⸣
33’	C 2’	[..] GAM
34’	C 3’	[.. GIG$^{?}$]-*su* GÍD
35’	C 4’	[..] GAM
36’	C 5’	[...GIG$^{?}$]-*su* DUGUD-*ma* GAM
37’	C 6’	[..GIG$^{?}$]-*su* GÍD-*ma na-ʾ-id*
38’	C 7’	[..GÍ]D-*ma* TIN
39’	C 8’	[..] GAM
40’	C 9’	[..] GAM
41’	C 10’	[..] ⸢LÚG⸣ NU ⸢TUK$^{?}$⸣

BREAK OF UNKNOWN LENGTH?

42’	D 1’	[.. ŠU ^{d}]XV
43’	D 2’	[.. ŠU ^{d}]XV
44’	D 3’	[.. ŠU] ⸢^{d}XV
45’	D 4’	[.. UD] ⸢x.KAM GAM
46’	D 5’	[...] ⸢TAG/*šum*$^{?}$⸣-*ma*$^{?}$ GAM
47’	D 6’	[..] GAM
48’	D 7’	[..*tur*$^{?}$]-⸢*ra* GAM
49’	D 8’	[...] ⸢x⸣ GIG TAG$_4$/kàt$^{?}$ (x)⸣

BREAK OF UNKNOWN LENGTH?

50’	E 1’	[.........................] ⸢x x x⸣ [..............................]

51’	E 2’	[.. ŠU] NAM?˺.[ÉRIM? (x)]
52’	E 3’	[DIŠ IGI 15-*šú i*]-*la-wi u i-su-šú nu*-˹*uš*˺ [(x)] ˹TIN?˺
53’	E 4’	[DIŠ IGI 150-*šú* KI].MIN GIG-*su* DUGUD-*ma* TIN
54’	E 5’	[DIŠ IGI-*šú šá* 150? *kap-ṣa-at*? *u i-s*]*a-šú nu*?-*uš-šá* ŠU XXX
55’	E 6ff.’	[DIŠ ... IGI 1]50-*šú kap-ṣa-at pu-us-su* / [... NUN]DUM-*su šá* 15 *na-šal-lu*?-*lu* / [...] ˹x *šá* 15 IM *ina ṣi-im-ri-šú* / [... *na*]-˹*ša*?˺-*a* NU ZU-*e* / [... ÚḪ]-*su ina* ŠUB-*e* / [...] *ana* EGIR SÌG-*iṣ*
56’	E 12ff.’	[..] ˹*lu šu-ru-u*’-*šú* / [... *šá* 1]50 *i-šag-gúm* / [...................................] x-*šú šá* 15 / [...] x x˺
	B ii 1ff.’	˹DIŠ IGI 15?˺-[*šú* ...] / ˹*ú-suk-ka* x (x)˺ [.............................] / *šá* 150 *i-šag-gum* ˹(x)? su? x˺ [...] / *šá* 15 IM NU KU$_4$-*ub* ˹*šá* x˺ [...] / *na-ṣa*-˹*pa*˺ NU ZU-*e u* ÚḪ˺-[*su* ...] / ˹ŠU? *mi-šit-ti*?˺ [...]
57’	B ii 7f.’	DIŠ IGI 150-*šú na-pal-kát-ma* IGI ˹15?˺-[*šú kap-ṣa-at* ....] / (empty) ˹15?˺ [*u* 150 GABA.RI SÌG-*iṣ*?]
	F 1 f.	[....................]-˹*pal*?˺-*kàt-ma* IGI 15-*šú kap-ṣa-at* / [...] ˹*mur*?˺-*din-nu ú*?-*qí*?/*qú*? 15 *u* 150 GABA.RI SÌG-*iṣ*
58’	B ii 9f.’	DIŠ IGI 15-*šú* GIG-*ma ka-la-a*-˹*at*˺ [......................................] / (empty) GEŠTU *šá* 150 MÚD ˹*ú*˺-*k*[*al* ...]
	F3f.’	[.....................] ˹GIG˺-*ma ka-la-a-at* ù ù ne? šit tú ram ma / [..................... 1]50 MÚD *ú-kal u ma*?-*diš*? *ana* KI-*nu im-qut*? *i-gaš*? GAM
59’	B ii 11’	DIŠ IGI 150-*šú* GIG-*ma* ˹*ka-la*˺-*a*[*t* ...]
	F 5’	[.....................] ˹GIG˺-*ma ka-la-a*?-*at u la ina-aš-ši* GAM
60’	B ii 12’	DIŠ IGI 15-*šú* SÌG-*át-ma* DUL-˹*ma*˺ [...]
	F 6’	[..... SÌ]G-*át-ma* DUL-*ma* NU BAD ŠU ^{d}AMAR.UTU *ana* UD 3.KÁM GAM
61’	B ii 13’	DIŠ IGI 150-*šú* SÌG-*át-ma* DU[L ...]
	F 7’	[............ SÌ]G-*át-ma* DUL-*ma* NU BAD ŠU ^{d}IŠKUR *ana* UD 4.KÁM GAM
62’	B ii 14’	˹DIŠ IGI 150˺-*šú* SÌG-*át-ma ka-l*[*a-a-at* ...]
	F 8‘	[.................................. *á*]*t-ma ka-la-a-at te-a-at u la ina-ṭal* GAM
63’	B ii 15’	[DIŠ IGI] ˹150?-*šú*˺ *kát-mat* [...]
	F 9’	[.....................................]-˹*mat*˺ GÍD-*ma* G[AM?]

64'	B ii 16'	[DIŠ IGI 15/150$^{?}$]-⌜*šú*⌝ *kât-mat-ma* [...]
	F 10'	[...]-*ma* NU BAD [...]
65'	B ii 17'	[xx(x)] ⌜x *ma*$^{?}$⌝ [...]
	F 11'	[..] ⌜x⌝ (empty) [x]
66'	F 12'	[..] (empty) ŠU DINGIR [x (x)]
67'	F 13'	[..] TUK-*ši* ŠU DINGIR [x (x)]
68'	F 14f.'	[...] ⌜x⌝ TAG$_{4}^{?}$.ME-*šú* ZÙ.GU[Z$^{?}$ x(x)] / [... ME]Š-*šú* ŠU DINGIR [x]
69'	F 16'	[.. *m*]*at*$^{?}$ ŠU DINGIR⌝ [x]

BREAK OF UNKNOWN LENGTH!

70'	C ii 1'	[.............]-⌜*šú* x⌝ [...]
71'	C ii 2'	DIŠ IGI.MIN-*šú* ⌜IM⌝.[GÚ ...]
72'	C ii 3'	DIŠ IGI.MIN-*šú* IM.G[Ú ...]
73'	C ii 4f.'	DIŠ IGI.MIN-*šú* IM.GÚ S[A$_{5}^{?}$ DIRI.MEŠ ...] / GIG BI TIN [...]
74'	C ii 6'	DIŠ IGI.MIN-*šú* MÚD DIRI.[MEŠ ...]
75'	C ii 7'	DIŠ IGI.MIN-*šú* MÚD DIRI.MEŠ x[...]
76'	C ii 8'	DIŠ IGI.MIN-*šú* MÚD DIRI.MEŠ x[...]
77'	C ii 9f.'	DIŠ IGI.MIN-*šú* MÚD DIRI.MEŠ [...] / IM.RI.⌜A$^{?}$⌝ [...]
78'	C ii 11'	DIŠ IGI.MIN-*šú* [...]

BREAK OF UNKNOWN LENGTH!

79'	D ii 1'	⌜DIŠ⌝ [...]
	G 1'	[DIŠ IGI.MIN]-⌜*šú* x⌝ [...]
80'	D ii 2'	DIŠ IGI.⌜MIN⌝-[*šú* ...]
	G 2'	[DI]Š IGI.MIN-*šú* ⌜GEN$_{7}^{?}$ x⌝ ⌜[...]

81’	D ii 3’	DIŠ IGI.MIN-*šú* [...]
	G 3’	[DI]Š IGI.MIN-*šú* GEN$_7^?$ ⸢ri/sag$^?$⸣-[...]
82’	D ii 4’	DIŠ IGI.MIN-*šú* Í[R ...]
	G 4’	[DIŠ I]GI.MIN-*šú* ÍR-*a* ⸢GE$_6$⸣ [...]
83’	D ii 5’	DIŠ IGI.MIN-*šú* Í[R ...]
	G 5’	[DIŠ IGI].⸢MIN⸣-*šú* ÍR-*a bir-d*[*u* ...]
84’	D ii 6’	DIŠ ⸢IGI⸣.[MIN-*šú* ...]
	G 6’	[DIŠ IGI.MIN-*šú*] ⸢ÍR TUK.T[UK-*a*$^?$ ...]
85’	G 7’	[DIŠ IGI.MIN-*šú* Í]R ŠUB.ŠUB-[*a*$^?$ ...]
86’	G 8’	[...] ⸢x x (x)⸣ [...]

BREAK OF UNKNOWN LENGTH!

87’	E ii 1’	⸢DIŠ IGI.MIN⸣-[*šú* ...]
88’	E ii 2f.’	DIŠ IGI.MIN-⸢*šú*⸣ [...] / GIG ⸢B[I/-*su*$^?$ ...]
89’	E ii 4’	DIŠ IGI.MIN-*šú bal*-[*ṣa-ma*$^?$ ...]
90’	E ii 5’	DIŠ IGI.MIN-*šú bal*-[*ṣa-ma*$^?$ ...]
91’	E ii 6’	DIŠ IGI.MIN-*šú na-bal*-[*ku-ta-ma*$^?$ ...]
92’	E ii 7’	DIŠ IGI.MIN-*šú na-bal*-[*ku-ta-ma*$^?$ ...]
93’	E ii 8’	DIŠ IGI.MIN-*šú* ŠUB-*ta*$_5$ *ina*$^?$ x [...]
94’	E ii 9’	DIŠ IGI.MIN-*šú* ŠUB-*ma* [...]
95’	E ii 10’	DIŠ IGI.MIN-*šú* ŠUB-*ma* [...]
96’	E ii 11’	DIŠ IGI.MIN-*šú* ŠUB-*ma* [...]
97’	E ii 12’	DIŠ IGI.MIN-*šú* ŠUB-*ma* [...]
98’	E ii 13f.’	DIŠ IGI.MIN-*šú* ŠUB-*ma* [...] / ⸢x x⸣ [...]

BREAK OF UNKNOWN LENGTH!

99’	H iii 1’	[DIŠ] ⸢IGI⸣.[MIN-*šú* ...]
100’	H iii 2ff.’	DIŠ IGI.MIN-[*šú* ...] / TA [GIG-*su it-tab-šú*$^{?}$ *ana* A.GA.NU.TIL-*le-e*] / GUR-*šu*[*m-ma*$^{?}$ *ina* UD BI.IZ AN-*e*$^{?}$ GAM$^{?}$]
101’	H iii 5’	⸢DIŠ⸣ [IGI.MIN]-⸢*šú it-te*⸣-[...]
102’	H iii 6’	DIŠ IGI.MIN-[*šú i*]*t-te*-⸢*né*⸣-[...]
103’	H iii 7’	DIŠ IGI.MIN-*šú* TA[G$^{?}$ ...]
104’	H iii 8f’	DIŠ IGI.MIN-*šú iṣ-ṣa-nun-d*[*a*$^{?}$ ...] / *u* UB.NIGIN.NA.BI ⸢DU$^{?}$⸣.[MEŠ$^{?}$ ...]
105’	H iii 10’	DIŠ IGI.MIN-*šú iṣ-ṣa-nun-da u* [...]
106’	H iii 11’	DIŠ IGI.MIN-*šú iz-za-ka* ni/q[á$^{?}$ ...]
107’	H iii 12f.’	DIŠ IGI.MIN-*šú ú-am-ma-a*[*ṣ* ...] / *ina* KIR$_{4}$-*šú* ⸢DU ⸢x⸣ [...]
108’	H iii 14’	DIŠ IGI.MIN-*šú bé-e*-[*ra* ...]
109’	H iii 15’	DIŠ IGI.MIN-*šú* DUGUD-*ma* [...]
110’	H iii 16’	DIŠ IGI.MIN-*šú* UG[U ...]
111’	H iii 17’	DIŠ IGI.MIN-*šú tar*-[...]
112’	H iii 18’	DIŠ IGI.MIN-*šú* ⸢x⸣ [...]

BREAK OF UNKNOWN LENGTH!

113’	I 1’	[DIŠ BABBAR$^{?}$ IGI.MIN-*šú* GU] ⸢SIG$_{7}$ GIB⸣.[MEŠ$^{?}$ ...]
114’	I 2’	[DIŠ BABBAR$^{?}$ IGI.MIN-*šú*] SIG$_{7}$ *ba-lil*$^{?}$⸣ [...]
115’	I 3’	[DIŠ BABBAR$^{?}$ IGI].⸢MIN⸣-*šú* BAL-*ut*-[*ma*$^{?}$ ...]
116’	I 4’	[DIŠ BABBAR$^{?}$ IGI].MIN-*šú* BAL-*ut-ma* AN.TA *u* [KI.TA ...]
117’	I 5’	DIŠ BABBAR IGI.MIN-*šú* BAL-*ut-ma* GÌR.MIN-*šú* SED.[MEŠ$^{?}$ ...]

118'	I 6'	DIŠ BABBAR IGI.MIN-*šú* BAL-*ut-ma* GÌR.MIN-*šú* ZI ⸢x⸣ [...]
119'	I 7'	DIŠ GE$_6$ IGI.MIN-*šú* BAL-*ut*-[*ma*$^{?}$ ...]
120'	I 8'	DIŠ GE$_6$ IGI.MIN-*šú* BAL-*ut-ma* GÌR.MIN-*šú ana* ŠÀ⸣-[*šú tur-ra*$^{?}$ ...]
121'	I 9f.'	DIŠ SA IGI.MIN-*šú* GEN$_7$ ŠU.GUR$^{?}$(SI) *kap-pu* [...] / *na-kid* [...]
122'	I 11f'.	DIŠ SA IGI.MIN-*šú* GEN$_7$ *ši-te-e* [...] / ŠU DINGIR-*šú lu* ŠU DINGIR UR[U-*šú* ...]
123'	I 13'	DIŠ SA IGI.MIN-*šú* DU.MEŠ-*ma šá* SAG.KI GAR-⸢*nu*⸣ [...]
124'	I 14'	DIŠ SA *kak-kul-ti* IGI 15-*šú* GE$_6$.MEŠ [...]
125'	I 15'	DIŠ SA *kak-kul-ti* IGI 150-*šú* GE$_6$.MEŠ [...]
126'	I 16'	DIŠ SA *kak-kul-ti* IGI.MIN-*šú* GE$_6$.MEŠ [...]
127'	I 17'	DIŠ SA *kak-kul-ti* IGI 15-*šú tar-ku* [...]
128'	I 18'	DIŠ SA *kak-kul-ti* IGI 150-*šú tar-ku* [...]
129'	I 19'	DIŠ SA *kak-kul-ti* IGI 15-*šú* ⸢*d*[*u*-ʾ-(*ú*)-*mu* ...]
130'	I 20'	DIŠ SA *kak-kul-ti* IGI 150-*šú* [...]
131'	I 21'	DIŠ SA *kak-kul-ti* IGI.MIN-*šú* [...]
132'	I 22f.'	DIŠ PIŠ$_{10}$ IGI.MIN-*šú* MÚ.ME[Š-*ha* ...] / MÚ.MEŠ-*ḫu* ⸢x⸣ [...]
	J 1'	[...] ⸢x⸣ [...]
133'	I 24'	DIŠ PA IGI.MIN-*šú* 2.T[A ...]
	J 2'	[.................................. À]M DAB.DAB-*tu*⸣ [x x x (x x)]
134'	I 25f.'	[DIŠ P]A IGI.MIN-*šú šá* 1[5 ....] / ŠU ^{d}[...]
	J 3'	[..] ⸢DAB$^{?}$⸣.DAB *u* KÚM *ṣar-ḫu* ⸢ku x⸣ [x x] / [....... ŠU ^{d}] ⸢XXX$^{?}$⸣ : ŠU ^{d}⸢UTU$^{?}$⸣
135'	I 27'	[DIŠ x x] ⸢IGI.MIN⸣-[*šú* ...]
	J 4'	[..........................] ⸢GU⸣ GIB ŠU ^{d}XXX : ŠU ^{d}UTU

136’ J 5’ [DIŠ ... S]A$^{?}$ SIG$_{7}$ GIB ŠU ^{d}XXX :$^{?}$ ŠU ^{d}UTU

137’ J 6’ [...] ˹x˺ ŠU ^{d}MAŠ˺

138’ J 7’ [...] ˹KIMIN$^{?}$ ^{d}AMAR$^{?}$˺.UTU

139’ J 8’ [...] ˹x˺ GAM

140’ J 9’ [...] (empty) GAM

141’ J 10’ [...] ˹x˺-*šú* DIRI/SA$_{5}$.ME GAM

142’ J 11’ [...] *tur-ra* GAM

Catchline

1 H iv 1’ [DIŠ GIG KIR$_{4}$-*šú* SA$_{5}$] TIN
J 12’ [..........................] (empty) [x]

Colophon H

1 H iv 2’ [... GABA.RI$^{?}$ ^{kur}]*ak*$^{?}$*-ka-de-e*

2 H iv 3’ [... *ma*$^{?}$]-*’-du-ú-ti*

3 H iv 4’ [...] *šá-ṭir is-sa-niq* ˹*ba*˺-˹*ri*

4 H iv 5’ [... ^{l}]^{ú}GAL A.ZU.MEŠ

5 H iv 6’ [...] *aš-šur*^{ki}

§ VIa A Note on the Physiognomic Omens *Alamdimmû* tablet 8

The passages in question are edited by B. Böck 2000: 110ff. (Lines: 61–72, 109–110), manuscripts B (82-5-22, 196a = CT 28 Pl. 28–29, Late Assyrian). Böck understands that the relevant passages are concerned with the human eyes. Nevertheless, there are strong warnings against Böck’s interpretation: the syllabic spellings of IGI in lines 23, 31, 73, 91, 95 and 111 (Böck 2000: 110, 112, 114) as *pa-nu/ni* rather suggest that these passages are concerned with the human face and not with the eyes. Therefore, they are not re-edited here.

Notes

§ I IGI 1

NC (BAM 514) According to Köcher 1980b: X note 11, AMT 20/2 does not belong to K 2570+ or to K 2970+, but the fragment has now been joined to Sm 1897, part of K 2970+, see Geller 1984: 293.

3f.' For a possible reconstruction of the two lines one might compare a similar prescription from the second tablet of the series, IGI 2: 156-7'.

6' The translation of *lipû*(Ì.UDU) 'fat' as a 'marrow' will be used when *lipû* refers to *eṣemtu* 'bone.' Additionally, the processing of the drug and its application might be guessed from IGI 1: 43'.

The identification of *lulû* (KÙ.GAN) as 'antimony' is uncertain. There are several other minerals as candidates for antimony, see Wasserman 2015: 610, and Schuster-Brandis 2008: 424.

For the interpretation of ARGAB^{mušen} as 'bat' see Civil 1984. The drug U$_5$.ARGAB^{mušen} is a common ingredient in eye therapy. Scurlock 2014: 336 note 104 rejects the translation 'bat guano' for *rikibtu* (CAD R 344f.) in favour of 'musk,' which might explain the unclear *rikibti ayyāli*, a problem recognized by Civil 1984: 7. However, occasionally in medical texts words for excrement are used instead of U$_5$, in combination with ARGAB^{mušen} (ŠE$_{10}$ in BAM 3 iv 4 [Civil 1984: 7] and ŠURUN in BAM 66 19). If these words are actual variants of U$_5$ designating excrement, then 'bat guano' still comes closest to a translation of U$_5$.ARGAB^{mušen}. The evidence cited above and the fact that the name does not appear in Irianna (especially Tablet 3) argues against *rikibti arkabi* being a 'Deckname' (Steinert 2015: 134 note 102). For a discussion of 'Deckname' see Rumor 2015: § 4.4ff. For drugs including *rikibtu*, see Chalendar 2018.

For the restoration, cf. IGI 2: 50'.

7' For a tentative reconstruction of the break, compare IGI 2: 115'. The reed straw *takkussu*(^{gi}SAG.KUD) is a medical instrument for drug application, blown into the eyes. Alternatively, the medical practitioner used a bronze tube, *uppi siparri* (MUD ZABAR). It is possible that ^{gi}SAG.KUD could be also rendered as *sakkuttu*, see CAD S 80.

8' A braid of wool is often used as a bandage for the head; compare for instance the same spelling from UGU 1, Ms. NI ii 8: *kun-ša*$_{25}$ ^{síg}GA.RÍG.AG.A KEŠDA, see below.

The reading KÉŠ is a more appropriate reading in a Sumerian context, but KEŠDA is a valid reading as a logogram.

https://doi.org/10.1515/9781501506550-012

For $SILA_4$ instead of KISAL, see comments to IGI 1: 29’ below.

NC i 8’ is damaged but compare it to NI i 22: *ana* SAG.DU-*šú* DUB-*ak*, and NI ii 9: [x SÌL]A Ì.GIŠ *ana* SAG.DU-*šú* DUB.

9’ *Sahlû* is a garden plant, according to Abusch and Schwemer 2011: 472 (with literature). Its identification is usually considered to be ‘cress,’ based on a similar term in other Semitic languages (e.g. Aramaic *tḥly’*), see Löw 1924/26, Flora 1, 506f..

10’ Kneading medical ingredients in the sap of a *kasû*-plant is a common technique, mentioned quite often in the first and second columns of UGU 1, see Ms. NI below. For the literature and discussion on the *kasû*-plant, see Heeßel and Al-Rawi 2003: 236 note i 2 and see Eypper 2019 arguing for *kasû* as tamarind.

The reading of the word ‘grain’ in Akkadian could be *še’u*(*m*) or *û*(*m*), see Weeden 2009.

11’ The stone *ašhar* is common in eye prescriptions, often crushed with other ingredients and mixed in fat, ghee and etc., in order to create a salve for daubing the eyes. It has been suggested (but not proven) that the mineral might be antimony, a product used in the production of kohl for the eyes, see Wasserman 2015: 609f. Furthermore, *tuškû* is a mineral used in the glass production, as well as in therapeutic texts, see CAD T 496.

12’ We suggest that KUŠ.EDIN is an abbreviation for KUŠ.ÙMMU(A.EDIN.LAL) = *nādu* meaning ‘waterskin’ for transporting and keeping water, as pictured in Persepolis reliefs. In medical contexts, it probably refers to waterproof leather (after Scurlock 2014: 480ff.). This kind of leather bandage could possibly keep ointments moist and fixed in place. Another possibility is to read *ina* KUŠ EDIN as *ina mašak serrēmi*, see Schwemer 2007: 111.

The term *šuhtu* could also refer to ‘rust,’ either of any residue of the copper worker or as ‘rust’ of the *tangussu*-kettle in l. 14 and elsewhere.

15’ The formulation 1-*šú* 2-*šú* 3-*šú* appears also in IGI 2: 3, 143’. This formulation appears also in a very fragmentary Middle Assyrian manuscript from Assur.

BAM 13: 4’	[.................................... 1-*šú* 2-*šú*] 3-*šú* [IGI.MEŠ-*šú* ....]
BAM 17: 5’	[... HE.H]E? UDU GABA 1-*šú* 2-*šú* ⸢3-*šú*⸣ IGI.⸢ME(Š)⸣-*šú* K[IMIN]
BAM 17: 6’	[...... H]E.HE UDU GABA 1-*šú* 2-*šú* 3-*šú* IGI.⸢ME(Š)⸣-*šú* K[IMIN]

Three fragments, VAT 11488 (BAM 13 = CDLI P285116) (+) VAT 10363 (BAM 17 = CDLI P285119) (+) VAT 16464 (BAM 25 = CDLI P285127), probably belong to the same multicolumned tablet (not noted by F. Köcher). The shape of the signs suggests early Neo-Assyrian or even Middle Assyrian dating. This formulation (1-*šú*

2-*šú* 3-*šú*) was a specific instruction for repeatedly applying medication to the eyes. It differs from other formulations, such as *ina ūme šalāšīšu līša tukaṣṣa*, 'You cool off (the head) with dough three times a day,' IGI 1: 24; 2 118,' or similar IGI 2: 144' etc.

16' For a possible reconstruction GI[G-*ma u ha-an-ṭa* ...], compare the previous prescription, IGI 1: 14'. Ms. NC i 16' only has D[IŠ? on Thompson's copy, (AMT 20/2), which cannot now be seen on the fragment.

17' The ruling on manuscript NC i 17' is reconstructed, and cannot be seen on the tablet itself.

18' One might restore the line according to IGI 2: 148'.

19' The reading ^{giš}*a*[*r-ga-nu* on Ms. NB i 4' is courtesy of Annie Attia. Note that the plant triad *sīhu*, *argānu*, and *barīrātu*, from UGU 2, BAM 482 ii 63' (Ms. NX), was used to cure inflamed and teary eyes caused by the hand of a ghost, 'deputy of Ištar,' see BAM 482 ii 11'. Furthermore, the triad appears in Irianna (Kinnier Wilson 2005a: 47), in anti-witchcraft texts (Abusch and Schwemer 2011: text 1.1: 31'; 7-10: 195'), and elsewhere, BAM 156: 17. The fixed sequence of the plant trio suggests that there is nothing to be reconstructed between *argānu* and *barīrātu* (see also Geller 2005: 5).

20' Spoons of different materials were used to apply cosmetics like kohl to the eyes, see Stol 2016b: 48f. For a kohl application, consult Wasserman 2015: 608ff. Different instruments which might have been used for medical or cosmetics purposes of the eyes are discussed in Sternitzke 2012. See also the tools from the queens' tombs at Kalhu, Hussein et al. 2016: 99 (IM 115425f.) plate 82, 155 (IM 126290), 163 (MM 2134), plate 179b, and Dalley and Postgate 1984: no. 151. Note that the reading of DÍLIM A.BÁR as *itqūr abāri* is uncertain and the interpretation of Parys 2014: 80, and Attia 2015: 100, regarding DÍLIM A.BÁR as *itqurtu* should not be excluded. A syllabic spelling, *it-qur-ti* 'spoon' appears once in IGI, but in a broken context, see IGI 3: 109'. Furthermore, Attia 2015: 100 *et passim* understands DÍLIM A.BAR as a salve, based on Stol 1989a: 166. This is certainly the case with DÍLIM A.BÁR in IGI 3: 94ff.,' also IGI 3: 105,' where it designates a salve made in a lead spoon. However, we interpret other instances of DÍLIM A.BÁR as a medical or cosmetic instrument, i.e. 'lead spoon,' with which the medical practitioner prepared the salve and/or applied kohl to the eyes, see also Scurlock 2014: 361. Pappi 2008: 572f. follows CAD and understands *itquru* as coming from DÍLIM A.BÁR, but without supporting evidence. For the use of lead in medical contexts, see the note of Arkhipov 2009.

The sign MAR on Ms. NC i 20' seems to be on line 20,' pace BAM 514, where it is on line 21'. In other words, we count one line less than Köcher. It might be that the prescription is written over two cuneiform lines, or that the numbering is erroneous, see also Attia 2015: 8: § 11.

21’ There is a certain pattern in the symptomology. First it is said that the eyes are ‘sick’, and then it is specified exactly in which way, e.g. ‘closed’ (lit. ‘covered’). The pattern can be seen also in the previous prescriptions IGI 1: 14f.’: GIG-*ma u ha-an-ṭa*, and furthermore in manuscripts: ND i 22: DIRI-*ma u* DU-*ak*; and NF ii’ 9’, *la-zi-iz-ma u ma-gal i-li-hi-ip*. For a description of double-clause symptoms, also in Hippocratic texts, see Geller 2001/02: 64ff.

The aromatic plant *kikkirânu* is associated with seeds of *burāšu* ‘juniper’ in Irianna, see Abusch and Schwemer 2011: 471.

22’ We prefer reading ^{ú}ÚKUŠ.LAGAB instead of ^{ú}KUŠ$_{8}$.LAGAB because of the gloss *ak-šu* in KADP 4 39, see Geller 2015: 35 note 11, 41.

23ff.’ The same treatment is to be found in IGI 2: 117ff.’, which raises the question why this common prescription was edited in two different tablets of the same Series. There are some small differences, like the exclusion of obvious phrases, e.g. Ms. ND ii 47 omits IGI.MIN-*šú* but adds more applications at the end of the prescription. Cf. the notes below on IGI 2: 117ff.’.

The sign -*š*]*ú*$^{?}$ on Ms. NC i 23’ is suggested by the copy of BAM 514 i 24’. The dividing line on Ms. NC i 25’ is reconstructed.

Geller’s collations of Ms. AB (BAM 159) are recorded in Parys 2014: 19f. It is worth noting that the Assur parallel (AB iv 6f.) is labelled as a *bulṭu latku* ‘tested remedy’ (see Steinert 2015), but not in the Nineveh IGI Series. This may be because a *bulṭu latku* in the Assur parallel (Ms. AB) implies testing for a practical application and hence not necessarily applicable in a Nineveh library context. In addition, there are signs to be seen on the line before Köcher’s copy on col. iv 1’, suggesting that the prescription starts from iv 3’, see plate 43.

24’ Read *tu-kàṣ-ṣa* and not *tu-kaṣ-ṣa*, as in Parys 2014: 19.

Against the copy in BAM 20 14’, NÍG in Ms. AA 13f.’ has the parameters a3, and not the usual a4 (for the parameters see Gottestein and Panayotov 2014).

25’ Note that the rest of manuscript ND ii 47 deviates, see also IGI 2: 119’.

Ms. AA 15’ has Ì.NUN$^{!}$ against the copy of Köcher (BAM 20: 15’), which led to a confusion in Parys 2014: 19 note 79: ‘Lu d’après la copie de Köcher : *šaman pūri*, huile de pot? mais ì.sur n’est pas exclu ni même ì šur.mìn.’ Also at the end of AA 17’ [(...) *bul-ṭ*]*u*$^{!}$ *lat-k*[*u*] is not clear on Köcher’s copy, BAM 20: 17,’ and see the note to ll. 23ff.’ above.

26’ This prescription suggests a degree of empirical experience, since chopping onion causes tearing which counteracts dryness in the eyes. Drinking onion in beer might cause tearing, but chopping onion certainly will; the active substance is a gas (propanethiol S-oxide) produced by the damaged onion which gets into the eyes. Note that the verb, *uhašša* 'he (the patient) should chop' is deliberately spelled syllabically in order to avoid confusion about who is doing what. Cf. the prescription in IGI 1: 15'.

27' The expression *lām patān* 'before eating' is distinct from *balu patān*, 'on an empty stomach.'

28' The exotic, amphibian drug 'bile of yellow-green *muṣa''irānu*-frog' appears in a therapeutic commentary SpTU 1/49: 2 = Scurlock 2014: 346ff., and additional literature at http://ccp.yale.edu/P348470. Outside Mesopotamia, bile from amphibians, among many other sorts of bile, is used in traditional Chinese medicine. For instance, dog's bile was used as eye drops for itchy and dry eyes, see Wang and Carey 2014: esp. 9959, and table 2. Interestingly, a treatment with frog's bile was used to counteract eye dryness in IGI 1: 26,' perhaps because of its moist properties. For references concerning the use of diverse frogs in medical texts, see Bácskay 2018b.

It remains unclear how to distinguish between the logograms ^{uzu}ZÍ and ZÍ, but ^{uzu}ZÍ might specifically indicate the 'gall bladder,' while ZÍ can refer either to bile or the bladder.

29' Note that the difference between GAZI and KISAL is only one vertical wedge. GAZI might not be a mistake for KISAL, but it could be a logogram for Akk. *kāsu*, 'a cup' used as a measurement and written logographically as GÚ.ZI. In other words, GAZI might be an alternative logographic orthography for GÚ.ZI. In the Babylonian Talmud Gittin 68b, Aramaic *ksy* for 'cups' designates a measurement. The logograms GAZI and KISAL also appear in places where the sign GÍN ('shekel') is found in duplicates and parallels. This has been seen by the CAD editors, who suggest that KISAL is a variant for GÍN (CAD Š/3: 99), which was rejected by Borger 2010: p. 330. However, GAZI can also be read as SILA$_4$ as a phonetic variant of SÌLA. Therefore, we might understand KISAL as SILA$_x$, and all of these values are renderings of SÌLA, which is a standard measure.

30f.' This fragmentary incantation seems to be used for activating *materia medica*, in a '*Kultmittelbeschwörung*.' It is uncertain how to read the signs on Ms. NA i 25' (BAM 510); one might consider *a-šar zēru ú-k*[*al-lu*...]. Cf. also the incantation in IGI 1: 65ff.,' which shows certain similarities to our line, and the generous spacing of the signs there possibly suggests no signs between *e* and *li*; thus, we tentatively reconstruct *e-li* as the correct reading.

32' Note that on Ms. AC (BAM 19), the sign form of BA in ^{ú}MAŠ.TAB.BA has parameters [a1b1c2], see Gottstein and Panayotov 2014: category 4. This sign form might suggest an early Neo-Assyrian or even Middle Assyrian dating.

For the spelling ᵘNUMUN on Ms. AmA ii 12' (BAM 165) see the discussion in Geller 2011: 340f. The layout of Ms. AmA does not fit the spacing of the inscribed text. We suggest that the tablet was manufactured, ruled, and formatted as a template for a different text genre, since the vertical middle dividing ruling of col. ii is completely redundant, as is the ruling after line ii 12'. An additional piece (VAT 11824, see the copy to the left) placed in the Museum's box in which Ms. AmA is found, certainly belongs to the same tablet, and might have been col. i' or ii' (not mentioned in Maul und Strauß 2011: no. 52). Note that this fragment also has a redundant ruling. It remains unclear, however, if the tablet originally had two or three columns per side. The remaining text suggests an incantation, but it remains unclear if it was also against the sick eye (ig]i? gig-ga in l. 5'). A tentative transliteration of VAT 11824 reads: 1'[...] x ⌜dugud⌝ x [...] 2'[...] x hé-íb-d[u$_{11}$...] 3'[...] *ṣe-ri* [...] 4'[... h]ul-gig záḫ ⌜a? x⌝[...] 5'[... ig]i? gig-ga x[...] 6'[...] x 1 kisal a ku[r? ...] 7'[... kisa]l? ⌜a⌝ k[ur? ...]. VAT 11824: 4' reminds one of the Assur Medical Catalogue l. 15, the third chapter of the treatise **IV NECK** (see Steinert, Panayotov, Geller, Schmidtchen, and Johnson 2018: 210: DIŠ *šum$_4$-ma* HUL.GIG *ana* L[Ú*? NU TE-*e*] '(One tablet): for hate magic [not to approach] a man.' This supposition is indirectly supported by the fact that ghost afflictions mentioned in Ms. AmA ii' 8,' 15' are a major cause for problems in the neck area. The expression hul-gig záḫ 'to eliminate hate magic' does not seem to be attested elsewhere.

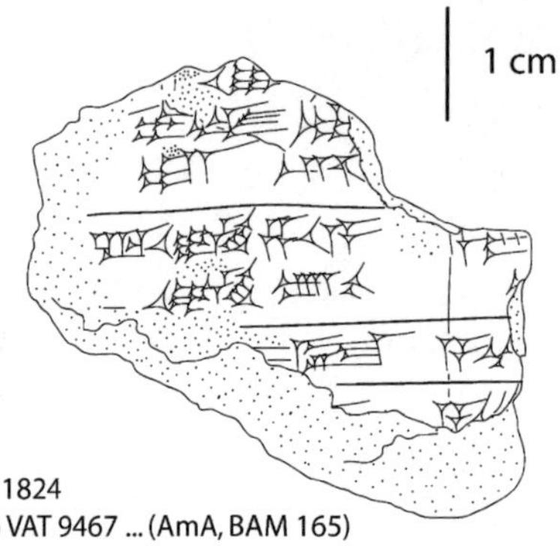

VAT 11824
(+) to VAT 9467 ... (AmA, BAM 165)

(copy S.V. Panayotov)

Ms. AA (BAM 20) is almost completely eroded. Against the copy in BAM 20: 1', there is hardly any space for more signs after ᵘKUR.R[A in Ms. AA 1', although ᵘKUR.KUR might have been written over the edge.

The reconstructed *atā'išu*-plant (ᵘKUR.KUR) was identified with 'white hellebore,' Thompson 1949: 151ff., see also Stadhouders 2012: 16 note 97, and Abusch and Schwemer 2011: 468, but any evidence for a convincing identification is lacking.

The plant *burāšu* is one of the most common drugs in Mesopotamian medicine, and probably belongs to a variety of junipers, see Stol 1979a: 16. According to Abusch and Schwemer 2011: 469, *burāšu* is 'probably a Phoenican juniper.' However, a precise botanical identification is uncertain since the term *burāšu* 'juniper' can possibly refer to different conifers of similar appearance, see in detail Besnier, Boutrolle, Chanut and Hawley 2015: esp. 120f.

For the identification of the reconstructed *nīnû* as a mint variety, see the argumentation of Kinnier Wilson 2005a: 50f. Furthermore, note that the name *nana* for mint or spearmint is still widespread in the Orient and around the African coast.

33' The reading BIL-*lu*$_4$ *u* Ì in Ms. AA: 5' (according to Köcher's copy BAM 20) has been corrected to ⌜BÍL-*lu*$_4$ *ina* Ì⌝.[UDU].

The *kammu*-tanning was used as a leather tanning agent, see Thompson 1949: 168-171; Scurlock 2008: 173f., and analysed as 'fungus' in CAD and Fincke 2011: 173. Postgate and Collon 1999: 8 elucidate this further: 'while on the subject of *kammu* it seems worth raising the possibility that these metal items used for fixing things to wood or perhaps leather were dome-headed nails or tacks and were called *kammu* because of their mushroom shape.' This comment might be based on how the authors imagine modern champignons, but there is little specific evidence to associate *kammu* with fungus. However, the word *kammu* has possible Aramaic cognates for 'truffle,' but only in Palestinian Aramaic, see DJBA: 262. 'Truffle' in Akkadian (*kam'atu*, *ka'u*, see Stol 2014) might be also cognate, if the identification is correct.

For *ribku* see line 78' below.

Al-Rawi copied the number '6' in Ms. sA (*IRAQ* 65, fig. 2), but the photo in *IRAQ* 65, p. 222, fig. 1, shows that '8' is also possible, which fits with the recipe instructions.

The syllabic spelling of *tuštabbal* in Ms. NA i 28' with the meaning 'to stir/mix ingredients' raises a general question whether to read HE.HE as *tuštabbal* or *taballal*.

34' Köcher's copy of BAM 19' shows KID BABBAR, which now has been corrected to Ú.BABBAR, thanks to the photo of EHE 330 provided kindly by M. Guichard.

36' NA i 31' and NC i 37' show an Old Babylonian spelling *šum*$_4$*-ma*. This might suggest that these two manuscripts were copied from the same *Vorlage*.

The LB parallel, Ms. xA 8 is very eroded, and we cannot follow Fincke's reconstruction, see Fincke 2009: 86.

37' Sheep's dung and milk of *musukkatu* are *Dreckapotheke* substances. Animal dung is quite widespread in folk medicinal practices, see Hatfield 2004: 146f. The milk of the *musukkatu* refers to the milk of a woman after childbirth, see Stol 2016b: 439f. On the etymology of *musukku* see Feder 2016: 112ff. The milk of a woman in maternity was a powerful drug, presumably because lactation was associated with fertility and new life. Mother's milk was used not only in Mesopotamia, but also in Ancient Egyptian, Coptic and Greco-Roman medicine, see Ritner 2000:

116. For a healing substance: 'milk of one who bore a male' in Ancient Egyptian see Pommerening 2015. In Dioscorides' *de materia medica* breast milk was used as a solvent for plants, and the salve was also applied to the eyes, see Osbaldeston and Wood 2000: 30. In the Babylonian Talmud breast milk from a nursing mother has been thought to come directly from the blood, which explains why a nursing mother does not menstruate, see Rosner 1995: 119.

On Ms. NC i 37,' one might also read GAZI^{sar} *tur-ár ki-b*[*a-tu* ...], based on comparision with Ms. NX ii 7 (BAM 482): GAZI^{sar} *tur-ár qēm kibti/kibāti* (ZÌ GIG), which is from the second tablet of the Nineveh UGU Treatise and has a similar healing context, see Attia and Buisson 2003: 67: 71.

As with the previous line, the LB parallel Ms. xA 9f. is very eroded, and we cannot follow Fincke's reconstruction, see Fincke 2009: 86.

38' There are two interesting details to be noted: instructions are to be carried out in the morning, and the root of the *rapādu*-plant is to be cut with a bronze knife. The plant for *rapādu*-disease is not common in eye disease contexts. From the LB period, we know of an incantation in an anti-withcraft context, recited over the *rapādu*-plant in order to activate its magical and medicinal properties, see Abusch, Schwemer, Luukko, and van Buylaere 2016: 100ff. This text has some noticeable similarities to Lady Drower's Mandaic 'A Phylactery for Rue' (Drower 1946).

Note that Fincke 2009: 86 reads *mu*]-⌜*kil*⌝ instead of [*ina še-r*]*ì*. As with the previous lines, the LB parallel, Ms. xA 10f., is very eroded, and we cannot follow Fincke's reconstruction.

39' The context suggests that after 'the root of the *rapādu*-disease plant' (l. 38') was cut, it was wrapped (NIGIN-*mi*) in a cord of red and white wool. See similar cases in AMT 4/6: 5': *ina* ^{síg}HÉ.MED.DA NIGIN-*mi* SAG.KI-*su tara-kás* (Scurlock 2006: no. 57). Ms. NB i 24' omits NU.NU between SÍG BABBAR and NIGIN-*mi*.

Concerning Ms. NC i 39f.,' compare the different readings in Fincke 2009: 86 note 22. Furthermore, Ms. xA 11f.' is almost completely eroded away.

40' The expression IGI.MIN-*šú* MÚD *šu-un-nu-ʾa* is also known from the Diagnostic Handbook, Tablet 22: 34-35 (Scurlock 2014: 187), see also MSL 9: 99.

The *egemgīru*-plant is attested in Aramaic as *gargira* and may be 'rocket,' DJBA 298, see also Kwasman 2015: 361, although the word may be etymologically related to the common term 'ginger.'

A reading *lēru* for SAHAR.KÙ.GI is suggested from Irianna III 523-533.

For the term *dišpu* (LÀL) 'honey' vs. 'date syrup,' see Stol 1994: 156f.

41' Ms. AE 3f. (BAM 18) has the sign Ù in place of the more common KIMIN or MIN, see Köcher 1963a: xv; Borger 2010: 409b; further Stol 2016a: 121b.

Note the learned spelling *me*$_{5}$-*sal-lì* for *eme-sal-lì*, a type of salt. The sign *me*$_{5}$(A) 'water' suggests that the substance is a fluid, compare also *me*$_{5}$(A)-SILIM in IGI 2: 195'; IM 202652 i 19. Also BAM 548: 12 has MUN *me*$_{5}$(A)-*sal-lim*. Accordingly, the 'fumigation' commentary BRM 4/32: 13 (see also the note below to IGI 1: 46') has an interesting entry: MUN *eme-sal-lì* MUN *šá lìb-bi* ÍD, '*emesallu* is a salt amidst the river' (Geller 2010: 169, and https:// ccp.yale.edu/P296515), suggesting that a saline solution is meant. *Emesallu* is one of the common ingredients in eye therapy, perhaps because it resembles the salty chemistry of human tears. Furthermore, a saline solution, acting as an antiseptic, is an ingredient of modern eye drops and eyes washes.

Ms. AB iv 25 has ⸢IGI.MIN-*šú*⸣ according to collations of BAM 159 (see Parys 2014). Furthermore, Parys 2014: 21 § 51 reconstructs 1/2 [GÍN] instead of 1/2 [KISAL]. Note that the Assur text Ms. AE 3f. (BAM 18) has the measurement SILA$_{4}$ instead of GÍN. See the note to l. 29' above.

42' On the bases of our text and collations, one might reconstruct BAM 13 (+): 3' as follows [... *ta-b*]*i-la ana* Š[À$^{?}$ IGI. MEŠ-*šú* MAR-*ru* ...]. For BAM 13 see above to IGI 1: 15.'

For the problematic equation of ŠIM.BI.SIG$_{7}$.SIG$_{7}$ see Forbes 1950: 267; Potts, et al. 1996; Jursa 2009: 158 note 51; Schuster-Brandis 2008: 405 fn. 663, 444-445; Middeke-Conlin 2014. ŠIM.BI.SIG$_{7}$.SIG$_{7}$ can be equated with *lēru, šīpu* or *dāmātu* (Irianna III 523-533, also CAD L 148a; Š/3 93b), but all these substances designate different pastes. The reading *dāmātu* is based on ^{ú}ŠIM.BI.SIG$_{7}$.SIG$_{7}$ = ^{ú}*da-ma-tú* in Irianna, cited above.

43' Compare also IGI 2: 53,' 70,' 145'. The spelling in the broken part of NC i 44' might be also *l*[*a-a-am* ...], as in IGI 1: 27'. Note that the expression, *la patān* usually refers to consuming *materia medica* on an empty stomach, but in many cases in the IGI-treatise, the patient has to be fasting before receiving external eye treatments.

45' Geller 2009: 5 equates ŠIM.BI.SIG$_{7}$.SIG$_{7}$ with the *ashar* stone, but see the commentary to l. 42' above.

46' Thompson 1949: 125f. bases the identification of *tarmuš* as 'lupins' on Semitic cognates, see also Abusch and Schwemer 2011: 473, but the identification with lupin is not secure. For Babylonian Aramaic, see DJBA 1235. The plant occurs often in combination with *imhur-līm* and *imhur-ešrā*, and in connection with fumigation prescriptions.

The tentative restoration *nikipta* [*zikara u sinniš*] is suggested by the fact that we have enough place for it (different in Geller 2009: 5), and that the plant *nikiptu* is often mentioned with male and female varieties, see CAD N/2 222). The *nikiptu*-plant is widespread in Mesopotamian medicine, and its importance and power is expressed through esoteric writings such as $^{\text{šim.d}}$MAŠ or $^{\text{giš.šim.d}}$NIN.URTA 'aromatic plant of the (warrior) god Ninurta,' in Parpola 1993: no. 323: 16; Finkel and Reade 2002: 39ff.; Searight, Reade and Finkel 2008: 35. Oil from *nikiptu* was a precious substance and was introduced from Babylonia into Egypt (Hoch 1994: 194f., nos. 260-261). Varieties of *nikiptu*-plant were used for fumigation and their appearance was commented upon in an ancient commentary on fumigation texts, see BRM 4/32: 11: 'Male *nikiptu*-plant is like tamarisk bark, firm and red, while female *nikiptu*-plant is (also) like tamarisk bark, but thin and yellow-green,' after Geller 2010a: 172; also Scurlock 2014: 340ff., photos and additional literature on https://ccp.yale.edu/P296515. See also Abusch and Schwemer 2011: 471, without conclusive evidence.

On Ms. NC i 47,' Köcher copied *-tú* instead of the clear *-tu*$_4$ in *ni-kip-tu*$_4$, which suggest that he copied the broken places with the help of his transliterations.

47' Schuster-Brandis 2008: 404f. identifies *aban tasniqti* as '(schwarzer) Kieselschiefer (?),' assuming that the name might refer to a touchstone used for testing gold. Compare the similar prescription in IGI 3: 39'. However, recently Kleber (2016b) has shown that the stone was not called *aban tasniqti* but rather *aban tašrīti*.

Human spittle is a powerful magical substance, which could be 'cast' like a spell and was associated with sorcery, see Stol 1991/92: 47; Abusch and Schwemer 2011: 3f. The Babylonian Talmud (bPes. 111a) refers to being protected from 'spilled' (i.e. bewitched) water by spitting into it or treating it with dust.

Schuster-Brandis 2008: 444f., suggests that *šimbizidû* (the reading is speculative) is possibly the substance from which *guhlu* was produced and tentatively identifies *šimbizidû* with 'Galenit/Bleiglanz (PbS) oder Weichmanganerz/Pyrolusit (MnO_2) (?),' see also Schuster-Brandis 2012: 178 with earlier literature. Stol 1989a: 165f. accepts the identification of *guhlu*, with *kohl* in Arabic but suggests that it was of lead origin and not made of antimony. See also Cadelli 2001 and Wasserman 2015: 610.

48' The drug MÚD *ša* ŠÀ ŠAH 'blood from a pig's 'heart/insides' seems to be unattested, but the usage of pig parts in magic and medicine is well-known, cf. Rumor 2015: 3.3.8; Irianna III 49ff.; or Abusch and Schwemer 2011: 112: 2: 4; Text 10.3: 1-10; George 2016: 118; 166f. (Old Babylonian).

50' For the reconstruction, see IGI 1: 42'. The spelling *t*]*a-zar-ri* is unusual since one would rather expect *tazarru* (as in IGI 1: 42'), since *zarû* is a /u/-class verb, and a

2nd person feminine form seems unsuitable in our context. We know, however, that the 3rd person singular durative of *zarû* can colour the final /u/ to /i/, as in *i-zar-ri im-ta*, cf. AHw 1516 (see Farber 2014: 84: 126, 155f., reading *iṣarri imta* 'she spatters venom'). For *zarû* in a metaphorical context see Cohen and Llop 2017: 109.

51' For the drug *šammi ašî*, see Abusch and Schwemer 2011: 472. There is a group of plants in the Vademecum designated as *šammi ašî* 'drug against the *ašû*-disease' (BAM 1 i 62ff. Attia and Buisson 2012: 27f., 37f., Scurlock 2014: 277). For the *ašû*-disease, see the note to IGI 1: 178'.

52' Often in Mesopotamian medicine, certain drugs were dissolved differently depending on the seasons summer or winter, see for instance Ms. AD 30 (BAM 22, Assur), or Ms. uA: 11 (SpTU 50, Uruk). There is empirical experience behind such practices, since certain liquids were more suitable as a solvent in cold or warm weather. Generally, it seems common to use the sap of the *kasû*-plant during the summer as a solvent or flush, as in Heeßel and Al-Rawi 2003: 225, § 7: 29; Geller 2007b: 8: 13; BM 30918 r.35; maybe also in the restored text by Scurlock 2014: 456: 59; George 2016: no. 74: 9f. Also note that A GAZI^{sar} is *mê kasî*, and not *mê kaṣûti* 'cold water,' as Stadhouders postulates in George 2016: 168.

For washing drugs see Goltz 1974: 27. Note also l. 20,' in which ingredients are pounded in the 'sun-heat' (*ṣētu*), which may be a parallel idea.

55' We have rendered KIMIN as *ašar šanîmma*, following Köcher's suggestion (1971: xxxii, BAM 417), modified without further argumentation by Böck 2003: 170 etc., as *ašar šanîm*. In this respect, Kinnier Wilson 2011: 12 advocates *ana ašri šanimma* for DIŠ KIMIN as 'alternatively' or 'additionally', which we follow, with the slight modification to *ana ašri šanîmma* (reference courtesy A. Attia, see also Note des éditeurs in *JMC* 31). Furthermore, the phrase *ašar*(KI) *šanîmma*(MIN) 'here again' for 'ditto' has a forerunner in HS 1883 (BAM 393, see Geller 2006) where each prescription is introduced by *àš-šár* 'where', *pace* the reading 400 for *šumma* by Fincke 2007: 138 fn. 54, and 6,40 for *šumma* by Abusch and Schwemer 2011: 65ff. CAD G 87, s.v. *girgiššu* b) corrects *àš-šár* for *šumma* without explanation. See also the comments to ASC 207 and HS 1883 in the introduction to 2nd Millennium BCE therapeutic prescriptions.

The crucial text mentioned by Köcher is the Nineveh tablet, K 10547 (CDLI P398747), which might be part of a two-colum tablet since it is rather thick, measuring ca. 6,2×5×3,4 cm.

Obverse$^{?}$

1'	Ú$^{?}$ ⌜MAH⌝ x [...]
2'	*šum-ma ina* x [..]
3'	LÀL Ì.GIŠ Ì.NUN.N[A ....]

4’ ZÌ EŠA KAŠ GEŠTIN *ina pa-an* MU[L ....]

5’ *mu-uh-ra* DINGIR HUL ⌜A⌝.[LÁ HUL ....]
6’ ^{d}MAŠ.TAB.BA ^{d}x [..]
7’ ***a-šar šá-nim-ma*** *tab-*⌜*ba*⌝- [.........................]
8’ *it-ti-ku-nu mim-ma le*[*m*$^{?}$-*nu*$^{?}$ ....]
9’ LUGAL *iš-šak-nu* DINGIR H[UL$^{?}$ ....]
10’ UDUG *lem-nu* GAL$_{5}$.LÁ H[UL$^{?}$ ....]
11’ GIDIM *lem-nu šá it-*[*-ti*$^{?}$*-ku*$^{?}$*-nu*$^{?}$ ....]
12’ ***a-šar šá-nim-ma*** P[A$^{?}$ ....]

13’ ⌜*an*⌝*-na-a* DUG$_{4}$.GA [......................................]
14’ ^{lú}MAŠ.MAŠ *ana* É T[U (.RA) *illak*$^{?}$ ....]
15’ [^{gi}]^{š}⌜ŠÀ.GIŠIMMAR⌝ ^{g}[^{iš}ŠINIG$^{?}$ ....]

For most of the reverse see Ambos 2013: 48-50. Note that there is no dividing line after rev.$^{?}$ 9’, in contrast to the other manuscripts, see Ambos 2013: 49.

56’ The restoration of Ms. NB ii 8’ [... Ú.BABBAR *ta-b*]*i-lam* is based on IGI 1: 42’.

57’ Plants mixed in coarse flour (*ina isqūqi*) might be imbibed or the mixture could be used for bandages, see UGU 2, Ms. NX ii 64’ (BAM 482).

The rendering ‘dog’s tongue plant,’ for the partly restored *lišān kalbi,* is a literal translation of the ancient name. Abusch and Schwemer 2011: 471 suggest the identification with *cynoglossum* ‘hound’s tongue,’ which is likely to be anachronistic.

The restoration at the end of Ms. NB ii 9’ is uncertain, instead of N[A]G there might be two signs.

58’ In Ms. NC ii 6’ one might think of reconstructing Ú.BABBAR ^{šim}GIG, based on Ms. (bB) 3, see IGI 2: 25.

60’ Compare also IGI 1: 58’ and IGI 2: 21.

61’ Differently in Fincke 2000: 150, 166. Compare also CAD Š/2 439. ‘if a man’s eyes have a deposit(?) of blood.’ The spacing on the copy BAM 22 r.27’ (Ms. AD) is wide and there is nothing after ⌜IGI⌝*-al,* while the signs Ú.BABBAR are broadenly written to fill the space. The lines on Ms. xA 16f.’ (Fincke 2009: 87, 89) are almost completely eroded.

62’ The reconstructed drug *kukru* is an aromatic plant often used in fumigation, originating (according to incantations) in the mountains, see Abusch and Schwemer 2011: 471; Stol 1979: 16ff. LB syllabic spellings suggest normalization as *kukru* instead of *kukuru*, see Jursa 2009: 162.

63’ For this line, compare also IGI 2: 24. The line on Ms. xA 18’ is almost completely eroded (Fincke 2009).

Concerning *šum*$_4$*-ma* AMA$^{?}$.MEŠ, compare also AMT 76/2: 3; AMT 98/3: 5.

ZA.NA = *passu* has a possible Aramaic equivalent in *pys* ‘small stone,’ see DJBA 901b. See further Attia 2015: 39 note 147, and the reference in Irianna III 250 to ZA.NA as *mūnu* ‘larva,’ i.e. something small. The word *passu* probably refers to the size of a pebble as a gaming piece. We prefer to translate *passu* ‘gaming piece’ as a ‘small disc,’ see Finkel 2007: especially 21, 31.

The variants in Mss. AD (BAM 22) and xA (CM 37) may represent the difference in climate between Assur in the north and Sippar or Borsippa in the south.

64’ Köcher’s copy of Ms. NC, BAM 514 ii 12’ reads ⌜1/2$^{?}$ GÍN GIŠ DI$^{?}$⌝ instead of the collated ⌜1/2$^{?}$ GÍN Ú$^{?}$⌝. Furthermore, the sign Ú instead of Köcher’s DI is strongly suggested by the fact that white plant and bat guano often occur together: see IGI I: 34’, 41’, 44’, 71’; IGI 2: 8, 23, [92’, restore Ú.BABBAR], 122’, 140’: IGI III 49’. Also, § IV 12’; § IV.6 (AMT 18/4) 2’ and 6’-7’. § V.1 (BAM 480) 23 [restore Ú.BABBAR]; ibid 68.

The line presumably suggests that this recipe could have been used for twenty days. Compare also IGI 1: 85’. However, this notation could also be hemerological, i.e. ‘this is the drug of day twenty’ used in a certain month. Babylonian Aramaic formulations are sometimes clearer as in the Babylonian Talmud Shab. 140a: ‘Go bring 3 shekels of *hyltt*’ over 3 days.’

65’ The following incantation is difficult to understand, despite some thematic similarities with the incantation from IGI 1: 30’. We consider *kīri balāti* ‘kiln of life’ to be a metaphor for the womb, which probably indicates that the incantation was borrowed from another context. The incantation suggests that the fetus is too large and cannot be delivered, in which case the physician is advised to withhold treatment. The translation ‘I hold back (treatment) completely’ reflects the idea that the situation is hopeless. Similar advice can be found in the Hippocratic Corpus, see Nutton 2004: 92f. and Golder 2007: 183f., and for a similar case in Babylonia, see Geller 2010a: 41.

67’ The expression *ina itti* in omens suggests the time of observation: *šumma ina itti eqli qiššû ša magal rabû innamer* ‘if an abnormally large melon is found in the field at the normal time,’ see CT 39/5: 59. This and similar entries concerning plants can be found in *Šumma ālu* 55: 71f.,’ 82f.’ (Freedman 2017: 102). The statement that the practitioner holds back treatment in hopeless or terminal cases is well documented in all systems of ancient medicine.

68’ The technical term *ka’inimma* (KA.INIM.MA) ‘invocation’ was read in Sumerian in the first millennium BCE, as can be seen in the syllabic writing in Finkel 1999:

230, cf. also Maul 2009: 80. On the other hand, Farber 2014: 319 argues that in the OB period KA.INIM.MA was possibly realized as *šiptum* 'incantation', which however may not reflect the first millennium reading of the phrase.

69' The copy BAM 514 ii 12' (Ms. NC) shows X GÌN.NA, instead of the collated ZA.GÌN.NA.

For the logogram ^{ú}HA or ^{ú}KU$_6$, there are two readings (*urânu* and *šimru*). Nevertheless, in combination with SUHUŠ one should read *urânu*, according to Irianna I 327: SUHUŠ ^{ú}*u*$_5$*-ra-ni*. Note the expression from Irianna I 330: ^{ú}*pa-ri-e* : ^{ú}HA *šá* KUR-*i*. Ms. NC ii 17' (BAM 514) might read SAHAR$^?$.URUDU$^?$, but the second sign is too broken to be certain.

The word *dudubi*(DÙ.DÙ.BI) actually refers to a medical application within therapeutic texts, rather than 'its ritual,' which belongs to a completely different environment (for discussion of the reading see Maul 2009: 69ff., especially 76). Supporting evidence for the meaning 'medical application' can be found in an unpublished Old Babylonian medical incantation in a private collection, which includes a section beginning with KÌD.KÌD.BI (var. of DÙ.DÙ.BI) and a final statement GU$_7$-*ma i-né-eš* 'he shall eat it and get better' (ASC 31: 7, rev. 7). It is clear from the context that we are not dealing with a ritual but a supplementary medical treatment. See below to IGI 1: 78'. Also note the use and omission of DÙ.DÙ.BI and KÌD.KÌD.BI in BAM 503 versus BAM 506, and BAM 508, reference A. Attia.

70' The term *agašgû* is considered to be an academic title that might refer to both the *asû* and the *āšipu/mašmašu*, see Geller 2010: 132, and Oshima 2014: 214. Occasionally, we are informed that the *agašgû* wrote medical tablets (Geller 2007b: 14, 18). Additional references to *asû* have been collected by Mayer 2016: 189f.

The phrase *huhahi lā bamâ huhahi lā bamâ* could be a magical spell extracted from syllabaries, with which the novice learned to write cuneiform, and this would include the *agašgû* as a possible novice physician. The memorable sequence hu-ha-hi is widespread in lexical lists, see http://oracc.museum.upenn.edu/dcclt. On the other hand, *la ba ma* might also reflect graphic values of similar sign shapes or a close phonetic relationship between labials. Syllables had magical significance and other syllables are used as short spells on amulets with apotropaic power (Wiggermann 2000: 220 note 14, and Salvini 2008: 83f.).

73' Compare with IGI 1: 155,' and see also Collins 1999: 222ff. Although this line is likely to be Sumerian, there may be an underlying Akkadian interpretation. One could alternatively speculate and read *til*$_7$*-pa-na* as a pun on *tilpānu* 'bow,' which could be a metaphor for the shape of the ear. In addition, the phrase *a-ga-pa-na* might be a pun of *agappi īni* for *kappi īni* 'eyelid.'

The phrase ú-hu-ur$^{!}$-sag might stand for ú-hur-sag-sar and *azupīru* or *azupirānu*; ú-hu-ur-sag-gi-na might also stand for a 'real mountain plant' with gi-na interpreted as 'firm, real.' On the other hand, the signs 'gi-na' in ú-hu-ur-sag-gi-na might be syllabic for gin$_7$, thus meaning 'like the mountain-plant,' which might be a pun on *azupirānu*, 'the *azupīru*-like plant.'

74' Instead of *kuš-ri-in*, one might consider another possible reading: *su-ri-in su-ri-in-ni*, referring to a plant *surinnu* known from Irianna II 90f.

The noun *šá-hi* might be treated here as *šahhû*, the garment worn by penitents which appears in IGI 3: 76,' with the idea being that Gula surrounds the patient's *šahhû*-gown worn by patients.

An alternative possibility is to treat *ša-hi* as 'my pig,' corresponding to a bilingual incantation where a piglet is used as a magical substitute, see Schramm 2008: 36: 65ff.; for a connection with the Babylonian Talmud see Geller 1991: 108.

75' For the healing goddess Gula, see Böck 2014, add the critical reviews of Zomer 2015 and Geller 2015.

For the sinew/tendon, see Attia 2000.

76' It remains unclear how to render TU$_6$.ÉN.É.NU.RU. For the sake of convenience it is listed in the glossary under *tê šipti*. The signs might be understood only as graphical markers, which were realized in Sumerian and/or in Akkadian, depending on the reader.

78' Köcher 1995: 212a suggested 'gummi arabicum' as an identification for *hīl abukkati*.

The word *kidkidbû*(KÌD.KÌD.BI) 'its ritual' has the meaning of a medical application in the therapeutic corpus. See above to IGI 1: 69'.

For *rabāku* meaning 'to decoct,' see Scurlock 2017: 286, and differently Böck 2014: 104; 2009: 116 'to moisten.' There are Semitic cognates equivalent to Akkadian *ribku*, e.g, *rbykh* 'pulp,' produced by mixing fine flour and hot water (Jastrow, *Dictionary* 1442). This would suggest that *rabāku* involves heating up the substances. Attia 2015: 100 provides several translations, 'délayer, touiller, malaxer,' but the present edition will use 'make an infusion' for *rabāku* and 'infusion' for *ribku*.

79' The fragmentary lines of Ms. NB ii 31,' 32' seem to employ rulings (see pl. 9), which are unnecessary, and were not copied by Köcher in BAM 513, Tafel 12. It could be, however, that those visible rulings are only for scribal orientation purposes, but the fragmentary state of preservation leaves us guessing.

Concerning ^{šim}BULUH.HI.A = *baluhhu*, Abusch and Schwemer 2011, 469 suggest an identification with *ferula gummosa* and it's resin as galbanum, but here in the

IGI treatise, it is a metaphorical designation of a symptom, like the word *murdinnu*, also used in eye disease contexts, see the note to IGI 2: 1. The designation ^{šim}BULUH.HI.A is likely to be a sticky or liquid discharge or secretion from the eye that resembles the colour of the *baluhhu*, and appears together with blood, see Panayotov 2017: 218, 238.

80’ We consider the spelling *di-gal*$_9$(KAL) to be a variant of *digalu* ‘vision.’ For the common expression *diglu kabit*, see AHw 169a and CAD K 15. Note a similar expression *digla ukabbirma* ‘I worsened (lit. thickened) (my) eyesight,’ postulated by the scholar, *Nabû-zukup-kēnu*, to describe his eyesight due to cuneiform script, see Geller 2010a: 135.

^{d}LAMA IGI.MIN-*šú* ‘pupil of his eyes’ is written with a divine determinative. ^{d}LAMA ‘tutelary goddess’ in this expression refers to someone looking into the pupil of another person’s eye and seeing his own reflection, see Panayotov 2017: 219. Note that the word ‘pupil’ comes from Latin *pupila* ‘doll,’ which represents a similar idea, see also IGI 2: 121’.

81’ Leaving drugs under stars was a symbolic action for presumably enhancing a drug’s potency, according to Reiner 1995: 48. On the other hand, to stay overnight was essential for the drug extraction, or ‘maceration,’ see Böck 2009: 112ff.

The *hu-li-ia-am* vessel was probably a funnel in the shape of a conical helmet, which is what the term *huliam* designates. Could this have Indoeuropean cognates (cf. German *Helm*)?

82’ For a discussion of *zibû* as *Nigella sativa* ‘black cumin,’ see Heiss et al. 2012/13: 151f. Note also Radner 2014: 574-578, who discusses the grinding tools used for black cumin.

83’ Annie Attia suggests transliterating *ša ta-áṣ-hu-tu*, which would be suitable to line 81’ above.

84’ After $^{\text{na4}}$ŠU.MÌN, both Mss. NA ii 21’ and NC ii 32’ read ŠID-*nu*, which makes little sense, which is why we prefer to emend the reading slightly to SILA$_{11}$-*aš*.

For *šumēnu*($^{\text{na4}}$ŠU.MÌN) see the discussion in CAD Š/III 272b.

86’ The aromatic *murru* might possibly to be identified with *Balsamodendron* or *Commiphora*, see Middeke-Conlin 2014: § 3.2.2 , but this remains highly uncertain.

87’ The reading *šanîš* for MIN is uncertain. For *šanîš* in commentaries, see Gabbay 2016: 74ff.. Cf. *šá-niš* in BAM 16 r.6. The sign MIN seems to designate an alternative to the prescription in l. 79. See also IGI 2: 140’.

The practice of blowing medication into the eyes might have continued in the Babylonian Talmud, Gittin 69a, where medication was blown into the eyes of a dog, or alternatively into a patient’s gullet.

88' The plant *urnû* might be identified with Ammi, see Abusch and Schwemer 2011: 473.

The dividing line after NC ii 36' is not on Köcher's copy BAM 514, pl. 20.

89' The combinations of igi bar, igi bar-bar, igi huš igi huš-huš look as if borrowed from lexical lists (http://oracc.museum.upenn.edu/dcclt). Lexical material has magical significance in incantations and on amulet spells, see notes to IGI 1: 70' and 125'. Compare the similar spell in AMT 46/1 ii 8': én igi du_8-du_8 min hul du_8-du_8 igi bar-ra du_8-du_8.

Note that in Ms. UA 5' (AuOrS 23/27) one might reconstruct the text differently: [igi.bar.ra huš.huš] as Arnaud 2007: 98'.

90' It is worth noting that all three duplicate manuscripts use the same orthographic conventions, lit. igi bar ná-a, 'the open eye sleeps.' See IGI 1: 99' and 111'. The term da-a might stand for dé-a; for dé = *tabāku, šapāku* see Udughul, in Geller 2007a: 266, and MSL 9: 179. Furthermore, the term da-a could also simply mean 'at the side.'

91' For the restoration, compare Geller 1984: 296, and IGI 1: 176, 187. The phrase *dāma šenâ* has been thoroughly discussed by Fincke 2000: 168f., see also AHw 1162b *šanāʾu*. For *pursītu* see the discussion of IGI 1: 187'.

For comparable metaphor in diagnostic omens, see Heeßel 2000: 355: 33.

92' Similar metaphorical expressions can be found in medical incantations anchored in the *Suālu* series from Nineveh, BAM 574 ii 21ff. (Cadelli 2000: 77, 97f.; Collins 1999: 166ff.). Unlike Farber 1998: 65 note 31, A.MEŠ *ša a-gal-pe-e* is analogous to *me-e hi-ri-ti a-la-pa-a*, 'algae-covered ditch water,' BAM 574 ii 22. See furthermore Köcher 1980b, p. x fn. 14, citing Irianna No. 44 II 7: A.MEŠ *a-ga-la-pe-e* : *a-ga-me*, 'the algae(-filled) waters = a lagoon (*agammu*); see also Herrero 1975: 43 and Kinnier Wilson 2005b: 7-8. In the context of eye illnesses, the image of algae (*agalapû*) in lagoon-water is metaphoric for the blurry appearance of the eye. The words *a(g)alapû* and *alapû* are phonetic variants, noted as such in the dictionaries (see AHw 1542a). See also the commentary to IGI 1: 187f.'

Karpat ṭābāti is a vessel for preserving vinegar, according to Civil 1996: 150: 326. As a part of the household discussed in *Šumma ālu* omens, see Sallaberger 1996: 89. The attestation in IGI shows that the term *karpat ṭābāti* was not only limited to lexical tradition or omens, adding to Sallaberger 1996: 53 note 237.

93' ^{d}GÌR should be read Šakkan, compare also AMT 52/1: 10 (edited in TuL No. 6), specifying this god living in the steppe. ^{d}GÌR has been identified as Nergal in Geller 2010a: 93 and Attia 2015: 15, § 55. Neverthless, Šakkan is more appropriate in this context, especially with animals and landscape metaphors. Šakkan is perceived as an entity which resides in the nostrils and prevents breathing freely, similar to the symptoms of a severe allergy, which can also cause blurring of vision through excess tears.

The 'seat' (Akkadian *kussû*) defines a place in the human body, where disease is to be located. In a Mandaic incantation (see Drower 1946, cited above), a demon sits on the eyes as well as other body organs, which is a metaphor for the settling of an illness affecting that organ, see Müller-Kessler 1999: 346f. (courtesy T. Kwasman). For more examples with 'seat' as disease location with teeth and lungs, see CAD B 251, and the discussion in Geller 2010a: 93, 110-11; 124, 189. See more in Collins 1999: 90, 91, 102. There are also parallels with Hippocratic medicine where 'seat' (Greek *keimena*) designates a disease location, see Geller 2001/02: 62.

Note the different spellings of *ina berīšina* vs. *ina berūšina*. Possibly the scribe shows his expertise in this way, or just renders the signs alphabetically, i.e. noting only the crucial consonants.

94' The expression *ina libbi annīte* 'in the middle of this' refers to the *pitiqtu* 'mud-wall' (see the previous line), which presumably connotes the nose. A connection between nose and eyes is established also in the Diagnostic Handbook Tablet 6: 19ff., see Scurlock 2014: 54. Imagery such as a mud-wall probably goes back to mythological prototypes. For example, the landscape of Enūma eliš is the face of Tiamat, from whose eyes (sources), rivers flow like tears, see Lambert 2013: 100ff.

On Ms. NC ii 42' (BAM 514), Köcher copied TU rather then LA.

95' For the interpretation of *qīštaki* as 'your fee,' see Geller 2010a: 93. Concerning the rendering of TI.LA-*ma* and TI-*ma* as *bulliṭīma*, note the syllabic spelling in AMT 93/3 11 (edited in TuL No. 32), in a medical incantation with the rubric KA.INIM.MA *šum-ma* LÚ Á GÙB-*šú i-šam-ma-am-šú*, 'Invocation: If a man is paralysed on his left arm.' Phrases requiring Gula's help against fees are known since the second millennium BCE, see Arnaud 2007: no. 16, p 60: 6ff.' [^d*gu-la be-let ba-la-ṭi* / [*bu*]-*ul-li-ṭi-ma* NÍG.BA *mu-uh-ri* 'O Gula, mistress of life/health, keep (me) healthy and receive your fee.'

97' Note that colours carry symbolic meaning: white wool is for the healthy eye, and red wool for the sick eye, see also IGI 1: 109'.

99' Farber 1998: 66 restores [igi.bar.gig.a igi].bar.da.a. Our restoration igi bar ná-a is based on IGI 1: 90' and 111'. Note that MUD in Mss. NA ii 36' and NB iii 3 is syllabic for MÚD, providing that 'blood' was realized as MÚD, rather than ÚŠ, see also Farber 1998: 66 note 34.

The orthography *ap/bâtu* appears with contradictory evidence in ll. 111 and 123, etc., but the evidence for *apâtu* appears to be dominant and more consistent, with *abâtu* being less common.

100' Compare IGI 1: 134'. The broken sign in the beginning of NB iii 4 might be NA or BA. One might read NINNU(50) NA NINNU(50) as an unorthodox writing of NENNI A NENNI. In addition, NA 50 might stand for *amēl Enlil/Marduk/Asalluhi.* One difficulty with this interpretation is the lack of a divine determinative, although a divine name written only with numbers without a divine determinative is not uncommon (e.g. 30 for Sîn). Nevertheless, 'the man of Enlil' could be a metaphor for Ninurta or Dāmu, gods frequently occurring as a pair with Gula.

The phrase *sa-niq qá-bu-ú šá* ^{d}*gu-la* is reminiscent of a personal name construction, see CAD S 139, e).

101' For a parallel passage see IGI 1: 120'. The phrase *šittama šinama ahhātu* might be a pun, meaning 'the two eyes are shores' (see *ahu* II 'side, shore of the sea') with a 'mountain' (i.e. the nose) in-between, a metaphor for the human face as a landscape. One possibility is to imagine the range of mountains between the sources of the Tigris and Euphrates.

On Ms. NB (BAM 513) iii 5, Pl. 10, the fragment Th 98942 does not align neatly with K 13398 because other fragments of this tablet were not properly glued before Th 98942 was discovered. There is no doubt, however, about the alignment of ll. 5ff., see also the copy in Farber 1998: 68.

102' The answer to the question' *manna lušpur*' 'Whom shall I send?' is likely to be either the patient or Gula herself; for the phrase see Farber 1990. Everything mentioned in this passage is happening on a cosmic level, until it finally filters down to the patient. The ultimate aim of this incantation is the cleansing of the patient's eyes. The notorious daughter of Anu is the evil demon Lamaštu (cf. Wiggermann 2000; Farber 2014), not mentioned in this context. Ironically, beside Lamaštu, there is a group of Anu's daughters who are quite helpful in incantations, cf. Farber 1989, and Collins 1999: 325. This may reflect the idea that even evil demons could be enlisted in the struggle against other kinds of evil such as witchcraft; see Schwemer 2018.

103' All verbal forms in lines 103ff.' are feminine plural referring to the 'daughters of Anu,' mentioned in the previous line. On a graphical level there is a pun between ^{na4}NÍR (= ZA.GÌN) and ^{na4}ZA.GÌN; see also IGI 1: 122'. For Akk. *uqnû*(^{na4}ZA.GÌN) see Schuster-Brandis 2008: 453, 460. According to Abusch and Schwemer 2011: 473, the term is not restricted to lapis lazuli proper, but can refer to other blue stones as well.

The *hulālu* stone can be identified as agate, thanks to an inscription on a pearl of agate, see Schuster-Brandis 2008: 436, 459.

104' We assume that *tâmtu rapaštu* refers more likely to broad lakes, as in the marshes or possibly Lake Van. However, 'sea' and 'lake' could be also metaphors for ritual baths.

105' The form *likeṣṣâ* (3. pl. f. precative D stem) may be of Babylonian origin, see von Soden 1995: § 105n, see also line 123' below.

107' In Ms. AX ii' 10' (KAL 7/12), we suggest reading E[N$^{?}$...] for *bēltu* and corresponding to the phrase *bēlet šipte* from the Nineveh parallels (Mss. NA-NC). Meinhold 2017: 42: r.Kol. 10' reads differently: *i[qbûnimma* ...], but based on incantations from other contexts.

For the healing fee paid to the goddess of Gula, see notes to IGI 1: 95 above.

109' Note the symbolic meaning of colours: red connotes a sick appearance and white a healthy one, see IGI 1: 97'.

The copy BAM 513 iii 8' does not show the broken *ša* after *an-nu-ú*, but the beginning of *ša* is visible on Ms. NB iii 12, pl. 10.

111' For similar introductory lines, see IGI 1: 89ff., 98ff., 119ff. Note that these three incantations start with the same phrases, which renders the incipits unfit for organizational purposes within catalogues.

112' For *pursītu*, see the commentary of IGI 1: 187'.

113' For *taltallû ša gišimmari* see Landsberger 1957: 19.

114' Collations reveal a correct reading *ari* instead of *zārî* in CAD T 104, 385, 435.

115' Winds here are portrayed as natural causes of eye disease, without any distinction between harmful and beneficial winds.

117' 7 *u* 7 is a variation of 7 a.rá 2. àm/min.na.meš, see CAD S 203. It simply means 14 but in rituals it seems that the ancients wanted to keep the symbolic number 7. Occasionally, 14 is written instead of 7 and 7, see IGI 1: 69'.

118' The variants between the Nineveh manuscripts and the Assur parallel text, AX i' 15' (KAL 7/12), might suggest that the logogram TI.LA could be realized as *ina'eš*.

The medical procedure is based on the idea that 'red' denotes diseased while 'white' denotes healthy. See Geller 2005 (BAM 7): 7, referring to a standard apothecary practice of prescribing red liquids against fevers and green liquids against stomach disorders, based on the perception of these colours as either aggressive (red) or soothing (green).

120f.’ Compare the passage with IGI 1: 101’. For *mārat Ani* and *manna lušpur* see notes to IGI 1: 102’.

121’ The metaphor of eyes as sisters separated by a mountain appears in ll. 101’ and 126,’ but this entry adds the phrase that the one sister cannot go to the side (lit. cheek) of its sibling, suggesting the hope that a single diseased eye cannot carry the pathology to the other eye.

122’ This incantation has a close variant in IGI 1: 103,’ but the vessels are different and we have a *tallu*-flask instead of *kannu*-jar. The stone *zagindurû* is a variation of lapis lazuli, see Schuster-Brandis 2008, 455, 460. The logogram $DURU_5$ means ‘moist’ and refers to the shiny appearance of the stone.

The costly stone vessels are intended to convey pure water to the diseased eyes, which may have been based upon unwritten but commonly accepted notions of stone vessels being less susceptible to transferable impurities than ceramic vessels. This topic was popular in the Babylonian Talmud, see Miller 2003.

123’ The line has an Old Babylonian forerunner, see Goetze 1955: 9, text A: 19-20, and text B: 17-18, also in Collins 1999: 279-286. The form *li-be-la-a* suggests a Babylonian origin, see von Soden 1995, § 105n, see also line 105’ above.

The writing *li-is-sa-pa-ni-im-ma* indicates the Gtn or Gt-stem, see AHw 1000a, but CAD S 10 eliminates the double /s/ by deleting the <-is> syllable.

125’ The phrases igi sùh and igi sùh-sùh seem to be borrowed from lexical lists. Such repetitive expressions have specific magical significance in incantations, see the note to IGI 1: 70’. See also igi sùh = *i-nu e-ši-tum*, igi sùh-sùh = *i-na-an e-ši-a* in Civil 1986: 25: 27f., further http://oracc.museum.upenn.edu/dcclt. Ms. NC iii 28’ has partly preserved i[gi ba]r?, but igi is not in the copy of BAM 514 iii 28’. The joining of K 14879 to Ms. NC is courtesy of E. Jiménez.

127’ The translation ‘brow’ for *kiṣirtu* is uncertain and could simply mean that a ‘knot’ (as a biform of *kiṣru*) is ‘knotted,’ as a metaphor for a furrowed or wrinkled brow.

128’ The copy BAM 513 iii 28’ has missed the broken /na/ in IM-*ši*-***n[a***-*ma*], see pl. 11, Ms. NB iii 32.

On Ms. NC iii 31,’ there is nothing in the break (ca. 1,5 cm wide) between IM-*ši-na-**ma*** on K 2456 + and ⌜***a***-*a*⌝-*ú* on K 14879, except for two round ‘firing’ holes.

130’ The phrase *at-ta pu-ṭur* ‘you indeed release’ refers to a god, whose name is broken. In AMT 74 ii 27, 29 and 31 (foot disease), the divinity is Šamaš, associated with the same phrase (*at-ta pu-ṭur Šamaš*). Here, however, we suggest restoring ⌜dAMAR?⌝.[UTU ...] for Marduk, which is indirectly supported by the fact that *pu-ṭur lem-nu* is the oft-cited incipit of an incantation to Marduk included in Udughul

Tablet 2, see Geller 2016: 60. The restoration *ṣu-lu-um pa-ni* was proposed by Geller 1984: 295, and substantiated by collations of Ms. NB iii 34 (BAM 513). The expressions *šār pāni ikil pāni ṣulum pāni* are all metaphors for emotions, lit. 'head-wind,' 'dark of face,' and 'black of face.'

131' Concerning the copy of Ms. NC iii 34,' note that BAM 514 is misleading, since the fragment K 2979 starts here.

132' The opening line of the incantation might tentatively be reconstructed from a parallel incantation (IGI 1: 89' etc.), but not the second line (IGI 1: 133').

134' The restoration of the word *sa-niq* is according to IGI 1: 100'.

135' It is uncertain whether ŠU.BI.GIN$_7$.NAM is to be read *kīma annî*, or just *šubiginnam*, since there is no decisive evidence for either reading.

136' Compare similar formulations in IGI 1: 91'. This fragmentary incantation again reinforces the idea of the dangers posed by dust and dirt in the eye, coming from both urban or agricultural environments.

138' The copy (BAM 514) of Ms. NC iii 41' is misleading (not MIN but SAHAR).

141' One might read ^{ú}HAR.HAR, but the Ú is too uncertain.

142' The begining of AMT 8/3 appears on Ms. NB iii 47a'.

143f.' For the tentative restorations, see IGI 1: 117' and 154'.

145' An alternative reading, not to be excluded, is *mi*]*m-ma lem-nu* (courtesy Annie Attia).

147' The meaning of ta-ma-ad-ra-áš is unclear. Attia 2015: 18 fn. 81 reads *arratu*(ÁŠ) *ta-ma-ad-ra*. Furthermore, it might again be a pun with syllables (see, for instance, notes to IGI 1: 70'), but ta-ma-ad-ra-áš does not seem to be borrowed from any lexical list. Another explanation would be that ta-ma-ad-ra-áš is a foreign word with magical significance, e.g. Elamite or Hurrian, like hu-tu-ul in IGI 1: 182'. The expression ta-ma-ad-ra has no equivalent form in Akkadian but might be a play on the verb *madāru*, see IGI 2: 196,' but only if one accepts a defective present tense (*tamaddarāšu* < *tamadrāš*), 'you spoil it.'

149' The beginning of K 13465 [AMT 18/1] is found on Ms. NA. The restoration is based on IGI 1: 135,' and similar.

150' Cf. Collins 1999: 224.

151f.' Compare Collins 1999: 166: 26 and CAD G 110a (*gišûtu* 'belch'). Furthermore, see Geller 2007a: 172: 153f. It is not often to find an Akkadian translation of the Marduk-Ea formula. The pattern of this incantation probably follows Šurpu V-VI: 30-32; VII 45ff., which is bilingual. Collins 1999: 224 restores [*īmurma Asalluhi ana*]

Ea abišu išass[*si*] / [*ša anāku id*]*û atta tīdi t*[*ē šipti*], and the tablet has enough space to accommodate the additional phrase.

154' There are clear traces on Ms. NC of *ina-eš* rather than TI-*uṭ*, unlike in BAM 514 iv 1. For 7 u 7 see the note to IGI 1: 117'.

155' The phrase gi bàn-da-zu 'your tiny reed' might refer to the reed-straw instrument *takkussu*(gišSAG.KUD), used to introduce medication into the eyes. See also IGI 1: 73' and 183'.

157' We consider the word pa-la as a phonetic reading of túgpàla 'royal robe,' which might be a metaphor for bandages, or refer to the reddish surface of the diseased eye.

160' See Landsberger 1967: 14b: ŠÀ (= *libbi*) *elleti gišimmari ina pīka teheppi ina qātika tepettil* «you beat (rip) (into fibres) the offshoot (leaves) of a clean date palm with your mouth (= teeth) and twist it (to thread) with your hand».

161' Ms. HA has BAD in front of GURUŠ, which is difficult to interpret.

163' There are thematic parallels with the so-called *merhu* incantation, see for further details IGI 1: 194ff.'

164' For wind as a metaphor for a natural cause of eye disease, see Collins 1999: 94 note 39, see also the note to IGI 1: 115'.

166f.' Ms. NB (BAM 513) has a different text format than Mss. NA and NC, combining two Sumerian phrases per line with interlinear Akkadian.

Note that Ms. NB iv 17 has *i-da-šú da-*⌈*al*⌉*-h*[*a*] 'his sides/arms are troubled,' which differs significantly from *i-na-šú da-al-ha* 'his eyes are troubled' in Mss. NA iv 10 and NC iv 15.

The Sumerian-Akkadian equations (lú-bi igi-bi lù-lù-a : *šá* LÚ *šu-a-tú i-na-šú da-al-ha*) seem borrowed from lexical lists, compare Civil 1986: 25: 27f.

168' The Sumerian literally means: lú-u$_{18}$-lu-bi ní-te-a-ni-šè ér gig ì-šéš-šéš 'that man weeps bitter tears for himself.'

169' The text here resembles the oft-repeated Marduk-Ea dialogue known from incantations, in which a god, in this case Nammu, notices the problem and receives an Apsû incantation, presumably from Ea. This may be an abbreviated version of this magical motif.

170' The sign LI in *le-qé-ma* on Ms. HA 43 looks Middle Assyrian, similar to signs from Tell Chuēra or Šēḫ Ḥamad, see Gottstein and Panayotov 2014: category 7, parameters a2c5.

The sign gá in gaz-gá is not clear, but see mùnu-gaz-gá, mùnu-al-gaz-gá for *Schrotmalz* in Stol 1989b: 324, see further Brunke 2011: 41.

173' The line suggests metaphors for washing the eye and removing foreign objects.

174' Ms. HA has im igi lú-geš sù-sù instead of [im ig]i lú-ka sù-sù. One might interpret a sandhi spelling here between geš and sù, and the value /ge/ as a syllabic variant for ka.

175' Ms. HA includes ritual prescriptions for the preceding incantations, in contrast to the Nineveh manuscripts. This might suggest that this Sultantepe manuscript (HA) had a more practical function than did the Nineveh library tablets.

176' For the word *pursindu*, see the commentary on IGI 1: 187' below.

177' It remains questionable whether *ana* IGI is to be normalised as *ana pāni* or *ana mahri*, although both phrases have the same meaning.

The reference to the mother / creator goddess Mami takes the eye complaint back to creation, with the eyes complaining about the imperfect nature of their formation.

178' The *ašû*-disease is associated with the head and the eyes, as explained in Fincke 2000: 100f. Scurlock 2014: 274 unconvincinlgy connects *ašû*-disease with pox. Attia and Buisson 2012: 37f. consider *ašû* to be a dermatological disease affecting the head; see Hausperger 2000: 442ff. There is a special plant *šammi ašî* used to counteract *ašû*-disease, see the note to IGI 1: 51'.

182' The phrase še lá refers to 'winnowed grain', see CAD Z 70, and http://oracc.museum.upenn.edu/dcclt/corpus. If so, then it denotes harm similar to the *merhu* metaphor, a kernel which enters the eye during harvest time, since small particles in the air can cause eye problems. Accordingly, the *merhu* incantation follows this one.

The expression igi lal refers to a 'diminished' eye (vision), since LAL can stand for *maṭû*, occurring with eyes, see CAD M 433a, IGI 2: 196,' and IGI 3: 51'. Furthermore, hu-tu-ul has been interpreted as a Hurrian verb 'to glorify,' see Attia 2015: 21 note 101, and Haas and Thiel 1978: 12f. fn. 22 (reference courtesy M. Stol), compare also to IGI 1: 147'. In addtition, hu-tu-ul was equated in lexical lists with *hatû ša murṣi* 'to strike, (said) of disease' (CAD H 151, MSL 17: 166 (tablet 7), p. 211 l. 15), i.e. afflicted.

Entries from lexical lists are used in these incantations with specific magical significance, as in the case of IGI 1: 70,' 89 etc., see notes above.

183' The phrase *ša-at-ti pa-na* is a pun on *pān šatti* 'beginning of the year,' i.e. spring.

184’ Ms. NC (BAM 514) iv 36ff. on pl. 18 is almost entirely eroded, since the copy, see Geller 1984.

185’ M. Stol suggests translating *birki immeri* as a ‘testicle of a sheep,’ see CAD K 74b.

187f.’ For the restorations see Collins 1999: 216 and Geller 1984: 296. We assume sufficient space in the break for *a*[*t-ti-na i-na pu*]*r-*⸢*si-mi-it*⸣. Landsberger 1958: 58 reconstructed only ÉN *ī*[*nū*] *pursimît*. The *pursītu* ‘bowl’ is a loanword from Sumerian ^{dug}BUR.ZI, see Sallaberger 1996: 98, 116. The word is metaphoric for an ‘eye blood vessel,’ having the meaning ‘veins/arteries’ in the Old Babylonian period, see Ziegler 2005: 4f.; see also Fincke 2000: 20, 226-228. The crucial metaphorical connection is that the *pursītu*-vessel and the eye both contain liquids, and perhaps their physical shape was not dissimilar (as in English ‘blood vessel’). In addition, *šaharru* (var. *šuharru*) ‘porous’ refers to a clay container, and the meaning was extended to eyes, suffused with blood and tears.

The word *taš-ša-ni* might also mean ‘to be blurred’ (courtesy Annie Attia), see also CAD Š/3 366.

The words *hāmū* ‘chaff’ and *alapû* ‘algae’ (next line) are equated with each other in an Irianna commentary (CAD A/1 336, lexical section of *alapû*). See also the notes to IGI 1: 92’.

For a spelling *ha-an-d*[*a-aš-pi-r*]*a*, see Landsberger 1958: 58 and CAD Š/3 266. However, since there does not seem to be sufficient space on the tablet, another possible reading would be *ha-an-d*[*a-bi-l*]*u*$^{?}$, also written $^{\text{na4}}$PEŠ$_4$.PEŠ$_4$. According to Röllig 1993: 451a, *handabillu* is a kind of shell, but this could refer to pebbles, because of the determinative NA$_4$.

For the interpretation of *šuršurru* as a small fruit, see von Soden 1971: 69: 176, but we understand *šuršurru* as a small fibre from plants that may enter the eye and cause inflammation.

189’ The word *tubkinnu* (in plural fem.) is used together with *huṣābu* ‘twig’ in *Maqlû* II 186, Abusch 2016: 73.

The Babylonian Talmud (bAZ 28a) has a wound prescription containing Dilmun dates (*’sn’* = Akk. *asnû*) and *nyqr’ mqylqlt,’* ‘twigs from the refuse heap.’ *Nyqr’* is a loan from Akkadian *niqru*, ‘salvaged wood.’

190f.’ For literature concerning the healing goddess Gula, see IGI 1: 75’ above.

Note that Asalluhi and Marduk are occasionally not identified with each other, see Geller 1985: 15. This question has been raised again in a new study by Johandi 2019.

192' For the phrase *iddīma anāku aššī* 'she casts (it) and I (the healer) carry (it) out,' see a discussion in Lambert 2008: 93ff. The two verbs here are preterite in form but present in meaning.

194' This historiola incantation has Old Babylonian forerunners, see Lambert 2013: 399f., which although different shares the same idea of the gods creating the *merhu*-kernel. For a discussion of *historiola*, see Frankfurter 2001. Stol 1989a: 165 is critical of the translation 'ergot' for *merhu*. The *merhu*, although divine in origin, represents a natural cause of illness, see Geller 2007c: 292.

The Old Babylonian forerunner in *JNES* 14: 15 translates the passage as follows: 'The earth - it is being said - the earth gave birth to mud, mud gave birth to the stalk, the stalk gave birth to the head-of-grain, the head-of-grain gave birth to the *merhu*. In the square field - 7 bur-measures (of surface) - of the god Enlil, (while) the Moon-god was reaping (and) the Sun-god was harvesting, the *merhu* entered into - it is being said - the eye of the lad' (see Panayotov 2017: 212f.).

The word *alallû* is a variant of the Middle Assyrian *elallû* 'a pipe,' and for the latter see Bagg 2000: 262, 365. The word is not to be confused with the *alālu* 'song,' see Rendu Loisel 2016: 103ff. Geller 2010a: 94 interprets *alallû* as 'water-carrier,' needed to bring water down to earth for creating vegetation. Since the theme is agriculture, the translation 'shaduf' might be more reasonable than 'pipe.' Compare also the 'water of the shaduf' (a a-lal-la) in IGI 1: 150,' to be understood in the same way in *Maqlû*, contra Abusch 2016: 217, 101'. Furthermore, *a-la-lu ur-da* might be a pun on alal-urud, PSD A III 159. See Maul 2013: 31b, ad 25:38 (reference courtesy M. Stol).

195' Lambert 2013: 399 reads *še-er-ʾu*$_5$. On the other hand, Borger 2010: 277 states that the reading *ʾu*$_5$ for HU is unnecessary.

200ff.' The name of the Nineveh treatise is given by Köcher in *BAM* vol. 6 ix as *šumma*(DIŠ) *amēlu*(NA) *īnāšu*(IGI.MIN-*šú*) *marṣā*(GIG) 'If a man's eyes are sick,' an incipit not known from Nineveh proper. We are informed about the name only from the Assur Medical Catalogue l. 8 (Steinert, Panayotov, Geller, Schmidtchen, and Johnson 2018: 210: DIŠ NA IGI.MIN-*šú* ⌜GIG⌝). We assume that Köcher took the name of the IGI Treatise from the Assur Medical Catalogue, on which he had been working (Panayotov 2018a: 89) but never explained this in the introduction to later BAM volumes.

§ II IGI 2

ND (BAM 515), K 15765 and K 15769 are small pieces joined to the colophon, but not yet on the copy, BAM 515. According to Köcher, BAM vol. 6: xii, the numerous joins on BAM 515 go back to Geers. Borger 1991: 41, however, states that J.V. Kinnier-Wilson is responsible for piecing together the fragments of BAM 515. Whoever made these joins did impressive work.

Photos of **uB (NBC 4211)** were kindly provided by Enrique Jiménez.

1 For *murdinnu* 'bramble' as a disease metaphor, see Panayotov 2017: 238ff. *Murdinnu* has an afterlife in Jewish Babylonian Aramaic cognates, also designating a kind of 'bramble' (Kwasman 2015: 361). In the title (incipit) of Tablet Two of IGI, the plural is used, 'If a man's eyes are full of *murdinnu*–brambles,' probably indicating many bramble-like shapes in the human eye. Annie Attia suggests that *murdinnu* might indicate granules (2015: 53-55). The associated incantation (én íd-da-ta ^{giš}tir gal-gal-la-ta) characterises *murdinnu*-bramble and *murdinnu*-disease as a stinging sensation, i.e. as if the eye was stung by a thorny *murdinnu*-'bramble'; see the notes on Ms. NF (BAM 520), l. 35' below.

The restoration NU DUH is uncertain, but suggested by IGI 2: 6 (also partly reconstructed), see also Attia 2015: 37.

2 The restoration [*ka-la*] ⸢UD-*me* is suggested from IGI 2: 5. The restoration at the end of the line is uncertain, but for similar cases see IGI 1: 72'; 2: 78'; 3: 30'.

According to Abusch and Schwemer 2011: 472, the aromatic plant, *suādu* might be identified with 'chufa' (yellow nutsedge), but not based on secure evidence.

3 For the formulation 1-*šú* 2-*šú* 3-*šú*, compare also IGI 1: 15'. Before the signs SAG KAL one might expect NA_4 (Attia 2015: 37) but collations cannot substantiate this restoration. In addition, the end of the sign before SAG could be TU, thus restoring *t*]*u-šaq-qal*$_4$, but this form does not seem to be attested.

Fat from the knuckles of different mammals is known in other (non-medical) contexts (literature in Mayer 2016: 227). Compare also the LB tablet BM 40737: 6' (Ms. xB in IGI 3): Ì.UDU ⸢*kur*⸣-*sin-na-a-tú* UDU.NÍTA 'fat of the knuckles of a male sheep.'

After MAŠ.DÀ, Köcher saw IGI.M[IN x] x on BAM 515 i 3, but now not visible. The final two signs on the line could possibly be read *u*]*b-bab*, i.e. 'the fat from a gazelle's ankle cleanses the eyes.'

4 Attestations of *irru* as a salve are rare, but see Attia 2015: 37: 'ensuite tu piles dans une crème au plomb.' See especially the connection of *irru* with *egû* 'kohl' in HH XI 303; MSL 7: 139, and the commentary to IGI 1: 20'. Note that the spelling *ir-ri* (l. 4) vs. *er-ri* (l. 2) above must refer to different words.

The plant *hūratu*(gišHAB), possibly a type of sumac, was used to produce red dye (literature in Borger 2010: 420 (no. 755), and Abrahami 2014: 295).

5 gišMAŠ.HUŠ with the gloss *u* gišŠINIG suggests editorial redacting which added an alternative plant for this prescription, possibly coming from a different manuscript. Thus, a medical practitioner might have used gišMAŠ.HUŠ or gišŠINIG, depending on the availability of either drug. It was common in ancient medicine to substitute a drug if one was unavailable or unaffordable.

The phrase *k*]*a-la* UD-*me* 3-*šú* KEŠDA *ú-kal-ma* ZI is differently understood in Parpola 1983: 249 note 11: 'you put it on three times a day, he keeps it on and gets up.'

7 The drug mixture refers to the whole passage, from IGI 2: 1 onwards.

8 Instead of IM.G[Ú.EN.NA] one might reconstruct IM.G[Ú.GAR.RIN.NA].

9 For the restoration *mur-d*[*in-ni* DIRI] compare IGI 2: 1. Note the deliberate syllabic spelling of *šum-ma*, which eliminates the confusion which DIŠ might otherwise have caused.

The word *ṭīpu* 'compress' might also have another meaning, 'drops,' based on a common Semitic root, as in Aramaic (Jastrow, *Dictionary* 533; DJBA 503). This interpretation makes more sense in eye disease therapy. The examples of *ṭīpu* in CAD Ṭ 112f. might belong to two different roots.

10 The restoration *ṭi-*[*pu šá* IGI.MIN] is suggested not only from parallel texts but also from the same manuscript, IGI 2: 57 (Ms. ND).

Note that the trio *šammu peṣû*, *aban gabî* and *ṭābat emesalli* is quite common in eye prescriptions.

11 The restoration [*ṭi-pu šá* IGI.MIN] in ND i 11 is based on the preceeding line, but [LAL *šá* IGI.MIN] is also not to be excluded, as suggested by the parallel Ms. AA 8.

12ff. We suggest that *giddagiddû* is a scholastic writing from *gīdu* 'sinews,' which might mean 'a long string,' on the model of im.gíd.a for (*im*)*giṭṭu* 'oblong tablet.' This interpretation is supported by the fact that *giddagiddû* is preceded by *murdinnu*, a visible symptom on the eye (see notes to IGI 2: 1). *Giddagiddû* is also mentioned in AMT 12/11: 4' (Sm 1156), now joined to UGU 1 (not in the copy, BAM 480 (UGU 1) K 2354+, see CDLI no. P365742). For lexical attestations of *giddagiddû*, see Veldhuis 2014: 165, and especially Attia 2015: 55f. *Giddagiddû* appears in the Emar text, Ms. EA (see manuscripts of IGI 1), and is attested in SEAL 5.3.8.1.

For a reference to 'short-sightedness,' see Köcher, Oppenheim, and Güterbock 1957-58: 65, line 14, note 15.

The copy of BAM 515 does not properly reproduce the sign KÁ. The scribe missed one wedge from the sign (in comparison with line 15). KÁ[!] has the parameters a3b3 (l. 12) and not the usual a3b4 (l. 15), see Gottstein and Panayotov 2014.

KIMIN in line 13 and 15 might well refer to the instruction: 'he goes to a strange house and calls at the door.' This is reminiscent of a snake namburbi, which has the ritual instruction of a man entering another house and having a sex with a strange woman, see Maul 1994: 285f. Our tentative suggestion for understanding this passage is that the patient acts according to the logic of namburbi-rituals, so that the man enters into a strange house and calls out at the door like the owner of the house (reconstructing *bēl bīti*), thereby assuming a new identity, which gives him the right to demand the removal of the *giddagiddû*-disease. Another namburbi-type ritual occurs below in IGI 3: 76.

16 For *lipištu* as 'sang gâté' see the discussion in Durand 2006: 65-71, and Attia 2015: 56, but there is no obvious evidence for *lipištu* meaning 'spoiled blood' in medical texts. We translate 'fleshy substance,' since the ideogram UZU.NU means 'fleshy form;' see more attestations in Mayer 2016: 234. Note that in l. 19 below, the symptom *šīru āliku* 'loose tissue' appears in a parallel position, suggesting that *lipištu* resembles some kind of fleshy tissue.

17 The gap cannot accomodate the restoration DIŠ NA [*ina* UGU I]GI.MIN, proposed by Scurlock and Andersen 2005: 193, 9.49.

19f. Compare to IGI 2: 22, but we are not sure if the restoration there can also apply to l. 19.

The plant GI.ZÚ.LUM.MA can alternatively be rendered as *buṣinnu*, *kūru* or *kurṣiptu*, see Abusch, Schwemer, Luukko, and van Buylaere 2016: 510, Abusch and Schwemer 2011: 469, and discussions in CAD K 572a and AHw 143a, 512a, 515b. For the restoration NUMUN GIŠ.GI.ZÚ.LUM.MA (the seed of this plant), see IGI 2: 196', 206'. Another possibility would be PA GIŠ.GI.ZÚ.LUM.MA (using the leaf of this same plant), based on IGI 3: 71,' also attested as a medication for the eyes in AMT 74 ii 18 and BAM 124 ii 45. (For *artu*(PA) as foliage, leaves, see Landsberger 1967: 16-17.) We suggest that GIŠ.GI.ZÚ.LUM.MA means 'date reed,' i.e. the small branches holding the dates, and the translation *buṣinnu* "wick", might support this idea. Other Akkadian correspondences to GI.ZÚ.LUM.MA, *kūru* 'the short one' or *kurṣiptu* 'butterfly', are descriptive metaphors for the plant botany. Mayer 2016: 227 suggests that *kurṣiptu* is the insect 'horse fly.' See also the note to 159' below.

23 The spacing on the tablet might allow for an additional sign before ^{šim}GIG.

24 On Ms. ND (BAM 515) i 24, Köcher copied HE.HE ⌜DÙ⌝, but collations reveal rather HE.HE Z[A, which fits the parallels. For the reading ZA.NA compare also IGI 1: 63'.

The term *erēnu* ‘cedar’ can correspond to several species of conifer, see Hansman 1976: 27-30.

25 On Ms. ND (BAM 515), ŠIM after DIRI in DIRI $^{\text{š[im}}$S]ES is not in Köcher’s copy of BAM 515, but the beginning of ŠIM is visible on the tablet.

26 In Ms. bB, the scribe left out the second vertical of HU in U$_5$, see also the copy, BAM 382: 3.

27 This line references a type of eye pathology which has the appearance of parasitic *qūqānu*-worms, see Panayotov 2017: 239. The ‘vulva of a pig’ is a descriptive name for a drug, like *biṣṣūr atāni* ‘vulva of a donkey’ in stone lists (for the latter see also Radner 2016: 119f.). According to Irianna III and commentaries, the mumbo-jumbo word *gurušgaraš* as ‘vulva’ is an alternative name for pig’s sperm: Irianna III 603f. *rihûtu guruṣu-guraṣu ša šahî* : *ri-hu-tú ša šahî*, see photos in http://ccp.yale.edu/P461289.

28 The restoration is according to IGI 2: 103’.

50’ The restoration is according to IGI 2: 53’. [GÌR.PAD].⌜DU LÚGUD⌝.DA might designate the ‘cannon’ bone.

54f.’ Ms. AD (BAM 22) offers a thematic parallel to this line:

(AD) 1-3’ ⌜IGI.MIN-*šú*⌝ *ip-pa-a ana* TI-*š*[*ú* ... ^{šim}]LI
^{giš}GÚR.GÚR *sah-lé-e* DÙ.A.B[I ...] ŠÀ ^{šim}LI
1-*niš* SÚD *ina* Ì.EREN *u* x [x x (x) HE.H]E MAR

54’ The verb *eṭû* in the Gtn, *i-te-né-ṭa-a* ‘they (the eyes) become constantly dim,’ is a synonym of *ekēlu* in the Gtn, see Schramm 2001: 50, 70, l. 88.

For *šipir*(KIN)-*šú* ‘its effect (i.e. of the disease),’ see also BAM 52: 67: NA.BI *ni-kim-tú* IM UD.DA GIG KIN-*šú i-la-bir-ma* ‘that man suffers from flatulence and fever, and the effect on him will be longlasting’; similarly in BAM 168: 2: NA.BI *ni-kim-ti* IM *u* UD.DA GIG KIN-*šú* SUMUN-*ma*.

56’ The restoration follows TDP 34:17, 144 iv 52; STT 89: 203; CT 23/44 r.5. For similar cases and treatments, see also Ms. NK (BAM 518: 6ff.), discussed in Attia 2015: 59.

57’ The restoration follows IGI 2: 10.

58f.’ For the passage, see also Parys 2014: § 54. Note that different manuscripts show the same symptomology but the drugs and applications differ. For instance, Ms. ND recommends burying the medical ingredients under the threshold for seven days, omitted in the other parallels. In other words, there are many ways to heal the same condition. For a possible restoration of line 59’ see IGI 2: 28, 103’. Ms. AB has significantly deteriorated since Köcher’s copy of BAM 159 iv, compared with plate 43.

61' We suggest that the verbal form in IGI.MIN-*šú a*[*r-pa* ...] is from *erēpu*, 'to become dusky.' For the restoration of the second half of the line, compare IGI 1: 14,' 16'. However, an alternative restoration IGI.MIN-*šú a*[*r-ma* ...] seems possible according to the catchline of BAM 3: DIŠ NA ⸢IGI.MIN-*šú*⸣ GISSU *ár-ma* 'If a man's eyes are covered with a film.'

Note also Ms. NW (BAM 439) 6' [...] x *ina* Ì *u* ⸢SAHAR⸣.URUDU [...].

62' For a discussion of *kibšu* 'fungus,' and the passage in question, see Fincke 2011: 173ff. Ms. NI replaces the 'old potsherd' (*haṣba labīra*) by a 'potsherd of perfumed oil' (*haṣab igulî*), a more cumbersome variant.

63' For the restoration of the line, see IGI 2: 68'.

Karān šēlebi 'fox-vine/grape' is etymologically related to the Arabic *inab-ath-thalab* 'fox grape,' exported from Iran to India under the Farsi name *sag-anjar* 'dog's grapes' (Hooper and Field 1937: 172). The term also appears in Aramaic *'inby ta'ala'* 'fox grape,' recorded in the Babylonian Talmud, Gittin 70a. The same figurative language can be found in the Bulgarian *cherno-kucheshko-grozde* 'black dog's grapes' (Vodenicharov and Petrov 2001: 231). These later names designate black nightshade or its fruits (*Solanum nigrum L.*, references above), but we cannot retrospectively conclude the same about Akkadian *karān šēlebi*, nor identify it with black nightshade.

65' Compare to IGI 2: 98,' and to CAD Ṭ 78.

Mss. sA and AD have virtually the same prescription as ND, but sA and AD were used for different eye conditions, as in IGI 2: 98' below. The final verb in ND is uncertain but might have a cognate Semitic root B'R (*Mandaic Dictionary* p. 51), or BᶜR (DJBA 228), both meaning 'to burn.' This might suggest an Akkadian *bahāru* in G stem 'to be hot.' This term (*bâru*) appears in a recipe for spleen disease, BAM 77: 24-25:

[*g*]*a-bid* GU_4 HÁD.A SÚD *ina* KAŠ ^{lú}KÚRUN.NA [*tara-bak b*]*a-a-a-ri ik-ta-na-su-us*
'Your dry out and pound ox liver and [decoct] it into tavern-beer and he should chew it while hot.'

67' NINDA *ši-ib-ri* is in the construct state, and NINDA replaces the otherwise expected ZÌ, see CAD Š/II 382. Note also that the following line includes different types of flour. However, neither *akla šibra* nor NINDA *ši-ip-ri* can be ruled out.

68' The *diqāru* was a large pot, used for cooking, see the texts and images in Gaspa 2007: 150ff. This sequence of ordinary powders or flours occurs frequently in ritual instructions for incantations.

70' There seems to be no place for the determinative NA_4 before AN.ZAH.GE_6. For *kutpû*(^{na4}AN.ZAH.GE_6), see the notes in Schuster-Brandis 2008: 398f. This entry is the first in a series of animal parts used as *materia medica*. The list includes:

sheep bone marrow (70'), turtle bladder (71'), (missing, 72'), lizard head (74'), sheep rib (75'), cow brain (77'), male pigeon brain (77'), and raven egg (79'). This kind of list of *materia medica* from animal parts is also found in recipes in the third section of the Syriac Book of Medicines.

71' For NÁ-*al*, there two possibilities: *tuštāl*, Š stem < *i/utūlu* 'to lie down' (AHw 1564), and *tušnâl*, Š stem< *nâlu* 'to lie down' (AHw 784), both having the same meaning. Note that in BAM 14: 6, the scribe wrote [*ina* MU]N DÀRA$^{?}$.MAŠ$^{?}$.DÀ$^{?}$-*al* instead of [*ina* MU]N NÁ-*al*, confusing the homophonous *nālu*(DÀRA.MAŠ.DÀ) 'deer' and *nâlu*(NÁ) 'to lie down.' See Köcher 1963a: xiv, who reads this bit differently as [*ina* MU]N DÀRA-*al*.

Pickling substances in salt certainly helped preservation and drying out of the drugs. For instance, both eyes of a carp could be pickled in salt as a part of a ritual for establishing the safety of a newly built well, see Moren Freedman 1998: 259: 49.

In Ms. AF read BAR ^{giš}NU.ÚR.MA instead of PA ^{giš}NU.ÚR.MA in BAM 23: 9'.

72' The reconstruction of Z[Í is uncertain but the traces resemble the sign in the previous line. A knife might be used to extract the gall bladder, then to pound it directly over a bronze knife.

73' With ŠU.SI-*ka* 'your finger,' the finger of the medical practitioner is meant. A similar application is known from Hattuša, see Fincke 2010: 12.

74' This prescription is far from clear. ZABAR might be an abbreviation of GÍR.ZABAR, see IGI 2: 72' and 79' According to IGI 2: 79', the knife was smeared with the ointment. That does not explain the problem with ŠU LÚ, which is why we exclude it, in order to get a reasonable translation. Another possibility is that ŠU.LÚ.ZABAR is a variant of NÍG.ŠU.ZABAR = *mušālu*, as suggested by the next line.

75' For GAG.TI TI, see CAD S 247, but the repetition TI TI might indicate the ribcage (*sikkat ṣēli*) rather than a single rib.

The term *mušālu*, otherwise unattested in medical texts, refers to a physician's instrument comparable to the lead spoon, see IGI 1: 20.

The adverb *kayyamānu* 'constantly' suggests that the procedure was done over a three-day period.

76' The scribe added one more vertical wedge at the end of DUL.

77' The word *muhhu* (UGU) can mean both 'cranium' and 'brain'. The latter meaning fits this particular context, since one is unlikely to crush a cow's cranium. For other occasions of *muhhu* (UGU) as a 'brain,' see Westenholz–Sigrist 2006: 2ff.

For *rīmtu* as 'wild cow' we follow the dictionaries, but there is no real evidence to support it. *Rīmtu* might also have meant water buffalo or a specific kind of domesticated cow.

78' Reconstruction after IGI 2: 75'. The logogram SAG.UŠ might be rendered *kayyānam*, since it is written syllabically in IGI 2: 82'.

79' For '[you pound] a raven's egg,' see the restoration in CAD P 320b. Raven's egg also appears in a recipe in the Syriac Book of Medicines as *b*^{c}*' d*^{c}*wrb,'* Budge 1913: 559:1.

82' Reconstruction after IGI 2: 74f.'

84' For ^{im}KAL.GUG and their pastes, see the discussion in Stol 1998: 347f.

86' The presumption of two prescriptions is deduced from the tablet's format.

87' The reconstruction NUMUN is not certain, but see IGI 1: 40'.

The /e/ in *úr-né-e*$^{?}$ does not seem to have the usual graphic parameters a3b2, but a2b2 (for the parameters see Gottestein and Panayotov 2014).

90' The scribe may have copied this line from earlier texts, judging by the spelling *qut-ram*(ÁG). Compare also IGI 2: 135'. It is noteworthy that one fumigates the eyes with lamp smoke.

91' For washing the patient's eyes see Goltz 1974: 91.

93 Note also Ms. NW (BAM 439) 6' [...] x *ina* Ì *u* ⸢SAHAR⸣.URUDU [...].

94 The beginning of the fragmentary line before *ina* ^{urudu}ŠE]N$^{?}$.TUR is broken away, but the tiny cuneiform fragment was found in a plastic bag in the British Museum, dated 10 June 2005.

For the restoration Ú.BABBAR see notes to IGI 1: 64'.

97' For the reconstruction of the beginning of the line, see IGI 2: 4. The verb *kašû* 'to cover over' fits the context, but the preterite is strange. Another option we opt for is *kašû* 'to increase, yield profit'. We follow Attia 2015: 44, who translates 'tu piles [...] (jusqu'à obtention) [d'une crème? au] plomb.'

98' The phrase *īnī kiṣâti* means 'skinned eyes' referring to the irritated area around the eyes. The dictionaries themselves are contradictory as to whether this condition refers to the *kiṣṣatu* 'skin disease' or to the adjective *kīṣu* 'flayed.' Attia 2015: 44 choses *kiṣṣatu*, but we prefer *kiṣâti* because of *ki-ṣa-a-ti* in Mss. AD and Sa. Note the wordplay between *īnī kiṣâti* and *sahlê kiṣâti*, indicating a sympathetic procedure more indicative of magic.

Note the Jewish Babylonian Aramaic noun GRD,' which can indicate grating / scraping of *materia medica* – e.g. Dilmun dates – (DJBA 299).

Compare the prescription with IGI 2: 65'.

DIŠ in Ms. AD simply means 'entry,' referring to a prescription.

99' URUDU SUMUN is a special ingredient. According to Irianna, it was an old piece of copper, sometimes buried under the soil for a certain period of time, see Irianna III 476b: *ep-ri* URUDU, SAHAR.URUDU Ì.GU$_{7}$.E : URUDU.SUMUN *šá qaq-qa-ru* GU$_{7}$-*šú* 'copper dust : old copper which the soil has eroded.' See also Irianna III 514: ZÌ.URUDU Ì.GU$_{7}$.E URUDU.SUMUN *šá qaq-qa-ru* GU$_{7}$-*šú*.

It is noteworthy how often rust or patina of metal substances feature in IGI as *materia medica*, which may bear some similarity to the predominance of collyrium or lead ingredients in Roman eye treatments.

101' The gloss provides a completely different ingredient, perhaps taken from another Vorlage.

103' The reconstruction is according to IGI 2: 28, 59'.

105ff.' This prescription does not refer to human eyes, since in therapeutic texts human eyes are designated with *īnīšu* 'his eyes' and not with *īnīšunu* 'their eyes.' The passage has ritual implications that Thompson compared with practices from the Syriac Book of Medicines, see Attia 2015: 45 fn. 179 (Thompson 1924 to be corrected to 1926), Budge 1913: 662; Gottheil 1899: 202.

sb prwg' dsnwnyt' w^{c}qwr ^{c}ynwhy w'swr bh 't' wšbwq lh bwnh tlt' ywmyn w'tyn 'mh wḥzyn lh d'ytwhy smy' w'zl' wmytyn ḥd mn ^{c}qr' wsym' ^{c}l ^{c}ynwhy wmtptḥn

'Take the chick of a swallow and pull out its eyes and bind a sign on it and leave it for three days. When its mother comes and sees it that it is blind, she goes and brings a certain root and places it on its eyes and they open.'

This close correspondence between IGI and the Syriac Book of Medicines is a significant example of *Wissenstransfer*.

108' The logographic orthography is not consistent (GIG.GIR and GIR.GIG). Many examples of *kurāru*-pustles appear in Böck 2003 and Wasserman 2007, see especially 59-60.

109' The tentative reconstruction [*tu*$^{?}$-*gal*$^{?}$-*lab*$^{?}$] is based on the phraseology of BAM 156 rev. 1; BAM 494 iii 24' (presumably also BAM 494 iii 55'), see Böck 2003: 170, 172, 176.

We suggest that ^{ú}BAL (l. 109) is a variant of ^{šim}BAL and refers to the *ballukku*-aromatic. In addition, Irianna III 359(308) equates ^{ú}BAL with the *bīnu*-tamarisk:

356 (305)	MÚD GUD MU AŠ AŠ AŠ	Ú *bi-nu*
357 (306)	Ú *dam-qa-tum*	Ú MIN
358 (307)	UZU UR.BAR.RA	Ú MIN

359 (308)	Ú BAL	Ú MIN
360	Ú NU.LUH	Ú MIN

An alternative possibility for ŠE$_{10}$ *up-pu-te* would be *ku-up-pu-te* 'pill-formed' (seeds), but not as Böck 2003: 180: 37, ⸢Ú⸣.[x (x)] ⸢x⸣-*ki-ki ku-ub-bu-te*.

110' We interpret Ù.TU as a verbal form *ūlidu*. For another interpretation as *alittu* see Böck 2003: 180: 38.

According to Köcher apud Böck 2003: 181, the entire line 110' refers to a Deckname, but this is not based on Irianna.

111' Pace *ṣa-bi-tam* in Böck 2003: 180: 39, the grammar requires a subordinative *la ṣa-bi-tú*, also suggested by the proceeding verb *la na-*⸢*aš-ku*⸣.

The restoration [ÉLLAG] of line 111' is uncertain, but there is a similar phrase attested in 2nd and 1st millennium BCE therapeutic, anti-witchcraft prescriptions. BAM 393 obv. 1-3 (2nd mill.): *kalīt kalūmim ša adīni šammam lā ihruṭam* 'the kidney of a lamb that has not eaten grass,' see Abusch and Schwemer 2011: 66, see also AMT 85/1: 7 (1st mill.): *kalīt kalūmi ṣehri ša adīna šammu lā ilemmu* 'the kidney of a young lamb that has not yet eaten grass,' see Abusch and Schwemer 2011: 93: 104''''-105''''. According to Stol 1993b: 107, it might be that *kalītu* means "rennet" in the context of a young suckling kid. The expression *ina nemsēte taqallu* refers to a big cooking vessel, where one could roast hooves, kidneys, grains and plants. Since *nemsētu* was normally used for washing (< *mesû*), we translate it as 'tub.'

112' For a discussion of the *baltu*-plant see Attia 2015: 105.

The qualification *ša ṭābti* 'salted' for drugs is known elsewhere in therapeutic texts, see CAD Ṭ 13f.

For ^{ú}GÚR.UŠ = *šarmadu*, see Böck 2003: 181 and Attia 2015: 110.

113' The first three drugs are misread in Böck 2003: 180: 41. ^{ú}KUR$_4$.GI.RIN.NA is a syllabic variant to ^{ú}KUR.GI.RIN.NA, see Attia 2015: 110, and add Irianna II 227; III 103. Böck 2003: 181: 41 assumes only one plant after *egemgīra*, but collation allows the restoration of [GI.DÙ]G.GA.

114' Read presumably UD.15.KÁM LAL.M[EŠ$^?$], see Attia 2015: 45, differently in Böck 2003: 181: 42.

115' For *amurriqānu* 'jaundice,' see Kämmerer 2000, but lacking references to sick eyes.

116' It is interesting to note that in l. 115' and 116' the diagnosis is repeated, where one might expect KIMIN 'ditto.' However, note that the scribe used different sign forms for SIG$_7$, with l. 116' showing a more Middle Assyrian form than the Late Assyrian form in l. 115,' see Panayotov 2015: fig. 7, compare also IGI 1: 42' (Mss.

NB i 28'; NC i 43'), IGI 1: 45' (Mss. NB i 31'; NC i 46'), and IGI 2: 116' (Ms. ND ii 44). These features might indicate that the scribe was copying from *Vorlagen* belonging to different periods.

117f.' The logogram SAG (rather than SAG.DU) in Ms. ND ii 45 (line 117') might be a Middle Assyrian spelling, see Deller 1985: 337ff.

Compare IGI 1: 23ff.' See also Worthington 2006: 33 i.18-19. In Ms. ND ii 46 (line 118') one would like to read [*ma-li*]-⸢*i*⸣ (see Attia 2015: 45) but the sign looks more like MI, and one would expect *malā* because of the dual IGI.MIN-*šú* (on the model of IGI 1: 99'; IGI 2: 19) The unclear word cannot be in construct with SAG.DU-*su* because of the lack of a genitive.

119' For *ú-za-ku-ú* see also AMT 91/5: 3': EN *ú-zak-ki-u* NAG.MEŠ 'you keep watering it (donkey milk), until it becomes clear' (see CDLI no. P394243).

121' For *á*[*r-ma*]*t*, see Fincke 2000: 231 notes 1715 and 1717. For *šišītu* 'a membrane,' see Attia 2015: 14 fn. 51, especially 66, which does not only appear in human eyes, but was also observed in animal birth anomalies (*izbu*), see Leichty 1970: x 26' (equally uncertain).

122' The translation of *errû* as 'colocynth' is uncertain (as with other plants). Ethnological data show that the colocynth was used medicinally in Iraq, see Townsend and Guest 1980: 191. On the other hand, Stol 1985: 85 proposed an identification as 'wild melon.'

Sahlânu is a variation of the plant *sahlû* or part of it, with the *-ānu* suffix giving a meaning of '*sahlu*-like,' which is a common formulation in plant names, e.g. *amurriqānu*, *šizbānu*, etc.

123' The number of drugs, 11$^{\text{(sic!)}}$, must be mistaken since there is not enough space for eleven drugs in the previous line.

124' For this reconstruction, compare IGI 2: 121,' 126,' which might repeat the symptoms, as in ll. 115' and 116'.

The white spot, or fleck, *pūṣu*, appears in an OB Love incantation, ⸢*i*⸣*-ir-ti ra-qá-*⸢*at*⸣ *i-na-a pu-ṣa-*⸢*tum ma*⸣*-li-*IḪ 'My chest is undeveloped (lit.: empty), my eyes are full of flecks!,' see SEAL Project 10.1.1.

For *Lamassat īnīšu* the anthropomorphic goddess of the eye, see IGI 1: 80'.

126' Compare IGI 2: 121,' 124'. The expression *digalšu kabit* appears in the LB text, BM 35512 rev. 19': DIŠ GIG *ina* KUŠ LÚ È-*ma* ⸢*pa*?*-ni*?⸣*-šú u* IGI.MEŠ-*šú* MÚ.MEŠ *di-ig-la k*[*a-bit* ...] 'If a lesion appears on someone's skin, and his face and eyes are inflamed (and) vision is heavy.' BM 35512 is designated as the 34th *nishu* from a Babylon recension of the compendium *Šumma amēlu muhhašu umma ukâl*, copied from a manuscript of the Dabibi house, see Bácskay 2015: 2 fn. 13.

128' The line is too fragmentary and nothing seems to fit, but we expect drugs, since the next line has SÚD MAR.

Attia 2015: 46 fn. 187 connects IM.DU. One might also think of *tuš-ba*[*t*] but we are uncertain about a star name.

130' The common translation 'mandrake' is uncertain, see also Abusch and Schwemer 2011: 471.

135' Because of the broken context, it is unclear what *šittu* means in this line. See also IGI 2: 90'.

137' For Ms. AF, compare also IGI 1: 121'. The different prescriptions of manuscript AF follow the same sequence as the Nineveh Ms. ND. Could it be that Mss. AF and ND have the same *Vorlage*?

The precise reading of NU.LUH is uncertain. According to Irianna III 360, it might correspond to the *bīnu* plant (a kind of tamarisk, see Panayotov 2018b: 207f.):

356 (305)	MÚD GUD MU AŠ AŠ AŠ	Ú *bi-nu*
357 (306)	Ú *dam-qa-tum*	Ú MIN
358 (307)	UZU UR.BAR.RA	Ú MIN
359 (308)	Ú BAL	Ú MIN
360	Ú NU.LUH	Ú MIN

According to Abusch and Schwemer 2011: 471, NU.LUH might be the *tīyatu*-plant. Borger 2010: 270 considers the reading for NU.LUH to be unknown. One additional troubling factor is the lack of an Ú determinative, in either manuscript, before NU.LUH. ILLU NU.LUH could potentially, mean 'unwashed resin,' and it could also be a wordplay with ILLU ^{šim}BULUH, which immediately follows. Nevertheless, we suggest that NU.LUH is shorthand for the *nuhurtu*-plant.

138' Thompson 1926: 55, CAD N/2 11f) interprets the time period as 18 months, modified by Böck 2004: no. 42 (without citing the earlier references); see more recently Attia 2015: 47 fn. 193.

139' For 15 ŠE ŠIKA see also IGI 2: 141'.

140' Compare also with IGI 1: 42' and IGI 2: 4. For *šanîš*(MIN) see Glossary.

141' One might also restore the line according to the parallel Ms. AF, but 15 ŠE Š[IKA is suggested by the same manuscript, ND ii 67, IGI 2: 139'.

142' Both manuscripts have ^{ú}*im-hur-lim* syllabically written. The name means 'it resists a thousand (ailments).' It occurs often in combination with *imhur-ešrā* and *tarmuš* in medical recipes as well as in fumigation.

143' For the formulation 1-*šú* 2-*šú* 3-*šú*, compare also IGI 1: 15'.

145' It is worth noting the close parallel from Hattuša (Ms. BoA). We do not agree with the reconstruction in Fincke 2010, since her proposed restoration [ú]ÚR.TÁ[L.TÁL [ú]UD NAGA.SI] has been unconvincingly adapted from our line (ND iii 11'), with the order of the drugs out of sequence. It is methodologically unsound to reconstruct a Hattuša text based on a much later Nineveh Ms.

148' Attia 2015: 48 also restores this line according to IGI 2: 110'. One might alternatively consider restoring GA [munus]Ú.ZÚG *šá* NITA Ù.TU … in § IV.5. Ms. NR (BAM 522) and NRa (K 19831): 5'.

149' Due to the fragmentary state of the line, it is unclear what is meant. The expression *šāru* (*w*)*aṣû* is known from medical texts, see CAD Š/2 137-38, and wind is a natural cause of eye disease.

151' The verb *tašaqqal* could also mean 'to weigh out drugs.'

153' The broken sign in the beginning looks more like ŠÀ than Ú, but this might be due to damage. However, *libbāni-aṣi* might be a variant for *libbi-iṣṣi*, a descriptive name for a part of the date palm, see Landsberger 1967: 1, 3: 351. For the reading [ú]*bāni-aṣi* see Thompson 1926: 34 and Attia 2015: 110. Note that *ubānu* occurs as a plant name connected to colocynths in Irianna, I 246: *ubānu*, UKUŠ.TUR[sar] = *ú-ba-nu*, cf. Irianna III 164, Irianna I 503. In this case UKUŠ.TUR might suggest that *aṣi* is a form of *wīṣu* 'small,' and *ubāni-aṣi* 'small finger-like (plant),' could designate something like a cornichon.

154' For the choice of reading HÁD.DU or È, see the discussion in Attia 2015: 48. We assume *tubbal* refers to condensing (lit. drying out) the saps of the plants mentioned on the previous line, see also IGI 2: 157'. The word *šihiltu* seems to be a hapax in CAD Š/2 415a, but it derives from *šahālu* 'to sift, filter, cognate with Aramaic *šḥl'* meaning 'strainer' or 'filter,' see DJBA 1127.

156' For the restoration A].MEŠ-*šú-nu*, see IGI 2: 153'.

159' For *katmā* 'closed' as a description of the eyes of a birth anomaly, see Leichty 1970: v: 38, x: 27'.

As mentioned above (note to IGI 2 19f.), the descriptive name 'field butterfly' (*kurṣipti eqli*) is an alternative name of a plant associated with GI.ZÚ.LUM.MA in Irianna II:

381 (351)	Ú GI.ZÚ.LUM.MA	Ú *kur-ṣib-ta* A.ŠÀ
382 (352)	Ú NUMUN GI.ZÚ.LUM.MA	Ú MIN
383 (353)	GI.ZÚ.LUM.MA	Ú *kur-ṣib-ta-nu*

See also Attia 2015: 110. In addition, Mayer 2016: 227 suggests that *kurṣipti eqli* is 'Brennessel.'

The reading ^{na4}BAR.DÙ.E is not unproblematic (see *PSD* B 117; and *MSL* 17: 154: 112 where BAR is read as MAŠ), but a reading *bardû* cannot be entirely ruled out.

160' For *šadâna ṣābita* see Schuster-Brandis 2008, 424f.; 'regarded as a stone of truth;' see also Abusch and Schwemer 2011: 472.

166f.' For the broken prescription compare IGI 2: 105'.

171f.' These broken two lines contained an incantation or a ritual prescription. A rendering of the signs as *i-mid* 'he leans on' is too interpretative for the broken context. As for the broken signs *x-hap-pi* one might compare *ú-hap-pa* 'he smashes' in AMT 105: 15 (third tablet of the Nineveh UGU series).

174' For the line see also IGI 2: 28, 58'.

185' Reconstruction [... *ina* IGI-*š*]*ú* GIG after Fincke 2000: 70 fn. 542, but collations do not confirm *šú* before GIG. See also Attia 2015: 50 fn. 212.

194' The restored translation '[You apply]' is tentative, see also IGI 2: 78,' 89,' 115,' 145,' 148'.

195' Compare the esoteric writing *me_5*-SILIM with *me_5-sal-lim* in BAM 18: 4 and the note to IGI 1: 41' above.

196' Fincke 2000: 123 discusses the verb *madāru*. In the *Mandaic Dictionary* 258, the root *mdr* means 'rotten,' and the same word in Jewish Babylonian Aramaic, DJBA 642, is used for rotten eggs. This might be an analogy with conjunctivitis, which produces unpleasant odours due to eye discharge. In omens, *madāru* can describe the gall bladder (CAD M/1 11). Alternatively, one might consider the reading *īnšu maṭi* 'his eyesight is weak,' see IGI 3: 51' and Geller 2007b: 14 fn. 77.

199' Compare IGI 1: 22,' IGI 2: 9,' as well as the catchline of BAM 3 iv 46: DIŠ NA ⌜IGI.MIN-*šú*⌝ GISSU *ár-ma* 'If a man's eyes are covered with a film.' The obscure word ⌜*šam-ha*⌝ can also be read ⌜^{ú}HA⌝, referring to *urânu*-plant, but a verbal form is expected.

200' Nothing is visible on the tablet now, but see Fincke 2000: 204 fn. 1530.

201' For the restoration *š*[*e-e-li*, see Fincke 2000: 297.

202' The sign MA in GISS[U-*ma* is not visible on the tablet now, but see Fincke 2000: 204 fn. 1530.

204f.' The two lines illustrate the use of two special kinds of milk. The first one is qualified as ZALAG.GA 'shiny/good quality,' and the second one is common in eye prescriptions, milk from a woman in maternity (see commentary to IGI 1: 37'). The lines do not distinguish between good quality or impure milk (of a woman in maternity), but stresses the usefulness of both substances. The restoration SÚD$^{?}$ in line. 205' follows IGI 2: 77'.

206' The restoration *si-ik-t*[*i* ŠE.SA.A HE.HE follows IGI 2: 146'. For the problematic reading of the plant of GI.ZÚ.LUM.MA see the note above to IGI 2: 19f.'

208' After the sign MAR and before the sign DIŠ one would expect a gloss, as in IGI 2: 70'; IGI 3: 37ff.'

209' The restoration ⌜*ṣi*⌝-[*ri-ih-ta*$_5$ DIRI is uncertain and follows Fincke 2000: 204 fn. 1531.

215' For the catchline to tablet 3, see notes to IGI 3: 1.

Ashurbanipal's Colophon, BAK No. 329

218' The verb *ēhuzzu* shows a doubling of the final consonant due to the subordinate lengthening of the stress, see von Soden 1995 (GAG): § 83d.

220' This colophon with the phrase *bultī ištu muhhi adi ṣupri liqtī ahûti* 'medical prescriptions from head to the (toe)-nail, non-canonical materials' is typical for serialized medical tablets, see Panayotov 2018a: 108f.

222' For the phrase *ana tāmarti šitassīya* see Geller 2010: 135-137.

§ III IGI 3

Tablet 3 appears to introduce a new theme – attributing causation of eye disease to the 'hand of the ghost,' although one cannot rule out the possibility that this theme may have appeared earlier in gaps in Tablet 2 which are not preserved.

1 Compare to IGI 3: 32,' 43'. The spellings IGI.MEŠ-*šú* (NE i 1; Ua r.8.) vs. the more common IGI.MIN-*šú* (NC iv 36; ND iv 45'; xA r.9) have the same meaning. A restoration, Ì.NUN in Ms. NE i 1 is possible (so Attia 2015: 71), but we cannot be certain, since it is based on Late Babylonian texts parallels, but not duplicate texts.

2 The usage of *burṣu* is similar to *birṣu* in AMT 85/2, similar to Akkadian *burku* and *birku* both meaning 'knee.' The latter is thematically comparable to (NF), BAM 520. Note that *barāṣu* and *barāqu* have similar meanings, 'to lighten, shine,' which might reflect the same phonetic change of /*ṣ*/ and /*q*/, as in Aramaic (with *'rṣ'* and *'rq'* both meaning 'earth').

3 *Annakku* designates a tin-bead, see Abusch and Schwemer 2011: 468.

4 *Mūṣu* is a natural stone as well as a stone discharged from the urinary passage, see Abusch and Schwemer 2011: 471; Geller 2005: 1 and passim. It could also be used in *materia medica*, see Geller 2015: 42, 44 (KADP 4: 57).

For *erû zikaru* 'male copper (bead),' see Schuster-Brandis 2008: 452.

6 According to Scurlock 2008a: 174, the phrase *kám-ma ina* UGU URUDU reflects the colouring of metal. The reading x lul in Scurlock 2006: no. 122 should be corrected to [*ta-š*]*a-pah*, as confirmed by Ms. NF i' 11'. Note that seeds in this recipe are treated as stones.

7f. The reconstruction [DIŠ KIMIN] NUMUN ... follows Scurlock 2006: no. 121. For line 8, Scurlock has [^{šim}L]I, but there is space on the tablet to restore [NUMUN ^{šim}L]I, also suggested from line 7.

9f. Ms. AH (BAM 209) preserves two eye prescriptions at the end of the reverse of the tablet, although these belong to another series. They are added after the catchline DUB 3.KÁM DIŠ NA SA.GÚ-*šú* [GU$_7$-*šú* ŠU.GIDIM.MA] 'Third tablet (of the treatise) 'If a man's neck tendons [hurt him: Hand-of-the-Ghost],' which parallels Nineveh BAM 473, 474, see Panayotov 2018a: 97f. A blank line intentionally separated the catchline on Ms. AH (BAM 209) from the additional eye prescriptions.

For these lines, see also Scurlock 2006: Texts 126 and 128, and a different interpretation by Attia 2015: 72, which we follow. There seems to be an association between 'lighting' (hence eyes) and a 'ghost,' see references in Scurlock 2014: 65, 174 (with modification): if his ears wiggle like the ears of a young goat, 'hand' of ghost (Diagnostik Handbook 8: 16); [if his body] gets hot and then cold, his attack(s) are numerous, his confusion state(s) are close together, he gets no rest days and night (and) his cry is like the cry of a goat, ['hand' of] a strange [ghost] has seized him in the wasteland (Diagnostik Handbook 18: 3f.).

The Gtn-stem of *šakānu* (concerning body parts) is well attested in the Diagnostik Handbook 10: 18; 16: 2f., 43.

11f. Ms. AH r.23'–25' (BAM 209) designates this fragmentary prescription as a salve (*tēqītu*) for 'ghost' afflictions, but it is not certain if these lines were duplicated in Nineveh.

Attia (2015: 72 fn 252) interprets DÙ A.BÁR as a lead salve. It is also equated in Irianna with ú.dílim.a.bár, Irianna II 367ff., ^{ú}dílim.a.bár, ^{ú}dù.a.bár, ^{ú}ku.a.bár, ^{ú}*mir-gi-ra-nu*, ^{ú}šà.ki.li : ^{ú}*as-har* (var. $^{\text{na4}}$*áš-har*) ú *ši-šá-hu* : ^{ú}min *ina Šubari* = KADP 11 iii 7-12, var. CT 37/28 i 1ff., cf. Irianna II 341.

14 The lonely ÍD sign might have belonged to sulphurs (PIŠ$_{10}$-^{d}ÍD or ÚH-^{d}ÍD), often employed in salves and fumigation.

24f.' Alternatively, one might consider *ki-sa* SÁ.S[Á and *a-da-pa-tu*$_4$ *in-i* as possible readings. For the interpretation of *a-da-pa-tu*$_4$ as *voile frangé* and other possibilities, see Attia 2015: 73 fn. 254.

26' Compare this rubric to the incantations in IGI 1: 91,' 99,' 111f.,' 123,' 176'; Ms. NK (BAM 518) 9'.

28' The first trace of the star name seems to be AŠ, suggesting either DILI.BAT (Venus) or GÍR.TAB (Scorpio).

30' The restoration is based on IGI 3: 54'. Compare also Ms. NI (BAM 480) ii 6, and IGI 2: 4.

31' Attia 2015: 73 fn. 256 understands *tu-šam-har* as «tu traites, tu opères de la même manière» (following CAD). The verb *hapāpu* probably means to rinse with drugs rather than water, since the Semitic root *ḥpp* means 'to shampoo the hair' or 'to rub', see DJBA 477f..

32' For a possible reconstruction of the end of the line, see the compound prescriptions for an amulet bag for *birrat īnī*, 'flashing of the eyes,' Attia 2015: 73 fn. 257; Schuster-Brandis 2008: 250 (= SpTU 22+ 1-14) and *Kette* 60: *mūṣu* ZÁLAG *sû* AN.ZAH AN.ZAH.BABBAR AN.ZAH.GE$_6$ KÙ.GAN SUHUŠ ^{giš}NAM.TAR NÍTA. See also SpTU 22+ 12-14, Fincke 1998: 30 (courtesy Annie Attia).

33' Note that SUHUŠ ^{giš}NAM.TAR NÍTA (*Kette* 60) is similar in PA ^{giš}NAM.TAR NÍTA, in our line. Since leaves of the plants *taramuš imhu-līm imhur-ešrā* immediately follow in *Kette* 60 (Schuster-Brandis 2008: 250), these may have originally appeared in our line.

34' The star of Gula, as goddess of healing, may be meant, see also IGI 1: 81'. The line distinguishes between minerals (NA_4.MEŠ) and plant-based drugs (Ú.HI.A), which is not often the case in prescriptions. The reference to minerals may refer specifically to *Kette* 60, as suggested in the preceeding notes.

35' The explanatory translation 'in a leather bag' is taken from Schuster-Brandis 2008: 250 and *Kette* 60. The verb *pašāšu* suggests a more aggressive treatment than *eqû*, reflecting the difference in substances being used.

36' The expression ITI.1.KÁM refers to the first month, *Nisannu*, see § 5.4, AMT 5/3 i 11,' Ms. NZ, in the edition. The expression D[Ù-*ma*] ⸢*i*⸣-*šal*-⸢*lim*⸣ is similar to DÍM-*ma* AL.SILIM at the end of each clause on STT 300, see Geller 2014: chapter III.

37' The plant *bulālu* seems to be a foreign word for either *irrû* or *ankinute*, see Irianna I 268, 560: ᵘ*bu-la-lu* : ᵘ*an-ki-nu-te* / ᵘ*ir-ru ina šú-ba-ri* (CT 37/32 iv 31). According to this, *ankinute* is a descriptive name *irrû*, corresponding to the Subarian *bulālu*. Del Olmo Lete (2007: 217) treats *bulālu* as a Semitic word designating plants and stones, but we cannot find any justification for this. In addition, the personal name *Bulālu* is likely to be a plant name (like Rose, Lily, and Violet), see references in Panayotov 2018b: 196 note 13. A similar phrase appears in BM 40183+ rev. 7 and 12, and SpTU 3, No. 83 rev. 27 (courtesy M. Stol and I. Finkel).

38' The mountain lapis lazuli was a precious stone, often mentioned among objects sent as a gift to kings during the Amarna period, cf. for instance EA 11 r.24; EA 15: 13; EA 16: 11; EA 22 i 49 and 56; EA 25 ii 21ff. EA 27: 22. We prefer a literal translation 'mountain lapis lazuli' instead of the more interpretive 'genuine lapis lazuli' in CAD.

39' For the *muššaru*-stone see Schuster-Brandis 2008: 433.

40' We suggest that *ṣurri ṣalmi* 'black flint' might be 'obsidian,' but Schuster-Brandis 2008: 457 thinks that the stone might be *Bergkristall*.

41' It is difficult to know if the *mirgu*-plant or *mirqu*-powder is meant. Since there is no determinative, and it appears to be in the status constructus, we have opted for powder.

42' ⸢MUŠEN.HABRUD?⸣ is uncertain. IGI 3: 40 suggests, however, that the pill (or fat) comes from a bird. Another possible reading could be $BURU_5$.HABRUD, or $BURU_5$ ÍD for *erib nāri* 'river locust.' See the list in Landsberger 1934: 39ff.

49' For UD.DA TAB.BA as *ṣēta hamiṭ* 'sun-fever', attested in Old Babylonian medicine, see BAM 393, Geller 2006: 7.

50' Note that the prescription is very similar to IGI 1: 41'.

51' The spelling *ma-a-ṭi* might represent linguistic interference from Aramaic (*m*ᶜ*ṭ*).

52’ Köcher (BAM 516 ii 9’) saw traces of Ú in [Ú].BABBAR, now lost. The gloss $^{\text{ŠIM.HAB}}$ introduced together with a *Glossenkeil* for ÚKUŠ.LAGAB represents a variant reading taken from another manuscript.

The *ṭūru*-plant as ‘opopanax’ has been discussed by Stol 1979a: 71ff.

53’ Köcher copied a clear ***ina*** LÀL.KUR in BAM 516 ii 10’, but *ina* was already marked as damaged by Thompson in AMT 17/4: 10. Collation gives the correct reading as DIŠ.

The tentative restoration Z[A$^{?}$.NA$^{?}$ *te*$^{?}$*-p*]*u-uš* is based on similar expressions, as in IGI 1: 63’ (reconstructed from parallels); IGI 2: 24’.

For the *ušû*-plant see in detail Stol 1979a: 34ff. ^{ú}ESI appears in contexts with daubing, see BAM 7 no. 26 iii 12 (BAM 96); BAM 7 no. 28: 99 (BAM 104); BAM 7 no. 35: 11 (BAM 99). ^{ú}ESI may be the logogram for the *ašû*-plant, since *ušû* appears as a variant for the *ašû*-disease, TDP 184 r.1 (CAD A/II 476). Note also that NUMUN ^{giš}ESI is equated with the *ašû*-plant in BAM 1 i 63 (Scurlock 2014: 277). Therefore, one might postulate that the terms *ašû* and the *ušû* are allomorphs for the same plant.

60’ For the reconstruction of the line, compare with IGI 2: 5. Annie Attia remarks that SAG-*k*]*a ú-kal* is also possible.

62’ The surface of the tablet is very rubbed but the reading adopted here (⸢^{d}IŠKUR *ra-hi-iṣ*⸣) is well attested and fits the signs. The gloss shows, however, that the scribe was editing different versions of the same prescription.

Instead of ⸢^{d}IŠKUR *ra-hi-iṣ*⸣, Köcher read ^{d}IŠKUR *ša* HAR. Gilles Buisson has collected references to ^{d}IŠKUR *ša* HAR in secondary literature, see Schwemer 2001: 686 fn. 5626; Feliu 2003: 242, but these are likely to be based on Köcher’s misreading of the gloss.

66’ Note the Old Babylonian orthography ^{d}*Iš*$_{8}$*-tár* compared to ^{d}15 of line 63’ above. This difference again suggests editorial work from heterogeneous sources from various periods.

68ff.’ The reading DIŠ NA *ši-*[*li* ...] is suggested by l. 70,’ rather then reading DIŠ NA IGI.[MIN-*šú* ...]. For *šīlu*, see the discussion in Attia 2015: 83ff. The expression *šīlu šaddu* appears to borrowed from extispicy contexts, see Biggs 1974: 354.

71’ The verb *sekēru* is discussed in Kleber 2016a, referring to gold production.

73f.’ The eye-disease *Sîn-lurmâ* is treated in detail in Stol 1986. The passage finds close parallels in KUB 37/4: ‘If a man’s eyes [...] at night and [*day* ...] he does not see [...] – it’s name is ..., see Abusch, Schwemer, Luukko, and van Buylaere 2016: 9f. with the discussion of previous literature and reconstructions. The authors also mention the close similarities of KUB 37/4 with KUB 37/2 and KUB 4/55 (Mss. BoB and BoC in the present edition). Note that ^{d}30-*lu-ur-ma-a* is an esoteric writing with the possible meaning, 'Sîn has indeed become slack towards me.'

In the Babylonian Talmud, Gittin 69a, night and day blindness is described with the Akkadian loanword ŠBRYRY, a Š-form of *barāru*, see AHw 1547. For discussions of the passage see also Geller 1991: 107. The Aramaic text reads as follows: b.Git. 69a:

lšbryry dlyly' nyty šwdr' brq' wnysr ḥd' krᶜ' mynyh wḥd' krᶜ' mklb' wnyṭrpw ynwqy ḥsp' 'btryh wlymrw lyh 'š' (var. 's') klb' 'ks' trngl' wlygby šb 'wmṣy mšbᶜh bty wlytbynhw nyhlh bṣynwr' ddš' wnyklynhw bqlqwly dmt' btr hky lpšwṭ šwdr' brq' wnymrw hky šbryry dplwny br plwnyt' šqynh lplwny br plwnyt' wlyhrw lklb' bbbyt' dᶜynyh

'For night blindness, let one take rope of animal hair, let him tie (it) to one leg from him (the patient) and one leg of a dog, and infants beat potsherds behind him, and they say to it, "be off, dog, depart, cock!" and they collect 7 pieces (of meat) from 7 houses and let it be given to him on the door pivot and he (the patient) should eat it at the town garbage dump. After this, (one needs) to remove the animal rope and say this, 'O Sabriri-blindness of So-and-so, remove it from So-and-so, and one should snort at the dog in the pupil of its eye.'

lšbryry dmm' lyty šbᶜh swmqy mgww' dḥywt' wnyṭwynhw 'ḥsp' d'wmn' wlytyb 'yhw mgw'y w'ynyš 'ḥryn' m'br'y wnym' lyh ᶜwyr' hb ly d'ykwl wnym' lyh h'yk ptyḥ' sb 'ykwl wbtr d'kyl lytbryh lḥsp' d'y l' hdry ᶜylwyh

For day blindness, let one take seven red (pieces) from the insides of an animal and let him roast them over the potsherd of an 'expert' (*ummānu*) and let this one sit inside and another man outside, and let the blind one say, 'give me that I should eat (them) and the sighted [lit. open(-eyed)] should say to him, 'take, eat'. After it is eaten, let one smash the potsherd, so that it should not return to him.

75' The anatomical part *makūtu* is not only found with the liver, but also associated with the belly *makūt libbi*, see Böck 2000: 54, 162f.: 181. The meaning of *gabīdu* for 'liver' is open to further analyses, see Militarev and Kogan 2000: 127, and Jeyes 1989: 184. The expression *makūt gabidi* also occurs in the spleen-disease recipe BAM 77 (see the note to IGI 2: 65' above).

77' I.e. the cloth is positioned between the man and the sun.

79f.' For the passage see also Attia 2015: 77. The verb *muhra* indicates that the bread has to be received. However, note that *muhra* might also refer to to a request, see line IGI 3: 85'.

For *namra īni* as 'clear of eye,' and *balṣa īni* as 'dim of eye' see Stol 1986: 297. The expressions *namra īni and balṣa īni* are negative terms associated elsewhere with criminals, see Malku I 87f. (Hrůša 2010: 37); see also Mayer 2005: 160. These low-life protagonists in the Akkadian text reflect the character of the corresponding Aramaic recipe, in which the subject is addressed insultingly as a 'dog' or 'cock' and has to consume the donated food on a garbage heap.

Note that the SAG.HUL.HA.ZA-demon can cause *īnāšu bulluṣā* 'staring / dim eyes' as described in *Šumma ālu*, see Fincke 2000: fn. 653.

81' The beginning of the line has been reconstructed after IGI 3: 75'.

82' The writing ^{lú}TUR.MEŠ may also be the adjective *ṣehru* 'small.' Based on the occurrence of ^{lú}TU.RA and MAŠ.MAŠ from ll. 79'-80,' we might propose a restoration [*ina* ZAG-*ka ana* IGI MAŠ.M]AŠ ^{lú}TUR.MEŠ *tu-pa-har-ma*, 'you assemble children [at your right side in front of the] *mašmašu*.' One clue may be in Ms. Bo9: 30' [...] x ZAG-*ka a-na* IGI-*šu tu*-⌜*up*$^{?}$⌝-x-[x]. It is uncertain how to restore the rest of *tu*-⌜*up*$^{?}$⌝-x-[x], but this may be a form of *pahāru*.

83' In the beginning of this line, there is sufficient room to restore *muhra balṣā īni* or *muhra namrā īni*, based on ll. 79,' 80'.

87f.' ŠU.SI *ha-še-e* is not found in CAD U/W 5, but in CAD H 144b. The restoration of ⌜7$^{?}$⌝ is tentative, but the number 7 does occur in the Aramaic version, see IGI 3: 73f.' For similar Aramaic terms see Geller 1991: 105.

Note that 7 pieces of meat are eaten at the door in the Talmud version. Furthermore, one might think of restoring *askuppu* 'threshold' or *ṣerru* 'door-pivot' in the break before [...] ^{giš}IG, parallel to *bṣynwr' ddš'* in the Aramaic text, see IGI 3: 73f.' and Geller 1991: 106.

89' The broken [...] x PA might stand for [... *s*]*a-pa*, the *sappu* 'bowl.' For *kerṣu* as a variant to *herṣu*, see Stol 1986: 297 fn. 19.

93' It may not be entirely coincidental that the reverse of the tablet (col. iv) begins with a series of recipes ascribed to the 'hand' of the physician (*asû*), consisting of similar-looking recipes for an ointment (*tēqītu*), infusion (*ribku*), and a softening salve (*napšaltu lubku*), containing both plant and minerals. This may have been a separate collection of recipes from a new source other than those on the obverse of the tablet.

DÍLIM A.BÁR refers to a 'lead spoon'-salve, and not to the actual medical instrument, See the discussion above, IGI 1: 20'.

94' The reading ES[IR ...] is courtesy of Annie Attia. According to Stol 2010: 48, 60, ESIR = *iṭṭû* 'bitumen' can indicate both liquid and dry substances. In medicine, however, dry bitumen (*kupru* see IGI 3: 106' below) was usually preferred. Because a salve has been made, it is plausible to suggest that liquid bitumen was used in this case, which can be added to references in Stol 2010: 60 fn. 155 and 156.

96' For the label that a cure was tested by the hand of the *ummânu*-expert, see Geller 2010a: 193.

105' Note that the scribe used two different logographic writings for *abāru*, A.GAR$_5$ and A.BÁR.

106' See the note on IGI 3: 94' above.

109' The sign following *it-qur-ti* might be IR, the beginning of *irru*, another word for a salve, see IGI 2: 4.

§ IV.1 NF (BAM 520)

NF (BAM 520) Köcher (BAM VI: xiv fn. 21) suggested that K 9503+ (Ms. NF, BAM 520) might belong to K 2448+(BAM 473), and to K 11723 (AMT 14/2), the latter being an indirect join. Concerning K 2448+(BAM 473), Köcher's suggestion is not possible, since the rulings between columns on Ms. NF (BAM 520) were made by a twisted thread, while the rulings between columns on K 2448+(BAM 473) were incised with a stylus or another sharp instrument. Note that Ms. NN (K 6329) and Ms. NO (K 8211+K 4609a (+) BM 98589+ ...) seem to be duplicates.

1' Presumably not to be read as TI = *iballuṭ* since it is not the end of the prescription. Köcher copied NI before TI, but it is too uncertain, according to collations.

4' An orthography *te-qì* is not expected for the first millennium BCE, but it makes good sense; the spelling *te-qì* might be a relic of the Old Babylonian period, see MSL 4: 45–127. Another example of Old Babylonian orthography might be the syllabic writing *ka-a-a-man-nam-ma*, see Ms. NF i' 12'.

9' The translation 'carnelian' covers only one of the stones named *sāmtu* (^{na4}GUG), see the discussion in Schuster-Brandis 2008: 413f.

10' Ms. (NE) i 4f. shows space for more stones, but they can not be reconstructed according to NF i' 10,' since these texts are not actual duplicates.

11' For *ta-ša-pah* 'you drip' see MSL 9: 85 sub 117d.

13' For seeing light-flashes, see also Ms. NT (K 2557: 4': DIŠ NA *ina* IGI.MEŠ-*šú bir-ṣi* I[GI.IGI-*mar* ...] 'If a man [constantly sees] light-flashes in his eyes [*and* ...]'). The tentative reconstruction is based on Fincke 2000: 241 fn. 1792, with small differences.

The parallel Ms. uC i 18f. suggests that IGI-*ru* represents a Gtn-form (*i-ta-nam-ma-ru*), although one might have expected IGI.IGI-*ru*.

14’ The restoration [*anāku ša Ištar u Nanāya*?] is tentative and based on the parallel, Ms. uC i 19f. This type of phraseology probably originates in Sumerian incantations, such as Udug-hul 3: 124, in which the exorcist claims himself to be the ‘man of Namma, the man of Nanše,’ see BAM 8 (Geller 2016): 114; see also ibid. 274 (UH 7: 115-120), in which the exorcist claims to belong to Ea, his consort Damkina, Enlil, Lugalurra, and Marduk. It is not clear in the present passage whether the patient or practitioner makes this declaration.

15’ For the expression *ana* GÙB-*ka* GUB-*zu*, compare Scurlock 2006: 264. Normally one would read *ina pēmti*(NE) ‘over charcoal’ (Farber 2014: 207), but in the present context *išātu*(IZI) ‘over a fire’ fits better. Annie Attia suggests KI.MA]H ‘tomb’ instead of *ana* ZA]G?.

17f.’ The restoration of the lost herbal ingredients is based on the common occurrence of the plant trio *bīnu*, *maštakal*, and *libbi gišimmari*, see Panayotov 2018b: 203ff.

19’ The restoration follows Maul 1994: 462.

20’ The restoration follows Caplice 1967: 297.

21’ The restoration follows parallels in Maul 1994: 462.

26’ A useful discussion of the demon *mukīl rēš lemutti* ‘supporter-of-evil’ can be found in Farber 1974. The restoration is based on Ms. NF 25’.

27’ For similar ritual actions on the roof with the same expression (*l*[*u* NI]TA *lu* MUNUS *ina* ⌜ÙR⌝ *tu-še-li-ma*), see the pub ritual (Panayotov 2013: 291: 9).

29’ The spreading of the small heaps of flour might suggest that the healer wanted to check for footprints of demons entering the window. This procedure is known from the Babylonian Talmud (Ber. 6a), which instructs someone to sprinkle fine ash around his bed, and in the morning he will see footprints of demons looking like the feet of a cock.

30’ A reading NU *i-bit-tu-šu*, ‘They shall not spend the night,’ could make equally good sense here, but a transitive use of the verb *biātu* ‘spend the night’ is unexpected.

31’ Köcher in BAM 520 ii 7’ seems to have seen DU after the LU, but collations reject this reading.

33’ In Köcher 1980: xiv, Ms. NL iv 2’ and BAM 39 2’ are listed as parallels (mit abweichendem Rezept). Scurlock’s usage of BAM 520 to reconstruct BAM 39 is not methodologically sound (2014: 485, 725), since these texts represent different contexts without matching wording.

For *lahābu* as 'to whimper' see Farber 2014: 247f., a commentary to Lamaštu II 165. The spelling *i-li-hi-ib* might also originate from *la'ābu* with an intransitive meaning, 'to be infected.'

34' For 'maltster-water' see Stol 1989b: 328. In Ms. (XA) ii' 11f.', all the signs after ^{giš}ŠE.Ù.SUH$_5$ are uncertain and have not been translated. Another possible segmentation would be TUK-*a* SAR.MUNU$_6$ instead of TUK A SAR.MUNU$_6$, (courtesy Annie Attia).

35' The gap at the end of the line (Ms. NF ii' 11') might have contained the expression, ^{giš}KIŠI$_{16}$ *ša e-li pi-ti-iq-ti* È 'acacia that sprouts over the wall' (CAD A/2 409a; CAD P 437a, b). Note the variants 10$^?$ KISAL ^{giš}KIŠI$_{16}$ (in Ms. NF ii 11') compared to *ina* Ì.GIŠ ^{giš}KIŠI$_{16}$ (in Ms. XA ii' 12f.'). It is obvious that the scribes understood the signs differently.

36' Scurlock 2017: 286 states that the incantation én ur-sag ^{d}asal-lú-hi 'found a home in *Utukkû lemnūtu* 10' (for the Udug-hul material see Geller 2007b: 8: 19 and Geller 2016: 325, incipit of Tablet 10). This statement is not quite accurate since both incantations start with the same incipit but gradually differ afterwards, which is often the case with medical incantations (see for instance: IGI 1: 89ff; IGI 1: 98ff; IGI 1: 110ff; IGI 1: 119ff and etc.). The incantation in question (on NF ii 12ff' and parallels) is not a standardized incantation but a medical incantation, with a broad spectrum of variants suggesting oral transmission. The incantation in Ms. AJ (BAM 216): 12'-15' was used with fumigants against ghost afflictions, causing eye trouble. Note also that K 11969 might be related, since it reads in l. 6': én ur-sa[g ...], see Kocher BAM V, xxxvi.

We do not follow the translation of Zomer 2018.

38' Köcher's copy of Ms. NM (BAM 508) has l[íl instead of k[i in this line.

40' Ms. AI: 14 reads nam-ma-kal, which might be a late syllabic writing for nam-á-gál. Based on the parallels, this is an epithet for the god Nabû. Furthermore, dumu-sag ^{d}ag-ke$_4$ is an allusion to the common phrase dumu-sag ^{d}en-ki-ke$_4$ from UH 2: 9-10 (Geller 2016).

In Mss. NO and AI, the sign /tal/ is a phonetic variant of /tar/. An alternative translation of the passage would be: 'O my son, the fate has been decided, can the man not see?'

42' Note that the incantation **ur-sag ^{d}asal-lú-hi igi-bi hé-pà** can be combined with another, **én íd-da-ta** (Thompson 1937b: 32), or used separately:

a) the incantation **én ur-sag ^{d}asal-lú-hi** following **én íd-da-ta**: Ms. **NM** (BAM 489+; Nineveh); Ms. NN (K 6329); Ms. NO (K 8211+(+); Nineveh). In Ms. AI (LKA 145; Assur), **én íd-da-ta** precedes **én ur-sag ^{d}asal-lú-hi** without a dividing line, indicating that the Assur scribe considered the whole text to be an incantation. See plate 44.

b) **én ur-sag ^{d}asal-lú-hi** used alone: Ms. NF (possibly IGI 4, BAM 520; Nineveh), **én ur-sag ^{d}asal-lú-hi** stands alone, but afterwards the tablet is broken, with the possibility that **én íd-da-ta** followed it; Ms. XA (BM 123362, Nineveh or Assur?), **én ur-sag ^{d}asal-lú-hi** stands alone, but the beginnings of cols. i’ and iv’ are lost, where **én íd-da-ta** might have been present.

c) **én íd-da-ta** used alone: BAM 386 iii 7ff.’ (Late Babylonian, see Farber 1982: 596, **én íd-da-ta** stands alone, but the tablet afterwards is broken, thus used in combination with **én ur-sag ^{d}asal-lú-hi** cannot be excluded. The reference in Köcher 1971 (BAM IV): xxvii, that BAM 386 iii 7’-21’ parallels K 2566+ (UGU 3) iii: 25’-32,’ is partly misleading. K 2566+ is a parallel to Ms. NG (K 4023+), where the passage in question is preserved; SpTU 4/129 vi 30ff.’ (Late Babylonian, Uruk); Ms. NG iii 17’ (K 04023+, UGU 3; Nineveh); Ms. NGa iii’ 1’ (K 14698 presumably duplicates UGU 3 from Nineveh, but it is too fragmentary to judge); Ms. NH iii 6’ (BAM 486 may duplicate UGU 3 from Nineveh, but it is also too fragmentary to judge).

1 Incantation: from the river, from the great forests!

AI 1	én íd-da-ta ^{giš}tir gal-gal-la-ta
NG iii 17’	én íd-da-ta tir gal-gal-⸢la-ta⸣ →
NH iii’ 6’	⸢én íd⸣-da-ta tir gal-gal-l[a-ta ...]
NM i’ 29’	én ⸢íd-da⸣-ta ^{giš}tir gal-gal-la-ta →
BAM 386 iii 7’	én íd-da-ta ^{giš}t[ir ....]
SpTU 4/129 vi 30’	⸢én⸣ íd-da-ta ^{giš}tir gal-gal-la-⸢ta⸣

2 The (forest-)habitat of the ‘stag horn’ is exalted (and) distant, it removes (^{AI} the thorns of) the *murdinnu*-bramble!

AI 2	tir si-dàra-bar mah-mah ul-ul : gír-gír geštin-gír-ra mu-un-kar
NG iii 17f.’	tir ⸢si-dàra⸣-bar ⸢mah-m[ah] / ul-ul ^{giš}geštin-gír mu-un-⸢kar-e⸣→
NH iii’ 6f.’	[.......................................] / ⸢ul⸣-ul ^{giš}geštin-gír mu-un-ka[r-e]
NM i’ 29f.’	^{giš}tir si-dàra-bar mah m[ah] / ul-⸢ul⸣ ^{giš}geštin-gír mu-un-kar-re→
BAM 386 iii 8f.’	tir dàra-ba[r ....] / ul-ul ^{giš}geš[tin ....]
SpTU 4/129 vi 31f.’	⸢tir⸣ si-dàra-bar mah-mah / ⸢ul⸣-ul ^{giš}geštin-⸢gír mu⸣-un-kár-⸢re⸣

3 The acacia thorn causes pain – snakes causing swelling.

$^{\text{(var. AI, SpTU)}}$ It hurts like an acacia thorn – the snakes cause swelling.

AI 3 gír gin$_7$ ì-gu$_7$-e muš-muš šu mú-mú-e-dè
NG iii 18f.' ⸢^{giš}kiši$_{16}$⸣ ì-gu$_7$-⸢e muš⸣ [muš] / šu mú-mú-e-dè →
NH iii' 7f.' [.....................................] / [šu mú-m]ú-⸢e-dè⸣ →
NM i' 30f.' ^{giš}kiši$_{16}$ ì-gu$_7$-⸢e⸣ / muš-⸢muš⸣ ki mú-mú-e-dè →
NO ii' 1' [.....................................d]è$^?$
BAM 386 iii 10f.' ^{giš}kiš[i$_{16}$ ....] / muš-mu[š ....]
SpTU 4/129 vi 33' ⸢^{giš}gír⸣ ì-gu$_7$-e$^!$(^{copy}KAL) muš-muš šu mú-mú-e-dè

4 The pure 'arrow'(-drug, Akk. *mulmullu*) of the pure eastern mountains can heal the breast for the patient,

AI 4 mul-mul kur kur-ra sikil-la : gaba ì-til-la tu-ra-šè
NG iii 19' mul-mul ⸢kur kur⸣-r[a sik]il$^?$-e gaba ⸢ì⸣-ti-la ⸢tu-ra⸣-[...]
NH iii' 8' ⸢mul⸣-mu[l ....]
NM i' 31f.' mul-mul kur kur-ra sikil-l[a] / gaba ì-ti-⸢la⸣ tu-ra-šè →
NN ii' 1' [..] r[a ....]
NO ii' 2f.' [...] ⸢mul$^?$⸣ [..................... l]a / ⸢gaba⸣ ti-la ⸢tu⸣-[ra]-šè
BAM 386 iii 12f.' mul-m[ul ....] / gaba ì-ti-[.......................]
SpTU 4/129 vi 34f.' mul-mul kur kur-ra ⸢sikil⸣-la / gaba ì-ti-la kur-r[a x] x

5 One refers to the rescued one as 'blameless' (lit. absolved of guilt)!

(var. AI, SpTU) One does not know (how to) absolve the guilt of the patient!

AI 5 du$_8$ nam-tag-ga ^{lú}⸢tu⸣-ra nu-un-zu-a
NG iii 20' du$_8$ nam-tag-ga lú-kar-ra mu-un-⸢sa$_4$-a⸣ →
NM i' 32' du$_8$ nam-tag-ga lú-kar-ra ⸢mu-un-sa$_4$⸣-[a]
NN ii' 2' [........................$^{l]ú}$⸢kar⸣-ra ⸢mu⸣-u[n-.........]
NO ii' 4' du$_8$ nam-tag-ga lú-⸢kar⸣-ra ⸢mu-un-sa$_4$⸣-a
BAM 386 iii 14' du$_8$ nam-ta[g ....]
SpTU 4/129 vi 36' du$_8$ nam-tag-ga lú-kár-ra mu-un-sa$_4$-a

6 Found on the threshold, the 'arrow'(-drug) is garden grown (i.e. cultivated) / (var. AI) is a (wild)-growing thorn (i.e. not cultivated).

AI 6 zag-gar gag-ti gír bùlug-gá
NG iii 20' zag-du$_8$ gar ^{giš}⸢x⸣-ti ⸢$^{giš?}$⸣k[iri$_6^?$ ...]
NGa iii' 1' ... x x x ...
NM i' 33f.' zag-du$_8$ gar ⸢gag ti⸣ ^{giš}kiri$_6$ bùlug-g[á] →
NN ii' 3' [........] x ⸢gar gag⸣-ti ^{giš}kiri$_6$ bùl[ug ...]
NO ii' 5' zag-du$_8$ giš$^?$ gar$^{?\ \text{OVER ERASURES}}$ gag-ti ^{giš}kiri$_6$ bùlug-g[á]
BAM 386 iii 15' zag-du$_8$ gar [.......................................]

SpTU 4/129 vi 37' zag-du$_8$ gar gag-ti ^{giš}kiri$_6$ bùlug-gá

7 May the evil demon come to an end. May the evil Ala-demon come to an end. May the evil ghost come to an end.

AI 7 udug-hul hé-til a-lá hul hé-til gidim hul hé-til
NG iii 21' udug-hul hé-til a-lá hul hé-til ⸢gidim⸣ h[ul h]é-til →
NGa iii' 2' [............. hé-t]il a-lá hul hé-til g[idim$^?$........]
NM i' 33f.' udu[g-hul] h[é ....] / gidim ⸢hul hé-til⸣ →
NN ii' 4' [..... hu]l hé-til a-lá hul min gidim h[ul ....]
NO ii' 6' udug-hul hé-til a-lá hul min gidim hul mi[n]
BAM 386 iii 16f.' udug-hu[l.........................] / gidim hu[l ......]
SpTU 4/129 vi 38' udug-hul hé-til a-lá hul min gidim hul min

8 May the evil Galla-demon come to an end. May the evil god come to an end and the evil Maškim-demon come to an end.

AI 2 gal$_5$-lá hul hé-til dingir hul maškim hul hé-til
NG iii 21f.' gal$_5$-lá ⸢hul hé-til⸣ / dingir hul hé-til maškim hul hé-til →
NGa iii' 3' [...................................... h]ul hé-til máškim hul hé-til →
NM i' 34f.' ⸢gal$_5$⸣-l[á ....]
NN ii' 5' [.......... hu]l min dingir hul min maškim hu[l ....]
NO ii' 7' gal$_5$-lá hul min dingir hul min maškim hul min
BAM 386 iii 17f.' [..] / maškim hul m[in ....]
SpTU 4/129 vi 39' gal$_5$-lá hul min dingir hul min maškim hul min

9 May the Kamadme-demon come to an end. May the Kamadme-demon come to an end. May the Kamad-me-lagab-demon come to an end.

AI 9 ^{d}kamad-me hé-til ^{d}kamad-me-a hé-til ^{d}kamad-me-lagab hé-til
NG iii 22f.' ^{d}⸢kamad-me⸣ hé-til ^{d}kamad-me-a hé-til / ^{d}kamad$_{10}$-me-lagab hé-til →
NGa iii' 4' [..^{d}ka]mad$_x$-me-lagab hé-til →
NM i' 35' ^{d}kam[ad-me ....]
NN ii' 6' [... ka]mad$_x$-me hé-til ^{d}kamad$_x$-me-a hé-til ^{d}kamad$_x$-me-lagab hé-til
NO ii' 8' ^{d}kamad$_x$-me hé-til ^{d}kamad$_x$-me-a hé-til ^{d}kamad$_x$-me-lagab hé-til
BAM 386 iii 19' ^{d}kamad$_x$-me [...]
SpTU 4/129 vi 40' ^{d}kamad$_x$-me min ^{d}kamad$_x$-me-a [min ^{d}]kamad$_x$-me-lagab min

10 May you be adjured in heaven, may you be adjured on earth. Incantation spell.

NG iii 23' zi-an-⸢na hé-pà zi-ki⸣-a hé-pà tu$_6$-én
NGa iii' 4' zi-an-na hé-p[à ....]

NM i' 36' zi-an-na h[é ....]

NN ii' 7' [... a]n-na hé-pà zi-ki-a hé-pà

NO ii' 9' zi-an-na hé-pà zi-ki-a hé-pà

BAM 386 iii 20' zi-an-na hé-p[à ....]
SpTU 4/129 vi 41' ⸢zi⸣-an-na hé-pà zi-ki-a hé tu$_6$-én

11 Invocation for 'headache.'
NG iii 24' ka-inim-ma ⸢sag-ki⸣-dab-ba-ke$_4$
NGa iii' 5' [ka-i]nim-ma [............................]
NZa rev. 1' [..................... s]ag-ki-da[b-........]
SpTU 4/129 vi 42' ka-inim-ma sag-ki-dab-ba-kam

12 Its ritual: you spin together red (and) white wool. You thread on *stag's horn* (and) date stone.

12 DÙ.DÙ.BI *šīpāti sāmāti šīpāti peṣâti ištēniš taṭammi qaran ayyali aban suluppi tašakkak*
NG iii 25' DÙ.DÙ.BI SÍG SA$_5$ SÍG BABBAR 1-*niš* NU.NU ⸢SI$^?$ DÀRA$^?$.MAŠ$^?$⸣ NA$_4$ ZÚ.LUM.MA È
NGa iii' 5' [... SÍ]G SA$_5$ SÍG BAB[BAR ....]
NZa rev. 2' [... DÀ]RA.MAŠ NA$_4$ ⸢ZÚ⸣.L[UM.MA É]

13 You tie seven and seven knots. Whenever you make a knot you shall recite the incantation (above). You bind it on his both temples, then he should recover.

13 *sebet u sebet kiṣrī takaṣṣar ēma taktaṣru šipta tamannu ina nakkaptīšu tarakkasma iballuṭ*
NG iii 26' 7 KA.KEŠDA KEŠDA *e-ma* KEŠDA ÉN ŠID-*nu ina* ⸢SAG.KI⸣.[MIN-*š*]*ú tara-kás-ma* AL.TI
NGa iii' 6' [7 KA.KEŠD]A$^?$ KE[ŠDA ....]
NZa rev. 3' [... SAG.K]I.MIN-*šú tara-kás-ma* ⸢AL.TI⸣

Notes to lines: **2)** For the term *murdinnu* 'bramble' see notes to IGI 2: 1. **3)** šu mú is a compound verb (Karahashi 2000: 163) and non-finite here (lit. for causing swelling). **4)** The writing mul-mul might refer to a plant ^{ú}mul-mul as well, see Irianna. **9)** According to Borger 2010: dìm is dim$_9$, but note that George 2018 reads dìm as kamad. For convenience we render dim$_{10}$ as kamad$_x$.

For the sake of convenience, we provide a transliteration of col. iii' of Ms. **XA** (BM 123362), see plates 47-48.

XA iii' 1	[..................] x ^{ú}IGI-*lim* ^{ú}HAR.HAR ^{ú}*aš-ka-a-d*[*ù* ....]
XA iii' 2	[..................] x NUMUN ^{giš}ŠINIG NUMUN ^{giš}MA.NU [.............]
XA iii' 3	[.................. K]A$^{?}$ 7 ^{ú}TÁL.TÁL-*nu*$^{?}$ *ina* SAG.KI-*šú* KEŠ[DA ......]
XA iii' 4	[............^{šim}GÚ]R.GÚR ^{šim}LI ÚH-^{d}ÍD ⸢KA.A.AB⸣.B[A ....]
XA iii' 5	[.............. ^{i}]^{m}KAL.⸢GUG⸣ 1-*niš ta-sàk ina* ^{urudu}⸢ŠEN⸣.T[UR ....]
XAiii' 6	[.............. É]N$^{?}$ ⸢7-*šú*⸣ *ana* UGU ŠID-*nu* LAL.LA[L-*ma ina-e*]*š*
XA iii' 7	[...] x ⸢^{na4}KA.GI⸣.NA.DAB.BA ^{na4}⸢AN.ZAH⸣ ⸢^{na4}AN.ZAH.BABBAR⸣
XA iii' 8	[........................^{na4}DU]R.⸢MI.NA.BÀN.DA⸣ Ú.DILI UR.BI SÚ[D]
XAiii' 9	[........................ É]N$^{?}$ ⸢7-*šú*⸣ *ana* ŠÀ ŠID-*nu* SAG.⸢KI⸣-*šú* IGI [...]
XA iii' 10	[.. *ana* T]I-*šú* TAG.TAG-*ma ina-e*[*š*]
XA iii' 11	[.. PI]Š$_{10}$-^{d}ÍD ⸢NA$_{4}$$^{?}$ GÌŠ⸣.ŠAH ^{giš}G[I]
XA iii' 12	[.. N]IR Ì.HUL Ì KU$_{6}$ 1-*niš* HE.HE-⸢*ma*⸣
XA iii' 13	[.. *a*]*n-ni-ta* 7-*šú* ŠID-*nu-ma ina-e*[*š*]
XA iii' 14	[..^{n}]^{a4}*mu-ṣa ni-kip-tú* KA *tam-*⸢*tì*⸣
XA iii' 15	[.. Š]À$^{?}$⸢IGI.MIN⸣-*šú* ŠÉŠ-⸢*ma* TI⸣
XA iii' 16	[...] x HE.HE EŠ.MEŠ-*su-ma* ⸢TI⸣
XA iii' 17	[... E]Š.MEŠ-*su-ma* ⸢TI⸣
XA iii' 18	[...] ⸢TI⸣

§ IV.2 Ms. NK (BAM 518)

3f.' The use of human bone as *materia medicia* (an example of Dreckapotheke) occurs in K 3628+ (Scurlock 2014: 6 22), but also in the Syriac Book of Medicines as *grm' dbrnš'* (Budge 1913: 582: 3). See also BRM 4/32: 20 (cf. Geller 2010a: 169) for the use of a human skull and human flesh. It is unusual, however, to use the skull as a bowl for recipe ingredients. On the other hand, later Aramaic incantations in exceptional cases used human skulls in place of magic bowls, which reflects on Akk. *kallu* 'bowl' as a medium for writing incantations in ink, rather than as a receptacle for magical or medical ingredients; for these Aramaic skull inscriptions, see Levene 2006.

6' The phrase, IM TI.MEŠ // *šāra leqâ* literary means 'his eyes took (in) wind,' which is interpreted as 'swollen' here. Attia 2015: 59 translates 'ils sont pris par du vent.'

7' There is insufficient space to restore [*ina*$^{?}$ KAŠ$^{?}$], on Köcher's copy, BAM 159 (Ms. AB), see also Parys 2014: 20 fn. 80.

Köcher 1980b: xiii fn. 19 transcribes *qēm kasî qalûti* for ZÌ GAZI^sar^ BÍL.MEŠ (in BAM 159 = Ms. AB iv 9f.'), but an alternative might be *qēm kasî taqallu*, as suggested by BÍ]L-*lu* on Ms. NK 7'.

8' There appears to be nothing in the break before Ú.BABBAR, see IGI 2, ND i 10, and Attia 2015: 38.

9' As in line 7,' the wind is a natural cause of suffering, bringing dryness and eye irritation with foreign particles.

10ff.' Compare IGI 2: 68. There is not enough space in Köcher's copy, BAM 159 (Ms. AB) i 13f.' for ZÍ ^ú^[ŠE.NÚ/DÙ].A, compare also l. 7'. In the break of line 12 one might reconstruct *qēm kasî*, based on BAM 159 (Ms. AB) i 13f.,' and slightly differently ([ZÌ ^šim^MAN.DU (GAZI^sar^) 1]-*niš*) in Parys 2014: 20. In addition, signs in the middle part of Ms. AB iv 15f' (copy BAM 159 iv 15') have been completely lost since Köcher's copy, compare BAM 159 iv with plate 43.

Many of the powders (or flours) mentioned in this text can also be found in a Late Babylonian tablet in the British Museum (BM 66942), which consists of a list of similar ingredients used for external application for an unspecified ailment. Overlap between BAM 518 and BM 66942 includes various powders, such as ZÌ GAZI^sar^ BÍL.MEŠ, ZÌ ŠE.SA.A, ZÌ GÚ.GAL and ZÌ GÚ.TUR. Of interest, however, is the practical notation at the end of the late tablet: *a-na ka-ṣa-ri šum-ma ti-*[*bu*]*-tú ina* KAŠ *šum-ma* DAGAL.MEŠ *ina* A GAZI^sar^ SILA$_{11}$-*aš* LÁ-*ma* TI-*uṭ*, 'in order to make a concentrate, if (powders / flours) rise, you knead it in beer, if broad (i.e. flat, like pita-bread) - in tamarind-juice. You bandage it on and it gets better.'

§ IV.3 Ms. NP (BAM 517)

8' The sign RI might be the end of *tazarri*, see IGI 1: 50'.

§ IV.4 Ms. NQ (BAM 521)

4' The signs might represent either ⌜^ú^⌝TÁL.T[ÁL ...], the *urânu*-plant, or [... *ta-ṭa*]*p-pi x* [...] 'you apply,' see BAM 158 iii 26.

5' An alternative to *dimta*(ÉR) *ittanaddâ*(ŠUB.ŠUB-*a*) would be *dimta*(ÉR) *nadâ*(ŠUB-*a*), see Fincke 2000: 136, and ibid. p. 97 fn. 746. The context of 'constantly giving off tears' is well known also from the UGU Treatise, Tablet 1, BAM 480 (Ms. NI), see Worthington 2005: 7: 3. See also BAM 518: 9, Ms. NK above.

8' The reconstruction after Ms. NA i 30' is hypothetical. See also BAM 19: 13' and BAM 16: 3,' courtesy Annie Attia.

9' For similar ingredients and healing context, see UGU 2, BAM 482 (Ms. NX ii 65').

For *šikari rēštû* vs. *šikaru* see Abusch and Schwemer 2011: 36a, but *šikari rūšti* might be better reading, based on *šaman rūšti* (Ì.(GIŠ).SAG).

10' This prescription appears to occupy more lines on the three-columned Assur tablet (BAM 159, Ms. AB) than on fragmentary Nineveh fragments, e.g. Ms. NQ (BAM 521). In the Assur manuscript, this prescription was known as a 'tested eye salve of Hammurapi,' Ms. AB (BAM 159) iv 22: *te-qit* IGI.MIN.MEŠ *šá* ^{m}*Ha-am-mu-ra-pí lat-ku*, which is similar to BAM 382 (Parys 2014: 10f., 20, 57). See also the note to § IV.6. Ms. NS (AMT 18/4) 2'. The expression *natāla muṭṭu* 'reduced vision' should be compared to *digil īnīšu maṭi* (IGI 3: 51').

§ IV.5 Ms. NR (BAM 522) and NRa (K 19831)

3' For parallels see also BAM 22 r.25 and Fincke 2009: 86: 15' (Ms. xA CM 37, IGI 1, § I.3).

5' The signs DÙ-*uš* on Köcher's copy BAM 522 should rather be read as ^{munus}Ú.ZÚG ⸢*šá* NITA⸣ ⸢Ù⸣[.TU ...], cf. K 8080: 10 (join to K 3612, AMT 46).

8' The copy in BAM 522 shows *te-s*[*ek-ker*] but a better reading is *te-p*[*i*, see also IGI 2: 65 and compare CAD E 247f.

§ IV.6 Ms. NS (AMT 18/4)

2' BAM 382: 9ff. has a shorter prescription excluding the clause with the sun-god, employing the same ingredients as *te-qit* ^{m}*Ha-am-mu-ra-pí* 'eye salve of Hammurapi,' reminiscent of Ms. AB (BAM 159) iv 22, see the notes on Ms. § IV.4. NQ (BAM 521) 10,' above.

4' The measuring of drugs in front of the divine judge Šamaš advocates precision in choosing the correct amount.

5' See also Ms. NB (BAM 513) ii 5' [....... *ta-bi-l*]*am ta-ṭe-ep-pi*. The statement in CAD T 25b that AMT 18/4: 5 duplicates BAM 159 iv 21 and BAM 513 ii 5 (Ms. NB) is partly misleading, the passages are different, but all ending with the expression *tābīla teṭeppi* 'you apply (it) in a dry state.'

§ IV.7 Ms. NT (AMT 85/2)

2’ The precise meaning of *mi-na-at* UZU is unclear (‘parts of flesh’), but see BAM 231 i 12

3’ References to the months Abu (5) and Tebet (10) have symbolic value: 5th month vs. 10th month. Exorcist almanacs explain that certain months and days were particularly important for healing measures. For instance, for the month Abu (5), the magico-medical monthly guide STT 300 prescribes therapy against witchcraft, *Anfallskrankheiten* and ghosts. For the month of Tebet (10), social rituals are prescribed, but also anti-witchcraft measures, as well as protective rites against *Lilû* and *Lilith* demons (Geller 2014: 47ff.). For a parallel see BM 55281: 13-18 (ghosts).

4’ See also AMT 87/3 ii’ 6’: DIŠ NA *bir-ṣa* IGI.IG[I-*mar* ...]. For IGI.IGI-*mar* see in detail Fincke 2000: fns. 1608, 1786. See also Kette 56 in Schuster-Brandis 2008: 74 *et passim.*

5’ The reading *mu-u*[*š* in Scurlock 2006: No. 129 and Scurlock 2008b: 197 should be modified to *mu-ú*[*r-tap-pi-du*, see CAD M/2 228, AHw 325 under *harbūtu*, and further Stol 1993: 73 fn. 63.

6’ For possible reconstructions of the plant description, see Scurlock 2006: Nos. 104, 264, 265.

9’ KU.KU → *uṭṭatu* ‘grain’ is regularly used to indicate a small measure of drugs, see the discussion in Borger 2010: No. 808 and add CAD U/W 356, s. v. *uṭṭatu*.

§ IV.8 Ms. NU (AMT 14/3)

AMT 14/3 possibly belongs to AMT 14/2 (K 11723, CDLI no. P399417, see Thompson 1926: 47-48), but the shape and size of signs seem similar to K 2611, Ms. NX (UGU 2) below. Further parallels to AMT 14/3 are cited at the BabMed website: http://www.geschkult.fu-berlin.de/e/babmed/Corpora/AMT/AMTX14-3/index.html.

5’ Compare the treatment to IGI 3: 35’.

8’ Note the spelling A ^{giš}ŠINIG (l. 6’) vs. A.MEŠ ^{giš}ŠINIG (l. 8’), both standing for *mê bīni* ‘tamarisk sap.’

10’ For a parallel, see BAM 183: 4, pointed out by Thompson 1926: 47, but not the reference in Köcher 1963b: xx, that BAM 183: 4–5 parallels IGI 2: (BAM 515) iv 31.

12’ The dividing line is superfluous, but it seems that the scribe insisted on visually separating the long diagnostic part (ll. 11’-12’) from the therapy (ll. 13’-16’).

16’ The phrase ^{d}*Ea li-ni-ih-ka* ‘may Ea appease you’ occurs within the incantation *ezzētunu šamrātunu dannātunu gaṣṣātunu* ‘raging, furious, strong, cruel’ in Maqlû V: 136 (Abusch 2016: 146: 136; see also Muššuʾu, Böck 2007: 295: 178; Wiggermann 1992: 33), although not as part of the incipit. However, the phrase appears in a bilingual incipit in a medical context: K 8447+ (CDLI P397634): 1f. én bir-b[i] $^{d+}$en-ki hé-en-hun-gá / *ka-li-tu*$_4$ ^{d}*é-a li-ni-ih-ki* ‘Incantation: O (hurting) kidney, may Ea soothe you!’ For the reverse of K 8447+ see Abusch, Schwemer, Luukko, and van Buylaere 2016: text 7.11, Ms. J.

17’ The broken-off lines must contain the incantation mentioned in 16’.

§ IV.9 Ms. NV (AMT 18/3)

1ff.’ Despite the impression given by the copy in AMT 18/3, the beginning of the tablet is lost. We render ^{ú}HA as *urânu* and not *šimru*, since the plant *urânu* was employed against skin diseases (KADP V 35-39, see Scurlock 2017: 280), matching the *kiṣṣatu*-skin disease mentioned in line 1’.

3’ There may have not been a direct borrowing between Greek *ναφθα* and Akkadian *napṭu*, although this is the usual assumption. According to Greek lexicons the term is borrowed from Persian *naft*. But there is an alternative Persian homonym *nafṭ* ‘bitumen’ which is morphologically closer to Akkadian *napṭu*, with both Akkadian and Persian terms being unrelated to the Greek; see the online Steingass, Persian Dictionary (1895), 1414, 1416 (http://dsal.uchicago.edu/dictionaries/steingass/).

5’ The sign before UD.14.KÁM might be GAR.

7’ It is not clear what ŠU.GIDIM.MA *šá-ni* ^{d}*Iš*$_8$*-tár* means. The expression *šani* often appears in the explanatory drug-list *Šammu šikinšu*. The comment in Stadhouders 2011: 4, that ‘*Šammu šikinšu* shows a tendency to digress on the disease’s cause by attributing it to a deity’s avatar of ill will through the phrase *Šēdu šanê* DN,’ does not actually explain the meaning or function of *šanû*, often translated as ‘deputy.’

§ IV.10 Ms. NW (BAM 439)

4’ The interpretation of this line is tentative, but the theme is comparable to IGI 1: 91’. Instead of *lā paris* (NU KUD-*is*) ‘not stopped,’ one might also consider ...-*nu tanakkis* (KUD-*is*) ‘you shall incise ...’

6’ For the common ingredients Ì and SAHAR.URUDU see also IGI 2: 61f.’, 93’.

§ IV.11 Ms. NZb (AMT 17/2)

1ff.' Borger 1975: 280 connects the first lines (ll. 1'-5') to K 2402 + 17'-23' (Finkel 1998: 93ff.). Although some phrases are similar, any real connection seems excluded.

5' Following ^{ú}*kur-ka-nu-u* (lit. 'a duck-like plant'), we read *tál-p[ap*, 'you wrap up,' since a reading BABBAR.DILI seems unlikely because of the lack of a NA_4 determinative.

6' The verb *abāku* B references body parts like the liver, see CAD A/1 8.

7' Note the clear Assyrian vocal harmony in *e-mur-šú-ma*. The broken divine name (^{d} ...) might have been *Ištar* (^{d}15).

8' Instead of *naq me-e* one might think of *nakmû* 'roasting implement,' since the passage shares similarities with K 6057 + (CDLI no. P396340) ii 22f. [*a*]-⌜*a*⌝ *iṭ-hi-ka nak-mu-*⌜*ú*$^{?}$⌝ [...] / [*a*]-⌜*a iṭ*⌝*-hi-ka mas-da-ra* [...] 'The cautery may not approach you, ... the 'knife may not approach you'; see Böck 2014: 19 fn. 66. For the *masdara* 'knife,' see Stol 2007b: 238.

12' Thompson in AMT 17/2 copied *na-ás-puh lu*, but the reading cannot be confirmed by remaining traces of the signs.

§ V.1 UGU 1 (BAM 480)

1 BÀR is used for BAR, with Stol 1993a: 94 and Scurlock 2014: 335, different in Worthington 2005: 7: 1. Note especially the commentary SpTU 1/47: 8f.: IGI-*šú i-ṣa-par* : BAR : *ṣa-pa-ru* / BAR : *za-a-ru* 'his eye winks: BAR (means) 'to wink,' (but) BAR (also means): to twist.' Compare also K 2418+ iv 11: *īnšu iṣappar* in Kinnier Wilson and Reynolds 2007: 81 (CDLI P394418), which is the fifth tablet from the Nineveh treatise dealing with neck complaints and related matter, see Panayotov 2018a: 98.

2 For the term *murdinnu* 'bramble' see notes to IGI 2: 1.

7 Compare to IGI 2: 55'.

10 The hypothetical translation is based on parallels in Worthington 2005: 16. For the passage, see also the Assur counterpart BAM 3 i 15ff.

CAD U/W 249 renders *urṣu* as 'pestle' (against AHw), which is unlikely to be correct in the light of this passage, where the mouth or opening likely refers to the bowl.

11 For *lā šulputū* as 'sprinkled', compare AMT 50/3 r.(?) 5, see CAD Ṭ 5.

12 The reconstructed line is based on BAM 3 ii 15ff. NAG-*šú* might be also read *tašaqqīšu* 'you have him drink (it),' instead of *išattīšu*. Nevertheless, both have the same result.

22 For the expression *ina bīti ša tarāna išû* 'in a room, which has a canopy,' see line 73 on Ms. NI below. In another case, the patient is advised to sit in a reed hut, see BAM 323: 95 (Scurlock 2006: 306).

25 Against BAR in Scurlock 2014: 308: 25 and Worthington 2005: 8: 25, the collated reading is PA. See also line 30 below, where PA is used.

26 The dividing line is uncertain, since the surface is too broken.

30 Compare BAM 12: 11.

31 For GUR-*ma* HÁD.A, see SpTU 1/44: 9 and 11 (GUR-*ma* HÁD.DU/A). Note that there is a possibility that GUR-*ma* can be normalized as *ta-šá-ni-ma*, since this syllabic spelling is well attested in medical texts, see CAD Š/1 388b. Note that in a late bilingual gur$_{10}$-gur$_{10}$ corresponds to *šanû* (Geller 2016: 90: 3), which could have been based on an awareness of GUR as a logogram for *šanû*.

32 Note that ^{ú}HAB might be also read *hûratu* (normally ^{giš}HAB), since the determinatives GIŠ and Ú might be interchangeable. See ^{giš}HAB, for instance, in BAM 515 (Ms. ND) i 4.

34 [GAR]-⸢*an*⸣ seems to be what Köcher wanted to read on BAM 488, but it is not now legible on the tablet.

42 The restoration is according to BAM 480 i 31, as proposed by Scurlock 2014: 308: 42,' p. 335 fn. 89. See also IGI 2: 56'.

44 For the hypothetical reconstruction, compare IGI 2: 147'.

46 Against the copy BAM 480 i 46, read GA instead of LUH.

47 It is noteworthy that the end of the line is duplicated in Nimrud (Ms. KA 8', see the Mss. to IGI 2): [... L]ÀL.KUR-*i šu-hat* KUG.GI ⸢MAR⸣ *te-qí*.

54 For the *marišmalû*-plant see Stadhouders 2018.

56 See also IGI 2: 134, 147'.

57 The plant *supālu* is written with the logogram ^{ú}ZA.BA.LAM. For another writing, ^{ú}NIGIN^{sar}, see Abusch and Schwemer 2011: text 2.5, 1.: 12,' and Stol 2016: 121, No. 804.

58 Contrary to Kocher's copy BAM 480 i 58' and the reading KURUN in Worthington 2005: 9: 58' and Scurlock 2014: 309: 58', read KAŠ Š[EG$_{6}$.G]Á and compare line 49 above.

64 This tentative restoration is based on UGU 2 (BAM 482), Ms. NX iii 6.

66 An alternative reading might be *tu-pa-ṣa*, a D-stem durative with ventive from *pa'āṣu*.

67 Compare to IGI 2: 71', 157'.

69 There is insufficient space at the beginning of the line for the sign EME, as in Scurlock 2014: 310 or Worthington 2005: 9; the first fragmentary sign begins with a vertical wedge suitable for ŠE$_{10}$.

71 For a similar treatment with a lead spoon-salve, see IGI 3: 54'.

72 Against the provocative reading in Worthington 2005: 9, and Scurlock 2014: 310 (SUD ^{ú}SÍG.GA.RÍG.GA^{sar}), the sign is clearly KUN and not SUD, as in the copy of BAM 480 ii 8, thus rendering *kun-ša*$_{25}$ ^{síg}GA.RÍG.AG.A KEŠDA.

73 The line calls for sitting in a dark room, which could be beneficial for a patient's eyes if sensitive to light. Compare the expression to line 22 from above. A. Attia suggests that 'people with migraine feel better when they lie down in the dark! Maybe the canopy is only to protect from the sun, or the sky or the stars?'

74 Note that Worthington 2005: 9: 74', and Scurlock 2014: 310: 10 read IN.DAR. We prefer IN.GÙN, see Panayotov 2016a: 63 fn. 9. In addition, Bácskay 2018a: 64 note 74 suggests IN.DAR instead of IN.DAR.<RA> for an adjectival form of *pa'āṣu* 'to crush'.

79 The restoration *ina* GA ⸢SILA$_{11}^{?}$-*aš*$^{?}$⸣ [SAR-*ab* KI]MIN follows the phraseology of ll. 80-82 and was proposed by Scurlock 2014: 311: 15.

80 Scurlock 2014: 311: 16 reads ^{ú}U$_5$[.ARGAB^{mušen} ...] instead of ^{ú}*u*$_5$-*r*[*a-na*. Her reading can be excluded since U$_5$.ARGAB^{mušen} is not a plant and does not require a Ú determinative.

82ff. For a connection between *samānu*-disease and eye complaints, see igi-gig á-zág : *mu-ru-uṣ i-ni a-sak-ku sa-ma-nu* 'disease of the eye, Asakku, and Samāna,' (Udughul tablet 6 in Geller 2016: 230: 57).

The prescription in Ms. NI ii 19-20 is fragmentary but may be tentatively reconstructed from a parallel Assur text, see BAM 3 i 20-21. Another parallel text is Ms. NZ (AMT 5/3) i 8'-9'.

What follows next is fragmentary: [DIŠ NA U]GU-*šú* UD.DA.TAB-*m*[*a* IGI.M]IN$^{?}$-⸢*šú*⸣$^{?}$ ⸢*i-bar*⸣$^{?}$-*ru-ra ù* MÚD DIRI-⸢*a*⸣. The second part of the incipit is reminiscent of the catchline of AO 11447, but in reverse order: DIŠ NA IGI.MIN-*šú* MÚD DIRI LÁ-*ma u i-bar-ru-ru* (Geller 2007b: 14).

§ V.2 UGU 2 (BAM 482)

1 The formulation *dimta ukâl* '(the eye) contains tears' suggests an excess of tears as an abnormal physical state.

Note that in ii 20 - ii 27 all prescriptions start with *sahlê* and similar substances, but with a new ingredient added in each case. This may be evidence for some kind of experimental process, looking for active ingredients or an active combination of ingredients.

2 For the restoration B[A.BA.ZA M]UNU$_6$ see also lines ii 25, 27 below.

4 The difference between AL.ŠEG$_6$.GÁ and ŠEG$_6$.GÁ is not clear, but could be 'boiled' versus 'boiling.'

7f. See the Assur UGU 1 counterpart, BAM 3 iii 28-30, in Worthington 2006.

9f. This recipe has the same symptomology and ingredients but a slightly different application if compared to BAM 3 iii 31-33, see Worthington 2006.

11' Fincke 2000: 140 fn. 1069 and 1070 recognized the similarity between Ms. NX (BAM 482 ii 62') and the Diagnostic Handbook. ŠU.GIDIM.MA *šá-ni* ^{d}*Iš$_8$-tár* ('hand of the ghost, deputy of Ištar'). This reflects another affliction similar to *qāt*(ŠU) *Ištar* in IGI 3: 63'. See also notes to § IV.9. Ms. NV (AMT 18/3): 7' above.

12' The syllabic spellings of the plants in this line show clearly that the accusative can be expressed by *u*- instead of *a*-ending, as expected in texts of this period.

18' There is a partly erased U sign after SAG.KI-*šú*.

19' Presumably the line refers to an unspecified temple (left or right), since the previous lines dealt separately with the left and the right temples.

20' Normally one excepts SÚD after *ina* Ì ^{giš}EREN, and not before it.

§ V.3 Ms. NY (BAM 494 II 53-57 AND AMT 25/8)

The fragment contains medical incantations and therapeutic prescriptions presumably against 'blurred' eyes. The small fragment (AMT 25/8) duplicates BAM 494, see Bácskay and Simkó 2017: Ms. M.

1ff.' For this and the next line see IGI 1: 165-167.

3' The reading *a-šá-a* might also refer to the *ašû*-disease, see Bácskay and Simkó 2017: 11, Ms. H$_{\text{obv. 10'}}$.

4' For the reading Ú *aš-lì*, see Bácskay and Simkó 2017: 14; the reading Ú *aš-ši* in Ms M. is possible but doubtful, since normal spelling of the '*ašû*-disease-plant' is Ú *a-ši-i*.

Furthermore, MAŠ.TAB.BA might be an alternative spelling for the *ašû*-disease, as proposed by Köcher, see Bácskay and Simkó 2017: notes to ii 30.

5f.' The incantation remains obscure, see also see Bácskay and Simkó 2017: 14.

§ V.4 Ms. NZ (AMT 5/3)

3' The reading N]U is clear from collations, although different on the copy AMT 5/3. Compare UGU 3 (K 2566 = AMT 102) 2: *ina* IGI *ṣi-in-di ù* ÉN NU KUD-*as* '(if the ... disease) does not cease despite bandage(s) and (an) incantation,' Scurlock 2006: no. 133.

4' See also BAM 480 ii 12, Ms. NI, courtesy Annie Attia.

7' Compare to Ms. NI (BAM 480) ii 12f.

10' Compare to Ms. NI (BAM 480) ii 19f.

11' Occasionally therapeutic texts pay special attention to specific months; some examples are collected by Stol 1991/92: 58 fn. 102.

21' The shape of the signs Ì.GIŠ looks more Babylonian than Assyrian.

22' Note that the sign $MUNU_6$ normally has the parameters a1b1c7. However, the sign here has an additional *Winkelhaken* over the GAD sign, having the parameters a1b1c8. For the parameter system, see Gottstein and Panayotov 2014.

§ V.5 Ms. NZa (AMT 13/5 + 14/5)

Prescriptions for head ailments caused by the 'hand of a ghost.' This fragment might be a part of the Nineveh treatise UGU 3, see K 07642 (AMT 102ff.) or K 11578 (BAM 485).

9' The spelling *e-zu-uš* is problematic, as is the alternative *e-zu-úz*.

10' For the precise plucking method *ina nasāhīšu Šamaš lā īmaru* 'the plant has not seen the sun when it was torn out' see also CT 14/23: 7, and BAM 1 i 7 (Scurlock 2014: 398ff., and 273ff.).

The suggestion *ú-ṣa-a*[*m-mad*?] is tentative, since we would expect a second person verbal form.

§ VI Diagnostic Medical Omens Concerned With Sick Eyes (Diagnostic Handbook, *Sakikkû* Chapter 5)

The restoration of the title follows the incipit of the commentary SpTU I, No. 31, as well as the catchline on Tablet 4.

55' It is tempting to restore *nāhiru* 'nostril' (on the right side) which cannot take in air (lit. 'wind'), since the connection between lungs and respiration is not clearly mentioned in texts and may not have been clearly recognised. See also l. 56'.

56' The verb *šagāmu* 'to roar' might mean 'to ring' in this context, referring to an abnormal sound in the ears.

89' The symptom *balṣu* 'staring' occurs in IGI 3, in a medical namburbi-type ritual.

104f.' Assyriologists understand that circling eyes is idiomatic for vertigo. However, A. Attia points that 'what is idiomatic is the fact that everything is rolling around the patient, his eyes don't move!'. For instance, A. Attia refers to https://www.ncbi.nlm.nih.gov/pmc/articles/PMC2696792/.

Glossaries and Logograms with Cuneiform Signs

Uncertain Readings and Words

bappak (syllabic): NY 5’
GI.ZÚ.LUM.MA ‘date reed plant’ → *zēr/arti* GI.ZÚ.LUM.MA
huhahi (syllabic): IGI 1: 70’
ITI.1.KAM ‘one month’: IGI 3: 36’
SILA$_x$(KISAL) ‘SILA-measure’: IGI 2: 85’; NF 35’ → SILA$_4$!(KISAL)
SILA$_4$!(KISAL) ‘SILA-measure’: IGI 1: 8’, 12’, 29’, 41’ → SILA$_x$(KISAL)
ŠU.BI.AŠ.ÀM ‘ditto’: IGI 1: 158’, 162’
ŠU.BI.GIN$_7$.NAM ‘ditto’: IGI 1: 124’, 131’, 135’, 149’, 156’; IGI 3: 84’
tamadraš (syllabic) ‘magical spell’: IGI 1: 147’
TU$_6$.ÉN.É.NU.RU: IGI 1: 76’
UD.1.KAM ‘first day’: NZ 11’
UD.3.KAM ‘third day’: IGI 1: 9’, 200’; IGI 2: 1, 6, 75’, 78’, 114’
UD.9.KAM ‘nine days’: IGI 1: 85’
UD.14.KAM ‘fourteen days’: NV 5’
UD.15.KAM ‘fifteen days/fifteenth day’: IGI 2: 114’
UD.20.KAM ‘twenty days’: IGI 1: 64’; NU 6’
UD.21.KAM ‘twenty first day’: IGI 3: 36’
upak (syllabic): NY 5’, 6’

Hurrian

hu-tu-ul ‘to glorify?’: see notes to IGI 1: 182’

Numbers

1 → *ištēn*
1-*niš* → *ištēniš*
1-*šú* → *ištiššu*
2-*ma* → *šitta*
2-*šú* → *šinīšu*
2,30 or 150 → *šumēlu*
3 → *šalāš*
3-*šú* → *šalāšīšu*
4 → *rebû*
5 → *hamiš, hamšat*

https://doi.org/10.1515/9781501506550-013

6 → *šediš*
7 → *sebe*
8 → *samānat*
9 → *tiše, tišît*
10 → *ešeret*
11 → *ištēššeret*
14 → *erbēšeret*
15 → *imittu, hamiššer*
20 → *šarru*, logogram MAN
30 → dİ30, *Sîn*
40 → d40, *Ea*
150 or 2,30 → *šumēlu*

Dividing and Ditto Signs

: 'a dividing sign': IGI 1: 34', 35', 47', 135', 155', 156', 158', 164', 165', 166', 167', 168', 169', 170', 171', 172'; IGI 2: 5, 20, 21, 70', 74', 101', 116', 141'; IGI 3: 37', 38', 39', 52'
KIMIN → *ašar šanîmma* 'ditto'
MIN → *šanîš* 'alternatively, ditto'
ŠU.BI.AŠ.ÀM (ŠU, no. 567) → ŠU.BI.AŠ.ÀM in Uncertain Readings and Words
ŠU.BI.GIN$_7$.NAM (GIM, no. 686) → ŠU.BI.GIN$_7$.NAM in Uncertain Readings and Words

Divine Names

Adad (dIŠKUR) 'the weather god Adad': IGI 3: 62'
Anu (syllabic) 'the sky god Anu': IGI 1: 102', 120', 121', 134'
Asalluhi (syllabic) 'God of incantations, son of Ea': IGI 1: 94', 106', 191'; NF 36'
Dāmu (syllabic) 'god Dāmu': IGI 1: 95', 106'; NF 40' → *dāmu* 'blood'
dLAMA.MEŠ → *lamassatu* 'pupil of the eye'
dŠE.TIR → *ašnan* 'grain'
Ea (syllabic and d40) 'god Ea': IGI 1: 94', 106', 151'; IGI 3: 85'; NU 16'
Enki (d*En-ki*) 'god Enki': NF 37', 38'
Enlil (d*En-líl*) 'god Enlil'; NF 13'
Gula (d*Gu-la*) 'the goddess of healing, Gula': IGI 1: 75', (76'), 95', 100', 106', 107', 191', 192'; IGI 2: 221'; NZb 1'
Ištar (d15, d*Iš$_8$-tár*, d*Iš-tar*) 'the goddess Ištar': IGI 3: 63', 66'; NF 14'; NV 7'
Mami 'the mother goddess Mami': IGI 1: 177',
Marduk (dAMAR.UTU) 'the king-god Marduk' IGI 1: 130', 151', 191'; NF 37'
Nabû (dAG) 'god Nabû': IGI 2: 217'; NF 40'
Nammu (dEngur) 'the goddess Nammu': IGI 1: 169', 173'

Nanāya (dNa-na-a) 'the goddess Nanāya: NF 14''
Ningirimma (dNin-g̃irima) 'mistress of incantations': IGI 1: 95', 107', 191'
Ninlil (dNin-líl) 'the goddess Ninlil, consort of Enlil': NF 13'
Ninurta (dNin-urta) 'god Ninurta': IGI 2: 221'; NF 39'
Sîn (d30) 'the moon god': IGI 1: 197', 198'
Šakkan (dGÌR) 'the god Šakkan': IGI 1: 93'
Šamaš (dUTU) 'the sun god': IGI 1: 197', 198'; IGI 3: 77'; NF 19', 28'; NS 4'; NZa 10' → *ṣīt šamši*
Šazu (dšà-zu) 'the god Šazu, lit. the one who knows the inside, an incarnation of *Marduk*: NF 37', 38'
Šeriš ($^{d}GU_{4}$) 'the ox god' → *kabūtu*
Šulpaea (syllabic) 'god Šulpaea': IGI 3: 62'
Tašmētu (syllabic) 'goddess Tašmētu': IGI 2: 217'

Month Names

Nisannu (itiBÁRA) 'month Nisannu': NZ 11'
Abu (itiNE) 'month Ab': NT 3'
Ṭebētu (itiAB) 'month Tebet': NT 3'

Personal names

Aššur-bāni-apli (m*Aš-šur*-DÙ.A) 'Ashurbanipal': IGI 2: 217'

Akkadian Words

Notes:

- References are given even if reconstructed from broken bits.
- *Materia Medica* is printed in bold.
- The relevant parallels of the Nineveh IGI are not listed in the glossary.
- Mss. **NI** (V.1 UGU 1 = BAM 480) and **NX** (V.2 UGU 2 = BAM 482) are indexed by Worthington 2005; 2007, and Attia and Buisson 2003. The Mss. in chapter VI Diagnostic Medical Omens Concerned with Sick Eyes (Diagnostic Handbook, Sakikkû Chapter 5) will be indexed in the forthcoming publication of Eric Schmidtchen. Therefore, these texts are excluded from the present glossary, in order to omit unnecessary repetition.
- Akkadian follows *CDA* and not *CAD*.

A

abāku (syllabic) 'overturned, reversed'
G-stem: *ab-ku*: NZb 6'
abālu (HÁD.DU) 'to dry'
G-stem: *ablat*(HÁD.DU): IGI 2: 71', 157'; *ītablu*(HÁD.DU): IGI 2: 71', 157'
D-stem: *tubbal*(HÁD.DU): IGI 2: 74', 154', 168'; *tu-bal*: NZa 10'
abālu (syllabic) 'to stir ingredients' < *wabālu*
Št^2-stem: *tuš-tab-bal*: IGI 1: 33'
aban gabî (NA$_4$ *ga-bi-i*) 'alum': IGI 1: 35'; IGI 2: 8, 10, 57', 66'; NK 8'; NR 2', 7'
aban hurāṣi (NA$_4$ KUG.GI) 'golden bead'; NT 10'; NZb 4'
aban sābi (NA$_4$ *sa-a-bi*) '*sābu*-stone': NZb 4'
aban tašrīti (NA$_4$ BAL) '*tašrītu*-stone': IGI 1: 47'; IGI 3: 4
abāru (A.GAR$_5$) 'lead': IGI 2: 198'; IGI 3: 95', 105' → *irri* / *itqūr abāri*
abnu (NA$_4$) 'stone, bead': IGI 3: 34', 37' → ***aban hurāṣi/mūṣi/sābi***; ***qēm aban suluppī***
abu (AD) 'father': IGI 1: 151'
abu → Month Names
abû → *apû*
abukkatu (LI.TAR/DUR) '*abukkatu*-plant' → *hīl abukkati*
adappu (syllabic) 'canal': IGI 3: 25'
adi (EN) 'until': IGI 2: 71', 119', 157', 220'; IGI 3: 54'
agalapû (syllabic) '*agalapû*-lagoon': IGI 1: 92'
agašgû (A.GA.ÁŠ.GA) 'novice (physician)': IGI 1: 70'
agubbû (A.GÚB.BA.A) 'holy water vessel': IGI 3: 76'; NF 17'
ahātu (syllabic) 'sister': IGI 1: 101', 121', 126'
ahāzu (syllabic) 'to take, acquire'
G-stem: *e-hu-uz-zu*: IGI 2: 218', 219'
ahê (syllabic) 'by itself, separately': IGI 2: 161'
ahennû (syllabic) 'separately, individually': IGI 1: 82', 117', 143', 180'; IGI 2: 136'
ahû (syllabic and BAR) 'stranger': IGI 2: 12; 'non-canonical (material)': IGI 2: 220'
ai (*a-a*) 'not', vetitive particle: NZb 9', 10'
akalu (NINDA) 'loaf of bread': IGI 2: 67'; IGI 3: 78'
akālu (syllabic and GU$_7$) 'to eat, consume, hurt, cause pain'
G-stem: *e-kal*: IGI 1: 74'; *ik-kal-ki-na-ši*: IGI 1: 113'; *ikkalma*(GU$_7$-*ma*): IGI 2: 131'; *ikkal*(GU$_7$): IGI 3: 82', 88'; *ikkalšu*(GU$_7$-*šú*): NV 6'
aktam (^{ú}*ak-tam* and ^{ú}*at-kám*) '*aktam*-plant': IGI 1: 18'; IGI 2: 125', 195'; IGI 3: 72'; NR 4'; NV 1'
alādu (Ù.TU) 'to give birth' < *walādu*
G-stem: *ullad*(Ù.TU): IGI 1: 67'; *ūlid*(Ù.TU): IGI 1: 195'; *ūlidu*(Ù.TU): IGI 2: 110', 148'; NR 5'; *ul-du*: NRa 3' → ***larsīni ša halli lahri ša šumēli ša māšī ūlidu, šizbi musukkati ša zikara ūlidu***
alāku (syllabic and DU) 'to go (+ ventive to come)'

ana pān (*ana* IGI) 'in front of': IGI 1: 177'; IGI 3: 28', 77'
anāku (syllabic) 'I, me': IGI 1: 100', 152', 192'; NF 14'
annakku ($^{\text{na4}}$AN.NA) 'tin': IGI 3: 3; NF 10'
annânam (syllabic) 'this here; from now on': IGI 3: 36'
annītu (syllabic) 'this': IGI 1: 94'; IGI 3: 87'
annû (syllabic and ŠEŠ) 'this, these': IGI 1: 62', 64', 85', 97', 109'; IGI 2: 10, 11, 26; IGI 3: 5, 29', 34', 43'; NF 11'; NS 3'; NU 14'
annuharu (syllabic) '*annuharu*-mineral': NZ 23'
anzahhu ($^{\text{na4}}$AN.ZAH) '*anzahhu*-glass (bead)': NT 8'
apsû (syllabic) 'underground water': IGI 1: 171'
aptu (syllabic) 'window': NF 29'
ap/bû (syllabic) 'cloudy, veiled (said of eyes)': IGI 1: 90', 99', 111', 123', 138', 176'; IGI 3: 26'; NK 9'; NQ 5', 10'; NS 1'
ap/bû (syllabic) 'to become cloudy, veiled (said of eyes)'
G-stem: *tab-ba-a*: IGI 1: 112'; *ip-pa-a*: IGI 2: 54'
arādu (syllabic) 'go down, descend, plunge' < *warādu*
G-stem: *ú-ri-du*: IGI 1: 104'; *ur-da*: IGI 1: 194'
arāmu (syllabic) 'to cover'
G-stem: *ár-mat*: IGI 2: 121', 124'
arāpu → *erēpu*
ardatu (^{munus}KI.SIKIL) 'young woman, maiden': IGI 1: 159', 161' < *wardatu*
argānu (^{giš}*ar-ga-nu*) '*argānu*-plant': IGI 1: 19'
arhu (ITI) 'month': IGI 2: 138', 144'
āribu (UGA^{mušen}) 'raven': IGI 2: 106' → ***pel āribi***
arkabu (ARGAB^{mušen}) 'bat' → ***rikibti arkabi***
arki (EGIR) 'after(wards)': IGI 2: 53', 79'
arkīšu (EGIR-*šú*) 'afterwards': IGI 3: 30', 54'
arkītu (EGIR-*tì*) 'afterwards' → *ina arkīti*
arku (GÍD.DA) 'long (of sheep's bones)': IGI 2: 53'
arqu (SIG$_7$) 'yellow-green': IGI 1: 28' → *muṣa''irānu*
arqūtu (SIG$_7$-*su*) 'freshness', as qualification for 'fresh-green' plants (*arqūssu*, lit. 'concerning his freshness'): IGI 1: 10', 21', 80'; IGI 2: 63', 153'; NU 7'
arti bīni (PA ^{giš}*bi-ni*) 'leaf of tamarisk': IGI 2: 144'
arti ēri (PA ^{giš}MA.NU) 'leaf of *ēru*-tree'; IGI 2: 144'
***arti* GI.ZÚ.LUM.MA** (PA GI.ZÚ.LUM.MA) 'leaf of date reed': IGI 3: 71'
arti lipāri (PA ^{giš}MI.PÀR) 'leaf of *lipāru*-tree': IGI 3: 71'
arti pillî zikari (PA ^{giš}NAM.TAR NÍTA) 'leaf of male *pillû*-plant': IGI 3: 33'
arti šunê (PA ^{giš}ŠE.NÚ.A) 'leaf of *šunû*-tree': IGI 3. 70'
arti titti (PA ^{giš}PÈŠ) 'fig leaf': IGI 3: 70'
artu (PA) 'foliage, leafs' → *arti bīni*/*ēri*/GI.ZÚ.LUM.MA/*pillî zikari*/*šunê*/*titti*
aru (syllabic) 'stalk, chaff': IGI 1: 114'

ashar (^{na4}*aš-har*, ^{na4}*áš-har*, presumably not ŠIM.BI.SIG$_7$.SIG$_7$ → *dāmātu*) '*ashar*-stone': IGI 1: 11', 13', 38', 58', 60', 72'; IGI 2: 21; IGI 3: 5, 104'; NR 2', 4'

askuppu (KUN$_4$) 'threshold': IGI 2: 28, 59', 103'

asu (^{šim}GÍR) '*asu*-aromatic' → ***šaman asi***

asû (^{lú}A.ZU) 'physician': IGI 3: 105'; NF 42' → *qātu*

asûtu (A.ZU-*ti*) 'medical skill': IGI 1: 192'

aṣû (syllabic and È-*a*) 'to go, come out' < *waṣû*

G-stem: *ittaṣâ*(È-*a*): IGI 1: 79'; *a-ṣa-at*: IGI 2: 17; *uṣṣâ*(È-*a*): IGI 2: 149'; *aṣû*(È): NW 4'

Gt-stem: *lit-ta-ṣi*: IGI 1: 174'

Š-stem: *ana ... šu-ṣi-i*: IGI 2: 98'; *tušeṣṣēma*(È-*ma*): IGI 1: 39'; *tušeṣṣi*(È): NU 9'

ašāgu (^{giš}KIŠI$_{16}$) '*ašāgu*-acacia': NF 35' → ***šuruš ašāgi***

ašar šanîmma (KIMIN) 'ditto': IGI 1: 55', 56', 86'; IGI 2: 13, 15, 152'; IGI 3: 38', 39', 40'; NF 5', 6', 33'; NS 5', 7'; NU 7'; NZ 6', 7' → *ana ašri šanîmma*

ašgikû (^{na4}ÁŠ.GI$_4$.GI$_4$) '*ašgikû*-stone': NT 7'

ašītu (syllabic) 'blurring (of the vision)': IGI 1: 80'

aškāpu (^{lú}AŠGAB) 'leatherworker' → ***kammu ša aškāpi***; ***šuhtu ša aškāpi***

ašlu (syllabic) 'rush' → ***zēr ašli zikari***

ašnan (^{d}ŠE.TIR) 'grain' → ***qēm ašnan***

aššum (syllabic) 'because of': IGI 1: 94'

Aššur (AN.ŠÁR^{ki}) 'Assyria': IGI 2: 217'

ašû (syllabic) 'blurred said of eyes (vision)': IGI 1: 90', 99', 111', 123', 137', 167', 176'; IGI 2: 17; IGI 3: 26'; NK 9'; NQ 5', 10'; NS 1'; NY 3'

ašû (syllabic) 'to be blurred said of eyes (vision)'

G-stem: *taš-šá-a*: IGI 1: 112'; *a-šá-a*: IGI 1: 178'

ašû (syllabic and MAŠ.TAB.BA) '*ašû*-disease'; NY 4'

ašūhu (^{giš}Ù.SUH$_5$) '*ašūhu*-pine': NF 18', 21'

atā'išu (^{ú}KUR.KUR) '*atā'išu*-plant': IGI 1: 32', 62'; IGI 2: 66', 189': IGI 3: 97', 99', 102'; NR 6'; NU 10'

attā (syllabic) 'you' (2 m. sg. pron.): IGI 1: 130', 152'

attī (syllabic) 'you' (2 f. sg. pron.): IGI 1: 76'

attina (syllabic) 'you' (2 f. pl. pron.): IGI 1: 187'

awīlu → *amēlu*

awurriqānu → *amurriqānu*

ayabba (A.AB.BA) 'sea': IGI 1: 103'

ayyu (syllabic) 'which': IGI 1: 128', 129'

azugallūtu (syllabic) 'the medical knowledge/art': IGI 2: 221'

B

ba'ālu (syllabic) 'to be large'

G-stem: IGI 1: 67'

bābu (KÁ) 'entrance-door': IGI 2: 12, 14
bakû (syllabic) 'to weep'
G-stem: *i-bak-ki*: IGI 1: 168'; *i-bak-ka*: IGI 1: 177'
balālu (HE.HE) 'to mix'
G-stem: *taballal*(HE.HE): IGI 1: 11', 13', 28', 40', 46', 57', 63'; IGI 2: 6, 18, 24, 53', 76', 78', 92', 94', 113', 120', 123', 125', 146', 150', 152', 154', 155', 165', 192', 193', 194', 206', 215'; IGI 3: 1, 48', 53', 69', 72', 83'; NF 20', 23'; NK 12'
balāṣu → *balṣu*
balāṭu (syllabic and TI(.LA)) 'life': IGI 1: 65', 66', 75'
balāṭu (syllabic and TI(.LA)) 'to live, heal, recover'
G-stem: *ba-laṭ*: IGI 1: 76'; *i-bal-lu-uṭ*: IGI 1: 161'; *iballuṭ*(TI): IGI 1: 13'; IGI 2: 99', 123', 125', 136', 138': IGI 3: 43', 61', 65', 67', 72'; NF 14'; NU 5', 6'; NV 3'; NZ 10'
D-stem: *bulliṭīma*(TI.(LA)-*ma*): IGI 1: 95', 107'; *ú-bal-liṭ*: IGI 1: 159' ; *ana bulluṭīšu*(TI-*šú*) 'in order to heal it': IGI 2: 19, 22, 55', 137' IGI 3: 3; NQ 11'; NS 1'; (*ana bulluṭi*) NU 8', 12'; NV 7'; *ana ... bul-lu-ṭi*: IGI 2: 98'; *bul-li-ṭi-ma*: NZb 1'
ballukku ($^{\check{s}im}$BAL / $^{\check{s}im}$MUG) '*ballukku*-aromatic': IGI 2: 69', 109'; NK 16' → ***šaman ballukki***
balṣu (syllabic) 'staring': IGI 3: 80', 86'
baltu ša ṭābti (syllabic) 'salted *baltu*-(thorn) plant': IGI 2: 112'
balṭu (syllabic and TI.LA) 'healthy': IGI 1: 97', 118', 181'; 'freshly': IGI 2: 68'
balû → *belû*
baluhhu ($^{\check{s}im}$BULUH) '*baluhhu*-aromatic': NZ 9'; '*baluhhu*-granule (in the eye)': IGI 1: 79' → ***hīl baluhhi***
bāmâ (syllabic) 'in half': IGI 1: 70'
bāqilu (SAR.MUNU$_6$; for MUNU$_6$.SAR) 'malster' → ***mê bāqili***
barāru (syllabic) 'to flicker (said of eyes)'
G-stem: *bar-ra*: IGI 2: 58'; *i-bar-ru-ra*: NZ 8'
barīrātu (syllabic) '*barīrātu*-sagapenum': IGI 1: 19'
barû (syllabic and IGI.KÁR) 'to collate (a tablet); to check (a remedy)'
G-stem: *abrēma*(IGI.KÁR-*ma*): IGI 2: 221'; *ba-ri*: IGI 3: 96'
bāṣu (syllabic) 'sand': IGI 1: 113'
bašālu (ŠEG$_6$(-*šal*)) 'to be cooked'
Š-stem: *tušabšal*(ŠEG$_6$(-*šal*)) 'to cook, boil': IGI 1: 18', 35'; IGI 3: 100'; NQ 8'
bašāmu (syllabic) 'to create'
G-stem: *ba-ša-mu*: IGI 1: 194'; *ba-áš-mu*: IGI 2: 221'
bašlu (syllabic and ŠEG$_6$.GA) 'boiled'; NW 2'; NZ 25' → *ṭābātu*
bâtu (syllabic) 'spend the night (under a star)'
Š-stem: *tuš-bat*: IGI 1: 81'; IGI 3: 34'; NF 19', 22'; NU 7'
bēltu (EN) 'mistress': IGI 1: 95', 107', 191', 192'
belû (syllabic) 'to end, terminate'
G-stem: *li-be-la-a*: IGI 1: 123'
beri/u- → *ina beri/u-*

berqu (NIM.GÍR) 'lighting': IGI 3: 9
billatu (syllabic and DIDA) 'beer mash': IGI 2: 168'; NZ 15'; NZ 18'
bīnu (syllabic and ^{giš}ŠINIG) 'tamarisk': IGI 1: 80'; IGI 2: 5; IGI 3: 23', 51'; NF 17', 21' → ***arti/dām/mê/zēr bīni***
biri → *beri*
birki immeri (*bir-ki* UDU) 'sheep testicle (lit. 'knee')': IGI 1: 185'
bi/urṣu (syllabic) 'flash of light': IGI 3: 2; NF 13', 17', 20', 23'; NT 4'
bītu (É) 'house': IGI 2: 12, 14; NF 19'; 'domestic': NS 4'
bulālu (syllabic) '*bulālu*-plant': IGI 3: 37'
bulṭu (syllabic and TI) 'cure, remedy, medical prescription': IGI 1: 76'; IGI 2: 220'
buqlu (MUNU$_6$) 'malt' → ***qēm buqli***
burāšu (^{šim}LI) 'juniper': IGI 2: 5, 16; IGI 3: 11, 55', 77', 93'; NF 34'; NU 3'; NV 4'; NZ 9' → ***qēm/zēr burāši***
burṣu → *birṣu*
būrtu (PÚ) 'well' → ***mê būrti***
buṣinnu (syllabic) 'a wick': IGI 2: 90'

D

dagālu (syllabic) 'to see, look'
Gtn-stem: *id-da-nag-ga-la*: IGI 3: 2
dalāhu → *dalhu*
dalhu (syllabic and LÙ.LÙ) 'troubled': IGI 1: 123', 166', 184'; IGI 2: 215'; IGI 3: 1; NR 6'
daltu (^{giš}IG) 'door': IGI 3: 88'
dām bīni (MÚD ^{giš}*bi-ni*) 'tamarisk 'blood' (i.e. resin)': NW 5'
dām erēni (MÚD ^{giš}EREN) 'cedar 'blood' (i.e. resin)': IGI 2: 24
dām kurṣipti alpi ṣalmi (MÚD *kur-ṣib-ti* GU$_4$ GE$_6$) 'blood of a black ox-fly': IGI 2: 214'
damqu (SIG$_5$) 'good' → ***himēti damiqte***
dāmātu (ŠIM.BI.SIG$_7$.SIG$_7$) '*dāmātu*-paste': IGI 1: 42', 45'
dāmu (syllabic, MÚD or MUD) 'blood': IGI 1: 36', 40', 45', 48', 61', 68', 71', 74', 75', 77', 79', 99', 178'; IGI 2: 25; NR 3', 5', 6', 10'; NW 4'; NZ 4'; NZa 8' → ***dām kurṣipti alpi ṣalmi***; ***dāma ša libbi šahî***; *pursīt dāmi*; 'blood' of a plant (i.e. resin)' → ***dām erēni/bīni***
dāmu ša libbi šahî (MÚD *ša* ŠÀ ŠAH) 'blood from a pig's 'heart': IGI 1: 48'
dannu (KALA.GA) 'strong': IGI 1: 81'
daqqiqu (syllabic) 'tiny' → ***zēr šammi daqqiqi***
diga/ilu → *diglu*
digil īnī (*di-gi-il* IGI.MIN) 'eyesight': IGI 3: 51'
diglu (syllabic) 'vision': IGI 1: 80'; IGI 2: 124', 126' → *digil īnī*
dimtu (ÉR) 'tear(s)': IGI 1: 79', 137'; IGI 2: 58', 121'; NK 10'; NQ 5', 10'; NS 1'; NV 6'; NZa 8' → *naqû*

diqāru (^{dug}ÚTUL) '*diqāru*-pot': IGI 2: 63', 68'

dišip šadê/î (LÁL.KUR.RA, LÀL.KUR(-*e/i*)) 'mountain honey': IGI 1: 40', 64'; IGI 2: 18, 62', 120', 154', 163'; IGI 3: 50', 53', 69'; NS 7'

dišpu (LÀL) 'honey': IGI 2: 20, 51', 148', 195'; IGI 3: 48', 67'; NF 16'; NS 4' → ***dišip šadê, dišpu peṣû***

dišpu peṣû (LÀL BABBAR) 'white honey': IGI 2: 195', 215'; IGI 3: 1

dudubi (DÙ.DÙ.BI) 'its ritual, medical application': IGI 1: 69', 72', 97', 109', 117', 124', 131', 135', 143', 146', 148', 149', 154', 156', 158', 162', 180', 185'; IGI 3: 27', 84', 87'; NF 44'; NZb 3'; NY 7'

E

ebbu (syllabic and DADAG) 'pure': IGI 1: 103', 122'; NF 23'

edēpu (syllabic) 'to blow, inflate'
  D-stem: *ud-du-pu*: IGI 1: 174'; *ud-du-pa-a-ma*: NK 9'

edû (syllabic) 'known': IGI 2: 14

edû (syllabic) 'to know'
  G-stem: *i-di/du-u*: IGI 1: 152': *ti-di*: IGI 1: 152'

egemgīru (syllabic and ^{giš}NÍG.GÁN.GÁN) '*egemgīru*-plant': IGI 2: 113' → ***zēr egemgīri***

egû (syllabic) 'to become lazy/tired'
  G-stem: *e-gu-ma*: IGI 1: 30'$^{?}$

ēkallu (É.GAL) 'palace': IGI 2: 217', 222'

elēnu (UGU-*nu*, AN.TA) 'above': IGI 1: 127'; IGI 2: 64'

eli (syllabic and UGU) 'on, over, above': IGI 1: 31'; IGI 2: 72', 119'; IGI 3: 68' → *muhhu*

ellu (KÙ) 'clean, holy': IGI 1: 160', 173'; NT 9' → ***libbi elleti gišimmari***

elû (syllabic) 'go up, get out, ascend'
  G-stem: *li-la-a*: IGI 1: 198'
  Š-stem: *šu-li-i*: IGI 1: 193', 199'; *tušellâmma*(E$_{11}$-*ma*): IGI 2: 28, 59', 79', 103'; NR 8'; *tu-še-li-ma*: NF 27'

ēma (syllabic) 'whenever': IGI 1: 69', 97', 109', 117', 144', 154', 186'; IGI 3: 89'; NU 15'

emēdu (syllabic) 'to lean on, apply'
  D-stem: *tu-mad*: IGI 2: 185'
  Št-stem: *tuš-te-mid*: IGI 1: 83'

emesallu (^{mun}*eme/me*$_{5}$(A)-*sal*(-*lì*), ^{mun}*eme-sal-la*, A.MEŠ-*sal*, *me*$_{5}$(A)-SILIM, ^{mun}*eme-sala*) '*emesallu*-saline solution': IGI 1: 41', 61', 82', 86'; IGI 2: 8, 10, 23, 57', 116', 146', 195'; IGI 3: 50', 52', 58'; NK 8'; NQ 12'; NS 2', 7'; NW 3'

emmu (syllabic) 'hot': IGI 2: 3

enqu (syllabic) 'expert': IGI 1: 75'

enūma (UD-*ma*) 'when': IGI 1: 17'; IGI 2: 71', 157'; IGI 3: 2; NF 13'; NT 12'

enzu (UD$_{5}$) 'goat': IGI 3: 10 → ***šizbi enzi***

eperu (SAHAR) 'dust': IGI 1: 138'

epēšu (syllabic and DÙ(-*šú*/*uš*)) 'to do, make'
G-stem: *tēpušu*(DÙ-*šú*): IGI 1: 17'; *teppuš*(DÙ-*uš*): IGI 1: 63'; IGI 2: 24; *teppušma*(DÙ-*ma*): IGI 3: 36', 45'; NT 3'; *te-pu-uš*: IGI 3: 53'; *e-pu-uš*: IGI 1: 152'
Gtn-stem: *tēteneppuš*(DÙ.DÙ-*uš*): IGI 1: 9' ; *tēteneppuš*(DÙ.MEŠ): IGI 1: 85'
epû (syllabic) 'bake'
G-stem: *te-ep-pi*: IGI 2: 65'; *te-pi*: NR 8'
eqû (syllabic and MAR) 'to daub, instil'
G-stem: *teqqi*(MAR): IGI 1: 11', 14', 15', 20', 33', 34', 35', 38', 40', 41', 44', 45', 46', 47', 49', 58', 60', 63', 64'
IGI 2: 4, 18, 20, 21, 24, 50', 51', 60', 61', 64', 66', 70', 71', 72', 73', 74', 75', 81', 83', 84', 93', 95', 99', 101', 102', 103', 104', 116', 119', 123', 127', 129', 139', 141', 142', 143', 144', 146', 147', 148', 150', 151', 154', 155', 157', 158', 161', 162', 164', 167', 168', 170', 173', 178', 187', 192', 193', 194', 208'
IGI 3: 6, 16', 17', 19', 30', 50', 53', 54', 95', 103'; NF 7', 12'; NP 2'–5', 7', 8'; NR 2', 4', 5'; NS 4', 8'; NU 6', 9'
te-(eq)-qí: IGI 1: 2', 4', 17', 22', 25', 28', 39', 41', 69'
IGI 2: 53', 85'–88', 97', 107', 114', 180', 182'–184', 186'
IGI 3: 69'; NF 2', 3', 16'
Gtn-stem: *tēteneqqi*(MAR.MEŠ): IGI 1: 13', 55'; IGI 2: 7, 55', 99', 125', 136'; IGI 3: 43', 61', 65', 67', 83'; *te-te-né-eq-qí*: IGI 1: 54'; *te-te-né-qí*: IGI 2: 82', *te-te-neq-qí*: IGI 2: 120'
erbēšeret (14) 'fourteen': IGI 1: 69'
erbēt (4) 'four': NK 13', 14'
erēbu (KU_4-*ub*) 'enter, go down, set (for sun)'
G-stem: *īrub*(KU_4-*ub*): IGI 1: 93', 198'; *e-re-bi*: NF 28'
erēnu (EREN) 'cedar tree'; NF 34': → ***dām*/*šaman erēni***
erēpu, *arāpu* (syllabic) 'to cloud over, grow dark'
G-stem: *e*/*i-ru-pu*: IGI 1: 30'; *ar-pa*: IGI 2: 61'
erēru 'to dry out'
G-stem: *ir-ri-ra*: IGI 2: 99'
erru I (syllabic) 'parched': IGI 2: 2
errû (^{ú}ÚKUŠ.LAGAB) '*errû*-colocynth': IGI 2: 122'; IGI 3: 52' → ***inib errî***
eršu (^{giš}NÁ) 'bed': NF 31'
ēru (^{giš}MA.NU) '*ēru*-tree': NF 18' → ***arti*/*šuruš*/*zēr ēri***
erû (URUDU) '*erû*-copper'; IGI 3: 6; NF 12' → ***erû labīru*, *hīl erî***
erû ($TI_8^{\text{mušen}}$) '*erû*-eagle': → ***muhhu ša erî***
erû labīru (URUDU SUMUN) 'old copper': IGI 2: 99',
erû zikaru (URUDU NITA) 'male copper (bead)': IGI 3: 4
esēpu (syllabic) 'to collect'
G-stem: *te-sip*: IGI 2: 28, 174'
eṣēdu (syllabic) 'to harvest'
G-stem: *e-ṣi-id*: IGI 1: 197'; *ina e-ṣe-di-šú*: IGI 1: 197'

eṣemti amēlūti (GÌR.PAD.DU NAM.LÚ.U_{19}.LU) 'human bone': NK 3'
eṣemtu (GÌR.PAD.DU/DA) 'bone': IGI 1: 6'; NZ 22' → ***eṣemti amēlūti*, *lipi eṣemti arikti*, *lipi eṣemti*, *lipi eṣemti kurīti immerim*, *lipi eṣemti kurīti ša immeri*, *lipi eṣemti immeri*, *lipi eṣemti ṣabīti*, *muhhu ša eṣemti kurīti immeri***
eṣēpu (syllabic) 'to twine thread (two-ply)'
G-stem: *te-eṣ-ṣi-ip*: IGI 1: 185'
ešeret (10) 'ten': IGI 1: 8', 12'; NF 35'
eṭemmu (GIDIM) 'ghost': NT 5'; NU 12'; NZb 8' → *harbātu*
eṭlu (GURUŠ) 'young man, lad': IGI 1: 159', 161', 198'
eṭû (syllabic) 'to become dark'
Gtn-stem: *i-te-né-ṭa-a*: IGI 2: 54'
ezzu (syllabic) 'anger': NZa 9'

G

gabīdu (syllabic) 'liver': → ***makūt gabīdi* (*ša imēri*)**
gabû (syllabic and IM.SAHAR.NA_4.KUR.RA) '*gabû*-alum': IGI 2: 161' → ***aban gabî***
galābu (syllabic and SAR(-*ab*)) 'to shave'
D-stem: *tugallab*(SAR-*ab*): IGI 1: 24'; NZ 21'; *tu-gal-lab*: IGI 2: 7, 109', 118'
giddagiddû (GÍD.DA.GÍD.DA, GÍD.DA.GÍD-*du*, GÍD.GÍD) '*giddagiddû*-fibers': IGI 2: 12, 13, 15
gišimmaru (^{giš}GIŠIMMAR) 'date palm': NF 18', 21' → ***libbi elleti gišimmari*, *šuruš gišimmari zikari*, *taltallû ša gišimmari***
gišrinnu (GIŠ.ÉRIN) 'scale'; NS 4'
gulgullu (syllabic) 'skull' → *kalli gulgul amēli*
gūqānu → *qūqānu*
gūru ša qanî (*gu-ra šá* GI) 'reed leaf': IGI 2: 109'
gurušgaraš ša šahî (*gu-ru-uš-ga-ra-aš ša šahî*) 'vulva of a pig': IGI 2: 27

H

habburru (syllabic and HÉNBUR) 'sprout': IGI 1: 195', 196' → ***habbur še'i***
habbur še'i (HÉNBUR ŠE.AM) 'grain-sprout': IGI 1: 10'
hallu (syllabic) 'hind leg' → ***larsīni ša halli lahri ša šumēli ša māšī ūlidu***
hallūru (GÚ.GAL) 'chickpea' → ***qēm hallūri***
hamāṭu (syllabic) 'to burn, inflame'
G-stem: *ha-an-ṭa*: IGI 1: 14'; IGI 2: 9; *hamiṭ*(TAB.BA): IGI 3: 49'; NS 6'
hamiš → *hamšat*
hamiššer (15) 'fifteeen': IGI 2: 139', 141'
hamšat, hamiš (5) 'five': IGI 1: 29', 44'; IGI 2: 92'

hāmū (syllabic) 'chaff': IGI 1: 187', 193'
handabillu (syllabic) '*handabillu*-shell': IGI 1: 188'
hapāpu (syllabic) 'to rinse'
  D-stem: *tu-ha-pap*: IGI 3: 31'
harāṣu (syllabic) 'to break off, cut into'
  G-stem: *ta-har-ra-aṣ*: IGI 3: 81', 90'$^{?}$
harbātu (syllabic) 'abandoned land'; NT 5' → *eṭemmu*
harištu (syllabic) 'woman in labour': IGI 1: 104'
haṣab igulê (ŠIKA *ì-gu-le-e*) 'potsherd of fine salve': IGI 2: 134'
haṣab nurmî (ŠIKA ^{giš}NU.ÚR.MA) 'pomegranate peel': IGI 2: 116'
haṣab ṭābti (ŠIKA MUN) 'flake of salt': IGI 2: 194'
haṣbu labīru ša kibša išû (ŠIKA LIBIR.RA *šá ki-ib-ša*$^{?}$ TUK-*ú*) 'old fungus-ridden potsherd': IGI 2: 62'
haṣbi šammi peṣî (ŠIKA Ú.BABBAR) 'peel of white plant': IGI 2: 139'
haṣbu (ŠIKA) 'potsherd, sherd, peel, flake': IGI 2: 141'; NZ 17' → ***haṣab nurmî/ṭābti/igulê, haṣbu labīru ša kibša išû, haṣbi šammi peṣî***
hašālu (GAZ) 'to crush'
  G-stem: *tahaššal*(GAZ): IGI 1: 16'; IGI 2: 56', 153', 162', 168'; IGI 3: 5, 72'; NF 11'
hašhūru (^{giš}HAŠHUR) 'apple': IGI 1: 47'; NF 18', 21'
hašlu (syllabic) 'crushed': IGI 1: 170'
hašû (syllabic) 'to chop (foodstuffs)'
  D-stem: *ú-haš-šá*: IGI 1: 26'
hašû (^{ú}HAR.HAR) '*hašû*-thyme': IGI 3: 100'; NU 4', 10'
haṭṭi rē'î (^{ú}NÍG.GIDRU) 'shepherd's-staff plant' → *zēr haṭṭi rē'î*
hepû (syllabic) 'to break'
  G-stem: *te-he-pi*: IGI 1: 160'
herṣu (syllabic) 'cut (in the liver)': IGI 3: 89'
hesû (syllabic) 'to squeeze out drugs'
  D-stem: *tu-ha-sa*: IGI 1: 80'; IGI 2: 63'
hīl abukkati (ILLU LI.TAR/DUR) 'gummy resin of *abukkatu*-plant': IGI 1: 78'; IGI 2: 208'; IGI 3: 13, 27'
hīl baluhhi (ILLU ^{šim}BULUH) 'resin of *baluhhu*-aromatic': IGI 2: 138'
hīl erî (ILLU URUDU) 'exudation of copper': IGI 1: 13', 82', 87'
hīl nuhurti (ILLU NU.LUH) 'resin of *nuhurtu*-plant': IGI 2: 137'
hīl tīyati (ILLU ^{ú}*ti-iá-tu*) 'resin of *tīyatu*-plant': IGI 3: 52'
hīlu (ILLU) 'resin' → ***hīl abukatti/baluhhi/erî/nuhurti/tīyati***
himēti damiqte (Ì.NUN SIG$_5$-*te*) 'good quality ghee': IGI 1: 16'
himētu (Ì.NUN(.NA)) 'ghee': IGI 1: 11', 13', 14', 25', 28', 33', 34', 35', 38', 41', 42', 44', 45', 46', 58', 60', 72', 84'; IGI 2: 18, 21, 51', 55', 58', 66', 70', 72', 76', 79', 81', 99', 119', 120', 139', 141', 142', 143', 144', 148', 150', 152', 157', 163', 165', 168', 198', 215'; IGI 3: 1, 38', 48', 50', 67', 69', 83', 103'; NF 16'; NR 4', 8'; NS 8'; NW 5' → ***himēti damiqte***
hulālu ($^{\text{na4}}$NÍR) 'banded agate (onyx)': IGI 1: 103', 122'

huliam (syllabic) '*huliam*-vessel': IGI 1: 81', 83'
huluhhu (^{na4}AN.ZAH.BABBAR) '*huluhhu*-slag (bead)': IGI 3: 33'; NT 8'
hurāṣu (KUG.GI) 'gold'; NF 20'→ ***aban hurāṣi***
hūratu (^{giš}HAB) 'dyeing sumac': IGI 2: 4
huṣābu (syllabic) 'twig': IGI 1: 189', 193'

I

ī, *ya* (syllabic) 'my': IGI 1: 66', 74'; IGI 2: 219', 220'
idru (syllabic) '*idru*-saltpetre': NZ 13'
igāru (É.GAR$_8$) 'wall' → ***ṣurār igāri***
igulû (syllabic) 'fine ointment': → ***haṣab igulê***
ikil pāni (syllabic) 'darkness of face, gloom': IGI 1: 130'
iklu (syllabic) 'gloominess, darkness' → *ikil pāni*
iltānu (IM.2) 'north wind': IGI 1: 115'
imbu' tâmti (KA.A.AB.BA) 'algae': NF 19', 22'; NU 3'
imēru (ANŠE) 'donkey': → ***makūt gabīdi ša imēri***
imhur-ešrā (^{ú}IGI-NIŠ) '*imhur-ešrā*-plant': NU 4'
imhur-līm (^{ú}IGI-*lim*) '*imhur-līm*-plant': IGI 2: 142'; NF 45'; NU 4'
imittu (ZAG, 15) 'right side': IGI 1: 146'; NV 6' → *īn imittīšu*; *ana imitti*
immeru (UDU, UDU.NÍTA) 'sheep, male sheep': IGI 1: 91'; IGI 2: 18 → ***birki immeri, kabūt immeri, lipi eṣemti immeri, lipi eṣemti kurî immeri, lipi eṣemti kurî ša immeri, lipi kalīti immeri, marat immeri, muhhu ša eṣemti kurî immeri, sikkat ṣēli immeri***
īn imittīšu (IGI(.MIN) ZAG/15-*šú*) 'man's (lit. his) right eye': IGI 2: 200'; NV 6', NZa 8'
īn šumēlīšu (IGI GÙB-*šú*) 'man's (lit. his) left eye': IGI 2: 202'
ina (AŠ and syllabic) 'in, on': IGI 1: 7', 10'–16', 18'–20', 22'–29', 33'–35', 37', 38', 41'–47', 52', 57', 58', 60', 62'–65', 67', 69', 72', 78', 79', 81', 84', 86'–88', 97', 109', 118', 144', 146', 148', 154', 161', 163', 168', 181', 186', 194', 200'
IGI 2: 1, 2, 4, 7, 16, 17, 18, 20, 21, 24, 28, 50', 51', 53', 54', 55', 56', 58', 59', 61'–66', 68', 69', 70'–78', 80'–82', 85', 86', 88', 93', 94', 97'–99', 101'–104', 111', 113', 116'–120', 123', 125', 139'–142', 144', 145', 148'$^{?}$, 150', 152'–155', 157'–159', 162', 163', 165', 167', 168', 174', 180', 181', 184', 185', 192'–195', 198', 205', 215', 221'
IGI 3: 1, 6, 28', 29', 31', 35', 36', 38', 39', 40', 44', 48', 50', 53', 56', 67', 69', 71', 72', 75', 76', 88', 100', 103'
NF 5', 11', 15', 16', 19', 20', 22', 27', 28', 33', 35', 44', 46'; NK 4', 7', 12'; NQ 8'; NR 3'–5', 7', 8'; NS 4', 7'; NT 3', 4', 6; NU 2'–4', 10', 13', 15'; NV 2', 4'; NW 5', 6'; NZb 11'; NZ 2', 10', 11', 18', 20'
'through, with': IGI 1: 7', 38', 84', 86'–88', 160', 173'; IGI 2: 2, 7, 73', 105', 115', 117', 132', 166', 201', 203'; 'over (charcoal)': IGI 1: 33'; IGI 2: 74', IGI 3: 64', 100', 103'; NK 5', NU 8'; NY 4'; 'from': IGI 1: 67', 174', 180', 188', 189'; IGI 2: 17; NU 9'; NW 4';

'under': IGI 1: 81'; IGI 2: 28, 59', 103'; IGI 3: 34'; NF 19', 22'; NU 7'; 'among': IGI 2: 219'; 'during, when': IGI 3: 28'; NZa 10'
→ *ina arkīti, ina beri/u-, ina libbi, ina pāni*

īnā/ī (IGI.MIN) '(both) human eyes': IGI 1: 4', 7', 10'–15', 17', 18', 20', 21', 22'–23', 25', 26', 28', 29', 32'–46', 48'–50', 56', 57', 59', 61', 63', 64', 68', 71', 72', 77', 78', 79', 80', 84'–88', 90', 91', 99', 105', 109', 111', 112', 123', 136'–138', 165'–167', 172', 184', 187', 193', 199', 200', 201'
IGI 2: 1–4, 7, 9–12, 16–19, 22, 24, 25, 27, 52', 53'–58', 60', 61', 63', 66', 69', 76', 78', 89', 91', 97'–99', 101', 105' (raven's eyes), 108', 115'–117', 119', 121', 123'–127', 132', 136', 137', 139', 142', 145', 148', 158', 159', 166', 169', 175', 181', 185', 190', 191' 194', 196', 199', 204', 207', 208', 213', 215', 216'
IGI 3: 1, 2, 6, 8, 9, 26', 30'–32', 35', 37', 39', 43', 49'–51', 53', 54', 57', 61', 67', 68', 70', 75', 78', 81', 83', 98', 103'
NF 7', 12', 16'; NK 6'–9', 15'; NP 7'; NQ 5', 7', 8', 10'; NR 2', 3', 5', 6', 10'; NS 1', 4', 6', 8'; NT 4'; NU 5', 6'; NV 1'; NZb 6'; NZ 4', 8'; NZa 8';
'vision': IGI 2: 17
→ *digil īnī, lamassat īnī, libbi īnīšu, rēš īnī*

ina arkīti (*ina* EGIR-*tì*) 'afterwards': IGI 2: 4'

ina beri/u- (syllabic) 'in between': IGI 1: 93', 101', 120', 126',

ina libbi (*ina* ŠÀ) 'from the middle of': IGI 1: 79', 94'; 'into': IGI 2: 147'; NU 5', 9'

ina muhhi (*ina, i-na* UGU) 'over': IGI 3: 6; NF 12'

ina pāni (*ina* IGI) 'in front of': IGI 3: 9, NS 4'

inbu (GURUN) 'fruit' → ***inib errî***

inib errî (GURUN [ú]ÚKUŠ.LAGAB) 'fruit of *errû*-colocynth': IGI 1: 22', IGI 2: 162'

īnu (syllabic and IGI) f. 'eye': IGI 1: 96', 108', 116', 118', 124', 126' (eyes), 131', 135' (136'–138'), 145', 149', 153', 156', 158', 159', 161', 162', 163', 173', 174'–176', 179', 181', 198'; IGI 2: 54', 209'; IGI 3: 79', 80', 86'; NV 6'; 'insight': IGI 2: 218' → *īn imittīšu/šumēlīšu*

irri abāri (*ir-ri* A.GAR$_5$) 'lead salve': IGI 2: 4, 97'

isqūqu (ZÌ.KUM) 'coarse flour': IGI 1: 57'; NZ 22'

iṣṣūr hurri (MUŠEN.HABRUD) 'partridge': IGI 3: 42'

išātu (IZI) 'fire': NF 15'; NT 6'

iškūru (GAB.LÀL) 'wax': IGI 1: 33'; IGI 2: 53', 58'; IGI 3: 42', 97', 103'

iškūru peṣû (GAB.LÀL BABBAR) 'white wax': IGI 3: 100'

ištēn (1) 'one, first': IGI 1: 41', 201'; IGI 2: 54', 140', 141'; IGI 3: 49'; NS 6'; NT 8'–11'

ištēniš (1-*niš* and UR.BI) 'together': IGI 1: 78', 83', 154'; IGI 2: 23, 53', 87', 113', 123', 215'; IGI 3: 1, 5, 12, 48', 72', 83', 95'; NF 11'; NK 12'; NR 7'; NU 9'; NZ 18', 24'

ištēššeret (11) 'eleven': IGI 2: 123'; IGI 3: 34', 43'

ištiššu (1-*šú*) 'once' → *ištiššu šinīšu šalāšīšu*

ištiššu šinīšu šalāšīšu (1-*šú* 2-*šú* 3-*šú*) 'once, twice, three times': IGI 1: 15'; IGI 2: 3, 143'

ištu (syllabic) 'from': IGI 1: 164'; IGI 2: 220'

išû (TUK) 'to have': *išû*(TUK-*ú*): IGI 2: 62'

itqu ([síg]ÀKA) 'woollen tuft'; NU 10', 15'

itqūr abāri (DÍLIM A.BÁR) 'lead spoon(salve)': IGI 1: 20', 25'; IGI 2: 93', 119', 167'; IGI 3: 30', 54', 93', 105'
itqurtu (syllabic) 'a spoon': IGI 3: 109'
itti (syllabic, and KI) 'with': IGI 1: 178'; IGI 2: 52', 91'; IGI 3: 72'; NT 1'
ittu (syllabic) 'an ominous sign': IGI 1: 67'
ittû (syllabic) 'seeder-plough': IGI 1: 195'
iṭṭû (ESIR) 'liquid bitumen': IGI 3: 94'
itūlu (NÁ-*al*) 'to lie down' → *nâlu*
Š-stem: 'to pickle, cure': *tuštāl*(NÁ-*al*): IGI 2: 71'; NR 3'
izuzzu (syllabic and GUB) 'to stand, be present'
G-stem: *i-ši-za-nim-ma*: IGI 1: 198'; *izzazzu/ū* (GUB-*zu*): NP 1'; *izzizzu* (GUB-*zu*): NF 15'; NT 6'; *izziz*(GUB-*iz*): NR 3', 5', 10'
Š-stem: *tuš-za-as-su*: IGI 3: 78'

K

ka 'you, your': IGI 2: 73', 80'; NZb 9', 10' → *ki*
kabābu (syllabic) 'to burn'
D-stem: *tu-kab-ba-ab*: NF 15'; NT 6'
kabātu (DUGUD) 'to become heavy'
G-stem: *ikabbitūšu*(DUGUD-*šú*) IGI 1: 80'; *kabit*(DUGUD): IGI 2: 124', 126', 137'; *ikabbitā*(DUGUD): IGI 3: 68'
kabūt alpi (ŠURUN GU_4) 'ox dung': IGI 3: 72' → ***kabūt Šeriš***
kabūt Šeriš (ŠURUN $^{d}GU_4$) 'ox dung': NU 10' → ***kabūt alpi***
kabūt immeri (ŠURUN UDU) 'sheep dung': IGI 1: 37'
kabūtu (ŠURUN) 'dung' → ***kabūt alpi/immeri/Šeriš***
kadādu (syllabic) 'to rub in'
G-stem: *ta-kad-da-ad*: IGI 2: 2
kakkabu (UL and MUL) 'a star': IGI 1: 81', 189'; IGI 3: 34'; NF 19', 22'; NU 7'
kakkû (GÚ.TUR) 'lentil' → ***qēm kakkî***
kala → *kalû*
kala ūme 'every day': IGI 2: 2, 5; IGI 3: 60'
kalbānu (^{giš}MAŠ.HUŠ) '*kalbānu*-plant (lit. dog-like plant)': IGI 2: 5
kalbu (UR.GI_7) 'dog' → ***lišān kalbi***
kalgukku (^{im}KAL.GUG) '*kalgukku*-red paste': IGI 2: 84'; NF 19'; NU 2'
kalītu (ÉLLAG) 'kidney' IGI 2: 17$^{?}$ → ***kalīt lalî lakî ša šamma lā našku uṭṭata lā ṣabitu; lipi kalīti alpi; lipi kalīt alpi ṣalmi; lipi kalīti immeri; lipi kalīti sāmu***
kalīt lalî lakî ša šamma lā našku uṭṭata lā ṣabitu (ÉLLAG MÁŠ.TUR *la-ki-i ša* Ú *la na-aš-ku* ŠE.BAR *la ṣa-bi-tú*) 'kidney of young suckling goat which has not (yet) bitten a plant nor grasped a grain kernel': IGI 2: 111'
kalli gulgul amēli (*kal-li gul-gul* LÚ.U_{19}.LU) 'cranium of a human skull': NK 4'

kalû (^{im}KAL) '*kalû*-paste': NF 19', 22'
kalû (syllabic) 'to hold (back)'
G-stem: *ak-lá*: IGI 1: 67'
kalû (syllabic and DÙ.A.BI) 'everything, the whole of': IGI 3: 73', 74' → *kala ūme*
kamkadu (syllabic) '*kamkadu*-plant': IGI 2: 108'
kammu (syllabic) '*kammu*-tanning-fungus: IGI 2: 17; IGI 3: 6, 100', 105'; NF 12'; NR 7' → ***kammu ša aškāpi***
kammu ša aškāpi (*kam-mu šá* AŠGAB) '*kammu*-tanning-fungus of a leather worker': IGI 1: 33'; IGI 3: 102'
kamūnu (^{ú}GAMUN) 'cumin' NK 2'
kanaktu (^{šim}GIG) '*kanaktu*-aromatic': IGI 2: 23 → ***lipi kanakti***
kanānu → *qanānu*
kannu (^{dug}GAN) '*kannu*-jar': IGI 1: 122'
kannu (syllabic) 'seedling': IGI 1: 196'
kânu (GIN and syllabic) 'to establish, deposit, to set up'
D-stem: *ú-kin*: IGI 2: 222'; *tukān* (GIN-*an*): IGI 3: 76'; NF 17'
kapātu (syllabic) 'to roll together (into a pill)'
D-stem: *tu-kap-pat*: IGI 1: 27'
kappu (syllabic and PA) 'eyelid': IGI 2: 97', 98', 108'
karān šēlebi (^{ú}GEŠTIN.KA$_5$.A) 'fox-vine': IGI 2: 63', 73', 86', 100', 112', 120'
karānu (GEŠTIN.NA) 'wine': IGI 1: 57'
karpat ṭābāti (DUG A.GEŠTIN.NA) 'vinegar vessel': IGI 1: 92'
karpatu (DUG) 'a vessel': IGI 1: 103', 122'
kâru (syllabic) 'to rub'
G-stem: *ta-kar-ma*: IGI 1: 85'
kaspu (KÙ.BABBAR) 'silver': NF 20'
kasû (syllabic and GAZI^{sar}) '*kasû*-plant': IGI 1: 10', 32', 37', 170'; IGI 2: 9, 11, 66', 69', 119'; IGI 3: 41', 94', 97', 99', 102', 107'; NK 16'; NR 11' → ***mê/qēm kasî***
kaṣāru (syllabic and KEŠDA) 'to tie, knot'
G-stem: *takaṣṣar(u)*(KEŠDA): IGI 1: 69', 97', 109', 117', 144', 154', 186'; *kàṣ-rat*: IGI 1: 127'
D-stem: *tu-ka-ṣar*: IGI 1: 161'
kâṣu (syllabic) 'to skin, grate' → *kīṣu*
G-stem: *ta-ka-aṣ*: IGI 2: 65'
kaṣû (SED) 'cold': IGI 2: 114'
kaṣû (syllabic) 'to be cold'
D-stem: *tu-kàṣ-ṣa*: IGI 1: 24'; IGI 2: 94', 118'; *li-ke-eṣ-ṣa-a*: IGI 1: 105'
kašādu (syllabic) 'to reach'
G-stem: *ik-šu-du-ki-na-ši*: IGI 1: 190'
kašāru (syllabic) 'to fix'
G-stem: *kuš-ri-in*(*-ni*): IGI 1: 74'
kašû (syllabic) 'to increase, benefit'

G-stem: *ik-ši*: IGI 2: 97'
katāmu (syllabic and DUL) 'to cover objects, close the eye'
G-stem: *katmā*(DUL-(*ma*)): IGI 1: 21', 37', 85'; IGI 2: 76'; *takattamma*(DUL-*ma*): IGI 2: 64'; *kát-ma*: IGI 2: 159'
kayyamānamma (syllabic) 'regularly, again and again': IGI 3: 6; NF 12' → *kayyamān*, *kayyānam*
kayyamānu (SAG.UŠ) 'regularly, again and again': IGI 2: 75', 78' → *kayyamānamma*, *kayyānam*
kayyānam (syllabic) 'regularly, again and again': IGI 2: 82' → *kayyamānamma*, *kayyamānu*
ka'inimma (KA.INIM.MA) 'invocation': IGI 1: 68', 71', 77', 96', 108', 116', 124', 131', 135', 149', 153', 156', 158', 162', 175', 179', 184', 193', 199'; IGI 3: 26'; NZb 2'
ki 'your' (f.): IGI 1: 95', 107', 160' → *ka*
kīam (syllabic) 'so, thus': IGI 3: 82'; NF 13'
kibrītu ($PIŠ_{10}$-^{d}ÍD) '*kibrītu*-sulphur': IGI 3: 94', 105', 106'; NU 14'
kibšu (syllabic) 'fungus': IGI 2: 62'
kibtu (GIG) 'wheat' → ***qēm kibti***
kidkidbi (KÌD.KÌD.BI) 'its ritual': IGI 1: 78'
kikkirânu (^{šim}ŠE.LI) '*kikkirânu*-aromatic': IGI 1: 21'
kilaltān (syllabic) 'both': IGI 1: 39'
kīma (syllabic and GIN_{7}) 'like, as': IGI 1: 91', 92', 189', 190'; IGI 2: 12, 14, 67', 99'; IGI 3: 6, 8, 9, 10, 37', 93'; NF 12', 28'
kināši (syllabic) 'to you': IGI 1: 113'–115', 190'
kirbānu (syllabic) 'lump, clod': IGI 1: 188'
kīru (syllabic) 'oven': IGI 1: 65'
kišādu (GÚ) 'neck': IGI 3: 35', 76'; NU 4', 10', 16'
kiṣirtu (syllabic) 'thickening, brow': IGI 1: 127'
kiṣru (syllabic and KA.KEŠDA) 'knot': IGI 1: 69', 97', 109', 117', 144', 154', 186'; 'a bud': IGI 1: 196'
kiṣṣatu (syllabic) 'skin condition': NV 1' → *kīṣu*
kīṣu (syllabic) 'grated': (*sahlê kiṣâti*) IGI 2: 98'; 'flayed, skinned, description of the irritated area around the eyes': (*īnī kiṣâti*) IGI 2: 98' → *kâṣu*, *kiṣṣatu*
kiššatu (ŠÚ) 'world': IGI 2: 217'
kukru ($^{šim/giš}$GÚR.GÚR) '*kukru*-aromatic': IGI 1: 62'; IGI 2: 11, 16; IGI 3: 11, 41', 93', 97', 100', 104', 110'; NK 16'; NQ 12'; NS 2'; NU 3'; NZ 14', 16' → ***qēm kukri***
kullu (syllabic and DAB) 'to hold, contain, keep, retain'
D-stem: *ú-kal*: IGI 1: 85'; IGI 3: 60'; *ú-kal-ma*: IGI 2: 5; *ú-kal-la*: IGI 2: 12, 58'; NZ 4'; NZa 8'
kunšu (syllabic) 'wool braid': IGI 1: 8'
kunu (syllabic) 'your' (2 m. pl. gen. suff.): IGI 2: 13, 15
kupru (syllabic) '*kupru*-dry bitumen': IGI 3: 106'
kurāru (GIG.GIR) '*kurāru*-pustle': IGI 2: 108'

kurkānû (syllabic and ^{ú}KUR$_4$.GI.RIN.NA) '*kurkānû*-plant': IGI 2: 113'; NZb 5'
kurkû (KUR.GI^{mušen}) 'goose': → ***šaman kurkî***
kursinnu (syllabic) 'ankle, knuckle' → ***lipi kursinni ṣabīti***
kurṣipti eqli (*kur-ṣip-ti* A.ŠÀ) 'field butterfly': IGI 2: 159'
kurṣiptu (syllabic) 'butterfly' → ***dām kurṣipti alpi ṣalmi, kurṣipti eqli***
kurû (LÚGUD.DA) 'short': → ***lipî eṣemti kurīti, lipî eṣemti kurīti immeri, lipi eṣemti kurīti ša immeri, muhhu ša eṣemti kurīti immeri***
kussû (^{giš}GU.ZA) 'throne, seat': IGI 1: 93'
kūṣu (EN.TE.NA) 'winter': IGI 1: 63'; NK 14'; NR 7'
kutpû ($^{\text{(na4)}}$AN.ZAH.GE$_6$) 'black frit (bead)': IGI 2: 70', 85'; IGI 3: 3, 33', 38', 104', 106'; NF 9'; NT 8'

L

lā (syllabic and NU) 'no, not, without': IGI 1: 23', 36', 70', 94', 104', 128', 129', 145', 191', 200'; IGI 2: 1, 6, 14$^{?}$, 65', 99', 111', 117', 219'; IGI 3: 49', 66', 68', 70', 73', 74'; NF 17', 20', 23'; NS 6'; NW 4'; NZ 3'; NZa 10' → *lām, lā(m) patān*
labāku (syllabic) 'to be(come) soft'
  D-stem: *tu-la-bak* 'you soften up': IGI 2: 81',
labânu (syllabic) 'neck tendons': IGI 3: 75'
labāru (SUMUN) 'to be(come) old, long-lasting'
  G-stem: *ilabbirma*(SUMUN-*ma*): IGI 2: 54'
labātu → *lapātu*
labīru (LIBIR.RA) 'old': → ***erû labīru, haṣbu labīru ša kibša išû, šaman iṣṣūr hurri$^{?}$ labīri***
labtu (ŠE.SA.A) 'roasted grain': IGI 2: 6, 52'; IGI 3: 92' → ***qēm labti, sīkti labti***
lahābu (syllabic) 'grows'
  G-stem: *i-li-hi-ib*: NF 33'
lahru (U$_8$) 'ewe': → ***larsīni ša halli lahri ša šumēli ša māšī ūlidu***
lakû (syllabic) 'suckling': IGI 2: 111' → ***kalīt lalî lakî ša šamma lā našku uṭṭata lā ṣabitu***
lalû (MÁŠ.TUR) 'a kid, young goat': IGI 2: 111' → ***kalīt lalî lakî ša šamma lā našku uṭṭata lā ṣabitu***
lā(m) patān (syllabic) 'before eating/meal': IGI 1: 27', 43'; IGI 2: 145'
lām (syllabic) 'before': IGI 1: 115', 190', 194'; IGI 3: 29' → *lā, lā(m) patān*
lamassat īnī (^{d}LAMA(.MEŠ) IGI.MIN) 'pupil of the eye': IGI 1: 80'; IGI 2: 121', 124', 207'
lamû (NIGIN) 'wrap up'
  G-stem: *talammi*(NIGIN-(*mi*)): IGI 1: 39'; NU 10'
lapāpu (syllabic) 'to wrap, make a wad
  G-stem: *tál-pap*: IGI 1: 180'; NU 15'; NZb 5'; *ta-la-pap*: NU 15'
lapātu (syllabic) 'to touch'

D-stem: *ina la-ba-ti-šá*: IGI 1: 173’

larsīni ša halli lahri ša šumēli ša māšī ūlidu (*la-ar-sì-ni ša hal-li* U_8 *ša* GÙB *ša* MAŠ.TAB.BA Ù.TU) ‘a hoof of the left hind leg of an ewe which bore twin(s)’: IGI 2: 110’

larsīnu (syllabic) ‘a hoof’ → ***larsīni ša halli lahri ša šumēli ša māšī ūlidu***

lâšu (syllabic and $SILA_{11}$(*-aš*)) ‘to knead’

G-stem: *talâš*($SILA_{11}$*-aš*) IGI 1: 10’, 15’, 19’, 27’, 29’, 37’, 84’; IGI 3: 56’, 72’; NR 8’; NZ 5’–7’, 10’; *ta-la/là-aš*: IGI 2: 114’, 145’, 181’

latāku (syllabic) ‘to test (a remedy)’

G-stem: *la-te-ek*: IGI 3: 96’

lazāzu (syllabic) ‘to endure, persist’

G-stem: *la-zi-iz*: NF 33’

lemnu (HUL) ‘evil’: NU 12’

lemuttu (HUL-tì) ‘evil’ → *mukīl rēš lemutti*

leqû (syllabic and TI(*-i/qé*), ŠU.TI) ‘to take, accept, + ventive to bring’

G-stem: *teleqqe*(TI(*-qé*)): IGI 1: 83’, 185’; IGI 2: 101’; IGI 3: 87’; NF 15’; NT 6’; NU 13’; NW 5’; NZ 1’; *liqī*(TI-(*i*)): IGI 1: 95’, 107’; *i-le-qu-ni-ku*: IGI 1: 160’; *le-qé-ma*: IGI 1: 170’; *il-qa-a*: IGI 2: 106’; *leqâ*(TI.MEŠ): NK 6’

lēru (SAHAR.KÙ.GI) ‘*lēru*-paste’: IGI 1: 40’

lētu (syllabic) ‘cheek, side’ → *ana lēt*

libbi elleti gišimmari (ŠÀ KÙ-*ti* ^{giš}GIŠIMMAR) ‘clean date-palm offshoot’: IGI 1: 160

libbi īnīšu (ŠÀ IGI.MIN-*šú*) ‘inner part of patient’s eyes’: IGI 1: (26’), 36’, (42’, 50’, 56’, 72’, 84’, 86’–88’); IGI 2: (2, 76’, 78’, 89’, 115’, 145’, 158’), 159’, (169’), 190’, (194’); NU 5’

libbu (ŠÀ) ‘middle, midst of’; ‘internal organ/heart’; → *a*/*ina libbi*, ***dāmu ša libbi šahî***, *libbi īnīšu*, *ša libbi*

libbu (ŠÀ) ‘offshoot (of date palm)’ → ***gišimmaru***, ***libbi elleti gišimmari***

lipāru (^{giš}MI.PÀR, $^{giš}MI.PAR_4$) ‘*lipāru*-tree’ → ***arti lipāri***

lipi alpi (Ì.UDU GU_4) ‘ox fat’: IGI 3: 105’, 108’

lipi eṣemti (Ì.UDU GÌR.PAD.DU) ‘bone marrow’: IGI 1: 108’

lipi eṣemti arikti (Ì.UDU GÌR.PAD.DU GÍD.DA) ‘marrow of a long bone’: IGI 2: 53’

lipi eṣemti immeri (Ì.UDU GÌR.PAD.DU UDU) ‘marrow of a sheep’s bone’: IGI 2: 70’

lipi eṣemti kurīti (Ì.UDU GÌR.PAD.DU LÚGUD.DA) ‘marrow of a short bone’: IGI 1: 43’

lipi eṣemti kurīti immeri (Ì.UDU GÌR.PAD.DU LÚGUD.DA UDU) ‘marrow of a sheep’s short bone’: IGI 2: 50

lipi eṣemti kurīti ša immeri (Ì.UDU GÌR.PAD.DA LÚGUD.DA *ša* UDU) ‘marrow of a short bone of a sheep’: IGI 1: 6’

lipi eṣemti ṣabīti (Ì.UDU GÌR.PAD.DU MAŠ.DÀ) ‘gazelle bone marrow’: NU 9’

lipi kalīti alpi (Ì.UDU ÉLLAG GU_4) ‘ox kidney fat’: IGI 1: 95’; NK 4’

lipi kalīt alpi ṣalmi (Ì.UDU ÉLLAG GU_4 GU_6) ‘kidney fat of a black ox’: IGI 3: 6; NF 11’

lipi kalīti immeri (Ì.UDU ÉLLAG UDU.NÍTA) ‘sheep’s kidney fat’: IGI 1: 33’; IGI 2: 53’

lipi kalīti sāmu (Ì.UDU ÉLLAG SA_5) ‘reddish kidney fat’: IGI 1: 20’

lipi kanakti (Ì.UDU ^{šim}GIG) '*kanaktu*-aromatic fat': IGI 1: 32', 62'; IGI 2: 25, 66'; IGI 3: 97'
lipi kursinni ṣabīti (Ì.UDU *kur-sin-ni* MAŠ.DÀ) 'fat from a gazelle's knuckle': IGI 2: 3
lipi nēši (Ì.UDU UR.MAH) 'fat from a lion': IGI 3: 52'
lipi qanî (Ì.UDU GI.MES) 'pith of reeds': IGI 3: 41'
lipi sāqi ṣabīti (Ì.UDU *sa-a-qí* MAŠ.DÀ) 'fat of a gazelle's thigh': IGI 2: 147'
lipi ṣallamti (Ì.UDU MUŠ.GE$_6$) 'fat from a black snake': IGI 3: 51', 69'
lipištu (syllabic) 'fleshy substance': IGI 2: 16
lippu (syllabic) 'wad, tuft: IGI 1: 180'; NU 15'
lipû (Ì.UDU) 'fat': IGI 1: 11', 82'; IGI 2: 17$^?$, 22, 96', 158', 194'; IGI 3: 103'; 'bone marrow; pith of plants, aromatic fat' → ***lipi*** ...
lipû sāmu (Ì.UDU SA$_5$) 'red fat': NR 3'
liqtu (syllabic) '(textual) material': IGI 2: 220'
lišān kalbi (^{ú}EME.UR.GI$_7$) 'dog's-tongue plant': IGI 1: 57' → ***mê/zēr lišān kalbi***
līšu (NÍG.SILA$_{11}$.GÁ) 'dough': IGI 1: 24'; IGI 2: 118'; IGI 3: 93'
lu (syllabic) 'or': IGI 2: 24
lū ... *lū* (syllabic) 'either ... or': IGI 3: 9, 10; NF 27'; NU 11', 12'
lubku → ***napšalti lubki***
lulû (KÙ.GAN) '*lulû*-antimony': IGI 1: 6'; IGI 2: 70'; IGI 3: 33'
lumnu (HUL) 'evil': NF 17', 20', 23'

M

ma'da → *mādu*
ma (enclitic particle) 'and (then, thus)': IGI 1: 13', 23', 26'$^?$, 36', 38', 39', 79', 84', 85', 95', 105', 107', 118', 123', 151', 154', 163', 169', 181', 186', 192', 198'; IGI 2: 5, 6, 7, 12, 14, 28', 54', 59', 64', 79', 97', 99', 103', 117', 121', 123'–126', 131', 136', 137', 221'; IGI 3: 6, 9, 35', 36', 43', 45', 54', 57', 61', 65', 67', 68', 70', 72', 82', 85', 87', 88', 90', 95'; NF 12', 14', 16', 20', 21', 23', 27', 33', 35'; NK 6', 9'; NR 3', 5', 8', 10'; NS 5'; NT 3'; NU 5', 6', 8', 12'; NV 3', 6'; NZb 1', 7'; NY 4'; NY 7a'; NZ 10'; NZa 8', 9'
enclitic particle marking nominal sentence: IGI 1: 14', 21', 25', 26'$^?$, 30'$^?$, 101', 126', 128', 129'$^?$; IGI 2: 22; affirmative: IGI 1: 170–172', 178'; IGI 2: 13, 15, 199', 200', 202'; → *ašar šanîmma*
madāru (syllabic) 'to be rotten'
G-stem: *ma-di-ra*: IGI 2: 196'
mādu, *ma'da* (syllabic) 'many, very much': IGI 1: 23'; IGI 2: 65', 99', 117' → *mēṣa mādu*
magal (syllabic) 'very much, greatly': NF 33'
magāru(ŠE.GA) 'to be favourable'
G-stem: *magir*(ŠE.GA): IGI 1: 183',
mahāru (syllabic) 'to face, oppose, accept'
G-stem: *mu-uh/úh-ra*: IGI 3: 79', 80', 85'; *lim-hu-ra*: IGI 3: 85'
Š-stem: *tu-šam-har*: IGI 3: 31'

mahru (IGI) 'in front': NF 29' → *ālik mahri*
makūt gabīdi (syllabic) 'pole' of a liver': IGI 3: 81, 89
makūt gabīdi ša imēri (*ma-ku-ut ga-bi-di ša* ANŠE) ''pole' of a donkey liver' IGI 3: 75'
makūtu (syllabic) 'pole': → ***makūt gabīdi* (*ša imēri*)**
mala (syllabic) 'as much as': IGI 2: 221'
malāku (syllabic) 'to advise':
  G-stem: *a-ma-lik*: IGI 1: 67'
malmališ (syllabic) 'equally, in equal amounts': IGI 1: 11', 46', 83'; IGI 2: 18, 29, 51', 78', 92', 154', 155'; IGI 3: 53'
malû (syllabic and DIRI(.MEŠ)) 'to be(come) full of'
  G-stem: *malâ*(DIRI-(*a*/*ma*)/ DIRI.MEŠ): IGI 1: 23', (*malâma*) 36', 45', 68', 71', 77', 79', 99', 200'; IGI 2: 1, 9, 19, (*malâma*) 22, 25, 27, 115'–117', (*malâma*) 121', 139', 207', 213'; IGI 3: 18'$^{?}$; NZa 8'; *lim-la-ni-im-ma*: IGI 1: 105'; *mali*(DIRI): IGI 2: 209'
mamma (syllabic) 'somebody', with negation 'nobody': IGI 2: 219'
manna (syllabic) 'whom': IGI 1: 102', 121'
mannu (syllabic) 'who': IGI 1: 159'
manû (ŠID(-*nu*)) 'to recite'
  G-stem: *tamannu*(ŠID(-*nu*): IGI 1: 69', 97', 109', 117', 144', 154', 186'; IGI 3: 88'; NU 16'
maqātu (syllabic) 'to fall, drop'
  Gtn-stem: *mi-ta-qu-ta-ni*: IGI 1: 190'
marāqu (syllabic) 'to grind'
  G-stem: *ta-mar-raq*: IGI 1: 62'; NR 7'
marāṣu (GIG) 'to be sick'
  G-stem: *marṣā*(*ma*) (GIG.(GA)-(*ma*)): IGI 1: 10', 12', 14', 21', 23', 26', 32', 34', 35', 57', 59', 79', 201'; IGI 2: 117', 121', 124', 126', 137'$^{?}$, 204', 216'; IGI 3: 78'; NQ 7', 8';
  marṣat(GIG-*at*): IGI 1: 159'
marat immeri (ZÍ UDU.NÍTA) 'bile of a sheep': IGI 1: 62'; 'gall-bladder of a sheep': NR 3'
marat raqqi (ZÍ BAL.GI^{ku6}) 'gall bladder of *raqqu*-turtle: IGI 2: 71'
marṣiš (syllabic) 'bitterly': IGI 1: 168'
marṣu (^{lú}TU.RA) 'sick man': IGI 3: 79', 80'
marṣu, (f.) *maruštu* (GIG.GA(.A)) 'sick': IGI 1: 96', 108', 109', 116', 118', 124', 131', 135', 149', 153', 156', 158', 162', 165', 175', 179', 181'; IGI 2: 185'
mārtu (DUMU.MUNUS) 'daughter': IGI 1: 102', 120', 121'
martu (ZÍ and ^{uzu}ZÍ) 'gall bladder, bile': IGI 1: 28'; IGI 2: 72'$^{?}$ → ***marat immeri*/*raqqi***
mašāšu (syllabic) 'to wipe off'
  G-stem: *ta-maš-aš*$^{?}$: IGI 2: 18
mašku (KUŠ) 'leather bag': IGI 3: 35'$^{?}$
māš*(*t*)*u (^{ú}MAŠ.TAB(.BA)) '*māš*(*t*)*u*-twin plant': IGI 1: 32'; IGI 3: 97', 99', 102'
māšu (MAŠ.TAB.BA) 'a twin': → ***larsīni ša halli lahri ša šumēli ša māšī ūlidu***
mašmašu (MAŠ.MAŠ) '*mašmašu*-healer': IGI 3: 78'–80'

mašqītu (syllabic) 'potion'; NF 32'
maštakal ($^{\text{(ú)}}$IN.NU.UŠ/ ^{ú}IN$_6$.ÚŠ) '*maštakal*-plant': IGI 1: 18', 46', 57'; IGI 3: 51'; NF 17', 21'; NU 14' → ***mê/zēr maštakal***
maqātu (syllabic) 'to fall, drop down'
Gtn-stem: *mi-ta-qu-ta-ni*: IGI 1: 190'
mātu (syllabic and KUR) 'land, earth': IGI 1: 194'; IGI 2: 217'
maṭû (syllabic) 'to diminish (of eye sight)'
G-stem: *ma-a-ṭi*: IGI 3: 51'
D-stem: *mu-uṭ-ṭu*: NQ 11'; NS 1'
mayyālu (KI.NÁ) 'bed': IGI 3: 70'
mazā'u (syllabic) 'to press, squeeze'
G-stem: *ta-ma-za-a'*: IGI 2: 145'
mê bāqili (A SAR.MUNU$_6$) 'maltster-water': NF 34'
mê bīni (A ^{giš}ŠINIG) 'tamarisk sap': NU 6', 8'
mê būrti (A PÚ) 'well water': NF 21'
mê kasî (A GAZI^{sar}) 'sap of a *kasû*-plant': IGI 1: 10', 27', 29', 52', 63'; IGI 2: 113'; IGI 3: 31', 72'; NK 12'; NW 2'
mê karān šēlebi (A ^{ú}GEŠTIN.KA$_5$.A) 'fox-grape sap': IGI 2: 100'
mê lišān kalbi (A ^{ú}EME.UR.GI$_7$) 'sap of dog's tongue-plant': IGI 2: 100'
mê maštakal (A ^{ú}IN$_6$.ÚŠ) 'sap of *maštakal*-plant': IGI 2: 100'
mê nurmî (A ^{giš}NU.ÚR.MA) 'sap of pomegranate': IGI 3: 47'; NY 7'
mê uhūli qarnānî (A NAGA.SI) 'sap of horned *uhūlu*-alkali': IGI 2: 91
mer'u → *merhu*
merhu, *mer'u* (syllabic) '*merhu*-kernel': IGI 1: 197'–199'
mêsallim → ***emesallu***
mesû (LUH(-*si*)) 'to wash'
G-stem: *temessi*(LUH-(*si*)): IGI 1: 15', 22', 52'; IGI 2: 80', 91', 119', 153', 154'; IGI 3: 53'; NR 8'; NU 6'; *imsû*(LUH-*u*): IGI 1: 104'
mēṣa mādu (syllabic) 'completely (lit. little and much)': IGI 1: 67'
mešēltu ($^{\text{na4}}$BAR.DÙ.E) '*mešēltu*-whetstone': IGI 2: 159'
mimma (syllabic) 'anything': IGI 1: 193'
minâ (syllabic) 'what': IGI 1: 152'
minâtu → *minītu*
minītu, (pl.) *minâtu* (syllabic) 'limbs, physique': IGI 3: 68', 91'; NT 2'
mirqu (syllabic) '*mirqu*-powder$^{?}$': IGI 3: 41'
mišlu (1/2) 'half': IGI 1: 8', 41', 64'; IGI 3: 50'; NS 7'
mû (A(.MEŠ)) 'water': IGI 1: 15', 22', 31', 63', 92', 103'; IGI 2: 2, 24, 80', 119', 153', 154', 180'; IGI 3: 34', 71'; NR 8'; NZb 8' → ***mê bāqili/bīni/būrti/kasî/karān šēlebi/lišān kalbi/maštakal/nurmî/uhūli qarnānî***; *naqû*
muhhu (UGU) 'cranium, brain, top': IGI 2: 77', 220'; 'top, upper part, surface': IGI 2: 108', 121', 124' → *ana/ina muhhi*; ***muhhu ša erî***; ***muhhu ša eṣemti kurīti immeri***, ***muhhu ša rīmti***, ***muhhu ša summati zikari***

muhhu ša erî (UGU *ša* TI_8 mušen) 'brains of an *erû*-eagle': IGI 2: 205'
muhhu ša eṣemti kurīti immeri (UGU *ša* GÌR.PAD.DU LÚGUD.DA UDU) 'marrow of a short sheep-bone': IGI 3: 46'
muhhu ša rīmti (UGU *ša* SÚN-*tì*) 'wild cow's brain': IGI 2: 77'
muhhu ša summati zikari (UGU *ša* TU mušen NITA) 'brain of a male pigeon': IGI 2: 77'
mukīl rēš lemutti (*mu-kíl*-SAG HUL-*tì*) 'supporter-of-evil': NF 26', 32'; NU 11' → sag-hul-ha-za
murdinnu, amurdinnu (syllabic) '*murdinnu*-bramble (as an eye condition)': IGI 1: 200'; IGI 2: 1, 9
murru (šimSES) 'bitter-plant': IGI 1: 86'; IGI 2: 8, 22, 25, 148'?; IGI 3: 102'; NQ 11'; NR 5'; NS 2'; NV 4'
murṣu (syllabic) 'illness': IGI 1: 169'
murtappidu (syllabic) 'wandering, roving': NT 5' → *eṭemmu*
musukkatu (syllabic and munusÚ.ZÚG) 'a woman in maternity' → ***šizbi musukkati***
muṣa''irānu (BIL.ZA.ZA) '*muṣa''irānu*-frog': IGI 1: 28' → *arqu*
mūṣu (syllabic) '*mūṣu*-stone': IGI 3: 4, 32', 37', 42', 104'; NF 9'; NU 8'
mušālu (syllabic and ŠU.LÚ.ZABAR?) 'bronze palette, mirror': IGI 2: 74', 75', 78', 82'
muššaru (na4MUŠ.GÍR) 'sardonyx': IGI 3: 39'; NF 10'
mūšu (GE_6) 'night': IGI 1: 36'; IGI 3: 28', 73', 74'; NF 28', 31'

N

nabalkutu (BAL-*at*) 'to cross over, change sides'
N-stem: *tabbalakkat*(BAL-*at*) 'you transfer': IGI 2: 86'
nabāsu (sígHÉ.MED/ME.DA) 'red wool': IGI 1: 39'; NZ 12'
nablu (syllabic) 'flame, meteor': IGI 1: 190'
nādu (KUŠ.EDIN) 'waterskin': IGI 1: 12'
nadû (syllabic and ŠUB) 'to put, apply, cover, set, install, recite, cast out (an incantation), to drip tears'
G-stem: *tanaddi*(ŠUB(-*di*)): IGI 1: 20', 72'; IGI 2: 2, 73', 74', 134'; IGI 3: 30', 34', (*tanaddīma*) 35', 54', (*tanaddīma*) 95'; NF (*tanaddīma*) 21'; NU 5'; *nadâ*(ŠUB-*a*): IGI 1: 92'; *it-ta-di*: IGI 1: 93'; *i-di-ma*: IGI 1: 171', 192'; *li-in-na-di*: NF 28'
Gtn-stem: *tattanaddi*(ŠUB.MEŠ): IGI 1: 12'; *tattanaddīšu* (ŠUB.ŠUB-*šú*) IGI 3: 71'; *tattanaddi*(ŠUB.ŠUB-*di*): IGI 2: 78'; NF 29'; *ittanaddâ*(ŠUB.ŠUB-*a*): NK 10'; NQ 5', 10'; NS 1'
naglabu (syllabic and GÍR.ŠU.I) 'barber's knife, scalpel': IGI 1: 190'; IGI 2: 201', 203' → *ṣurru*
nâhu (syllabic) 'to come to rest, appease, be still'
G-stem: *li-ni-ih-ka*: NU 16'
D-stem: *a-na nu-úh-hi*: IGI 2: 193'
nakāpu (syllabic) 'to push away'

D-stem: *ú-na-kap*: IGI 1: 80'

nakāsu (KUD) 'to cut'

G-stem: *tanakkis*(KUD): IGI 1: 38'

nakkaptu (SAG.KI) 'head-temple': IGI 1: 12', 13', 29', 39', 69', 144', 146', 148', 154', 161', 186'; NV 6'; NZa 8', 10' to

naklu (syllabic) 'elaborate': IGI 2: 220'

nâlu (NÁ-*al*) 'to lie down' → *itūlu*

Š-stem: 'to pickle, cure': *tušnâl*(NÁ-*al*): IGI 2: 71'; NR 3'

namāru (ZALAG.GA) 'to be(come) bright, shine'

G-stem: *namrā*(ZALAG.GA): IGI 2: 204'

namru (syllabic) 'bright, clear, shining': IGI 2: 218'; IGI 3: 79', 86'

napāhu (syllabic and BÚN, MÚ(-*ah*)) 'to blow; to light up, ignite'

G-stem: *tanappah*(BÚN): IGI 1: 7', 86'–88'; IGI 2: 115'?; *tanappah*(MÚ-*ah*): IGI 1: 56'; IGI 2: 132', infinitive: *ina napāhi* 'at sunrise': NZb 11': *nap-hat*: NV 6'

D-stem: *nu-up-pu-ha*: IGI 2: 56'; *nuppuhāma*(MÚ.MEŠ-*ma*): NK 6'

napāšu (syllabic) 'to ease off, to breathe'

G-stem: *na-pa-še*: IGI 1: 94'

napharu (PAP) 'total': IGI 2: 9; IGI 3: 34'

napšalti lubki (syllabic) 'softening ointment': IGI 3: 101' → *lubku*

napṭu (Ì.KUR.RA) 'naphtha': NV 3'

napû (SIM) 'to sift'

G-stem: *tanappi* (SIM): IGI 2: 56'; IGI 3: 72'

naqû (BAL-*qî*) 'to pour out (tears, water)'

G-stem: *dimta inaqqi*(BAL-*qî*): NV 6'; *naq me-e*: NZb 8'; *i-naq*?-*qi*?: NZb 8' → *dimtu, mû*

narmaktu (syllabic) 'bath': NF 32'

nāru (syllabic and dÍD) 'river': IGI 1: 113', 188',

nasāhu (syllabic and ZI) 'to tear out, remove'

G-stem: *inassah*(ZI): IGI 2: 5; *nasāhi*(ZI): IGI 2: 124'; *inassaha*(ZI-*ha*): IGI 2: 138'; *i-na-sah*: IGI 2: 176'; *ana nasāhīšu*(*ana* ZI-*šú*): IGI 3: 11; *ina nasāhīšu*(*ina* ZI-*šú*): NZa 10'

N-stem: *innassah*: NY 4'

naṣābu (syllabic) 'to suck'

G-stem: *i-na-ṣab*: IGI 1: 75'

našāku (syllabic) 'to bite'

G-stem: *na-aš-ku*: IGI 2: 111' → ***kalīt lalî lakî ša šamma lā našku uṭṭata lā ṣabitu***

- *nâši* (syllabic, 1 pl. dat. pron.) 'for us': IGI 1: 178'

našû (syllabic and ÍL) 'to carry, lift, + ventive to bring, carry along, pick up'

G-stem: *liš-šá-*(*a*)*-ni*: IGI 1: 103', 122'; *ta-aš-šá-ni*: IGI 1: 187'; *taš-ša-ni*: IGI 1: 189'; *áš-ši*: IGI 1: 192'; *inašši*(ÍL-(*ši*)): IGI 3: 70', (*inaššīma*) 78'

natāku (syllabic) 'to drip

D-stem: *tu-na-tak/ták*: IGI 1: 18', 48'; IGI 2: 76', 89', 148', 158', 169', 175'

naṭālu G (IGI-*al*) 'to see'
G-stem: *inaṭṭal*(IGI-*al*) IGI 1: 61'; *ina-ṭa-la*: IGI 3: 49'; NS 6'; *i-na-aṭ-ṭa-la*: IGI 3: 66'; *na-ṭa-la*: NQ 10'; NS 1'
nawāru → *namāru*
nemsētu (syllabic) 'tub': IGI 2: 111'
nêšu (syllabic) 'to get better'
G-stem: *ina-eš*: IGI 1: 25', 26', 118', 154', 181', 186'; IGI 2: 7; IGI 3: 6, 90'; NF 12', 16'; NY 7a'
nēšu (UR.MAH) 'lion' → ***lipi nēši***
- *ni* (syllabic) 'us': IGI 1: 178'
- *ni* (syllabic) 'me': IGI 1: 74'
nignakku (NÍG.NA) 'incense burner': IGI 3: 77'
nikiptu (syllabic) 'nikiptu-plant': NU 2' → *zikaru, sinništu*
nikiptu zikar u sinniš (*ni-kip-tu*$_4$ NÍTA *u* MUNUS) 'male and female *nikiptu*-plant': IGI 1: 46'; NF 18'
niksu (syllabic) 'cut off': IGI 1: 91'; NW 4'
- *ni*(*m*) → - *a*(*m*)
nīnû ($^{\acute{u}}$KUR.RA) '*nīnû*-mint': IGI 1: 32', 61'; IGI 2: 22, 25; IGI 3: 41', 97', 99', 102'; NK 3'; NQ 12'; NR 6'; NS 3'
niqqu (syllabic) 'fig seed': IGI 1: 114'
niqû (UDU.SISKUR) 'offering': IGI 3: 45'
Nisannu → Month Names
nisqu (syllabic) 'high level': IGI 2: 218'
nuhurtu (NU.LUH(.HA^{sar})) '*nuhurtu*-plant': IGI 3: 55', 99' → ***hīl nuhurti***
nurmû (^{giš}NU.ÚR.MA) 'pomegranate' → ***haṣab/qilip/mê nurmî***
nūru (syllabic) 'lamp(-light)': IGI 2: 90'; IGI 3: 9

P

pa'āṣu (syllabic) 'to crush'
G-stem: *ta-pa-a-aṣ*: IGI 2: 102'
D-stem: *tu-pa-âṣ*: NZa 10'
pa'ṣu (syllabic) 'crushed': IGI 2: 96'
pahāru (syllabic) 'to bring together, gather'
D-stem: *ú-pa-har*: IGI 1: 197'; *ina pu-hu-ri-šú*: IGI 1: 197'; *tu-pa-har*: IGI 3: 82'
palāsu (syllabic) 'to notice'
N-stem: *ip-pa-lis-su-ma*: IGI 1: 151'
pānu (IGI, IGI.MEŠ) 'front, face'; 'top': IGI 2: 64'; NZa 8'; 'in front': NF 19'; *pāna pāni:* IGI 1: 59'; → *ana pān, ikil pāni, ina pāni, pānūšu iṣṣanundū* (→ *ṣâdu*), *ṣulum pāni, šār pāni, šatti pāna*
papparhû (BABBAR.HI^{sar}) '*papparhû*-purslane': IGI 1: 19'

parāku (syllabic) 'to block, lie across, park'
G-stem: *pa-rik*: IGI 1: 101', (*parikma*) 126'
parāsu (KUD) 'to cease, stop'
G-stem: *paris*(KUD-*is*): NW 4'
N-stem: *ipparras* (KUD-*as*): NZ 3'
parzillu (AN.BAR) 'iron'; NT 9'
passu (ZA.NA) 'collyrium stick (lit. game disk)': IGI 1: 63'; IGI 2: 24; IGI 3: 53'
pašāru (syllabic) 'be released, saved':
N-stem: *na-ap-ši-ir*: IGI 1: 66'
pašāšu (ŠÉŠ) 'to smear, anoint'
G-stem: *tapaššaš*(ŠÉŠ(-*aš*)) 'you smear': IGI 2: 79'; IGI 3: 35', 37', 39';
(*tapaššassuma*(ŠÉŠ-*su-ma*)) NF 20', 23'; NU 5'; *tapaššassu*(ŠÉŠ-*su*): NV 3'
patālu, petēlu (syllabic) 'to twist'
G-stem: *te-pe-til*: IGI 1: 160',
patānu (syllabic) 'to eat' → *lā(m) patān*
patāqu 'to build (a mud wall)'
G-stem: *pat-qat*: IGI 1: 93', 120', 127'
patar siparri (GÍR.ZABAR) 'bronze knife': IGI 1: 14', 38'; IGI 2: 72', 79', 195'
paṭāru (DU$_8$) 'to loosen'
G-stem: *tapaṭṭaršuma*(DU$_8$-*šú-ma*) IGI 1: 38'; IGI 2: 7; *pu-ṭur*: IGI 1: 130'; *lā paṭāri*(NU DU$_8$): IGI 1: 191'; *tapaṭṭar*(DU$_8$-(*ár*)): IGI 1: 200'; IGI 2: 1, 6; IGI 3: 30', 54'
pel āribi (NUNUZ UGA^{mušen}) 'raven's egg': IGI 2: 79'
pelû (NUNUZ) 'egg' → *pel āribi*
pēmtu (NE) 'charcoal': IGI 1: 33'; IGI 2: 74'; IGI 3: 64', 100', 103'; NK 5'; NU 8'; NY 4'
peṣû (BABBAR) 'white': → ***dišpu peṣû, iškūru peṣû, šammu peṣû, šīpātu peṣâtu***
petēlu → *patālu*
petû (BAD-(*te*)) 'to open'
G-stem: *ipetti*(BAD): IGI 1: 23'; IGI 2: 117'; *tepette*(BAD-*te*) 84'; *i-pet-tu*: NF 30'
pillû zikaru (^{giš}NAM.TAR NÍTA) 'male *pillû*-plant': IGI 2: 130' → ***arti pillî zikari***
piqannu (A.GAR.GAR) 'droppings' → *piqan ṣabīti*
piqan ṣabīti (A.GAR.GAR MAŠ.DÀ) 'gazelle droppings': IGI 2: 177'; IGI 3: 72'
pitiltu (ŠU.SAR) 'string': IGI 1: 76'
pitiqtu (syllabic) 'a mud wall': IGI 1: 93', 120', 127',
pû (syllabic and KA) 'mouth, opening': IGI 1: 160'; NY 7a'
pursimītu → *pursīt dāmi*
pursindu → *pursīt dāmi*
pursītu (^{dug}BUR.ZI) '*pursītu*-bowl': IGI 1: 3'; IGI 2: 156' → *pursīt dāmi*
pursīt dāmi (*pur-si-it* / *pur-si-in-di* / *pur-si-mi-it* MÚD / *da-a-mi*) 'blood vessel in the eye':
IGI 1: 91', 112', 136', (*pursindi dāmi*) 176', (*pursimīt dāmi*) 187'
pūṣu (BABBAR) 'white spot': IGI 2: 124'
pūtu (SAG.KI) 'forehead': IGI 3: 8'; NF 46'

Q

qablu ($MURUB_4$) 'middle': IGI 1: 180'
qabû (syllabic and DUG_4.GA) 'to say, speak'
G-stem: *taqabbi*(DUG_4.GA): IGI 1: 31'; *qá-bu-ú šá*: IGI 1: 100', 134'; *i-qab-bi*: IGI 3: 79', 80'; NF 14'; *i-qab-bu-u*: IGI 3: 82', 83'; *liq-bi*; NF 13', (NT 4')
qadūtu šikāni (IM.GÚ.EN.NA) 'river silt': IGI 2: 8
qalû (syllabic, BIL-*la*, BIL-*lu*, BÍL,) 'to roast'
G-stem: *ta-qal/qàl-lu*: IGI 1: 33'; IGI 2: 111', 112'; IGI 3: 103'; *taqallu*(BÍL): IGI 2: 198'; *taqallu*(BÍL-*lu*): NK 7'; *taqallu*(BIL-*lu*): NZ 24'
qalû (BÍL) 'roasted': IGI 2: 68'
qanānu, kanānu (syllabic) 'to roll up'
D-stem: *ú-qa-an-na-an*: IGI 1: 75'
qanû (GI) 'reed' → ***gūra ša qanî, lipi qanî, qanû ṭābu***
qanû ṭābu (GI DÙG.GA) 'sweet reed': IGI 2: 113'
qaqqad ṣurāri (SAG.DU EME.ŠID) 'lizard's head': IGI 2: 74'
qaqqadu (SAG.DU, SAG) 'head': IGI 1: 8', 23', 24'; IGI 2: 6, 7, 117', 118'; NV 1'; NZ 19' → ***qaqqad ṣurāri***
qarnu (SI) 'horn' → ***uhūlu qarnānû***
qatāru (syllabic) 'to fumigate'
G-stem: *tu-qat-tar-šu*: NK 5'; *tuqattaršuma*(SAR-šú-ma): NY 4'
qātu (syllabic and ŠU) 'hand': IGI 1: 104', 160', 173'; IGI 2: 80'; IGI 3: 66', 88', (*qāt ummâni*) 96', (*qāt asî*) 105' → *asû*; *qāt Ištar/Šulpaea/Adad rāhiṣ*; *ummânu*
qāt Ištar (ŠU ^{d}15, ^{d}*Iš*$_8$-*tár*) 'hand of Ištar': IGI 2: 63', 66'
qāt Adad rāhiṣ (ŠU ^{d}IŠKUR *ra-hi-iṣ* (gloss of *Šulpaea*)) 'hand of Adad, the rain maker': IGI 2: 62'
qāt Šulpaea (ŠU ^{d}*Šul-pa-è-a*) 'hand of Šulpaea': IGI 2: 62'
qatû (TIL.LA) 'to come to an end, finish'
D-stem: *uqatta*(TIL.LA): IGI 1: 70'
qēm aban suluppī (ZÌ NA_4 ZÚ.LUM.MA) 'powder of date stones': IGI 1: 27'
qēm ašnan (ZÌ ^{d}ŠE.TIR) 'cereal flour': IGI 2: 52'
qēm buqli (ZÌ $MUNU_6$) 'malt flour': NZ 22'
qēm burāši (ZÌ ^{šim}LI) 'powder of juniper': NK 11'
qēm hallūri (ZÌ GÚ.GAL) 'chickpea powder': IGI 1: 29'; IGI 2: 68'; NK 10', 13'
qēm kakkî (ZÌ GÚ.TUR) 'powder of lentil': IGI 2: 68'; NK 10', 13'
qēm kasî (ZÍ GAZI^{sar}) 'powder of *kasû*-plant': IGI 1: 29'; IGI 2: 68'; NK 7', 12'
qēm kibti (ZÌ GIG) 'wheat flour'; NZ 15', 17'
qēm kukri (ZÍ ^{šim}GÚR.GÚR) 'powder of *kukru*-aromatic': IGI 2: 56'; NK 6', 11'
qēm labti (ZÌ ŠE.SA.A) 'flour of roasted grain': IGI 1: 200'; IGI 2: 1, 11, 56'; IGI 3: 72'; NK 7', 11'
qēm suādi (ZÌ ^{šim}MAN.DU) 'powder of *suādu*-aromatic': NK 12'
qēm šunê (ZÌ ^{giš}ŠE.NÚ.A) 'powder of *šunû*-tree': NK 11'

qēmu (ZÌ) 'flour, powder' → ***qēm aban suluppī, qēm ašnan, qēm hallūri, qēm labti, qēm kasî, qēm kukri, qēm šunê, qēm burāši, qēm buqli***
qerbu (syllabic) 'interior, inside': IGI 2: 222'
qerēbu (syllabic) 'to come close:
D-stem: *li-qer-ri-bu*: IGI 1: 76'
qeršu (syllabic) 'stripe of meat': IGI 2: 3
qilip nurmî (BAR ^{giš}NU.ÚR.MA) 'pomegranate peel': IGI 2: 115'
qilip šūmī (BAR SUM^{sar}) 'peel of garlic': NU 14'
qilpu (BAR) 'skin of plant, fruit, peel' → ***qilip nurmî/šūmī***
qīštu (NÍG.BA) 'fee': IGI 1: 95', 107'
qudru (^{ú}KI.^{d}IŠKUR) '*qudru*-plant' → ***zēr qudri***
qūqānu, gūqānu (syllabic) '*qūqānu*-worm': IGI 2: 27
qutāru (syllabic) 'fumigation': IGI 3: 8
qutru (syllabic) 'fume, smoke': IGI 2: 90', 135'

R

rabāku (syllabic) 'to make an infusion'
G-stem: *tara-bak*: IGI 1: 78', 200'; IGI 2: 1, 56', 63', 68', 84', 99'; NK 7'
rahāṣu (syllabic) 'to make rain, drench' → *tahāhu*
G-stem: *ra-hi-iṣ*: IGI 3: 62'
Gtn-stem: *ir-ta-na-haṣ-ma*: NF 35'
rakāsu (syllabic *tara-ká/às*, and KEŠDA) 'to bind, bandage body parts'
G-stem: *tarakkas*(KEŠDA): IGI 1: 8', 109', (*tarakkasma*) 118', (*tarakkasma*) 154', (*tarakkasma*) 181', (*tarakkasma*) 186'; IGI 2: 2, 3, 188'; *tarakkassu*(KEŠDA-*su*): IGI 1: 97'; 144'; NF 46'; *tara-ká/às*: IGI 1: (*tarakkasma*) 39', 59', 69'; *ru-kus-ma*: IGI 1: 172'; *tar-ku-si*: IGI 1: 178'
ramāku (syllabic and TU$_5$) 'to bathe, soak'
G-stem: *tara-muk*: IGI 1: 81'; *tarammukšu*(TU$_5$-*šú*): NF 19'; *irammuk*(TU$_5$): NU 6'
ramānu (syllabic) 'self': IGI 1: 168'
rapādu (^{ú}*ra-pa-di*) 'plant for *rapādu*-disease' → ***šuruš šammi rapādi***
rapšu (syllabic and DAGAL(-*te/i*)) 'wide, great': IGI 1: 104'; IGI 2: 217' → *tâmtu*
raqqu(BAL.GI^{ku6}) '*raqqu*-turtle' → ***marat raqqi***
rašû (TUK) 'to acquire, to develop (a disease)'
G-stem: *iraššâ*(TUK-(*a*)): IGI 1: 145'; NV 1'; *zūta irašši*(TUK): NF 34' → *zūtu*
rebiat (IGI.4.GÁL.LA) 'one-fourth': IGI 2: 84'; IGI 3: 50'; NS 3', 7'
rebû (4) 'fourth': IGI 2: 2, 7
rēš īnī (SAG IGI.MIN) 'upper part of the eyes or eyelids': IGI 1: 84'
ribku (syllabic) 'mixture, infusion': IGI 1: 33'; IGI 2: 7, 99'; IGI 3: 43', 98', 103'
rikibti arkabi (U$_5$.ARGAB^{mušen}) 'bat guano': IGI 1: 6', 34', 41', 44', 61', 64'; IGI 2: 8, 23, 26, 92', 122', 140', 141', 144', 152', 197'; IGI 3: 49'; NQ 11'; NS 2', 6'

riksu(KEŠDA) 'binding': IGI 2: 5; IGI 3: 60'
rīmtu (SÚN) 'wild cow': → ***muhhu ša rīmti***
rūqu (syllabic and SÙ.UD.DA) 'distant': IGI 1: 164'; IGI 3: 9
rūštu (SAG) 'top quality, premium': → ***šaman rūšti, šikar rūšti***
ru'tītu (ÚH-^{d}ÍD) '*ru'tītu*-sulphur (lit. river spittle)': IGI 3: 94'
ru'tu (ÚH) 'spittle': IGI 1: 47'

S

sābu (^{na4}*sa-a-bu*) '*sābu*-stone'; NT 10'
sahlânu (syllabic) '*sahlânu*-plant': IGI 2: 122' → *sahlû*
sahlû (syllabic and ZÀ.HI.LI.(A)$^{(sar)}$) '*sahlû*-plant': IGI 1: 9', 15', 29', 32', 35', 51', 200'; IGI 2: 1, 6, 22, 26, 65', 68', 98', 191'; IGI 3: 55', 94', 97', 99', 104', 107'; NK 3', 14'; NQ 8'; NR 6'
sâku (SÚD and syllabic) 'to pound'
G-stem: *tasâk*(SÚD): IGI 1: 6', 7', 9'–11', 13'–16', 18', 20', 22', 27', 34', 35', 38', 40', 41', 42', 43'–47', 54', 55', 58', 60', 64', 72', 78', 82', 87', 88'
IGI 2: 4, 16, 18, 20, 21, 23, 24, 29, 50'–53', 55', 58', 60'–62', 64', 66', 67', 69'–72', 74'–77', 79', 83'–88', 93', 97', 99', 101'–104', 107', 108', 113', 115', 116', 119', 123', 125', 127', 129', 132', 133', 139', 140'–144', 146'–148', 154', 155', 157'–159', 161', 162', 164', 165', 167'–169', 173', 180', 183', 184', 186', 187', 195', 205'
IGI 3: (*tasâkma*) 6, 12, 38'–40', 48', 50', 53', 59', 65', 67', 95', 100', 103'; NF 5', (*tasâkma*) 12', 16'; NP 2'–5'; NQ 12'; NR 2', 4', 5'; NS 4', 8'; NU 3', 5', 7', 9'; NV 2'–4'; NW 6'; NZ 2'
ta-sàk: IGI 1: 16', 19', 25'; IGI 2: 87', 107', 178', 186'
salā'u, šalā'u (syllabic) 'sprinkle water'
G-stem: *lis-la-ni-im-ma*: IGI 1: 105'
samānat (8) 'eight': IGI 1: 33'; IGI 2: 9, 138'
sāmtu (^{na4}GUG) 'carnelian': NF 9'
sāmu (SA_5) 'red': IGI 1: 36'; IGI 3: 18'$^{?}$, 37' → ***lipi kalīti sāmu, lipû sāmu,*** *šīpātu sāmātu*
sanāqu (syllabic) 'to check, execute'
G-stem: *sa-niq*: IGI 1: 100', 134'; *as-niq*: IGI 2: 221'
sapānu (syllabic) 'to dissolve, soften, flatten'
G-stem: *ta-sa-pan*: IGI 1: 63'; NR 7'
sâpu (syllabic) 'to draw water'
G-stem: *li-sa-pa-a-ni*: IGI 1:103'
Gtn-stem: *li-is-sa-pa-ni-im-ma*: IGI 1: 123'
sāqu (syllabic) 'thigh' → ***lipi sāqi ṣabīti***
sarāmu (syllabic) 'to cut'
G-stem: *ta-sa-rim*: IGI 2: 90'

sebe (7) 'seven': IGI 1: 97', 109', 144'; IGI 2: 28, 59', 95', 103', 138'; IGI 3: 27', 54', 78', 87', 102'; NF 44', NS 3'; NU 14'
sebet u sebet (7 u 7) 'seven and seven': IGI 1: 117', 154', 186'
sekēru (ÚŠ) 'to heat'
  G-stem: *tesekker*(ÚŠ-*ker/er*): IGI 3: 71'; NF 35'
sekru (syllabic) 'warmed-up': IGI 2: 113'
sêru (syllabic) G-stem 'to smear, spread onto'
  G-stem: *te-ser*: IGI 1: 12'
sīhu ([giš]*si-ha*) '*sīhu*-artemisia': IGI 1: 19'; NV 7'
sikillu ([ú]SIKIL) '*sikillu*-plant': NF 18', 45'
sikkat ṣēli immeri (GAG.TI.TI UDU) 'lamb chop': IGI 2: 75'
sīkti labti (*si-ik-ti* ŠE.SA.A) 'powder of roasted grain': IGI 2: 146', 206'
sillurmû, Sîn-lurmâ (syllabic and [d]30-*lu-ur-ma-a*) 'night/day blindness': IGI 3: 73'–75', 81'
simmu (syllabic) 'wound, sore': IGI 1: 163', 165'
Sîn-lurmâ → *sillurmû*
sinništu (MUNUS) 'female': IGI 1: 46', 67'; NF 18', 27' → ***nikiptu***
siparru (ZABAR) 'bronze' → *patar siparri, uppi siparri*
suādu ([šim]MAN.DU) '*suādu*-aromatic': IGI 2: 2 → ***qēm suādi***
suluppu (ZÚ.LUM.MA) 'date': IGI 3: 22', 51' → ***qēm aban suluppī***
summatu (TU[mušen]) 'pigeon': → ***muhhu ša summati zikari***
sumuktu (syllabic) '*sumuktu*-dirt': IGI 1: 139'
supālu (syllabic and [ú]ZA.BA.LAM) '*supālu*-juniper': *su-pa-la*: IGI 1: 21'
sūqu (SILA) 'street': IGI 1: 138', 188'

Ṣ

ṣabātu (syllabic and DAB) 'to seize, grasp, afflict'
  G-stem: *ṣa-bi-tú*: IGI 2: 111'; *iṣbassu*(DAB-*su*): IGI 3: (*iṣbassuma*) 9, 10; NF 26', 32'; NU (*iṣbassuma*) 12'; NZa (*iṣbassuma*) 9'
ṣabītu (MAŠ.DÁ) 'gazelle' → ***lipi kursinni ṣabīti***, ***lipi sāqi ṣabīti***, ***piqan ṣabīti***, ***lipi eṣemti ṣabīti***
ṣâdu (syllabic) 'to turn around, with *pānu* 'to have a vertigo'
  Gtn-stem: *pānūšu i-ṣa-nun-du*: NZa 9'
ṣahātu (SUR(-*at*)) 'to press out, draw liquid into vessel'
  G-stem: *taṣahhat*(SUR(-*at*)): IGI 1: 3', 81'; IGI 2: 156'; NU 7'
  D-stem: *ṣu-uh-hu-ta*: IGI 2: 63'
ṣalālu (syllabic and NÁ) 'to sleep'
  G-stem: *i-ṣa-lal-ma*: IGI 1: 36'; *iṣallal*(NÁ): IGI 3: 68'
ṣalāpu (syllabic) 'to cut open, dissect'
  G-stem: *ta-ṣa-lip*: IGI 1: 28'

Št-stem: *šu-te-eṣ-li-pa-a-tu*: IGI 1: 112’
ṣallāmtu (MUŠ.GE$_6$) ‘black snake’ → ***lipi ṣallāmti***
ṣallu (syllabic) ‘sleeping, resting’: NF 31’
ṣalmu (GE$_6$) ‘dark, black’: IGI 3: 40’ → ***dām kurṣipti alpi ṣalmi, lipi kalīt alpi ṣalmi, ṣurru ṣalmu***
ṣamādu (LAL(-*id*)) ‘to bandage’
G-stem: *taṣammid*(LAL(-*id*)): IGI 1: 10’, 13’, 15’, 18’, 19’, 22’, 29’, 35’, 37’, 48’, 78’, 200’; IGI 2: 1, 4, 6, 56’, 68’, 145’, 181’; IGI 3: 56’, 72’; NK 7’, 12’, 15’; NP 6’; NV 5’; NZ 5’, (6’, 7’), (*taṣammidma*) 10’
G-stem: *taṣṣanammid*(LAL.MEŠ): IGI 2: 114’
D-stem: *ú-ṣa-am-mad*$^?$: NZa 10’
ṣehru ($^{(lú)}$TUR) ‘a chick’: IGI 2: 106’; ‘a child’: IGI 3: 82’
ṣētu (UD.DA) ‘sun-heat’: IGI 1: 20’; IGI 2: 9; IGI 3: 49’; NS 6’
ṣillû (^{giš}DÁLA) ‘needle’: IGI 2: 105’, 166’
ṣillu (syllabic and GISSU) ‘shadow/film (on/in the eye)’: IGI 1: 23’, 80’, 92’; IGI 2: 117’, 121’, 199’, 200’, 202’, 207’, 209’
ṣimdu (syllabic) ‘bandage’: IGI 1: 76’
ṣirihtu (syllabic) ‘inflammation’: IGI 1: 105’; IGI 2: 209’
ṣīt šamši (^{d}UTU.È) ‘sunrise’: IGI 3: 29’
ṣubātu (TÚG) ‘cloth’: IGI 2: 28, 174’; NF 23’
ṣulum pāni (syllabic) ‘dark of face, anger’: IGI 1: 130’
ṣumlalû (^{šim}GAM.MA) ‘*ṣumlalû*-aromatic’; NZ 9’
ṣupru (UMBIN) ‘(toe-)nail’: IGI 2: 220’
ṣurār igāri (EME.ŠID É.GAR$_8$) ‘wall-lizard’: IGI 2: 74’
ṣurāru (EME.ŠID/DIR) ‘lizard’ → ***qaqqad ṣurāri, ṣurār igāri, zê ṣurāri***
ṣurru (syllabic and ^{na4}ZÚ) ‘flint (knife)’: IGI 1: 190’; → *ṣalmu, naglabu*
ṣurru ṣalmu (^{na4}ZÚ GE$_6$) ‘black flint = obsidian’: IGI 3: 40’

Š

ša (syllabic) ‘her, its’: IGI 1: 104’, 114’, 121’, 173’
ša (indirect genitive particle) ‘of, from’: IGI 1: 6’, 33’, 61’, 92’, 100’, 102’, 105’, 113’, 114’, 121’, 134’, 146’, 148’, 188’, 191’, 193’, 199’; IGI 2: 10, 11, 18, 26, 27, 57’, 77’, 90’, 108’, 124’, 135’; IGI 3: 96’, 98’, 101’, 103’; NF 13’, 14’; NK 8’; NR 5’; NZ 11’; NZa 9’; ‘because’: IGI 1: 137’: ‘regarding’: IGI 1: 166’; ‘against’: IGI 3: 32’, 43’, 46’ → ***baltu ša ṭābti, dāmu ša libbi šahî, gūru ša qanî, gurušgaraš ša šahî, kalīt lalî lakî ša šamma lā našku uṭṭata lā ṣabitu, larsīni ša halli lahri ša šumēli ša māšī ūlidu, kammu ša aškāpi, makūt gabīdi ša imēri, muhhu ša erî, muhhu ša eṣemti kurīti immeri, muhhu ša rīmti, muhhu ša summati zikari***, *ša libbi*, ***šuhtu ša aškāpi, šuhtu ša tangussi***

šamaškillu (SUM.SIKIL) ‘*šamaškillu*-onion’: IGI 1: 26’

šamāṭu (syllabic) ‘to tear down, strip away’

G-stem: *ta-šam-ma-aṭ*: IGI 2: 95’

šammi ašî (Ú *a-ši-i*) ‘*ašû*-disease-plant (against ‘*ašû*-disease’)’: IGI 1: 51’; IGI 2: 192’; IGI 3: 41’, 94’; NQ 3’, 12’; NS 3’

šammu (Ú) ‘plant, drug’: IGI 1: 33’, 62’, 64’; IGI 2: 7, 9, 26, 57’, 106’, 109’, 123’; IGI 3: 5, 29’, 43’, 98’, 101’, 102’; NF 11’; NS 3’; NU 14’ → ***kalīt lalî lakî ša šamma lā našku uṭṭata lā ṣabitu, šammi ašî, šammu ēdu, šammu peṣû, šuruš šammi rapādi***

šammu ēdu (Ú.DILI) ‘single plant’; NU 3’, 14’

šammu peṣû (Ú.BABBAR) ‘white plant’: IGI 1: 22’, 34’, 41’, 42’, 44’, 56’, 58’, 61’, 82’, 86’, 87’, 88’; IGI 2: 8, 10, 23, 25, 57’, 58’, 66’, 70’, 73’, 92’, 113’, 114’, 122’, 145’, 196’; IGI 3: 50’, 52’, 104’; NK 8’; NQ 11’; NR 6’; NS 2’, 7’; NV 2’ → ***haṣbi šammi peṣî***

šamnu (Ì(.GIŠ) ‘oil’: IGI 2: 61’, 62’, 71’, 74’, 86’, 88’, 93’, 116’, 162’, 184’, 193’; IGI 3; NF 5’; NU 2’, 9’; NV 2’; NW 6’ → ***šaman asi, šaman ballukki, šaman erēni, šaman iṣṣūr hurri labīri***$^{?}$, ***šaman kurkî, šaman pūri***

šamnu (Ì.GIŠ, Ì+GIŠ) ‘sesame oil’: IGI 1: 8’, 12’, 26’, 44’, 54’; IGI 2: 64’, 73’, 77’, 84’; IGI 3: 35’, 83’, 100’; NU 5’; NV 2’; NZ 2’, 21’ → *rēštû*

šamû (syllabic and AN(-*e*)) ‘sky/heaven’: IGI 1: 102’, 121’, 163’, 164’

šanā’u (syllabic) ‘to block (off)’

G-stem: *še-en-a*: IGI 1: 91’

D-stem: *šu-un-nu-’a*: IGI 1: 40’

Dt-stem: *ul-ta-ta-ni-’a*: IGI 1: 79’

šanîš (MIN) ‘alternatively’: IGI 1: 87’, 88’, 183’; IGI 2: 140’, 141’; ‘ditto’: IGI 2: 13, 133’, 140f.’, 163’, 195’

šanû (syllabic) ‘second’: IGI 2: 216’; ‘deputy of Ištar’: NV 7’

šapāhu (syllabic) ‘to sprinkle’

G-stem: *ta-ša-pah*: IGI 3: 6; NF 11’

šapāku (DUB(-*ak*)) ‘to pour’

G-stem: *tašappak*(DUB(-*ak*)) IGI 1: 8’, 83’; IGI 2: 52’; *ta-šap-pak-ma*: NY 7a’

šapāru (syllabic) ‘to send’

G-stem: *lu-uš-pur*: IGI 1: 102’, 121’; *ta-šap-pár*: IGI 1: 160’

šaplānu (KI.TA-*nu*) ‘below’: IGI 1: 127’

šaptu (NUNDUM) ‘lip’: IGI 3: 90’

šaqālu (syllabic) ‘to weigh’

G-stem: *ta-ša-qàl*: IGI 2: 151’

šaqû (NAG) ‘to give to drink’ → *šatû*

šarāku (syllabic) ‘to present, give’

G-stem: *iš-ru-ku-šú*: IGI 2: 217’

šarāpu (syllabic) ‘to burn’

G-stem: *ta-šár-rap*: IGI 2: 135’

šarmadu (^{ú}GÚR.UŠ) ‘*šarmadu*-plant’: IGI 2: 112’

šarru (LUGAL and 20) ‘king’: IGI 2: 217’, 219’

šārtu (SÍG) 'hair': IGI 2: 17
šāru (IM) 'wind': IGI 1: 128', 129', 163', 174', 178'; IGI 2: 149'; NK 6', 9' → *šār/ikil/ṣulum pāni*
šār pāni (syllabic) 'head wind, resistance': IGI 1: 130'
šasû (syllabic and GÙ-*si*) 'to call, cry out'
G-stem: *al-si-ki-na-ši*: IGI 1: 114', 115'; *i-šá-as-si*: IGI 1: 151'; *išassi*(GÙ-*si*): IGI 2: 12, 14
Gtn-stem: *ši-ta-si-ia*: IGI 2: 222'
šâšu (syllabic) 'of him': IGI 2: 107'
šâšunu (syllabic) 'those': IGI 2: 123'
šatti pāna (syllabic) 'spring': IGI 1: 183' → *pānu*
šatû (NAG) 'to drink'
G-stem: *išatti*(NAG): IGI 1: 26', 57'; IGI 3: 35', 72'
šâti → *šuātu*
šaṭāru (syllabic) 'write'
G-stem: *áš-ṭùr*: IGI 2: 221'
še'u (ŠE) 'grain' → ***habbur še'i***
šediš (6) 'six': IGI 1: 29'
šēlu (syllabic) 'sharp': IGI 2: 201'
šemû (syllabic) 'to hear'
G-stem: *še-me-ma*$^{?}$: IGI 3: 85'; *liš-ma-a*: IGI 3: 85'
šer'ānu (SA(-*a-nu*)) 'sinew/tendon': IGI 1: 75'
šerhu (syllabic) 'furrow': IGI 1: 195'
šērtu (syllabic) 'morning': NZb 11'
šēru (syllabic and UZU) 'flesh': IGI 1: 74'; IGI 2: 19, 22, 25, 26; IGI 3: 45', 75' NT 2'
šēru (syllabic and Á.GÚ.ZI.GA) 'morning': IGI 1: 38', 81'; IGI 3: 29', 76'; NF 19', 22'
šeššet → *šediš*
šibru (syllabic) 'broken': IGI 2: 67' → *akalu*
šihiltu (syllabic) 'filtered liquid': IGI 2: 154'
šikaru (KAŠ) 'beer': IGI 1: 15', 18', 26', 200'; IGI 2: 1, 56', 181'; IGI 3: 35', 72'; NK 7'; NR 7
šikar rūšti(KAŠ.SAG) 'premium beer': NQ 9'
šiknu (syllabic) '(blood) deposit (in the eye)': IGI 1: 61'
šīlu (syllabic) 'perforation of the eye(lid)': IGI 3: 68', 70'
šimbizidû (ŠIM.BI.ZI.DA and *šim-bi-zi-dam*) '*šimbizidû*-galena': IGI 1: 47'; IGI 3: 39'
-*šina* (syllabic) 'them, their, whom': IGI 1: 93', 101', 103', 120', 122', 126'–129', 177'; IGI 3: 68'
šina (syllabic) 'two': IGI 1: 101', 126', 177'
šīnāti amēlūti (KÀŠ *a-me-lu-ti*) 'human urine' NF 34'
šīnātu (KÀŠ) 'urine': IGI 2: 189'
šinīšu (2-šú) 'twice, two-ply': IGI 1: 185' → *ištiššu šinīšu šalāšīšu*
šīpātu peṣâtu (SÍG BABBAR) 'white wool': IGI 1: 39', 97', 117', 118', 143', 154', 180', 181'; NU 13'; NZb 3'

šīpātu sāmātu (SÍG SA_5) 'red wool': IGI 1: 109', 117', 118', 143', 154', 180', 181'; NF 44'; NZb 3'

šipru (syllabic and KIN) 'effect': IGI 2: 54'; 'skill': IGI 2: 219'

šiptu (syllabic and ÉN) 'incantation': IGI 1: 30', 65', 69', 70, 73', 89', 94', 95', 97', 106', 107', 109', 110', 115', 117', 119', 125', 132', 136', 144', 145', 147', 150', 154', 155', 157', 159', 163', 171', 176', 182', 186', 187', 191', 194'; IGI 3: 24', 85', 87'; NP 1'; NU 16'; NZb 6', 13'

šīpu (ŠIM.BI.KÙ.GI) '*šīpu*-paste': IGI 1: 7', 13'

šiqlu (GÍN) 'shekel': IGI 1: 29', 41', 64'; IGI 2: 55', 92', 140', 141'; IGI 3: 49', 50'; NK 13', 14'; NS 6', 7'

šišītu (syllabic) 'membrane': IGI 2: 121', 124', 139'

šitta (syllabic and 2) 'two': IGI 1: 101', 120', 126'

šittu (syllabic) 'remnant, rest': IGI 2: 135'

šizbi enzi (GA UD_5) 'goat's milk': IGI 1: 78'

šizbi musukkati (GA ^{munus}Ú.ZÚG) 'milk from a woman in maternity': IGI 1: 37', 47'; IGI 2: 155', 205': IGI 3: 39';

šizbi musukkati ša zikara ūlidu (GA ^{munus}Ú.ZÚG *šá* NITA Ù.TU) 'milk from a woman in maternity, who gave birth to a male': IGI 2: 148'?; NR 5'

šizbu (GA) 'milk': IGI 1: 19', 35'; IGI 2: 65', 69', 192'; NQ 8'; NZ 10'

šu 'his, its, him' (pronominal suffix): IGI 1: 7', 8', 10'–15', 17', 18', 20'–26', 28', 29', 31'–42', 44'–46', 48'–50', 56', 57', 59', 61', 63', 64', 68', 69', 71', 72', 77'–80', 84'–88', 93', 97', 105', 109', 114', 118', 144', 146', 148', 154', 166'–168', 174', 181', 184'–186', 197', 200', 201'; IGI 2: 1–7, 9, 12, 16–19, 22, 24, 25, 27, 52'–56', 58', 60', 61', 63', 66', 69', 76', 78', 89', 91, 97'–99', 101', 106', 108', 115'–119', 121', 123'–127', 132', 136', 137', 139', 142', 143', 144', 145', 158', 159', 169', 175', 181', 185', 190', 191', 194', 196', 199', 200', 202', 204', 207', 208', 213', 215', 216', 217'; IGI 3: 1–3, 6, 8, 9, 11, 30', 31', 35', 37', 39', 43', 49'–51', 53', 54', 57', 61', 67', 68', 70', 71', 75', 76', 78', 81', 83', 88', 90', 103'; NF 7', 12', 13', 16', 19', 20', 30', 33', 46'; NK 5'–7', 9', 15'; NP 7'; NQ 5', 8', 10', 11'; NR 2', 3', 5', 6', 10'; NS 1', 4', 6', 8'; NT 4'; NU 4'–7', 10', 12'; NV 1', 6', 7'; NW 4'; NZb 6', 7'; NY 4', 7a'; NZ 4', 8'; NZ 19'; NZa 8'–10'

šū (syllabic and BI) 'this same, that': IGI 1: 168'; IGI 2: 54'; IGI 3: 10, 49'; NS 6'

šuātu (syllabic and BI) 'that, this': IGI 1: 166', 169'; IGI 2: 54', 219'; IGI 3: 77', 84'

šubû (^{na4}ŠUBA) '*šubû*-stone': IGI 3: 4

šubultu (syllabic) 'head-of-grain': IGI 1: 196'

šugidimmakku (ŠU.GIDIM.MA) 'hand of a ghost': IGI 3: 2, 9, 10, 32', 43'; NV 7'

šuharru → *šaharru*

šuhtu (SAHAR.URUDU) 'copper patina': IGI 2: 51', 62', 64', 71', 93', 101'–104', 147', 154', 157', 158'; IGI 3: 53'; NW 6' → ***šuhtu ša aškāpi/tangussi***

šuhtu ša aškāpi (*šu-uh-ta ša* AŠGAB) 'patina from a leatherworker': IGI 1: 12'

šuhtu ša tangussi (SAHAR.URUDU *ša* ŠEN.TUR) 'patina of a copper *tangussu*-kettle': IGI 1: 14', 16', 61'; IGI 2: 95'

šukkulu (syllabic) D-stem: 'to wipe, rub: *tu-šak-kal*: IGI 2: 3

šumēlu (GÙB) 'left (side)': IGI 1: 148'; IGI 2: 110' → *īn šumēlīšu*, ***larsīni ša halli lahri ša šumēli ša māšī ūlidu***
šumēnu (^{na4}ŠU.MÌN) '*šumēnu*-mineral': IGI 1: 84'
šumma (DIŠ and *šum*$_4$*-ma*) 'if': IGI 1: 10', 12', 14', 16', 21', 23', 26', 32', 34'–36', 40', 45', 57', 59', 61', 71', 77', 79', 87'–88', 184', 200', 201'; IGI 2: 1, 9, 12, 16, 17, 19, 22, 25, 27, 53', 54', 56', 58', 60', 61', 63', 76', 115'–117', 121', 124', 126', 137', 139'–141', 147'–149', 159', 191', 196', 199', 200', 202', 204', 207', 209', 213', 215', 216'; IGI 3: 1, 9, 38'–40', 49', 51', 57', 66', 68', 70', 73'–75', 81'; NF 13', 15', 21', 26', 32', 33'; NK 6', 9'; NQ 5', 8', 10'; NR 3', 5', 6', 10'; NS 1', 6'; NT 4'; NV 1', 6'; NZ 19'; NZa 8'; 'when': IGI 1: 63'; NK 14'; NR 7'
šūmū (SUM^{sar}) 'garlic': IGI 1: 15' → ***qilip šūmī***
šunnu'ā → *šanā'u*
šunu 'their' (3 m. pl. gen.): IGI 1: 161', 180'; IGI 2: 105', 153', 156', 166'; IGI 3: 45'
šunû (^{giš}ŠE.NÚ.A) '*šunû*-tree': NF 18' → ***arti šunê***, ***qēm šunê***
šurru (syllabic) D-stem: 'to bow down, lean over': *šur-ra-ta*: IGI 1: 74'
šurrû (syllabic) 'beginning': IGI 1: 194'
šuršu (SUHUŠ) 'root' → ***šuruš ašāgi/ēri/gišimmari zikari/šammi rapādi/urâni***
šuršummū (syllabic) 'sediments/dregs of beer: IGI 1: 15'; NQ 9'
šuršurru (syllabic) '*šuršurru*-fibre$^{?}$': IGI 1: 188'
šuruš ašāgi (SUHUŠ KIŠI$_{16}$) 'root of *ašāgu*-acacia': NZa 9'
šuruš ēri (SUHUŠ ^{giš}MA.NU) 'root of *ēru*-tree': NU 13'
šuruš gišimmari zikari (SUHUŠ ^{giš}GIŠIMMAR NÍTA) 'root of male date palm': IGI 2: 160'
šuruš šammi rapādi (ŠUHUŠ Ú *ra-pa-di*) 'root of *rapādu*-disease-plant': IGI 1: 38'
šuruš urâni (ŠUHUŠ ^{ú}HA) 'root of *urânu*-plant': IGI 1: 69'
šuššu (IGI.6.GÁL.LA) 'one-sixth': IGI 1: 41'
šūtu (IM.1) 'south wind': IGI 1: 115'

T

tabālu (syllabic) 'take away, remove'
G-stem: *tab-la*: IGI 2: 13, 15
tābīla (syllabic) '(plant) in dry state': IGI 1: 42', 53', 56'; IGI 2: 4, 6, 140', 152'; NR 9'; NS 5'; 'eye dryness': IGI 1: 26'
tahāhu (syllabic) 'to drench' → *rahāṣu*
D-stem: *tu-tah-ha-ah*: IGI 1: 11'
tāhīzu (syllabic) 'teaching': IGI 2: 220'
takāpu (syllabic) 'to prick'
D-stem: *tu-ták-kap*: IGI 2: 105', 166'
takkussu (^{gi}SAG.KUD) 'reed-straw': IGI 1: 7'; IGI 2: 115', 132'
tallu (syllabic) 'flask': IGI 1: 103'
taltallû ša gišimmari (*tal-tal-lu-ú šá* ^{giš}GIŠIMMAR) 'pollen of date palm': IGI 1: 113'

tamāhu (syllabic) 'to grasp, seize'
N-stem: *it-ta-mu-uh*: NY 2'
tāmartu (syllabic) 'viewing': IGI 2: 222'
tâmtu (syllabic) ', sea, lake, ocean': IGI 1: 104' → *imbu' tâmti, rapšu*
tangussu (ŠEN.TUR) 'copper *tangussu*-kettle': IGI 2: 86', 94'; NU 3' → ***šuhtu ša tangussi***
tarāṣu (LAL) 'to spread out (a cloth)'
G-stem: *tatarraṣ*(LAL-*aṣ*): IGI 3: 77'
tarbaṣu (TÙR) 'animal stall': IGI 1: 138'
tarmuš (^{ú}*tar-muš₈*, ^{ú}*tar-muš*) '*tarmuš*-lupine': IGI 1: 46'; NU 4'
târu (GUR) 'to return, repeat'
G-stem: *itūr*(GUR): IGI 1: 80'; *tatârma*(GUR-*ma*): NZ 23'
D-stem: *tuttanār* (GUR.GUR): IGI 2: 119'
tê šipti (TU_6.ÉN) 'incantation spell': IGI 1: 67', 70', 95', 107', 123', 130', 134', 145', 152', 157', 161', 178', 183', 192', 198'; IGI 3: 86'; → tu_6-én; TU_6.ÉN.É.NU.RU → Uncertain Readings and Words
tebû (syllabic and ZI) 'to rise, throb'
G-stem: *it-ba-ki-na-ši*: IGI 1: 115'; *tebīma*(ZI-*ma*): NZa 8'
temēru (syllabic) 'to bury'
G-stem: *te-te-mer*: IGI 2: 28, 59', (*te-tem-mer*) 103'
tēqītu (syllabic) 'ointment': IGI 2: 26; IGI 3: 32'
tēqītu šalimtu (syllabic) 'healing ointment': IGI 3: 96'
tibnu (IN.NU) 'straw': IGI 1: 114'
tību (ZI) 'rising (of wind)': IGI 1: 129'
tinūru (NININDU) 'tannour-oven': IGI 2: 65', 98'; IGI 3: 71'; NF 35'; NR 8'
tiše, tišīt (9) 'nine': IGI 3: 44', 98', 101'
tittu (syllabic and ^{giš}PÈŠ) 'fig': IGI 1: 114'; NF 18', 21' → ***arti titti***
tīyatu (syllabic) '*tīyatu*-plant' → ***hīl tīyati***
tû (TU_6) 'incantation': IGI 1: 75'
tubkinnu (syllabic) 'hole, refuse heap': IGI 1: 189'
talupadu (syllabic) '*talupadu*-plant' → ***zēr talupadi***
tupšarrūtu (syllabic) 'scribal art': IGI 2: 218'
tuškû ($^{(na4)}$*tu-uš-ka-a*) '*tuškû*-mineral': IGI 1: 11', 82'; IGI 3: 104'

Ṭ

ṭābātu (A.GEŠTIN.NA) 'vinegar': IGI 1: 81'; IGI 2: 145'; (*ṭ. bašlāti*) NZ 25' → *karpat ṭābāti*
ṭābtu (MUN) 'salt': IGI 2: 17, 71', 112'; NR 3' → ***baltu ša ṭābti, haṣab ṭābti***
ṭābu (DU_{10}) 'sweet' → ***qanû ṭābu***
ṭābu (syllabic) 'good, friendly': NF 19'
ṭâbu (syllabic) 'to be good'
G-stem: *i-ṭàb*: IGI 1: 183'

ṭamû (NU.NU) 'to spin'
G-stem: *taṭammi*(NU.NU): IGI 1: 39', 97', 109', 117', 143', 154', 180', 185'; NZ 12'
ṭebētu → Month Names
ṭehû (TE) 'to be(come) near to, approach'
G-stem: *ṭehe*(TE-*e*): NF 17'; *iṭehhe*(TE): NF 20', 23'; *iṭ-hi-ka*: NZb 9', 10'
D-stem: *teṭehhīma*(TE-*ma*) 'you introduce': IGI 2: 98'
ṭênu (ÀRA) 'to grind up'
G-stem: *teṭên*(ÀRA-*en*): IGI 2: 190'
ṭepû (syllabic and TAB) 'to apply (drugs), add (ingredients)'
G-stem: *ta-ṭe-ep-pi*: IGI 1: 53'; *te-ṭe-ep-pí*: IGI 2: 67'; *te-ṭep-pi*: NS 5'
ṭerû (syllabic) 'to ooze'
G-stem: *iṭ-ri*: NR 3', 5', 10'; *ṭi-ri*: NR 6'
ṭīpu (syllabic) 'drop(s)': IGI 2: 9, 10, 11, 57', 67'; NK 8'
tuppu (syllabic and DUB) 'clay tablet': IGI 1: 201'; IGI 2: 216', 221'
ṭurru (DUR) 'a cord': IGI 1: 39', 97', 109', 118', 185'; NF 44'; NU 13'; NZ 12'
ṭūru (^{šim}HAB) '*ṭūru*-plant': IGI 2: 16; IGI 3: 52'

U

u (syllabic) 'and': IGI 1: 14', 21', 36', 39', 46', 54', 70', 84', 94', 95', 106', 117', 123', 138', 152', 154', 159', 161', 178', 185', 186', 190', 192', 193', 198'; IGI 2: 9, 17, 22, 25, 58', 61', 64', 77', 93', 98', 138', 214', 217', 221'; IGI 3: 8, 34', 50', 67', 83', 90', 100', 103'; NF 13', 14', 18', 31', 33', 34'; NK 10', 15'; NQ 5', 10'; NS 1', 8'; NT 2', 3'; NV 6'; NW 6'
ū (syllabic) 'or': IGI 2: 5 (gloss)
ubān hašê (ŠU.SI *ha-še-e*) 'lobe of the lung': IGI 3: 87'
ubāni-aṣi (syllabic) '*ubāni-aṣi* plant': IGI 2: 153'
ubānu (ŠU.SI) 'finger': IGI 1: 84'; IGI 2: 73'; IGI 3: 95'
uhūlu qarnānû ($^{(\text{ú})}$NAGA.SI) 'horned *uhūlu*-alkali': IGI 1: 10', 78'; IGI 2: 8, 91', 145'; IGI 3: 52', 53', 55', 94', 104'; NK 2'; NR 6'; NU 14'; NV 1' → ***mê uhūli qarnānî***
ul (syllabic and NU) 'no, not': IGI 1: 67', 94', 106', 115', 121', 152'; IGI 2: 149'; IGI 3: 30', 54'; NF 30'
ummânu (UM.ME.A) 'expert, sage': IGI 3: 96' → *qātu*
ummātu (syllabic and É.MEŠ, AMA.MEŠ) 'summer': IGI 1: 52', 63'; (NR 8')
ummu I (AMA) 'mother': IGI 1: 177'
ummu II (KÚM) '*ummu*-fever (lit. heat, summer)': IGI 1: 23', 105'; IGI 2: 117'; NF 33'
ūmu (UD-(*me/mi*)) 'day': IGI 1: 23', 24'; IGI 2: 7, 28, 59', 95', 103', 117', 118'; IGI 3: 44', 73', 74' → *kala ūme*
uppi siparri (MUD ZABAR) 'a bronze tube': IGI 1: 86'–88'
upputtu (syllabic) '*upputtu*-insect' → *zê upputte*
uqnâtu (^{ú}ZA.GÌN.NA) '*uqnâtu*-blue-plant': IGI 1: 69'
uqnû ($^{\text{na4}}$ZA.GÌN) 'blue stone, mostly lapis lazuli': IGI 1: 103'; IGI 3: 4

uqni šadê (^{na4}ZA.GÌN KUR.RA) 'mountain lapis lazuli': IGI 3: 38'
urânu (^{ú}HA) '*urânu*-plant': NV 2' → ***šuruš urâni***
urnû (^{ú}*úr-né-e*) '*urnû*-plant': IGI 1: 88'; IGI 2: 87'
urru (syllabic) 'day': IGI 1: 36'
ururu (syllabic) 'to parch'
  D-stem: *tur-ár*: IGI 1: 9', 16', 24', 27', 37'; IGI 2: 67', 70', 75', 102', 118', 146'
ūru (ÙR) 'roof'; IGI 3: 28'; NF 27'
ušû (^{ú}ESI) '*ušû*-plant': IGI 3: 53'
uṭṭatu (ŠE and ŠE.BAR / KU.KU) 'grain (also as a measure)': IGI 1: 44', 78'; IGI 2: 139', 141'; IGI 3: 27'; NT 9' → ***kalīt lalî lakî ša šamma lā našku uṭṭata lā ṣabitu***
uznu (GEŠTU) 'ear, understanding': IGI 2: 217'; NK 15'
uzun lalî (^{ú}UR.TÁL.TÁL) 'young goat's-ear plant': IGI 2: 145'

W

wabālu → *abālu*
walādu → *alādu*
warādu → *arādu*
wardatu → *ardatu*
waṣû → *aṣû*

Y

ya → *ī*
yā'uttun (syllabic) 'mine': IGI 1: 94', 106'

Z

zagindurû (^{na4}ZA.GÌN.DURU$_5$) '*zagindurû*-lapis lazuli': IGI 1: 122'
zakû (syllabic) 'to become clear'
  D-stem: *ú-za-ku-ú*: IGI 2: 119'
zalāqu (^{na4}ZÁLAG) '*zalāqu*-stone': IGI 3: 4; NF 9'; NU 5'
zanānu (syllabic) 'to rain'
  G-stem: *zu-un-na-ni*: IGI 1: 189'
zappi šahî (*zap-pí* ŠAH) 'pig's bristle'; NZ 20'
zâqu (syllabic) 'to blow'
  G-stem: *i-zi-qam-ma*: IGI 1: 163'
zarû (syllabic and MAR(-*ru*)) 'to scatter, spatter, sprinkle'
  G-stem: *tazarru*(MAR(-*ru*)) IGI 1: 26', 42'; IGI 2: 4, 6, 140'; NZ 24'; *ta-zar-ri*: IGI 1: 50'

zê ṣurāri ($ŠE_{10}$ EME.ŠID) 'lizard's excrement': IGI 1: 43', 78'
zê upputte ($ŠE_{10}$ *up-pu-te*) 'excrement of *upputte*-insect': IGI 2: 109'
zēr ašli (NUMUN $^{(ú)}$*áš-li*) 'seed of rush': IGI 3: 5, 7; NY 4'
zēr ašli zikari (NUMUN *áš-li* NITA) 'seed of male rush': IGI 3: 5
zēr bīni (NUMUN ŠINIG) 'seed of tamarisk': IGI 2: 16; IGI 3: 5, 7; NF 10', 45'; NT 11'
zēr burāši (NUMUN ^{šim}LI) 'seed of juniper': IGI 1: 32'; IGI 3: 8, 97', 102'
zēr egemgīri (NUMUN ^{giš}NÍG.GÁN.GÁN) 'seed of *egemgīru*-plant': IGI 1: 40'; IGI 2: 87'
zēr ēri (NUMUN ^{giš}MA.NU) 'seed of *ēru*-tree': IGI 3: 5, 7; NF 10'
***zēr* GI.ZÚ.LUM.MA** (NUMUN GI.ZÚ.LUM.MA) 'seeds of GI.ZÚ.LUM.MA-plant': IGI 2: 20, 196', 206'
zēr haṭṭi rē'î (NUMUN ^{ú}NÍG.GIDRU) 'seeds of shepherd's-staff plant': IGI 2: 112'
zēr lišān kalbi (NUMUN ^{ú}EME.UR.GI_7) 'seeds of dog's-tongue plant': IGI 2: 112', 122'
zēr maštakal (NUMUN $^{ú}IN_6$.ÚŠ) 'seeds of *maštakal*-plant': IGI 1: 24'; IGI 2: 118'
zēr qudri (NUMUN ^{ú}KI.^{d}IŠKUR) 'seeds of *qudru*-plant': IGI 2: 5
zēr šammi daqqiqi (NUMUN Ú *da-aq-qí-qí*) 'tiny$^{?}$ plant seeds': IGI 2: 109'$^{?}$
zēr talupadi (NUMUN ^{ú}*ta-lu-pa-di*) 'seeds of *talupadu*-plant': IGI 2: 109'
zēru (NUMUN) 'seed(s)': → ***zēr …***
zību (syllabic and GAMUN.GE_6) 'black cumin': IGI 1: 82'; IGI 3: 47', 52', 107'
zidubdubbû (ZÌ.DUB.DUB.BU) 'a heap of flour': NF 29'
zikaru (NÍTA, NITA) 'man, male': NF 27'; NR 5' → ***arti pillî zikari*, *muhhu ša summati zikari*, *nikiptu zikar u sinniš*, *pillû zikaru*, *šizbi musukkati ša zikara ūlidu*, *šuruš gišimmari zikari*, *zēr ašli zikari***
zû ($ŠE_{10}$) 'excrement' → ***zê ṣurāri***
zumru (SU) 'body': NF 33'
zūtu (IR) 'sweat'; NF 34' → *rašû*

Sumerian Words

a 'water': IGI 1: 150'
-a 'in': IGI 1: 164', 165', 174'; 'with' IGI 1: 173'
a-ga 'back': IGI 1: 73', 155'
a-lal-la 'shaduf': IGI 1: 150'
abzu 'underground water': IGI 1: 171'
ad-da 'father': NF 40'
an 'sky': IGI 1: 164'
bàn-da 'small/tiny': IGI 1: 155'
bar 'open': IGI 1: 89', 90', 98', 99', 110', 111', 119', 125', 132', 133'
bar-bar 'staring': IGI 1: 89', 98', 110', 119', 125', 132'
bar-ra 'opened': IGI 1: 89', 98', 110', 119', 125', 133'
-bi 'its, this, his': IGI 1: 157', 166'–169', 173', 174', 182'; NF 36'–39', 42'
da 'weak': IGI 1: 90', 99', 111'
di-ku_5 'judge': NF 42'
dumu 'son': NF 40'
dumu-sag 'first-born son': NF 40'
è 'to leave': IGI 1: 174'
én 'incantation': NF 36'
ér 'tears': IGI 1: 150'
ér šéš-šéš 'to pour out (tears), weep': IGI 1: 168'
gar 'to place/cause': IGI 1: 164', 165'
gaz-gá 'crushed': IGI 1: 170'
geštu 'ear': IGI 1: 73'
gi 'reed': IGI 1: 155'
gi-na 'to be firm/true, to be in order': IGI 1: 73', 133', 155', 157'
gig 'sick, bitter': IGI 1: 168', 175', 179'
gig-ga 'sore, lesion, wound': IGI 1: 163'–165'
gin_7 'like': IGI 1: 150'
gù dé 'to say, talk, speak': NF 40'
gub 'to stay, stand, be present': IGI 1: 65', 150'
hé-pà 'may adjure'; NF 36'–39'
hul 'evil, harmed': IGI 1: 90', 99', 111', 119'
hul-hul 'malevolent': 119'
huš 'reddish': IGI 1: 89', 98', 110', 157'
huš-huš 'crimson: IGI 1: 89', 98', 110', 132'
igi (and syllabic i-gi) 'eye': IGI 1: 73', 89', 90', 96', 98'–99', 108', 110', 111', 116', 119', 124', 125', 131'–133', 135', 149', 155', 158', 162–167', 169', 172–175', 179', 182'; NF 36'–39' (in rubrics, it is uncertain if not realized in Akkadian)
igi bar 'to see' NF 41
igi sì 'to see, look': IGI 1: 169'

ti-la ‘healthy’: IGI 1: 73’, 155’
tu-ra ‘illness; the sick’: IGI 1: 169’
tu_6-én ‘incantion spell’: IGI 1: 147’, 155’, 157’; NF 42’; NY 6’
tu_6-tu_6 sì ‘to recite an incantation: IGI 1: 171’
ú-hu-ur-sag-gi-na ‘the real mountain plant’: IGI 1: 73’
ur-sag ‘hero’: IGI 1: 155’; NF 36’–39’
zu ‘your’: IGI 1: 155’

Logograms with Cuneiform Signs

Notes:

- Cuneiform signs follow Neo-Assyrian forms as reflected in Nineveh.
- Logograms are also designated by the name and the number appearing in Borger 2010, *Mesopotamisches Zeichenlexikon* – in round brackets: e.g. (ŠU, no. 567). In case the logogram is missing in Borger 2010, it is marked with 'not in MZ.'

A

A.GA.ÁŠ.GA (not in MZ) → *agašgû* 'novice (physician)'
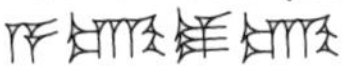
A.GAR.GAR (A, no. 839) → *piqannu* 'droppings (of gazelle)'
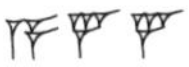
A.GAR$_5$ (A, no. 839) → *abāru* 'lead'
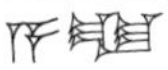
A.GEŠTIN.NA (A, no. 839) *ṭābātu* 'vinegar' → DUG A.GEŠTIN.NA
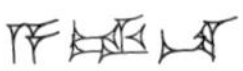
Á.GÚ.ZI.GA (Á, no. 560) → *šēru* 'morning'
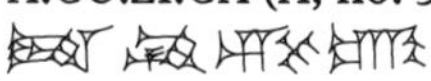
A.GÚB.BA.A (A, no. 839) → *agubbû* 'holy water vessel'
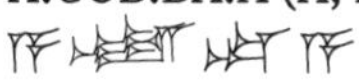
A.HA.TAR.DU = GÌRIMA (A, no. 839, Kap. II) → ^{d}*Nin-gìrima*
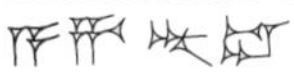
A(.MEŠ) (A, no. 839) → *mû* 'water'
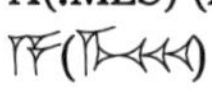
AMA.MEŠ (not in MZ) → *ummātu* 'summer'
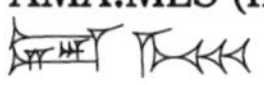
A.ZU-*ti* (not in MZ) → *asûtu* 'medical skill'
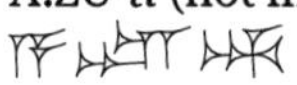
AN.BAR (AN, no. 10) → *parzillu* 'iron'
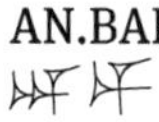
AN.ŠÁR^{ki} (AN, no. 10) → *Aššur* 'Assyria'
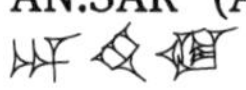
AN(-*e*) (AN, no. 10) → *šamû* 'sky/heaven'
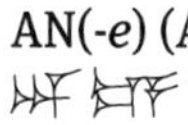
ANŠE (ANŠE, no. 353) → *imēru* 'donkey'
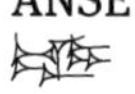
AN.ZAH.GE$_6$ (AN, no. 10) → *kutpû* 'black frit (bead)'
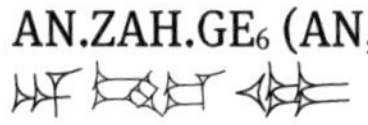

ÀRA (HAR, no. 644) → *ṭênu* 'to grind up'
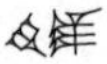

ARGAB^{mušen} (NÍG, no. 859) *arkabu* 'bat' → U$_5$.ARGAB^{mušen}
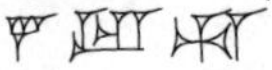

AŠ (AŠ, no. 1) → *ina* 'in, on'

B

BABBAR (UD, no. 596) → *peṣû* 'white'; *pūṣu* 'white spot'

BABBAR.HI^{sar} (UD, no. 596) → *papparhû* '*papparhû*-purslane'
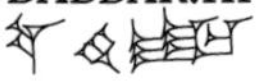

BAD (BAD, no. 113) → *petû* 'to open'

BAL (BAL, no. 5) → *naqû* 'to pour out (tears, water)'
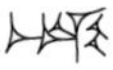 *nabalkutu* 'to cross over, change sides'

BAL.GI^{ku6} (BAL, no. 5) → *raqqu* 'turtle'
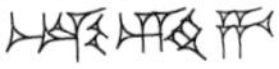

BAR (BAR, no. 121) → *ahû* 'stranger, non-canonical (material)'; *mišlu* 'half'
 *qilpu* 'skin of plant, fruit, peel'

BI (BI, no. 358) → *šū* 'this same, that'; *šuātu* 'that, this'

BIL (NE, no. 313) → *qalû* 'to roast'
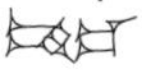

BÍL (BÍL, no. 312) → *qalû*(BIL)
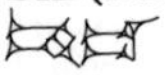

BIL.ZA.ZA (NE, no. 313) → *muṣa''irānu* '*muṣa''irānu*-frog'
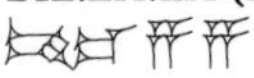

BÚN (BÚN, no. 54) → *napāhu* 'to blow; to light up, ignite'
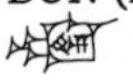

D

DAB (DIB, no. 813) → *ṣabātu* 'to seize, grasp, afflict'
 *kullu* 'to hold, contain, keep, retain'

DADAG (UD, no. 596) → *ebbu* 'pure'
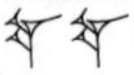

^{d}AG (AG, no. 127) → *Nabû* 'god Nabû'
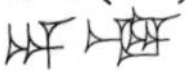

DAGAL (AMA, no. 392) → *rapšu* 'wide, great'
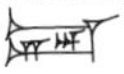

DIDA (BI, no. 358) → *billatu* 'beer mash'
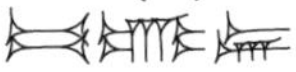

DÍLIM A.BÁR (LIŠ, no. 591) → *itqūr abāri* 'lead spoon(salve)'
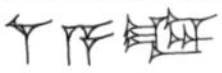

DIRI (DIR, no. 207) → *malû* 'to be(come) full of'
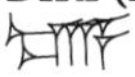

DIŠ (DIŠ, no. 748) → *ana* 'to, for, on, onto (also in compound prep.)'; *šumma* 'if'

^{d}*Nin-gìrima* (NIN, no. 887) → *Ningirimma* 'mistress of incantations'
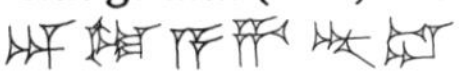

^{d}ŠE.TIR (ŠE, no. 579) → *ašnan* 'grain'
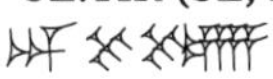

DU (DU, no. 350) → *alāku* 'to go (+ ventive to come)'

āliku 'moving, loose tissue in the eyes'

DÙ.A.BI (GAG, no. 379) → *kalû* 'everything, the whole of'
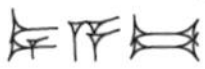

DÙ.DÙ.BI (GAG, no. 379) → *dudubi* 'its ritual, medical application'
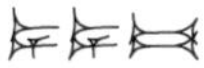

DÙ (GAG, no. 379) → *epēšu* 'to do, make'

DU$_{10}$ (HI, no. 631) → *ṭābu* 'sweet'

DU$_{8}$ (GAB, no. 298) → *paṭāru* 'to loosen'

DUB (DUB, no. 242) → *šapāku* 'to pour'
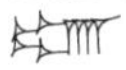

DUG (DUG, no. 499) → *karpatu* 'a vessel'
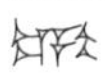

DUG A.GEŠTIN.NA (DUG, no. 499) → *karpat ṭābāti* 'vinegar vessel'
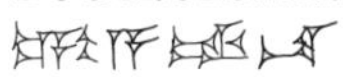

^{dug}BUR.ZI (BUR, no. 559) → *pursītu* '*pursītu*-bowl'
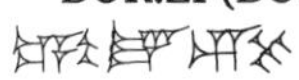

DUG$_{4}$.GA (KA, no. 24) → *qabû* 'to say, speak'
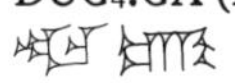

^{dug}GAN (GAN, no. 253) → *kannu* '*kannu*-jar'
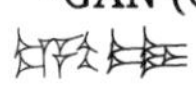

DUGUD (DUGUD, no. 704) → *kabātu* 'to become heavy'
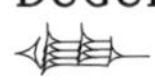

DUL (DUL, no. 720) → *katāmu* 'to cover objects, close the eye'

DUMU.MUNUS (TUR, no. 255) → *mārtu* 'daughter'

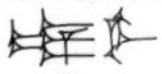

DUR (DUR, no. 178) → *ṭurru* 'a cord'

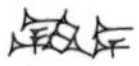

^{d}UTU.È (UD, no. 596) → *ṣīt šamši* 'sunrise'

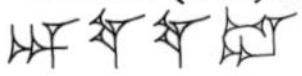

E

É (É, no. 495) → *bītu* 'house'

È (È, no. 596) → *aṣû* 'to go, come out'; *šakāku* 'to twist, thread (on a string)'

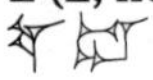

É.GAL (É, no. 495) → *ēkallu* 'palace'

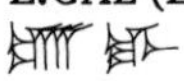

É.GAR$_8$ (É, no. 495) → *igāru* 'wall'

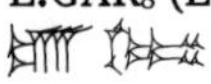

É.MEŠ (É, no. 495) → *ummātu* 'summer'

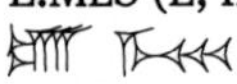

É.NU.RU (É, no. 495) → TU$_6$.ÉN.É.NU.RU

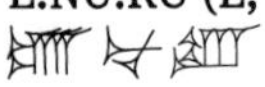

EGIR (EGIR, no. 356) → *arki* 'after(wards)'

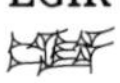

ÉLLAG (BIR, no. 643) → *kalītu* 'kidney'

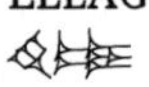

EME.DIR/ŠID (EME, no. 61) → *ṣurāru* 'lizard'

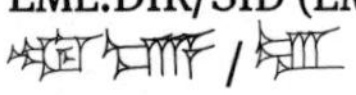

ÉN (ÉN, no. 870) → *šiptu* 'incantation'

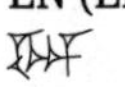

EN (EN, no. 164) → *adi* 'until'; *bēltu* 'mistress'

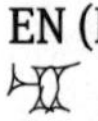

EN.TE.NA (EN, no. 164) → *kūṣu* 'winter'

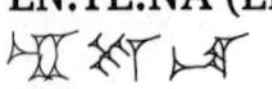

ÉR (A, no. 839) → *dimtu* 'tear(s)'

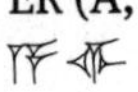

EREN (EREN, no. 818) → *erēnu* 'cedar tree'

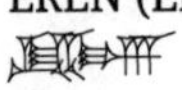

ESIR (A, no. 839) → *iṭṭû* 'liquid bitumen'

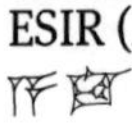

G

GA (GA, no. 491) → *šizbu* 'milk'

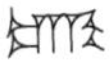

GAB.LÀL (GAB, no. 298) → *iškūru* 'wax'

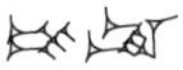

GAG.TI.TI (GAG.TI, no. 379) → *sikkat ṣēli* '(lamb) chop

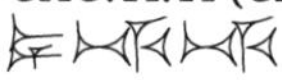

GAMUN.GE$_6$ (DIN, no. 119) → *zībû* 'black cumin'

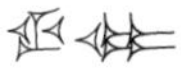

GAR (NÍG, no. 859) → *šakānu* 'to put, place, present'

GAZ (GAZ, no. 340) → *hašālu* 'to crush'

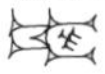

GAZI^{sar} (SILA$_4$, no. 408) → *kasû* '*kasû*-plant'

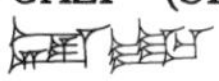

GE$_6$ (MI, no. 681) → *mūšu* 'night'; *ṣalmu* 'dark, black'

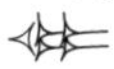

GEŠTIN.NA (GEŠTIN, no. 212) → *karānu* 'wine'

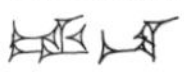

GEŠTU (PI, no. 598) → *uznu* 'ear, understanding'

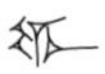

GI (GI, no. 141) → *qanû* 'reed'

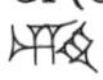

GIDIM (GIDIM, no. 830) → *eṭemmu* 'ghost'

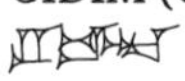

GI.ZÚ.LUM.MA (GI, no. 141) → Uncertain Readings and Words

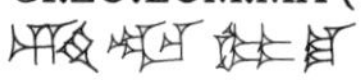

GÍD.DA (BU, no. 580) → *arku* 'long (of sheep's bones)'

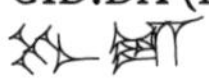

GIG (GIG, no. 705) → *marāṣu* 'to be sick'; *kibtu* 'wheat'

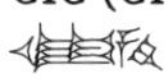

GIG.GA (GIG, no. 705) → *marṣu* 'sick'

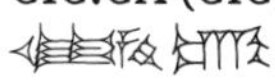

GIG.GIR (GIR, no. 558) → *kurāru* '*kurāru*-pustle'

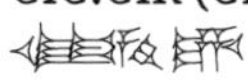

GIN (DU, no. 350) → *kânu* 'to establish, deposit, to set up'

GÍN (GÍN, no. 836) → *šiqlu* 'shekel'

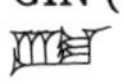

GIN$_7$ (GIM, no. 686) → *kīma* 'like, as'

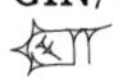

GÍR (GÍR, no. 6) → *patru* 'knife'

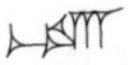

GÌR.PAD.DU/DA (GÍR , no. 6) → *eṣemtu* 'bone'

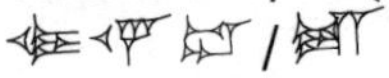

GÍR.ŠU.I (not in MZ) *naglabu* 'barber's knife, scalpel'

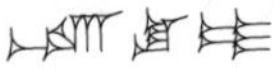

GÌRIMA → A.HA.TAR.DU

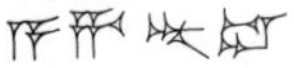

GISSU (GIŠ, no. 469) → *ṣillu* 'shadow/film (on/in the eye)'

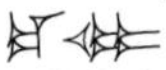

^{gi}SAG.KUD (SAG, no. 184) → *takkussu* 'reed-straw'

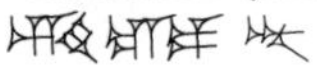

^{giš}DÁLA (IGI, no. 724) → *ṣillû* 'needle'

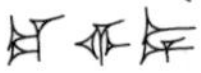

^{giš}ÉRIN (GIŠ, no. 469) → *gišrinnu* 'scale'

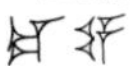

^{giš}GIŠIMMAR (SA$_6$, no. 571) → *gišimmaru* 'date palm'

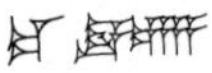

^{giš}GU.ZA (GU, no. 891) → *kussû* 'throne, seat'

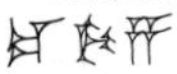

^{giš}GÚR.GÚR (GAM, no. 576) → *kukru* '*kukru*-aromatic'

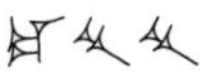

^{giš}HAB (LAGAB, no. 755) → *hūratu*'dyeing sumac'

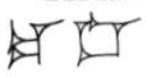

^{giš}HAŠHUR (HAŠHUR, no. 270) → *hašhūru* 'apple'

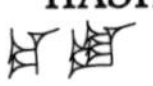

^{giš}IG (IG, no. 136) → *daltu* 'door'

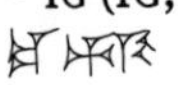

^{giš}MA.NU (MA, no. 552) → *ēru* '*ēru*-tree'

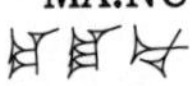

^{giš}MAŠ.HUŠ (MAŠ, no. 120) → *kalbānu* '*kalbānu*-plant (lit. dog-like plant)'

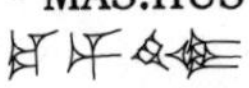

^{giš}MI.PÀR/PAR$_4$ (MI, no. 681) → *lipāru* '*lipāru*-tree'

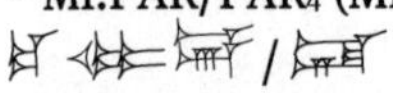

^{giš}NÁ (GIŠ, no. 469) → *eršu* 'bed'

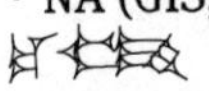

^{giš}NAM.TAR (NAM, no. 134) → *pillû* 'male *pillû*-plant'

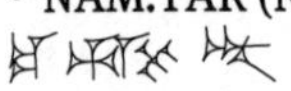

^{giš}NÍG.GÁN.GÁN (NÍG, no. 859) → *egemgīru* '*egemgīru*-plant'

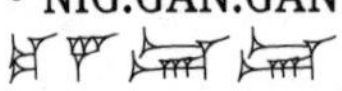

^{giš}NU.ÚR.MA (NU, no. 112) → *nurmû* 'pomegranate'

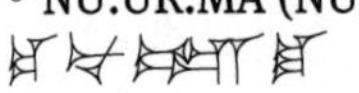

^{giš}PÈŠ (MA, no. 552) → *tittu* 'fig'

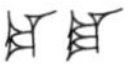

^{giš}ŠE.NÚ.A (ŠE, no. 579) → *šunû* '*šunû*-tree'

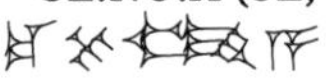

^{giš}ŠINIG (ŠINIG, no. 162) → *bīnu* 'tamarisk'

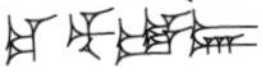

$^{\text{giš}}\text{KIŠI}_{16}$ (Ú, no. 490) → *ašāgu* '*ašāgu*-acacia'

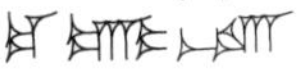

GÚ (GÚ, no. 176) → *kišādu* 'neck'

GÚ.GAL (GÚ, no. 176) → *hallūru* 'chickpea'

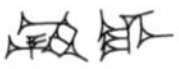

GÚ.TUR (GÚ, no. 176) → *kakkû* 'lentil'

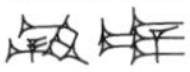

GU_4 (GU_4, no. 472) → *alpu* 'ox'

GU_7 (GU_7, no. 65) → *akālu* 'to eat, consume, hurt, cause pain'

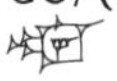

GUB (DU, no. 350) → *izuzzu* 'to stand, be present'

GÙB (KAB, no. 148) → *šumēlu* 'left (side)'

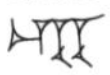

GUR (GUR, no. 180) → *târu* 'to return, repeat'

GURUN (GURUN, no. 503) → *inbu* 'fruit'

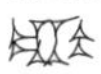

GURUŠ (KAL, no. 496) → *eṭlu* 'young man, lad'

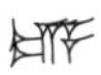

H

HÁD.DU (UD, no. 596) → *abālu* 'to dry'

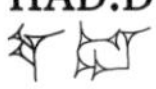

HE.HE (HI, no. 631) → *balālu* 'to mix'

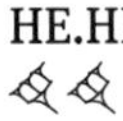

HÉNBUR (ŠE.GAG, no. 579) → *habburru* 'sprout'

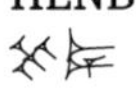

HUL (HUL, no. 733) → *lemnu* 'evil'

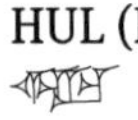

I

Ì(.GIŠ), Ì+GIŠ (NI, nos. 380, 436) → *šamnu* 'sesame oil'
𒉌(𒄑), 𒉌𒄑

Borger 2010: 325 transliterates Ì.ŠÉŠ mistakenly for Ì.ŠEŠ$_4$, see Stol 1979b: 177.

Ì.GIŠ.BUR (BUR, no. 559) → *šaman pūri* '*pūru*-oil'
𒉌𒄑𒁓

Ì.KUR.RA (NI, no. 380) → *napṭu* 'naphtha'
𒉌𒆳𒊏

Ì.NUN(.NA) (NI, no. 380) → *himētu* 'ghee'
𒉌𒉣(𒈾)

Ì.UDU (NI, no. 380) → *lipû* 'fat'
𒉌𒇻

IGI (IGI, no. 724) → *īnu* 'eye'; *naṭālu* 'to see'; *pānu* 'front, face'; *mahru* 'in front'
𒅆 amāru 'to see'

IGI.4.GÁL.LA (IGI, no. 724) → *rebiat* 'one-fourth'
𒅆𒐉𒅅𒆷

IGI.6.GÁL.LA (IGI, no. 724) → *šuššu* 'one-sixth'
𒅆𒐋𒅅𒆷

IGI.DU$_8$ (IGI, no. 724) → *amāru* 'to see'
𒅆𒂃

IGI.KÁR (IGI, no. 724) → *barû* 'to collate (a tablet); to check (a remedy)'
𒅆𒃻

IGI.SIG$_7$.SIG$_7$ (IGI, no. 724) → *amurriqānu* 'jaundice'
𒅆𒅊𒅊

ÍL (ÍL, no. 493) → *našû* 'to carry, lift, + ventive to bring, carry along, pick up'
𒅋

ILLU (A, no. 839) → *hīlu* 'resin'
𒀀𒆸

IM (IM, no. 641) → *šāru* 'wind'
𒅎

IM.1 (IM, no. 641) → *šūtu* 'south wind'
𒅎𒁹

IM.2 (IM, no. 641) → *iltānu* 'north wind'
𒅎𒈫

IM.3 (IM, no. 641) → *šadû* 'east wind'
𒅎𒐈

IM.4 (IM, no. 641) → *amurru* 'west wind'
𒅎𒐉

IM.GÚ.EN.NA (IM, no. 641) → *qadūtu šikāni* 'river silt'
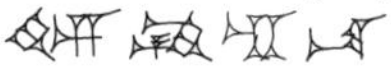
IM.SAHAR.BABBAR.KUR.RA (IM, no. 641) → *alluharu* '*alluharu*-mineral'
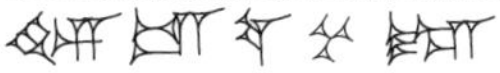
IM.SAHAR.NA_4.KUR.RA (IM, no. 641) → *gabû* '*gabû*-alum'
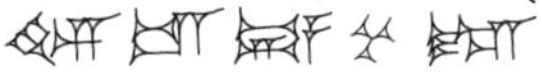
^{im}KAL (KAL, no. 496) → *kalû* '*kalû*-paste'
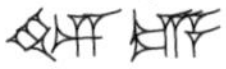
^{im}KAL.GUG (KAL, no. 496) → *kalgukku* '*kalgukku*-red paste'
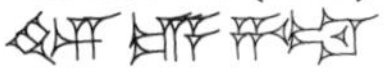
IN.NU (IN, no. 261) → *tibnu* 'straw'
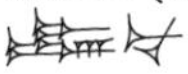
IN.NU.UŠ (IN, no. 261) → *maštakal* '*maštakal*-plant'
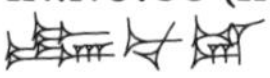
IR (IR, no. 437) → *zūtu* 'sweat'

ITI (ITI, no. 20) → *arhu* 'month'
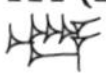
^{iti}BÁRA (ITI, no. 20) → *Nisannu* 'month Nisannu'
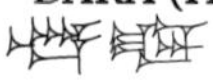
^{iti}NE (ITI, no. 20) → *Abu* 'month Ab'
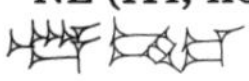
^{iti}AB (ITI, no. 20) → *Ṭebētu* 'month Tebet'
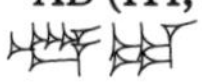
ITI.1.KÁM → ITI.1.KAM in Uncertain Readings and Words
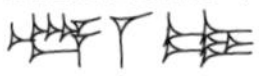
IZI (IZI, no. 313) → *išātu* 'fire'
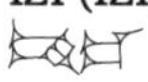

K

KÁ (KÁ, no. 222) → *bābu* 'entrance-door'
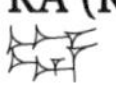
KA (KA, no. 24) → *pû* 'mouth, opening'
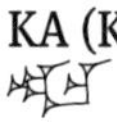
KA.A.AB.BA (KA, no. 24) → *imbuʾ tâmti* 'algae'
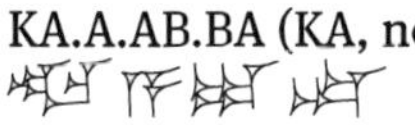
KA.INIM.MA (KA, no. 24) → *kaʾinimma* 'invocation'
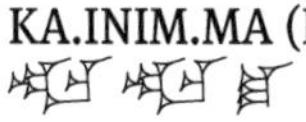
KA.KEŠDA (KA, no. 24) → *kiṣru* 'knots'
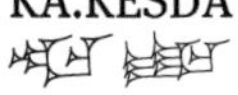

KALA.GA (KAL, no. 496) → *dannu* 'strong'
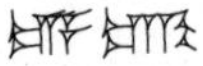
KÀŠ (KÀŠ, no. 384) → *šīnātu* 'urine'
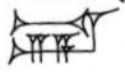
KAŠ (BI, no. 358) → *šikaru* 'beer'

KEŠDA (EZEN, no. 271) → *kaṣāru* 'to tie, knot'
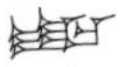
rakāsu 'to bind, bandage body parts'
KI (KI, no. 737) → *itti* 'with'

KI.NÁ (KI, no. 737) → *mayyālu* 'bed'
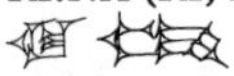
KÌD.KÌD.BI (AG, no. 127) → *kidkidbi* 'its ritual'
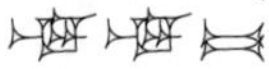
KIN (KIN, no. 815) → *šipru* 'effect'; 'skill'

KISAL (KISAL, no. 435) → see SILA$_{x/4}$(KISAL) Uncertain Readings and Words
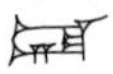
KÙ (KUG, no. 745) → *ellu* 'clean, holy'

KÙ.BABBAR (KUG, no. 745) → *kaspu* 'silver'
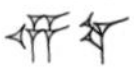
KÙ.GAN (KUG, no. 745) → *lulû* '*lulû*-antimony'
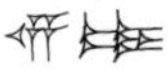
KUG.GI (KUG, no. 745) → *hurāṣu* 'gold'
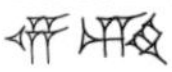
KU.KU (KU, no. 808) → *uṭṭatu* 'grain (also as a measure)'
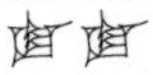
KU$_4$ (KU$_4$, no. 87) → *erēbu* 'enter, go down, set (for sun)'
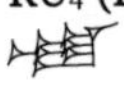
KUD (TAR, no. 9) → *nakāsu* 'to cut'; *parāsu* 'to cease, stop'

KÚM (NE, no. 313) → *ummu* '*ummu*-fever (lit. heat, summer)'; *emmu* 'hot'
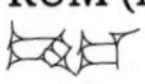
KUN$_4$ (I, no. 252) → *askuppu* 'threshold'
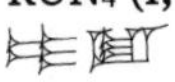
KUR (KUR, no. 578) → *mātu* 'land, earth'; *šadû* 'mountain'

KUR.GI^{mušen} (KUR, no. 578) → *kurkû* 'goose'
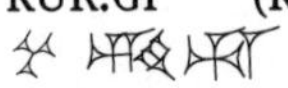
KUŠ (SU, no. 16) → *mašku* 'leather bag'
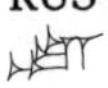

KUŠ.EDIN (not in MZ) → *nādu* 'waterskin'
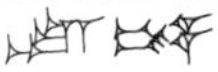

L

LAL (LAL, no. 750) → *ṣamādu* 'to bandage'; *tarāṣu* 'to spread out (a cloth)'

LÀL (LÀL, no. 170) → *dišpu* 'honey'

LÀL.KUR.(RA) (LÀL, no. 170) → *dišip šadê/î* 'mountain honey'
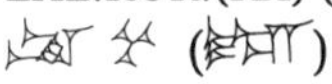

LI.DUR/TAR (LI, no. 85) → *abukkatu* '*abukkatu*-plant'
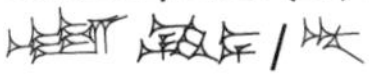

LIBIR.RA (LIBIR, no. 732) → *labīru* 'old'
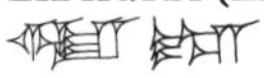

LÚ (LÚ, no. 514) → *amēlu* 'a man'
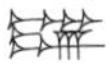

^{lú}A.ZU (A, no. 839) → *asû* 'physician'
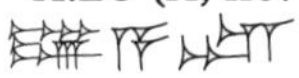

^{lú}AŠGAB (AŠGAB, no. 173) → *aškāpu* 'leatherworker'
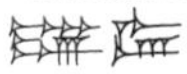

LUGAL (LUGAL, no. 266) → *šarru* 'king'
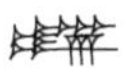

LÚGUD.DA (LAGAB, no. 755) → *kurû* 'short'
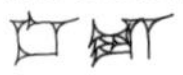

LUH (LUH, no. 494) → *mesû* 'to wash'
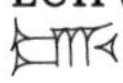

^{lú}TU.RA (TU, no. 86) → *marṣu* 'sick man'
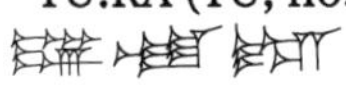

^{lú}TUR (TUR, no. 255) → *ṣehru* 'a chick'; 'a child'
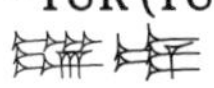

LÚ.U_{19}.LU (LÚ, no. 514) → *amēlu* 'a man'
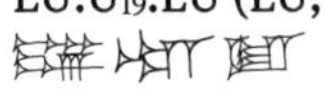

M

20 (MAN, no. 708) → *šarru* 'king'

MAR (MAR, no. 483) → *equ* 'to daub'; *zarû* 'scatter, spatter, sprinkle'
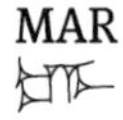

MAŠ.DÀ (MAŠ, no. 120) → *ṣabītu* 'gazelle'

MAŠ.MAŠ (MAŠ, no. 120) → *mašmašu* '*mašmašu*-healer'

MAŠ.TAB.BA (MAŠ, no. 120) → *māšu* 'a twin'

MÁŠ.TUR (MÁŠ, no. 130) → *lalû* 'a kid, young goat'

MIN (not in MZ) → *šanîš* 'alternatively'

MÚ (SAR, no. 541) → *napāhu* 'to blow; to light up, ignite'

MÚD (BAD, no. 113) → *dāmu* 'blood'
MÚD not ÚŠ, see the syllabic spelling in IGI 1: 118' (NB iii 3)

MUD (MUD, no. 137) → *uppu* 'tube'

MUL (MUL, no. 247) → *kakkabu* 'a star'

MUN (MUN, no. 168) → *ṭābtu* 'salt'

MUNU$_6$ (BÙLUG, no. 94) → *buqlu* 'malt'
(NF ii' 10') (NZ ii 10') NB.: many variants

MUNUS (MUNUS, no. 883) → *sinništu* 'female'

munusKI.SIKIL (KI, no. 737) → *ardatu* 'young woman, maiden'

munusÚ.ZÚG (Ú, no. 490) → *musukkatu* 'a woman in maternity'

MURUB$_4$ (MÚRU, no. 545) → *qablu* 'middle'

MUŠ.GE$_6$ (MUŠ, no. 585) → *ṣallāmtu* 'black snake'

N

NÁ (NÁ, no. 689) → *ṣalālu* 'to sleep, lie down'

NA (NA, no. 110) → *amēlu* 'a man'

NÁ (NÁ, no. 689) → *itūlu* 'to lie down'; *nâlu* 'to lie down'

NA$_4$ (NA$_4$, no. 385) → *abnu* 'stone, bead'

NA$_4$ BAL (not in MZ) → *aban tašrīti* '*tašrītu*-stone'

^{na4}AN.NA (AN, no. 10) → *annakku* 'tin'

^{na4}AN.ZAH (AN, no. 10) → *anzahhu* '*anzahhu*-glass (bead)'

^{na4}AN.ZAH.BABBAR (AN, no. 10) → *huluhhu* '*huluhhu*-slag (bead)'

^{na4}AN.ZAH.GE$_6$ (AN, no. 10) → *kutpû* 'black frit (bead)'

^{na4}ÁŠ.GI$_4$.GI$_4$ (ÁŠ, no. 548) → *ašgikû* '*ašgikû*-stone'

^{na4}BAR.DÙ.E (not in MZ) → *mešēltu* '*mešēltu*-whetstone'

^{na4}GUG (GUG, no. 858) → *sāmtu* 'carnelian'

^{na4}KA.GI.NA.DAB.BA (KA, no. 24) → *šadânu ṣābitu* 'magnetite'

^{na4}MUŠ.GÍR (MUŠ, no. 585) → *muššaru* 'sardonyx'

^{na4}NÍR (ZA, no. 851) → *hulālu* 'banded agate (onyx)'

^{na4}ŠU.MÌN (not in MZ) → *šumēnu* '*šumēnu*-mineral'

^{na4}ŠUBA (ZA, no. 851) → *šubû* '*šubû*-stone'

^{na4}ZA.GÌN (ZA, no. 851) → *uqnû* 'blue stone, mostly lapis lazuli'

^{na4}ZA.GÌN.DURU$_5$ (ZA, no. 851) → *zagindurû* '*zagindurû*-lapis lazuli'

^{na4}ZÁLAG (ERIM, no. 612) → *zalāqu* '*zalāqu*-stone'

^{na4}ZÚ (KA, no. 24) → *ṣurru* 'flint (knife)'

NAG (NAG, no. 64) → *šaqû* 'to give to drink'; *šatû* 'to drink'

NAGA.SI (NAGA, no. 293) → *uhūlu qarnānû* 'horned *uhūlu*-alkali'

NAM.LÚ.U$_{19}$.LU (NAM, no. 134 and 514) → *amēlūtu* 'human'

NE (NE, no. 313) → *pēmtu* 'charcoal'

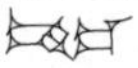

NÍG.BA (BA, no. 14) → *qīštu* 'fee'

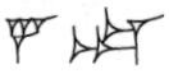

NÍG.NA (NÍG, no. 859 → *nignakku* 'incense burner'

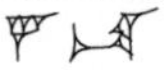

NÍG.SILA$_{11}$.GÁ (NÍG, no. 859) → *līšu* 'dough'

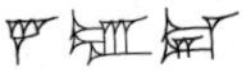

NIGIN (NIGIN, no. 804) → *lamû* 'wrap up'

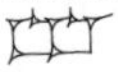

NIM.GÍR (NIM, no. 690) → *berqu* 'lighting'

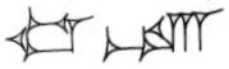

NINDA (NÍG, no. 859) → *akalu* 'loaf of bread'

NININDU (LAGAB×NÍG, no. 801) → *tinūru* 'tannour oven'

NITA (UŠ, no. 381) → *zikaru* 'man, male'

NÍTA (ARAD, no. 18) → *zikaru* 'man, male'

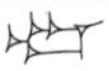

NU (NU, no. 112) → *lā* 'no, not, without'; *ul* 'no, not'

NU.LUH.HA^{sar} (NU, no. 112) → *nuhurtu* '*nuhurtu*-plant'

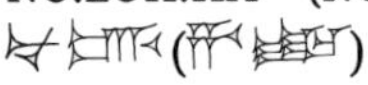

NU.NU (NU, no. 112) → *ṭamû* to spin'

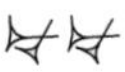

NUMUN (NUMUN, no. 117) → *zēru* 'seed(s)'

NUNDUM (NUNDUM, no. 31) → *šaptu* 'lip'

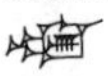

NUNUZ (NUNUZ, no. 614) → *pelû* 'egg'

P

PA (PA, no. 464) → *artu* 'foliage, leafs'; *kappu* 'eyelid'

PAP (PAB, no. 92) → *naphar* 'total'

PIŠ$_{10}$.^{d}ÍD (KI, no. 737) → *kibrītu* '*kibrītu*-sulphur'

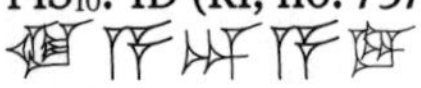

PÚ (TÚL, no. 786) → *būrtu* ‘well’

S

SA (SA, no. 172) → *šer’ānu* ‘sinew/tendon’

SA$_5$ (DIR, no. 207) → *sāmu* ‘red’
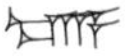

SAG (SAG, no. 184) → *qaqqadu* ‘head’; *rūštu* ‘first class, premium’
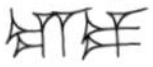 *rēšu* ‘upper part’

SAG.DU (SAG, no. 184) → *qaqqadu* ‘head’
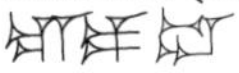

SAG.KI (SAG, no. 184) → *nakkaptu* ‘head-temple’; *pūtu* ‘forehead’
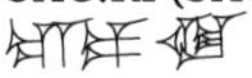

SAG.UŠ (SAG, no. 184) → *kayyamānu* ‘regularly, again and again’
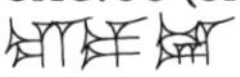

SAHAR (IŠ, no. 357) → *eperu* ‘dust’
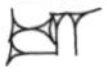

SAHAR.KÙ.GI (not in MZ) → *lēru* ‘*lēru*-paste’
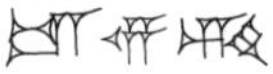

SAHAR.URUDU (IŠ, no. 357) → *šuhtu* ‘copper patina’
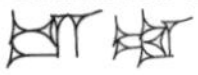

SAR (SAR, no. 541) → *galābu* ‘to shave’
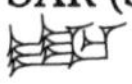

SAR.MUNU$_6$ (not in MZ) → *bāqilu* ‘malster’
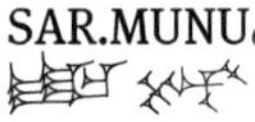

SED (SED, no. 155) → *kaṣû* ‘cold’
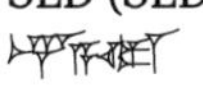

SI (SI, no. 181) → *qarnu* ‘horn’
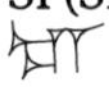

SÍG (SÍG, no. 816) → *šārtu* ‘hair’; *šīpātu* ‘wool’
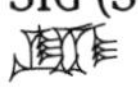

SIG$_5$ (SIG$_5$, no. 729) → *damqu* ‘good’
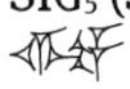

SIG$_7$ (SIG$_7$, no. 564) → *arqu* ‘yellow-green’; *arqūtu* ‘freshness’
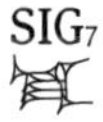

^{síg}ÀKA (ŠID, no. 485) → *itqu* ‘woollen tuft’
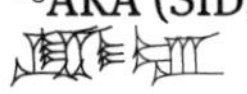

^{síg}HÉ.MED/ME.DA (GAN, no. 253) → *nabāsu* ‘red wool’
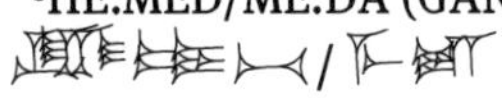

SILA (TAR, no. 9) → *sūqu* ‘street’

SILA$_x$(KISAL, no. 435) → see SILA$_x$(KISAL) Uncertain Readings and Words
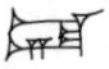

SILA$_4$ (SILA$_4$, no. 408) → see SILA$_4$!(KISAL) Uncertain Readings and Words
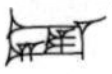

SILA$_{11}$ (ŠID, no. 485) → *lâšu* ‘to knead’
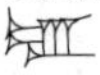

SILIM (DI, no. 736) → *šalāmu* ‘to be safe’

SIM (NAM, no. 134) → *napû* ‘to sift’
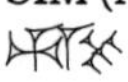

SU (SU, no. 16) → *zumru* ‘body’
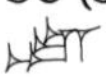

SÚD (ŠÌTA, no. 139) → *sâku* ‘to pound’
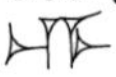

SUHUŠ (SUHUŠ, no. 351) → *šuršu* ‘root’
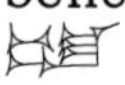

SUM.SIKIL (SUM, no. 292) → *šamaškillu* ‘*šamaškillu*-onion’
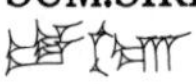

SUM^{sar} (SUM, no. 292) → *šūmū* ‘garlic’
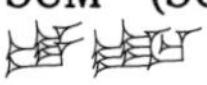

SUMUN (BAD, no. 113) → *labāru* ‘to be(come) old, long-lasting’; *labīru* ‘old’

SÚN (GUL, no. 682) → *rīmtu* ‘wild cow’
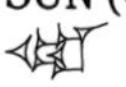

SUR (SUR, no. 151) → *ṣahātu* ‘to press out, draw liquid into vessel’

Š

ŠÀ (ŠÀ, no. 599) → *libbu* ‘middle, midst of’; ‘internal organ/heart’

‘offshoot (of date palm)’

ŠAH (ŠAH, no. 23) → *šahû* ‘pig’
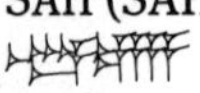

ŠE (ŠE, no. 579) → *še’u* ‘grain’; *uṭṭatu* ‘grain (also as a measure)’

ŠE.BAR (ŠE, no. 579) → *uṭṭatu* ‘grain (also as a measure)’
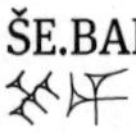

ŠE.GA (ŠE, no. 579) → *magāru* ‘to be favourable’
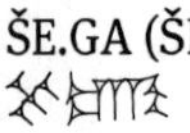

ŠE.SA.A (ŠE, no. 579) → *labtu* 'roasted grain'
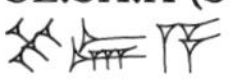
ŠE$_{10}$ (KU, no. 808) → *zû* 'excrement'

ŠEG$_6$(.GA) (NE, no. 313) → *bašālu* 'to be cooked'; *bašlu* 'boiled'
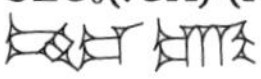
ŠEN.TUR (ŠEN, no. 17) → *tangussu* 'copper *tangussu*-kettle'
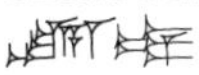
ŠÉŠ (ŠÉŠ, no. 821) → *pašāšu* 'to smear, anoint'
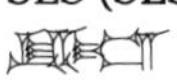
ŠEŠ (ŠEŠ, no. 535) → *annû* 'this, these'
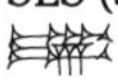
ŠID (ŠID, no. 485) → *manû* 'to recite'
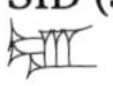
ŠIKA (LA, no. 89) → *haṣbu* 'potsherd, sherd, peel, flake'

^{šim}BAL (BAL, no. 5) → *ballukku* '*ballukku*-aromatic'
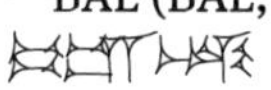
ŠIM.BI.KÙ.GI (ŠIM, no. 362) → *šīpu* '*šīpu*-paste'
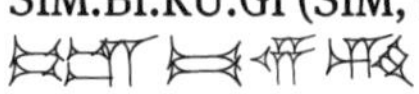
ŠIM.BI.ZI.DA (ŠIM, no. 362) → *šimbizidû* '*šimbizidû*-galena'
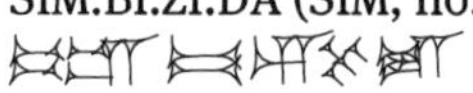
^{šim}BULUH (HAL, no. 3) → *baluhhu* '*baluhhu*-aromatic'
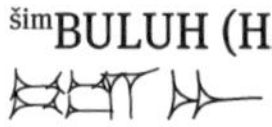
^{šim}GAM.MA (GAM, no. 576) → *ṣumlalû* '*ṣumlalû*-aromatic plant'
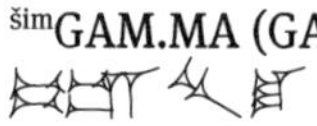
^{šim}GIG (GIG, no. 705) → *kanaktu* '*kanaktu*-aromatic'
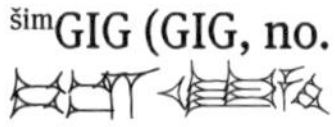
^{šim}GÍR (GÍR, no. 6) → *asu* '*asu*-aromatic'
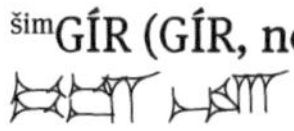
^{šim}GÚR.GÚR (GAM, no. 576) → *kukru* '*kukru*-aromatic'
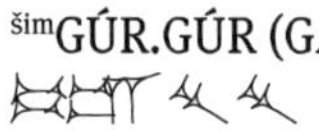
^{šim}HAB (LAGAB, no. 755) → *ṭūru* '*ṭūru*-plant'
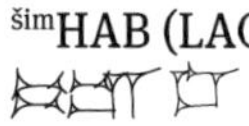
^{šim}LI (LI, no. 85) → *burāšu* 'juniper'
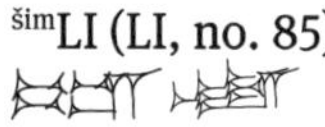
^{šim}MAN.DU (MAN, no. 708) → *suādu* '*suādu*-aromatic'
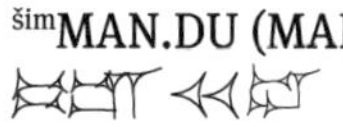
^{šim}MUG (MUG, no. 12) → *ballukku* '*ballukku*-aromatic'
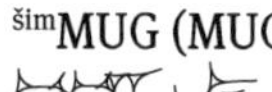
^{šim}ŠE.LI (ŠE, no. 579) → *kikkirânu* '*kikkirânu*-aromatic'
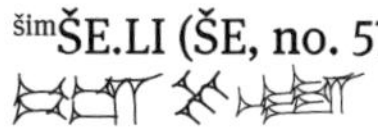

^{šim}SES (ŠEŠ, no. 535) → *murru* 'bitter-plant'
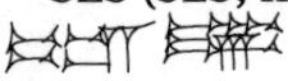

ŠU (ŠU, no. 567) → *qātu* 'hand'

ŠÚ (ŠÚ, no. 869) → *kiššatu* 'world'

ŠU.GIDIM.MA (ŠU, no. 567) → *šugidimmakku* 'hand of a ghost'
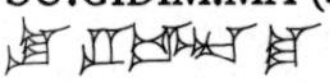

ŠU.LÚ.ZABAR (not in MZ) → *mušālu* 'bronze palette, mirror'
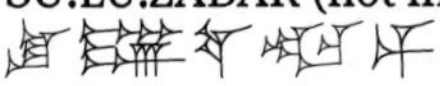

ŠU.SAR (ŠU, no. 576) → *pitiltu* 'string'
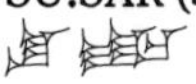

ŠU.SI (ŠU, no. 567) → *ubānu* 'finger'
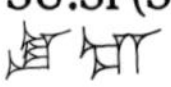

ŠU.TI (ŠU, no. 567) → *leqû* 'to take, accept, + ventive to bring'
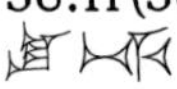

ŠUB (RU, no. 111) → *nadû* 'to put, apply…'
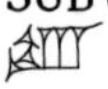

ŠURUN (U_8, no. 766) → *kabūtu* 'dung'
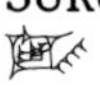

T

TAB (TAB, no. 209) → *ṭepû* 'to apply (drugs), add (ingredients)'
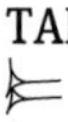

TE (TE, no. 589) → *ṭehû* 'to be(come) near to, approach'
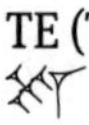

TI (TI, no. 118) → *balāṭu* 'to live, heal, recover'; *bulṭu* 'life'
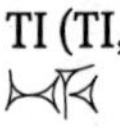

TI.LA (TI, no. 118) → *balāṭu* 'to live, heal, recover'; *balṭu* 'healthy'
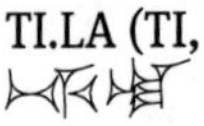

TI (TI, no. 118) → *leqû* 'to take, accept, + ventive to bring'
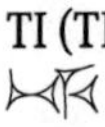

$TI_8^{mušen}$ (Á, no. 560) → *erû* '*erû*-eagle'
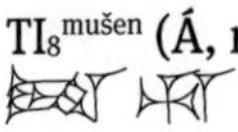

TU_5 (ŠU, no. 567) → *ramāku* 'to bathe, soak'
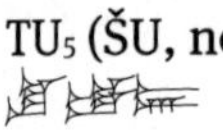

TU_6 (TU_6, no. 26) → *tû* 'incantation'
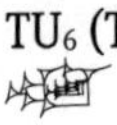

TU_6.ÉN (TU_6, no. 26) → *tê šipti*
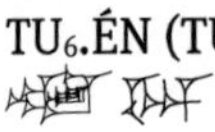

TU$_6$.ÉN.É.NU.RU → Uncertain Readings and Words
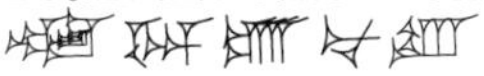
TÚG (TÚG, no. 809) → *ṣubātu* 'cloth'

^{túg}ŠÀ.HA (TÚG, no. 809) → *šahhû* '*šahhû*-cloth'
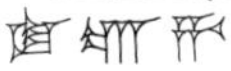
TUK (TUK, no. 827) → *rašû* 'to acquire, to develop a disease'
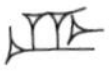
TU^{mušen} (TU, no. 86) → *summatu* 'pigeon'
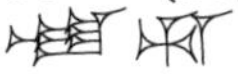
TÙR (TÙR, no. 146) → *tarbaṣu* 'animal stall'
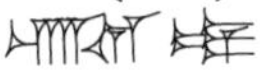
TUR (TUR, no. 255) → *ṣehru* 'small, young'

U

Ú (Ú, no. 490) → *šammu* 'plant, drug'
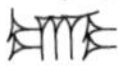
Ú.BABBAR (Ú, no. 490) → *šammu peṣû* 'white plant'
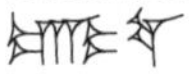
Ú.DILI (AŠ, no. 1) → *šammu ēdu* 'single plant'
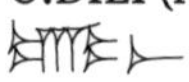
Ù.TU (Ù, no. 731) → *alādu* 'to give birth'
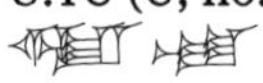
U$_5$.ARGAB^{mušen} (U$_5$, nos. 133 and 859) → *rikibti arkabi* 'bat guano'
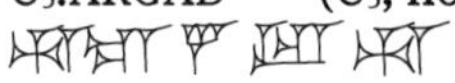
U$_8$ (U$_8$, no. 766) → *lahru* 'ewe'

UD (UD, no. 596) → *ūmu* 'day'; *enūma* 'when'
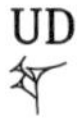
UD.1/3/9/14/15/20/21.KAM/KÁM/KAM* → Uncertain Readings and Words
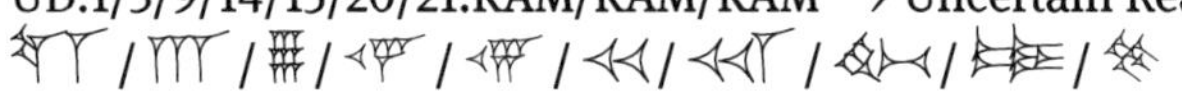
UD.DA (UD, no. 596) → *ṣētu* 'sun heat'
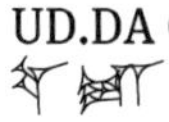
UD$_5$ (ÙZ, no 203) → *enzu* 'goat'
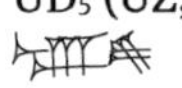
UDU (LU, no. 812) → *immeru* 'sheep'
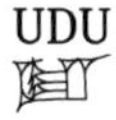
UDU.NÍTA (LU, no. 812) → *immeru* 'male sheep'
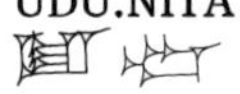

UDU.SISKUR (SISKUR, no. 696) → *niqû* 'offering'
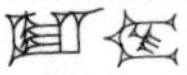

ᵘEME.UR.GI₇ (not in MZ) → *lišān kalbi* 'dog's tongue plant'
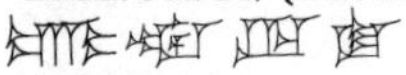

ᵘESI (KAL, no. 496) → *ušû* '*ušû*-plant'
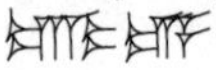

ᵘGAMUN (DIN, no. 119) → *kamūnu* 'cumin'
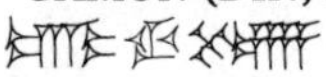

UGA^mušen (UGA, no. 490) → *āribu* 'raven'
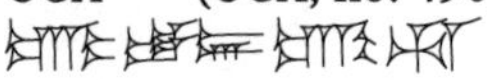

ᵘGEŠTIN.KA₅.A (not in MZ) → *karān šēlebi* 'fox-vine'
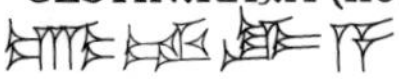

UGU (UGU, no. 663) → *eli* 'on, over, above'
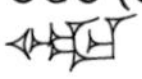
muhhu 'cranium, brain, top'; 'top, upper part, surface'

ᵘGÚR.UŠ (not in MZ) → *šarmadu* '*šarmadu*-plant'
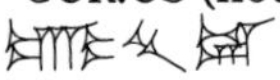

ÚH (ÚH, no. 611) → *ru'tu* 'spittle'
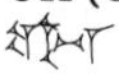

ÚH-ᵈÍD (ÚH, no. 611) → *ru'tītu* '*ru'tītu*-sulphur (lit. river spittle)'
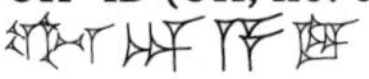

ᵘHA (HA, no. 856) → *urânu* '*urânu*-plant'
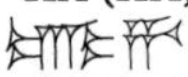

ᵘHAR.HAR (HAR, no. 644) → *hašû* '*hašû*-thyme'
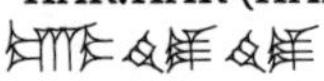

ᵘIGI-*lim* (IGI, no. 724) → *imhur-līm* '*imhur-līm*-plant'
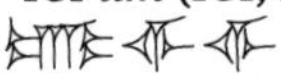

ᵘIGI-NIŠ (IGI, no. 724) → *imhur-ešrā* '*imhur-ešrā*-plant'
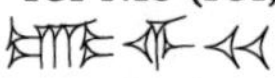

ᵘIN.NU.UŠ (IN, no. 261) → *maštakal* '*maštakal*-plant'
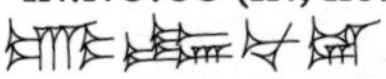

ᵘIN₆.ÚŠ (AŠ, no. 1) → *maštakal* '*maštakal*-plant'
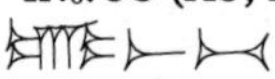

ᵘKI.ᵈIŠKUR (KI, no. 737) → *qudru* '*qudru*-plant'
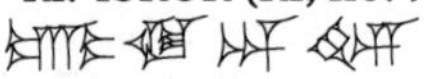

ᵘKUR.KUR (KUR, no. 578) → *atā'išu* '*atā'išu*-plant'
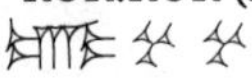

ᵘKUR.RA (Ú, no. 490) → *nīnû* '*nīnû*-mint'
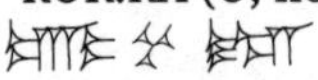

ᵘKUR₄.GI.RIN.NA (not in MZ) → *kurkānû* '*kurkānû*-plant'
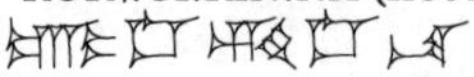 (LAGAB in ND ii 41 )

UL (UL, no. 698) → *kakkabu* 'a star'

^{ú}MAŠ.TAB.BA (MAŠ, no. 120) → *māš(t)u* '*māš(t)u*-twin plant'
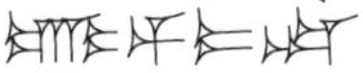

UMBIN (UMBIN, no. 160) → *ṣupru* '(toe-) nail'
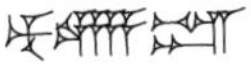

UM.ME.A (UM, no. 248) → *ummânu* 'wise man'
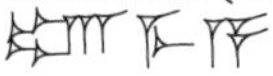

^{ú}NAGA.SI (NAGA, no. 293) → *uhūlu qarnānû* 'horned *uhūlu*-alkali'
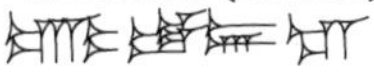

^{ú}NÍG.GIDRU (PA, no. 464) → *haṭṭi rē'î* 'shepherd's-staff plant'
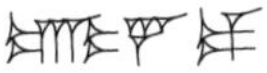

UR.BI (UR, no. 828) → *ištēniš* 'together'
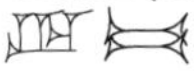

ÙR (ÙR, no. 411) → *ūru* 'roof'
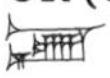

UR.GI$_7$ (UR, no. 828) → *kalbu* 'dog'
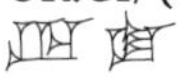

UR.MAH (UR, no. 828) → *nēšu* 'lion'
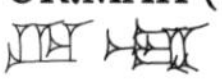

URUDU (URUDU, no. 230) → *erû* '*erû*-copper'

^{ú}SIKIL (EL, no. 899) → *sikillu* '*sikillu*-plant'
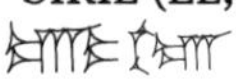

ÚŠ (BAD, no. 113) → *sekēru* 'to heat'

^{ú}ÚKUŠ.LAGAB (HÚL, no. 877) → *errû* '*errû*-colocynth'
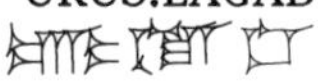

^{ú}UR.TÁL.TÁL (UR, no. 828) → *uzun lalî* 'young goat's-ear plant'
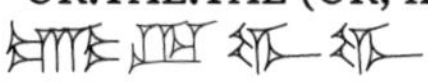

^{ú}ZA.BA.LAM (ZA, no. 851) → *supālu* '*supālu*-juniper'
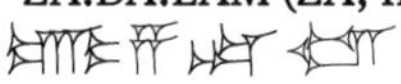

^{ú}ZA.GÌN.NA (ZA, no. 851) → *uqnâtu* '*uqnâtu*-blue-plant'
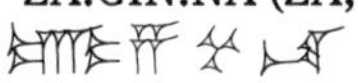

UZU (UZU, no. 311) → *šēru* 'flesh'
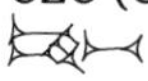

^{uzu}ZÍ (ZÍ, no. 259) → *martu* 'gall bladder'
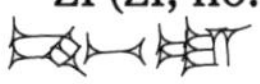

Z

ZÀ.HI.LI(.A^{sar}) (ZAG, no. 540) → *sahlû* '*sahlû*-plant'
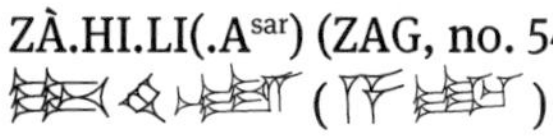

ZA.NA (ZA, no. 851) → *passu* ‘collyrium stick (lit. game disk)’
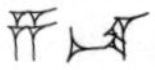

ZABAR (UD, no. 596) → *siparru* ‘bronze’
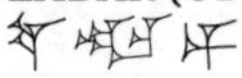

ZAG (ZAG, no. 540) → *imittu* ‘right side’
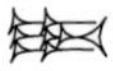

ZALAG.GA (not in MZ) → *namāru* ‘to be(come) bright, shine’
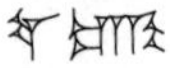

ZI (ZI, no. 140) → *nasāhu* ‘to tear out, remove’; *tebû* ‘to rise, throb’
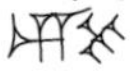 *tību* ‘rising (of wind)’

ZÍ (ZÍ, no. 259) → *martu* ‘bile’
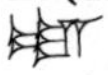

ZÌ (ŠÈ, no. 810) → *qēmu* ‘flour, powder’

ZÌ.DUB.DUB.BU (ŠÈ, no. 810) → *zidubdubbû* ‘a heap of flour’
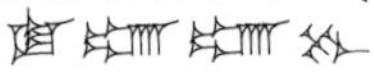

ZÌ.KUM (ŠÈ, no. 810) → *isqūqu* ‘coarse flour’
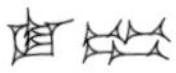

ZÚ.LUM.MA (KA, no. 24) → *suluppu* ‘date’
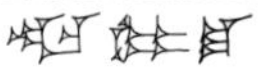

Abbreviations and Literature

Abbreviations, which have been used to a minimum, can be found at http://www.rla.badw.de/reallexikon/abkuerzungslisten.html.

Additional Abbreviations

DJBA	Sokoloff, M. 2002. *A Dictionary of Jewish Babylonian Aramaic of the Talmudic and Geonic Periods.* Ramat-Gan, Israel: Bar Ilan University Press; Baltimore: Johns Hopkins University Press.
Jastrow Dictionary	Jastrow, M. 1950. *A Dictionary of the Targumim, the Talmud Babli and the Yerushalmi, and the Midrashic Literature.* New York: Pardes Publishing House.
Mandaic Dictionary	Drower, E.S. and R. Macuch. 1963. *A Mandaic Dictionary.* Oxford: Clarendon Press.
SEAL	http://www.seal.uni-leipzig.de.
UH	Udug-hul incantations, see Geller 2016 below.

Literature

Abrahami 2014 = P. Abrahami. Wool in the Nuzi Texts. In *Wool Economy in the Ancient Near East and the Aegean. From the Beginnings of Sheep Husbandry to Institutional Textile Industry*, eds. C. Breniquet and C. Michel. Ancient Textiles Series 17. Oxford and Philadelphia: Oxbow Books: 283–309.

Abusch 2015 = T. Abusch, *The Witchcraft Series Maqlû*. Atlanta, Georgia: SBL Press.

Abusch 2016 = T. Abusch. *The Magical Ceremony Maqlû: A Critical Edition.* Ancient Magic and Divination 10. Leiden and Boston: Brill.

Abusch and Schwemer 2011 = T. Abusch, T. and D. Schwemer. *Corpus of Mesopotamian Anti-Witchcraft Rituals*, Volume 1. Ancient Magic and Divination 8/1. Leiden and Boston: Brill.

Abusch, Schwemer, Luuko, Van Buylaere 2016 = T. Abusch, D. Schwemer, M. Luukko, and G. Van Buylaere. *Corpus of Mesopotamian Anti-Witchcraft Rituals*, Volume 2. Ancient Magic and Divination 8/2. Leiden and Boston: Brill.

Ambos 2013 = C. Ambos. *Der König im Gefängnis und das Neujahrsfest im Herbst: Mechanismen der Legitimation des babylonischen Herrschers im 1. Jahrtausend v. Chr. und ihre Geschichte.* Dresden: Islet.

Annus 2019 = A. Annus. The Spiritual Dimensions of Healing Rituals in Ancient Mesopotamia. *Journal of Religion and Health*, https://doi.org/10.1007/s10943-019-00964-x.

Arkhipov 2009 = I. Arkhipov. L'usage médical du plomb à Mari. *Le Journal des Médecines Cunéiformes* 13: 48.

Arnaud 1987 = D. Arnaud. *Textes de la bibliothèque, transcriptions et traductions.* Recherches au pays d'aštata. EMAR 6/4. Paris: Editions Recherche sur les Civilisations.

Arnaud 2007 = D. Arnaud. *Corpus des textes de bibliothèque de Ras Shamra-Ougarit (1936–2000): en sumérien, babylonien et assyrien*. Aula Orientalis. Supplementa 23. Sabadell: Ausa.

https://doi.org/10.1515/9781501506550-014

Arnott 2002 = R. Arnott. Disease and Medicine in Hittite Asia Minor. In *The Archaeology of medicine : papers given at a session of the annual conference of the Theoretical Archaeology Group held at the University of Birmingham on 20 December 1998*, ed. R. Arnott. BAR international series 1046. Oxford: Archaeopress: 41–52.

Arnott 2004 = R. Arnott, Minoan and Mycenaean Medicine and its Near Eastern Contacts. In *Magic and Rationality in Ancient Near Eastern and Graeco-Roman Medicine*, eds. H.F.J. Horstmanshoff and M. Stol. Studies in Ancient Medicine 27. Leiden-Boston: Brill: 153–173.

Attia 2015 = A. Attia. Traduction et commentaires des trois premières tablettes de la série IGI. *Le Journal des Médecines Cunéiformes* 25: 1–120.

Attia and Buisson 2003 = A. Attia and G. Buisson. Si le crâne d'un homme contient de la chaleur, deuxième tablette. *Le Journal des Médecines Cunéiformes* 1: 1–24.

Attia and Buisson 2007 = A. Attia and G. Buisson. K 2392, un nouveau joint pour UGU 2. *Le Journal des Médecines Cunéiformes* 9: 47–48.

Attia and Buisson 2012 = A. Attia and G. Buisson. BAM 1 et consorts en transcription. *Le Journal des Médecines Cunéiformes* 19: 22–51.

Attinger 2008 = P. Attinger. La médecine mésopotamienne. *Le Journal des Médecines Cunéiformes* 11–12: 1–96.

Bácskay 2015 = A. Bácskay. Magical-medical prescriptions against fever: an edition of BM 42272. Le Journal des Médecines Cunéiformes 26: 1–32.

Bácskay 2018a = A. Bácskay. *Therapeutic Prescriptions against Fever in Ancient Mesopotamia.* Alter Orient und Altes Testament 447. Münster: Ugarit.

Bácskay 2018b = A. Bácskay. 'Seize a frog!' The use of the frog in medical and magical texts. *Le Journal des Médecines Cunéiformes* 32: 1–16.

Bácskay 2018c = A. Bácskay. The 34th Extract of the UGU Series from Babylon: An Edition of the Tablet BM 35512. In *Mesopotamian Medicine and Magic. Studies in Honor of Markham J. Geller*, ed. S.V. Panayotov and L. Vacín, with the assistance of Gene Trabich. Ancient Magic and Divination 14. Leiden and Boston: Brill: 93–115.

Bácskay and Simkó 2017 = A. Bácskay, and K. Simkó. Edition of BAM 494. The fifth tablet of UGU or a compilation of recipes against the skin diseases of the head. *Le Journal des Médecines Cunéiformes* 27: 1–71.

Bagg 2000 = A.M. Bagg. *Assyrische Wasserbauten: Landwirtschaftliche Wasserbauten im Kernland Assyriens zwischen der 2. Hälfte des 2. und der 1. Hälfte des 1. Jahrtausends v. Chr.* Baghdader Forschungen 24. Mainz am Rhein: Von Zabern.

Bauer 2007 = J. Bauer. Review of: van Dijk and Geller 2003. Ur III Incantations from the Frau Professor Hilprecht-Collection, Jena. *Bibliotheca Orientalis* 64: 175–179.

Beaulieu 1994 = P.-A. Beaulieu. *Late Babylonian Texts in the Nies Babylonian Collection.* Catalogue of the Babylonian Collections at Yale 1. Bethesda: CDL Press.

Beck 2015 = S. Beck. Sāmānu as a Human Disease. *Journal des Médecines Cunéiformes* 26: 33–46.

Besnier, Boutrolle, Chanut and Hawley 2015 = M.-F. Besnier, P. Boutrolle, C. Chanut and R. Hawley. On the Junipers of Ugarit. Part 2: The word *diprānu* and the genus junipers. *Orient & Méditerranée Archéologie* 16: 81–156.

Biggs 1974 = R. Biggs. A Babylonian Extispicy Text Concerning Holes. *Journal of Near Eastern Studies* 33: 351–356.

Borger 1967 = R. Borger. *Handbuch der Keilschriftliteratur. Band I, Repertorium der sumerischen und akkadischen Texte.* Berlin: Walter de Gruyter.

Borger 1975 = R. Borger. *Handbuch der Keilschriftliteratur Band II, Supplement zu Band I Anhang: zur Kuyunjik-Sammlung.* Berlin: Walter de Gruyter.

Borger 1991 = R. Borger. Ein Brief Sîn-idinnams von Larsa an den Sonnengott sowie Bemerkungen über "Joins" und das "Joinen". *Nachrichten von der Akademie der Wissenschaften in Göttingen. I. Philologisch-Historische Klasse 1991, Nr. 2.* Göttingen : Vandenhoeck and Ruprecht.
Borger 2010 = R. Borger. *Mesopotamisches Zeichenlexikon. Zweite, revidierte und aktualisierte Auflage.* Alter Orient und Altes Testament 305, 2. Auflage. Münster: Ugarit.
Böck 2000 = B. Böck. *Die babylonisch-assyrische Morphoskopie.* Archiv für Orientforschung, Beiheft 27. Wien: Horn, Austria Berger.
Böck 2003 = B. Böck. Hauterscheinungen in altmesopotamischer Divination und Medizin Teil 1: Das *kurāru*-Mal. *Aula Orientalis* 21: 161–184.
Böck 2004 = B. Böck. Anmerkungen zu zwei medizinischen Texten aus Assur. *Nouvelles Assyriologiques Brèves et Utilitaires* 2004-2: no. 42.
Böck 2007 = B. Böck. *Das Handbuch Muššu'u "Einreibung". Eine Serie Sumerischer und Akkadischer Beschwörungen aus dem 1. Jt. vor Chr.* Biblioteca del Próximo Oriente Antiguo 3. Madrid: Consejo Superior de Investigaciones Científicas.
Böck 2009 = B. Böck. On Medical Technology in Ancient Mesopotamia. In *Advances in Mesopotamian Medicine from Hammurabi to Hippocrates. Proceedings of the International Conference "Oeil malade et mauvais oeil," Collège de France, Paris, 23rd June 2006*, eds. A. Attia and G. Buisson. Cuneiform Monographs 37. Leiden–Boston: Brill: 105–128.
Böck 2014 = B. Böck. *The Healing Goddess Gula. Towards an Understanding of Ancient Babylonian Medicine.* Culture and History of the Ancient Near East 67. Leiden-Boston: Brill.
Bourguignon 2012 = A. Bourguignon. *Les emprunts sémitiques en grec ancien. Étude méthodologique et exemples mycéniens.* Thèse présentée en vue de l'obtention du grade académique de Docteur en Langues et lettres, sous la direction de Monsieur Philippe Talon. Université Libre de Bruxelles.
Brunke 2011 = H. Brunke. *Essen in Sumer: Metrologie, Herstellung und Terminologie nach Zeugnis der Ur III-zeitlichen Wirtschaftsurkunden. Geschichtswissenschaften* 26. München: Herbert Utz Verlag.
Budge 1913 = E.A.W. Budge. *Syrian Anatomy, Pathology and Therapeutics or "The Book of Medicines": The Syriac text, edited from a rare manuscript, with an English Translation, etc. Volume 2, English Translation and Index.* London et al.: Humphrey Milford-Oxford University Press.
Cadelli 2000 = D. Cadelli. *Recherche sur la Médecine Mésopotamienne: La Série šumma amêlu suâlam maruṣ.* Doctorat de l'Université de Paris I Panthéon Sorbonne.
Cadelli 2001, see Stol, Cadelli, and Milano 2001.
Caplice 1967 = R. Caplice. Namburbi Texts in the British Museum III. *Orientalia Nova Series* 36: 273–298.
Chalendar 2018 = V. Chalendar. Éléments de pharmacopée mésopotamienne : retour sur l'ingrédient *rikibtu*. *Le Journal des Médecines Cunéiformes* 32: 24–55.
Civil 1984 = M. Civil. 'On Some Terms for "Bat" in Mesopotamia.' *Aula Orientalis* 2: 5–9.
Civil 1986 = M. Civil. *Materials for the Sumerian Lexicon: Supplementary Series 1.* Roma: Pontificium Institutum Biblicum.
Civil 1996 = M. Civil. *HAR-ra = hubullu: Tablet X dug = karpatu.* In Sallaberger, W. *Der babylonische Töpfer und seine Gefäße nach Urkunden altsumerischer bis altbabylonischer Zeit sowie lexikalischen und literarischen Zeugnissen.* Mesopotamian History and Environment, Memoirs 3. Ghent: University of Ghent: 129–160.
Clancier 2009 = P. Clancier. *Les bibliothèques en Babylonie dans la deuxième moitié du Ier millénaire av. J.-C.* Alter Orient und Altes Testament 363. Münster: Ugarit.
Cohen and Llop 2017 = Y. Cohen and J. Llop. A Private Middle Assyrian Letter Sent by Pilta-ādur to Nabbānu (with an Aphorism drawn from the World of Medicine). *Zeitschrift für Assyriologie und Vorderasiatische Archäologie* 107: 105–110.
Collins 1999 = T.J. Collins. *Natural Illness in Babylonian Medical Incantations.* PhD. Dissertation. Chicago: University of Chicago.

Couto-Ferreira 2009 = E. Couto-Ferreira. *Etnoanatomía y partonomía del cuerpo humano en sumerio y acadio. El léxico Ugu-mu*. Tesi doctoral, Universitat Pompeu Fabra. Departament d'Humanitats.

Couto-Ferreira 2013 = E. Couto-Ferreira. The Circulation of Medical Practitioners in The Ancient Near East: The Mesopotamian Perspective. In *Mediterráneos: An Interdisciplinary Approach to the Cultures of the Mediterranean Sea*, eds. Sergio Carro Martín et al. Newcastle upon Tyne: Cambridge Scholars Publishing: 401–416.

Craik 2005 = E. Craik. The Hippocratic Treatise *peri opsios* (*de vedendi acie, On the Origan of Sight*). In *Hippocrates in Context: Papers Read at the XIth International Hippocrates Colloquium (University of Newcastle upon Tyne, 27–31 August 2002)*, ed. P. van der Eijk. Leiden: Brill: 191–207.

Craik 2015 = E. Craik. *The 'Hippocratic' Corpus: Content and Context*. Milton Park, Abingdon, Oxon; New York, NY: Routledge.

Coughlin 2016 = S. Coughlin. Physiology of Perception. In *The Soul is an Octopus: ancient ideas of life and the body*, ed. U. Kornmeier. Berlin: Berliner Medizinhistorisches Museum der Charité, Berlin: Excellence Cluster Topoi: 52–62.

Cunningham 1997 = G. Cunningham. *Deliver me from evil. Mesopotamian incantations 2500–1500 BC*. Studia Pohl, Series maior 17. Roma: Pontifcio Istituto Biblico.

Dalley and Postgate 1984 = S. Dalley and J.N. Postgate. *The tablets from Fort Shalmaneser. Cuneiform Texts from Nimrud* 3. London: British School of Archaeology in Iraq.

del Olmo Lete 2007 = G. del Olmo Lete. The Biconsonantal Semitic Lexicon. The Series /B-X-/*. *Aula Orientalis* 25: 201–235.

del Olmo Lete 2014 = G. del Olmo Lete. *Incantations and Anti-Witchcraft Texts from Ugarit. With a contribution by Ignacio Márquez Rowe*. Studies in Ancient Near Eastern Records 4. Boston and Berlin. Walter de Gruyter.

Deller 1985 = K. Deller. SAG.DU UR.MAH, >>Löwenkopfsitula, Löwenkopfbecher<<. *Baghdader Mitteilungen* 16: 327–346.

Drower 1946 = E.S. Drower. A Phylactery for Rue (an Invocation of the Personified Herb). *Orientalia Nova Series* 15: 324–346.

Durant 2006 = J.-M. Durand. Remarques sur le vocabulaire de quelques parties du corps. In *Médecine et médecins au Proche-Orient ancient. Actes du Colloque International organisé à Lyon les 8 et 9 novembre 2002, Maison de l'Orient et de la Méditerranée*, eds. L. Battini and P. Villard. BAR International Series 1528. Oxford: Oxford Hedges: 65–72.

Edel 1976 = E. Edel. *Ägyptische Ärzte und ägyptische Medizin am hethitischen Königshof. Neue Funde von Keilschriftbriefen Ramses' II. aus Boğazköy*. Rheinisch-Westfalischen Akademie der Wissenschaften G 205. Opladen: Westdeutscher Verlag.

Eypper 2019 = S. Choukassizian. *Kasû*(^{Ú}GAZI^{SAR}) Revisited. *Journal des Médecines Cunéiformes* 33: 35–49.

Falkenstein 1931 = A. Falkenstein. *Die Haupttypen der sumerischen Beschwörung*. Leipziger semitistische Studien, n. F., Bd. 1. Leipzig.

Farber 1974 = W. Farber. Saghulhaza *mukīl rēš lemutti*. *Zeitschrift für Assyriologie und Vorderasiatische Archäologie* 64: 87–95.

Farber 1981 = = W. Farber. Zur älteren akkadischen Beschwörungsliteratur. *Zeitschrift für Assyriologie und Vorderasiatische Archäologie* 71: 51–72.

Farber 1982 = W. Farber. Review of Franz Köcher, *Die babylonisch-assyrische Medizin in Texten und Untersuchungen*, Bd. V und VI. *Bibliotheca Orientalis* 39: 592–599.

Farber 1989 = W. Farber. *Schlaf, Kindchen, Schlaf! Mesopotamische Baby-Beschwörungen und –Rituale*. Mesopotamian Civilizations 2. Winona Lake: Eisenbrauns.

Farber 1990 = W. Farber. *Mannam lušpur ana Enkidu*: Some New Thoughts about an Old Motif. *Journal of Near Eastern Studies* 49: 299–321.

Farber 1998 = W. Farber. *māra/āt Anim* oder: Des Anu Töchterlein. In Singular und Plural, Text und Bild. In *Festschrift für Rykle Borger zu seinem 65. Geburtstag am 24. Mai 1994: tikip santakki mala bašmu,* ed. S. Maul. Groningen: Styx Publications: 59–69.
Farber 2014 = W. Farber. *Lamaštu. An Edition of the Canonical Series of Lamaštu Incantations and Rituals and Related Texts from the Second and First Millennia B.C.* Mesopotamian Civilizations 17. Winona Lake, Indiana: Eisenbrauns.
Feder 2016 = Y. Feder. Defilement, Disgust, and Disease: The Experiential Basis of Hittite and Akkadian Terms for Impurity. *Journal of the American Oriental Society* 136: 99–116.
Feliu 2003 = L. Feliu. *The God Dagan in Bronze Age Syria.* Culture and History of the Ancient Near East 19. Leiden and Boston: Brill.
Fincke 1998 = J.C. Fincke. SpTU III Nr. 85 joint zu SpTU II Nr. 22. *Nouvelles Assyriologiques Brèves et Utilitaires* 1988/26.
Fincke 2000 = J.C. Fincke . *Augenleiden nach keilschriftlichen Quellen. Untersuchungen zur altorientalischen Medizin.* Würzburger medizinhistorische Forschungen 70. Würzburg: Königshausen und Neumann.
Fincke 2003/04 = J.C. Fincke. The Babylonian Texts of Nineveh. Report on the British Museum's *Ashurbanipal Library Project. Archiv für Orientforschung* 50: 111–149.
Fincke 2007 = J.C. Fincke. Omina, die göttliche "Gesetze" der Divination. *Jaarbericht Ex Oriente Lux* 40: 131–147.
Fincke 2009 = J.C. Fincke. Cuneiform Tablets on Eye Diseases: Babylonian Sources in Relation to the Series DIŠ NA IGI^{II}-*šú* GIG. In *Advances in Mesopotamian Medicine from Hammurabi to Hippocrates. Proceedings of the International Conference "Oeil malade et mauvais oeil," Collège de France, Paris, 23rd June 2006,* eds. A. Attia and G. Buisson. Cuneiform Monographs 37. Leiden and Boston: Brill: 79–104.
Fincke 2010 = J.C. Fincke. KUB 4, 50: Ein medizinischer Text über Augenkrankheiten aus Ḫattuša. *Nouvelles Assyriologiques Brèves et Utilitaires* 2010/12.
Fincke 2011 = J.C. Fincke. Spezialisierung und Differenzierung im Bereich der altorientalischen Medizin. Die Dermatologie am Beispiel der Symptome *simmū matqūtu, kalmātu* (*matuqtu*), *kibšu, kiṣṣatu* und *gurištu.* In *The Empirical Dimension of Ancient Near Eastern Studies: Die empirische Dimension altorientalischer Forschungen,* eds. G.J. Selz and K. Wagensonner. Wien: Lit: 159–208.
Finkel 1976 = I.L. Finkel. *ḪUL.BA.ZI.ZI: Ancient Mesopotamian Exorcistic Incantations.* Ph. D. Faculty of Arts, University of Birmingham.
Finkel 1991 = I.L. Finkel. Muššu'u, Qutāru, and the Scribe Tanittu-Bēl. *Aula Orientalis* 9 (Fs. M. Civil): 91–104.
Finkel 1998 = I.L. Finkel. A Study in Scarlet: Incantations against Samana. In *Festschrift für Rykle Borger zu seinem 65. Geburtstag am 24. Mai 1994: tikip santakki mala bašmu,* ed. S. Maul. Cuneiform Monographs 10. Groningen: Styx Publications: 71–106.
Finkel 1999 = I.L. Finkel. On Some Dog, Snake and Scorpion Incantations. In *Mesopotamian Magic, Textual, Historical, and Interpretative Perspectives,* eds. T. Abusch and K. van der Toorn. Ancient Magic and Divination 1. Groningen: Styx Publications: 213–250.
Finkel 2004 = I.L. Finkel. Old Babylonian medicine at Ur: letter aux éditeurs. *Le Journal des Médecines Cunéiformes* 4: 26.
Finkel 2007 = I.L. Finkel. On the Rules for the Royal Game of Ur. In *Ancient Board games in perspective: papers from the 1990 British Museum colloquium, with additional contributions,* ed. I.L. Finkel. London: British Museum Press: 16–32.
Finkel 2018 = I.L. Finkel. On Three Tablet Inventories. In *Assyrian and Babylonian Scholarly Text Catalogues: Medicine, Magic and Divination,* ed. U. Steinert. Die babylonisch-assyrische Medizin in Texten und Untersuchungen 9. Berlin and Boston: Walter de Gruyter: 25–41.

Finkel and Reade 2002 = I.L. Finkel and J.E. Reade. 2002. On Some Inscribed Babylonian Alabastra. *Journal of the Royal Asiatic Society of Great Britain & Ireland* 12: 31–46.
Forbes 1950 = R.J. Forbes. *Metallurgy in Antiquity: A Notebook for Archaeologists and Technologists.* Leiden: Brill.
Foster 2005 = B.R. Foster. *Before the Muses. An Anthology of Akkadian Literature. Third Edition.* Bethesda: CDL Press.
Frankfurter 2001 = D. Frankfurter. Narrating power: the theory and practice of the magical historiola in ritual spells. In *Ancient Magic and Ritual Power*, (eds.) M. Meyer and P. Mirecki. Religions in the Graeco-Roman world 129. Leiden-Boston: Brill: 457–476.
Freedman 1998 = S. Moren Freedman. *If a city is set on a height: the Akkadian omen series Šumma alu ina mēlê šakin. Vol. 1, Tablets 1–21.* Occasional Publications of the Samuel Noah Kramer Fund, 17. Philadelphia: Samuel Noah Kramer Fund.
Freedman 2017 = S.M. Freedman. *If the city is set on a height: The Akkadian Omen Series Šumma Alu in Mele Šakin. Volume 3: Tablets 41–63.* Occasional Publications of the Samuel Noah Kramer Fund 20. Winona Lake: Eisenbrauns.
Gabbay 2016 = U. Gabbay. The Exegetical Terminology of Akkadian Commentaries. Culture and History of the Ancient Near East 82. Leiden and Boston: Brill.
Gaspa 2007 = S. Gaspa. Vessels in Neo-Assyrian documents: capacity measures and listing conventions. *State Archives of Assyria Bulletin* 16: 145–184.
Geller 1984 = M.J. Geller. Review of Franz Köcher, *Die babylonisch-assyrische Medizin in Texten und Untersuchungen*, Bd. V und VI. *Zeitschrift für Assyriologie und Vorderasiatische Archäologie* 74: 292–297.
Geller 1985 = M.J. Geller. *Forerunners to Udug-hul: Sumerian Exorcistic Incantations.* Freiburger altorientalische Studien 12. Stuttgart: Franz Steiner Verlag Wiesbaden.
Geller 1988 = M.J. Geller. New Duplicates to SBTU II. *Archiv für Orientforschung* 35: 1–23.
Geller 1991 = M.J. Geller. Akkadian Medicine in the Babylonian Talmud. In *A Traditional Quest. Essays in Honor of Luis Jacobs*, ed. D. Cohn-Sherbok. Sheffield: JSOT: 102–112.
Geller 2001/02 = M.J. Geller. West Meets East: Early Greek and Babylonian Diagnosis. *Archiv für Orientforschung* 48/49: 50–75.
Geller 2003 = M.J. Geller. Paranoia, the Evil Eye, and the Face of Evil. In *Literatur, Politik und Recht in Mesopotamien. Festschrift für Claus Wilcke*, eds. W. Sallaberger et al. Orientalia Biblica et Christiana 14. Wiesbaden: Harrassowitz: 115–134.
Geller 2005 = M.J. Geller. *Renal and Rectal Disease Texts.* Die babylonisch-assyrische Medizin in Texten und Untersuchungen 7. Berlin: Walter de Gruyter.
Geller 2006 = M.J. Geller. Les maladies et leurs causes, selon un texte médical paléobabylonien. *Le Journal des Médecines Cunéiformes* 8: 7–12.
Geller 2007a = M.J. Geller. *Evil demons canonical Utukkū Lemnūtu incantations: introduction, cuneiform text, and transliteration with a translation and glossary.* State Archives of Assyria Cuneiform Texts 5. Helsinki: Neo-Assyrian Text Corpus Project.
Geller 2007b = M.J. Geller. Textes médicaux du *Louvre*, nouvelle edition AO 11447, AO 7760 et AO 66774. Première partie. *Le Journal des Médecines Cunéiformes* 10: 4–18.
Geller 2007c = M.J. Geller. Incantations within Akkadian Medical Texts. In *The Babylonian World*, ed. G. Leick. New York and London: Taylor and Francis: 389–399.
Geller 2009 = M.J. Geller. Introduction to "Oeil malade et mauvais oeil". In *Advances in Mesopotamian Medicine from Hammurabi to Hippocrates. Proceedings of the International Conference "Oeil malade et mauvais oeil," Collège de France, Paris, 23rd June 2006*, eds. A. Attia and G. Buisson. Cuneiform Monographs 37. Leiden and Boston: Brill: 1–12.
Geller 2010a = M.J. Geller. *Ancient Babylonian Medicine. Theory and Practice.* Chichester: Wiley-Blackwell.

Geller 2010b = M.J. Geller. Augenkrankheiten. *Texte zur Heilkunde. Texte aus der Umwelt des Alten Testaments. Neu Folge* 5: 61–63.
Geller 2011 = M.J. Geller. Review of Maul and Strauss. 2011. Ritualbeschreibungen und Gebete I. *Zeitschrift für Assyriologie und Vorderasiatische Archäologie* 101: 339–344.
Geller 2014 = M.J. Geller. *Melothesia in Babylonia Medicine, Magic, and Astrology in the Ancient Near East.* Science, technology, and medicine in ancient cultures 2. Boston and Berlin: Walter de Gruyter.
Geller 2015a = M.J. Geller, Review of N. Heeßel, *Divinatorische Texte II.* Archiv für Orientforschung 53: 201–207.
Geller 2015b = M.J. Geller. Encyclopaedias and Commentaries. In *In the Wake of the Compendia. Infrastructural Contexts and the Licensing of Empiricism in Ancient and Medieval Mesopotamia*, ed. J.C. Johnson. Boston and Berlin: Walter de Gruyter: 31–45.
Geller 2015c = M.J. Geller. Review of Böck, B. 2014. *The Healing Goddess Gula. Towards an Understanding of Ancient Babylonian Medicine. Archiv für Orientforschung* 53: 160–163.
Geller 2016 = M.J. Geller. *Healing Magic and Evil Demons: Canonical Udug-hul Incantations. With the Assistance of Luděk Vacín.* Die babylonisch-assyrische Medizin in Texten und Untersuchungen 8. Boston and Berlin. Walter de Gruyter.
George 2013 = A.R. George. *Babylonian Divinatory Texts Chiefly in the Schøyen Collection.* Cornell University studies in Assyriology and Sumerology 18. Bethesda: CDL Press.
George 2016 = A.R. George. *Mesopotamian Incantations and Related Texts in the Schøyen Collection. Manuscripts in the Schøyen collection.* Cuneiform texts 8. Cornell University studies in Assyriology and Sumerology 32. Bethesda: CDL Press.
Goetze 1955 = A. Goetze. An Incantation against Diseases. *Journal of Cuneiform Studies* 9: 8–18.
Golder 2007 = W. Golder. *Hippokrates und das Corpus Hippocraticum. Eine Einführung für Philologen und Mediziner.* Würzburg: Königshausen and Neumann.
Goltz 1974 = D. Goltz. *Studien zur altorientalischen und griechischen Heilkunde: Therapie–Arzneibereitung – Rezeptstruktur.* Sudhoffs Archiv, Beihefte 16. Wiesbaden: Steiner.
Gottheil 1899 = R. Gottheil. Contributions to Syriac Folk Medicine. *Journal of the American Oriental Society* 20: 186–205.
Gottstein and Panayotov 2014 = N. Gottstein† and S.V. Panayotov. *Cuneiform Spotlight of the Neo- and Middle Assyrian Signs.* Dresden: Islet.
Graf 1997 = F. Graf. *Magic in the Ancient World.* Revealing antiquity 10. Cambridge: Harvard University Press.
Gurney 1953 = O.R. Gurney. Further Texts from Dur-Kurigalzu. *Sumer* 9: 21–34.
Gurney and Hulin 1964 = O.R. Gurney and P. Hulin. *The Sultantepe Tablets* II. Occasional Publications of the British Institute of Archaeology at Ankara 7. London: British Institute of Archaeology at Ankara.
Haas and Thiel1978 = V. Haas and H.J. Thiel. Die Beschrörungsrituale der Allaituraḫ(ḫ)i und verwandte Texte. Alter Orient und Altes Testament, Hurritologische Studien II. Neukirchen-Vluyn: Kevelaer, Butzon & Bercker.
Hannen 2014 = K. Hannen. *Bearbeitung und Kontext des medizinischen Textes VAT 13732.* Freie wissenschaftliche Arbeit zur Erlangung eines Bachelorgrades am Fachbereich Geschichts- und Kulturwissenschaften der Freien Universität Berlin im Bachelorstudiengang Altorientalistik.
Hatfield 2004 = G. Hatfield. *Encyclopedia of Folk medicine: old world and new world traditions.* Santa Barbara: ABC-CLIO Interactive.
Haussperger 2000 = M. Haussperger. Einige medizinische Anmerkungen zum Text BAM 3. In *Studi sul Vicino Oriente Antico dedicati alla memoria di Luigi Cagni*, ed. S. Graziani. Napoli: Istituto universitario orientale: 439–450.

Heeßel 2000 = N.P. Heeßel. *Babylonisch-assyrische Diagnostik. Alter Orient und Altes Testament* 43. Münster: Ugarit.
Heeßel 2001/02 = N.P. Heeßel. "Wenn ein Mann zum Haus des Kranken geht." Intertextuelle Bezüge zwischen der Serie *šumma ālu* und der zweiten Tafel der Series SA.GIG. *Archiv für Orientforschung* 48/49: 24–49.
Heeßel 2007 = N.P. Heeßel. The Hands of the Gods: Disease Names and Divine Anger. In *Disease in Babylonia*, eds. I.L. Finkel and M.J. Geller. Cuneiform Monographs 36. Leiden and Boston: Brill: 120–130.
Heeßel 2009 = N.P. Heeßel. The Babylonian Physician Rabâ-ša-Marduk. Another look at physicians and exorcists in the Ancient Near East. In *Advances in Mesopotamian Medicine from Hammurabi to Hippocrates. Proceedings of the International Conference "Oeil malade et mauvais oeil," Collège de France, Paris, 23rd June 2006*, eds. A. Attia and G. Buisson. Cuneiform Monographs 37. Leiden–Boston: Brill: 13–28.
Heeßel 2010 = N.P. Heeßel. 2010. Erkrankungen des Kopfes. In *Texte zur Heilkunde*, eds. B. Janowski and D. Schwemer. Texte aus der Umwelt des Alten Testaments, Neue Folge 5. Gütersloh: Gütersloher Verlagshaus: 46–52.
Heeßel 2018 = N.P. Heeßel. Identifying Divine Agency: The Hands of the Gods in Context. In *Sources of Evil, Studies in Mesopotamian Exorcistic Lore*, eds. G. Van Buylaere, M. Luukko, D. Schwemer, A. Mertens-Wagschal. Ancient Magic and Divination 15. Leiden and Boston: Brill: 135–149.
Heeßel and Al-Rawi 2003 = N.P. Heeßel and F.N.H. Al-Rawi. Tablets from the Sippar Library XII. A Medical Therapeutic Text. *Iraq* 65: 221–239.
Heiss, Stika, De Zorzi, Jursa 2012–2013 = A. G. Heiss, H.-P. Stika, N. De Zorzi, and M. Jursa. Nigella in the Mirror of Time: A Brief Attempt to Draw a Genus' Ethnohistorical Portrait. *Offa* 69/70: 147–169.
Herrero 1975 = P. Herrero. Une tablette médicale assyrienne inédite. *Revue d'Assyriologie* 69: 41–53.
Hrůša 2010 = I. Hrůša. *Die akkadische Synonymenliste malku=šarru. Eine Textedition mit Übersetzung und Kommentrar.* Alter Orient und Altes Testament 50. Münster: Ugarit.
Hoch 1994 = J.E. Hoch. *Semitic Words in Egyptian Texts of the New Kingdom and Third Intermediate Period.* Princeton: Princeton University Press.
Hooper and Field 1937 = D. Hooper and H. Field. *Useful Plants and Drugs of Iran and Iraq*. Botanical Series. Field Museum of Natural History 9/3. Chicago, Illinois: Field Museum of Natural History Chicago.
Hunger 1968 = H. Hunger. *Babylonische und Assyrische Kolophone*. Alter Orient und Altes Testament 2. Neukirchen-Vluyn: Kevelaer, Butzon & Bercker.
Hussein et al. 2016 = M.M. Hussein, M. Altaweel, and Mc. Gibson. *Nimrud: The Queens' Tombs.* Baghdad; Chicago: Iraqi State Board of Antiquities and Heritage: Oriental Institute of the University of Chicago.
Jeyes 1989 = U. Jeyes. *Old Babylonian Extispicy: Omen Texts in the British Museum.* Uitgaven van het Nederlands Historisch-Archaeologisch Institut te Istanbul 64. Istanbul: Nederlands Historisch-Archaeologisch Instituut te İstanbul.
Johandi 2019 = A. Johandi. *The God Asar / Asalluhi in the Early Mesopotamian Pantheon.* Tartu: University of Tartu Press.
Jones 1998 = W.H.S. Jones. *Volume IV: Nature of Man. Regimen in Health. Humours. Aphorisms. Regimen 1–3. Dreams.* Loeb Classical Library 150. Cambridge, MA: Harvard University Press.
Jursa 2009 = M. Jursa. Die Kralle des Meeres und andere Aromata. In *Philologisches und Historisches zwischen Anatolien und Sokotra Analecta Semitica. In Memoriam Alexander Sima*, eds. W. Arnold et al. Wiesbaden: Harrassowitz: 147–180.
Kämmerer 2000 = T. Kämmerer. Pathologische Veränderungen an Leber und Galle. Das Krankheitsbild der Gelbsucht. *Revue d'Assyriologie et d'archéologie orientale* 94: 57–93.

Karahashi 2000 = F. Karahashi. *Sumerian Compound Verbs with Body-Part Terms.* A Dissertation submitted to the Faculty of the Division of the Humanities in Candidacy for the Degree of Doctor of Philosophy: The Department of Near Easter Languages and Civilizations. Chicago, Illinois.

Kinnier Wilson 2005a = J.V. Kinnier Wilson. Notes on the Assyrian Pharmaceutical Series URU.AN.NA : *MAŠTAKAL. Journal of Near Eastern Studies* 64: 45–51.

Kinnier Wilson 2005b = J.V. Kinnier Wilson. On the Cryptogams in the lexical and related texts. *Le Journal des Médecines Cunéiformes* 6: 1–21.

Kinnier Wilson 2011 = J.V. Kinnier Wilson. A Journey through the Prescriptions. *Le Journal des Médecines Cunéiformes* 17: 1–24.

Kleber 2016a = K. Kleber. *Sekēru* – "to purify", not "to gild". *Nouvelles Assyriologiques Brèves et Utilitaires* 2016/3: 98–99.

Kleber 2016b = K. Kleber. On the ghost word *tasniqtu* "verification" and the stone called "beginning" in Hh. XVI, 189. *Nouvelles Assyriologiques Brèves et Utilitaires* 2016/4: 151.

Köcher 1963a = F. Köcher. *Keilschrifttexte aus Assur 1.* Die babylonisch-assyrische Medizin in Texten und Untersuchungen 1. Berlin: Walter de Gruyter.

Köcher 1963b = F. Köcher. *Keilschrifttexte aus Assur 2.* Die babylonisch-assyrische Medizin in Texten und Untersuchungen 2. Berlin: Walter de Gruyter.

Köcher, F. 1964. *Keilschrifttexte aus Assur 3.* Die babylonisch-assyrische Medizin in Texten und Untersuchungen 3. Berlin: Walter de Gruyter.

Köcher 1971 = F. Köcher. *Keilschrifttexte aus Assur 4, Babylon, Nippur, Sippar, Uruk und unbekannter Herkunft.* Die babylonisch-assyrische Medizin in Texten und Untersuchungen 4. Berlin: Walter de Gruyter.

Köcher 1980a = F. Köcher. *Keilschrifttexte aus Niniveh 1.* Die babylonisch-assyrische Medizin in Texten und Untersuchungen 5). Berlin and New York: Walter de Gruyter.

Köcher 1980b = F. Köcher. *Keilschrifttexte aus Niniveh 2.* Die babylonisch-assyrische Medizin in Texten und Untersuchungen 6. Berlin and New York: Walter de Gruyter.

Köcher 1995 = F. Köcher. Ein Text medizinischen Inhalts aus dem neubabylonischen Grab 405. In *Uruk – Die Gräber*, eds. R. M. Böhmer & F. Pedde & B. Salje. Ausgrabungen in Uruk-Warka Endberichte 10. Mainz: Philipp von Zabern: 203–217.

Köcher, Oppenheim and Güterbock 1957/58 = F. Köcher, F., A.L. Oppenheim, and H.G. Güterbock. The Old-Babylonian Omen Text VAT 7525. *Archiv für Orientforschung* 18: 62–80.

Krebernik 1984 = M. Krebernik. *Die Beschwörungen aus Fara und Ebla, Untersuchungen zur ältesten keilschriftlichen Beschwörungsliteratur.* Texte und Studien zur Orientalistik 2. Hildesheim; Zürich: G. Olms.

Kwasman 2015 = T. Kwasman. Loanwords in Jewish Babylonian Aramaic: Some Preliminary Observations. In *The Archaeology and Material Culture of the Babylonian Talmud*, ed. M. J. Geller. IJS Studies in Judaica 16. Leiden and Boston: Brill: 333–386.

Lambert 1957/58 = W.G. Lambert. Three Unpublished Fragments of the Tukulti-Ninurta Epic. Archiv für Orientforschung 18: 38–51.

Lambert 1965 = W.G. Lambert. A Middle Assyrian Tablet of Incantations. In *Studies in honor of Benno Landsberger on his seventy-fifth birthday, April 21, 1965*, eds. H. G. Güterbock and T. Jacobsen. Assyriological studies 16. Chicago: University of Chicago Press: 283–288.

Lambert 2008 = W.G. Lambert. The Classification of Incantations. In *Proceedings of the 51st Rencontre Assyriologique Internationale held at The Oriental Insitute of The University of Chicago July 18–22, 2005 ; dedicated to the memory of Erica Reiner*, eds. R.D. Biggs, J. Myers, and M.T. Roth. Series in Ancient Oriental Civilization 62. Chicago: The Oriental Institute of the University of Chicago: 93–97.

Lambert 2013 = W.G. Lambert. *Babylonian Creation Myths.* Mesopotamian Civilizations 16. Winona Lake: Eisenbrauns.

Lambert and Millard 1968 = W.G. Lambert and A.R. Millard. *Catalogue of the Cuneiform Tablets in the Kouyunjik Collection of the British Museum: Second Supplement.* London: Trustees of the British Museum.
Landsberger 1934 = B. Landsberger. *Die Fauna des Alten Mesopotamien nach der 14. Tafel der Series Har-ra = Ḫubullu.* Abhandlungen der Philologisch-historischen Klasse der Sächsischen Akademie der Wissenschaften 42. Leipzig. S. Hirzel.
Landsberger 1958 = B. Landsberger. Corrections to the Article an Old Babylonian Charm against Merḫu. *Journal of Near Eastern Studies* 17: 56–58.
Landsberger 1967 = B. Landsberger. *The Date Palm and its By-products according to the Cuneiform Sources.* Archiv für Orientforschung, Beiheft 17. Graz: Selbstverlag des Herausgebers.
Landsberger and Jacobsen 1955 = B. Landsberger and T. Jacobsen. An Old Babylonian Charm against Merhu. *Journal of Near Eastern Studies* 14: 14–21.
Langholf 1990 = V. Langholf. *Medical Theories in Hippocrates.* Berlin: Walter de Gruyter.
Leichty 1970 = E. Leichty. *The Omen Series Šumma Izbu.* Texts from Cuneiform Sources 4. Locust Valley, New York: J. J. Augustin.
Leichty 1986 = E. Leichty. *Catalogue of the Babylonian tablets in the British Museum 6, Tablets from Sippar, 1.* London, British Museum Press.
Löw 1924/26 = I. Löw. *Die Flora der Jüden.* Wien: R. Loewit Verlag.
Maul 1994 = S.M. Maul. *Zukunftsbewältigung. Eine Untersuchung altorientalischen Denkens anhand der babylonisch-assyrischen Löserituale (Namburbi).* Baghdader Forschungen 18. Mainz: Philipp von Zabern.
Maul 2009 = S.M. Maul. Die Lesung der Rubra DÙ.DÙ.BI und KÌD.KÌD.BI. *Orientalia Nova Series* 78. 69–80.
Maul 2013 = S.M. Maul. Ein altorientalischer Pferdesegen – Seuchenprophylaxe in der assyrischen Armee. *Zeitschrift für Assyriologie und Vorderasiatische Archäologie 103: 16–37.*
Maul and Strauß 2011 = S.M. Maul and R. Strauß. *Ritualbeschreibungen und Gebete I. Mit Beiträgen von D. Schwemer.* Keilschrifttexte aus Assur literarischen Inhalts 4. Wiesbaden: Harrassowitz.
Mayer 2005 = W.R. Mayer. Lexikalische Listen aus Ebla und Uruk. *Orientalia Nova Series* 74: 157–164.
Mayer 2016 = W.R. Mayer. Zum akkadischen Wörterbuch: A-L. *Orientalia Nova Series* 85: 181–235.
Middeke-Conlin 2014 = R. Middeke-Conlin. The Scents of Larsa: A Study of the Aromatics Industry in an Old Babylonian Kingdom. *Cuneiform Digital Library Journal* 2014.
Militarev and Kogan 2000 = A. Militarev and L. Kogan. *Semitic Etymological Dictionary. Vol I. Anatomy of Man and Animals.* Alter Orient und Altes Testament 278/1. Münster: Ugarit.
Miller 2003 = S.S. Miller. Some Observations on Stone Vessel Finds and Ritual Purity in Light of Talmudic Sources. In *Zeichen aus Text und Stein: Studien auf dem Weg zu einer Archäologie des Neuen Testaments*, eds. S Alkier and J. Zangenberg. Texte und Arbeiten zum neutestamentlichen Zeitalter 42. Tübingen: Francke: 402–419.
Müller-Kessler 1999 = C. Müller-Kessler. Dämon + *YTB'L* – Ein Krankheitsdämon. Eine Studie zu aramäischen Beschwörungen medizinischen Inhalts. In *Munuscula Mesopotamica. Festschrift für Johannes Renger*, ed. B. Böck et al. Alter Orient und Altes Testament 267. Münster: Ugarit: 341–354.
Nougayrol 1968 = J. Nougayrol. Textes suméro-accadiens des Archives et Bibliothèques Privées D'Ugarit. Ugaritica 5: 1–446.
Nutton 2004 = V. Nutton. *Ancient Medicine.* London and New York: Routledge.
Osbaldeston and Wood 2000 = T.A. Osbaldeston and R.P.A. Wood. *De materia medica: Being an herbal with many other medicinal materials: written in Greek in the first century of the common era: a new indexed version in modern English.* Johannesburg: IBIDIS.
Oshima 2014 = T. Oshima. *Babylonian Poems of pious sufferers: Ludlul Bēl Nēmeqi and the Babylonian Theodicy.* Tübingen: Mohr Siebeck.

Panayotov 2013 = S.V. Panayotov. A Ritual for a Flourishing Bordello. Bibliotheca Orientalis 70: 285–309.
Panayotov 2015 = S.V. Panayotov. 2015. The Gottstein System Implemented on a Digital Middle and Neo-Assyrian Palaeography. *Cuneiform Digital Library Notes* 2015/17.
Panayotov 2016a = S.V. Panayotov. Fragments of the Nineveh Medical Composition IGI join UGU. *Le Journal des Médecines Cunéiformes* 27: 59–67.
Panayotov 2016b = S.V. Panayotov. Addenda and Corrigenda to "Fragments of the Nineveh Medical Composition IGI join UGU, JMC 27. *Le Journal des Médecines Cunéiformes* 28: 66–67.
Panayotov 2017 = S.V. Panayotov. Eye Metaphors, Analogies and Similes within Mesopotamian Magico-Medical Texts. In *The Comparable Body. Analogy and Metaphor in Ancient Mesopotamian, Egyptian, and Greco-Roman Medicine*, ed. J.Z. Wee. Studies in Ancient Medicine 49. Leiden-Boston: Brill: 204–246.
Panayotov 2018a = S.V. Panayotov. Notes on the Assur Medical Catalogue with Comparison to the Nineveh Medical Encyclopaedia. In *Assyrian and Babylonian Scholarly Text Catalogues: Medicine, Magic and Divination*, ed. U. Steinert. Die babylonisch-assyrische Medizin in Texten und Untersuchungen 9. Berlin and Boston: Walter de Gruyter: 88–118.
Panayotov 2018b = S.V. Panayotov. Magico-Medical Plants and Incantations on Assyrian House Amulets. In In *Sources of Evil, Studies in Mesopotamian Exorcistic Lore*, eds. G. Van Buylaere, M. Luukko, D. Schwemer, A. Mertens-Wagschal. Ancient Magic and Divination 15. Leiden and Boston: Brill: 192–222.
Pappi 2008 = C. Pappi. Salbe, Salbengefäß (ointment, ointment container). *Reallexikon der Assyriologie und Vorderasiatischen Archäologie* 11: 572–574.
Parpola 1983 = S. Parpola. *Letters from Assyrian Scholars to the Kings Esarhaddon and Assurbanipal. Part II: Commentary and Appendices.* Neukirchen-Vluyn: Kevelaer: Butzon & Bercker.
Parpola 1993 = S. Parpola. *Letters from Assyrian and Babylonian scholars.* State archives of Assyria 10. Helsinki: Helsinki University Press.
Parys 2014 = M. Parys. Édition d'un texte médical thérapeutique retrouvé à Assur (BAM 159). *Le journal des médecines cunéiformes* 23: 1–88.
Pedersén 1985 = O. Pedersén. *Archives and Libraries in the City of Assur. A Survey of the Material from the German Excavations: Part* I. Acta Universitatis Upsaliensis. Studia Semitica Upsaliensia 6. Uppsala: Almqvist och Wiksell.
Pommerening 2015 = T. Pommerening. Milch einer Frau, die einen Knaben geboren hat. In *Proceedings of the Tenth International Congress of Egyptologists, University of Aegean, Rhodes, 22–29 May 2008, Vol. II.* eds. P. Kousoulis and N. Lazaridis. Leuven,Paris and Bristol, CT: Peeters: 2083–2095.
Postgate and Collon 1999 = J.N. Postgate and D. Collon. More stray Assur tablets. *State Archives of Assyria Bulletin* 13: 1–16.
Potter 2010 = P. Potter, *Hippocrates, Volume IX. Coan Prenotions. Anatomical and Minor Clinical Writings.* Loeb Classical Library 509. Cambridge, MA: Harvard University Press.
Potts et al. 1996 = D.T. Potts, et al. 1996. Guhlu and Guggulu. In *Festschrift für Hans Hirsch zum 65. Geburtstag gewidmet von seinen Freunden, Kollegen und Schüllern*, eds. A.A. Ambros and M. Köhbach. *Wiener Zeitschrift für die Kunde des Morgenlandes* 86. Wien: Institute für Orientalistik: 291–305.
Radner 2014 = K. Radner. Zagros Spice Mills: The Simurrean and the Hašimur Grindstones. In *From Source to History: Studies on Ancient Near Eastern Worlds and Beyond Dedicated to Giovanni Battista Lanfranchi on the Occasion of His 65th Birthday on June 23, 2014*, eds. S. Gaspa et al. Alter Orient und Altes Testament 412. Münster: Ugarit: 573–580.

Radner 2016 = K. Radner. Die beiden neuassyrischen Privatarchive. In *Ausgrabungen in Assur: Wohnquartiere in der Weststadt, Teil I*, eds. P.A. Miglus, K, Radner, and F.M. Stępniowski. Wiesbaden: Harrassowitz: 79–132, pls. 93–106.

Reade 1986 = J.E. Reade. Archaeology and the Kuyunjik Archives. In *Cuneiform Archives and Libraries: Papers read at the 30e Rencontre Assyriologique Internationale, Leiden, 4–8 July 1983*, ed. K.R. Veenhof. Uitgaven van het Nederlands Historisch-Archaeologisch Instituut te Istanbul 52. Istanbul: Nederlands Historisch-Archaeologisch Instituut te Istanbul: 213–222.

Reade 2016 = J.E. Reade. The Gates of Nineveh. *State Archives of Assyria Bulletin* 22: 39–93.

Reiner 1995 = E. Reiner. *Astral Magic in Babylonia*. Transactions of the American Philosophical Society, New Series 85/4. Philadelphia. American philosophical Society.

Rendu Loisel 2016 = A.C. Rendu Loisel. *Les Chants du monde: La paysage sonore de l'ancienne Mésopotamie*. Toulouse: Presses Universitaires du Mirail.

Riddle 1985 = J.M. Riddle. *Dioscorides on Pharmacy and Medicine*. History of science series 3. Austin: University of Texas Press.

Ritner 2000 = R.K. Ritner. Innovations and Adaptations in Ancient Egyptian Medicine. *Journal of Near Eastern Studies* 59: 107–117.

Rochberg 2016 = F. Rochberg. *Before Nature: Cuneiform Knowledge and the History of Science*. Chicago: The University of Chicago Press.

Rölling 1993 = W. Rölling. Muschel. *Reallexikon der Assyriologie und Vorderasiatischen Archäologie* 8: 450–451.

Rosner 1995 = F. Rosner. *Medicine in the Bible and the Talmud: Selections from Classical Jewish Sources*. Library of Jewish law and ethics 5. Hoboken: KTAV Pub. House; Yeshiva University Press.

Rudik 2011 = N. Rudik. *Die Entwicklung der keilschriftlichen sumerischen Beschwörungsliteratur von den Anfängen bis zur Ur III-Zeit*. Dissertation zur Erlangung des akademischen Grades Doctor philosophiae (Dr. phil.) vorgelegt dem Rat der Philosophischen Fakultät der Friedrich-Schiller-Universität Jena. Accessible at academia.edu.

Rumor 2015 = M. Rumor. *Babylonian Pharmacology in Graeco-Roman Dreckapotheke. With an Edition of Uruanna III 1–143 (138)*. Zur Erlangung des Doktorgrades eingereicht am Fachbereich Geschichts- und Kulturwissenschaften der Freien Universität Berlin im Juli 2015.

Rumor 2018 = M. Rumor. At the Dawn of Plant Taxonomy: Shared Structural Design of Herbal Descriptions in *Šammu šikinšu* and Theophrastus' *Historia plantarum* IX. In *Mesopotamian Medicine and Magic. Studies in Honor of Markham J. Geller*, ed. S.V. Panayotov and L. Vacín, with the assistance of Gene Trabich. Ancient Magic and Divination 14. Leiden and Boston: Brill: 446–461.

Rumor, in press = M. Rumor. The Identification of *Sikillu* as Σκίλλα through its Descriptions and Uses in Mesopotamian and Graeco-Roman Sources. In *Proceedings of the Workshop held at the 61st Rencontre Assyriologique Internationale*. Edited by J. C. Johnson. Winona Lake: Eisenbrauns.

Sallaberger 1996 = W. Sallaberger. *Der babylonische Töpfer und seine Gefäße nach Urkunden altsumerischer bis altbabylonischer Zeit sowie lexikalischen und literarischen Zeugnissen*. Mit einem Beitrag von M. Civil: HAR-ra = hubullu: Tablet X dug = karpatu. Mesopotamian History and Environment, ser. 2, memoirs 3. Ghent: University of Ghent.

Salvini 2008 = M. Salvini. Spigolature dai documenti cuneiformi di Tell Barri 'freddo, gelo, ghiaccio, uri, elefanti, leoni.' *La parola del Passato* 63: 76–101.

Scheil 1921 = V. Scheil. Catalogue de la collection Eugène Tisserant. *Revue d'Assyriologie et d'archéologie orientale* 18: 1–33.

Schmidtchen 2018 = E. Schmidtchen. *Mesopotamische Diagnostik. Die diagnostisch-prognostische Standardserie Sakikkû als ein Kernbereich des Beschwörungsexperten sowie eine Neuedition des zweiten Kapitels*. PhD, Freie Universität, Berlin.

Schramm 2001 = W. Schramm. *Bann, Bann! Eine sumerisch-akkadische Beschwörungsserie*. Göttinger Arbeitshefte zur altorientalischen Literatur 2. Göttingen: Seminar für Keilschriftforschung.

Schramm 2008 = W. Schramm. *Ein Compendium sumerisch-akkadischer Beschwörungen*. Göttinger Beiträge zum Alten Orient 2. Göttingen: Universitätsverlag Göttingen.

Schuster-Brandis 2008 = A. Schuster-Brandis. *Steine als Schutz- und Heilmittel. Untersuchung zu ihrer Verwendung in der Beschwörungskunst Mesopotamiens im 1. Jt. v. Chr.* Alter Orient und Altes Testament 46. Münster: Ugarit.

Schuster-Brandis 2012 = A. Schuster-Brandis. Stibium (Antimon). *Reallexikon der Assyriologie und Vorderasiatischen Archäologie* 13: 177–178.

Schwemer 1998 = D. Schwemer. *Akkadische Rituale aus Ḫattuša. Die Sammeltafel KBO XXXVI 29 und verwandte Fragmente*. Texte der Hethiter 23. Heidelberg: Winter.

Schwemer 2001 = D. Schwemer. *Die Wettergottgestalten Mesopotamiens und Nordsyriens im Zeitalter der Keilschriftkulturen. Materialien und Studien nach den schriftlichen Quellen*. Wiesbaden: Harrassowitz.

Schwemer 2005/06 = D. Schwemer. Lehnbeziehungen zwischen dem Hethitischen und dem Akkadischen. *Archiv für Orientforschung* 51: 220–234.

Schwemer 2007 = D. Schwemer. *Rituale und Beschwörungen gegen Schadenzauber. Keilschrifttexte aus Assur literarischen Inhalts 2*. Wiesbaden: Harrassowitz.

Schwemer 2013 = D. Schwemer. Gauging the Influence of Babylonian magic: The reception of Mesopotamian tradition in Hittite ritual practice. In *Diversity and standardization: perspectives on social and political norms in the Ancient Near East*, eds. E. C. Cancik-Kirschbaum et al. Berlin: Akademie Verlag: 145–171.

Schwemer 2018 = D. Schwemer. Evil Helpers: Instrumentalizing Agents of Evil in Anti-witchcraft Rituals. In *Sources of Evil, Studies in Mesopotamian Exorcistic Lore*, eds. G. Van Buylaere, M. Luukko, D. Schwemer, A. Mertens-Wagschal. Ancient Magic and Divination 15. Leiden and Boston: Brill: 173–191.

Scurlock 2006 = J. Scurlock. *Magico-Medical Means of Treating Ghost-Induced Illnesses in Ancient Mesopotamia* Ancient Magic and Divination 3. Leiden and Boston: Brill.

Scurlock 2008a = J. Scurlock. On some Terms for Leatherworking in Ancient Mesopotamia. In *Proceedings of the 51st Rencontre Assyriologique Internationale held at The Oriental Insitute of The University of Chicago July 18–22, 2005 ; dedicated to the memory of Erica Reiner*, eds. R.D. Biggs, J. Myers, and M.T. Roth. Series in Ancient Oriental Civilization 62. Chicago: The Oriental Institute of the University of Chicago: 171–176.

Scurlock 2008b = J. Scurlock. Some Mesopotamian Medicine for a Greek Headache. In *Studies in Ancient Near Eastern World View and Society presented to Marten Stol on the occasion of his 65th birthday, 10 November 2005, and his retirement from the Vrije Universiteit Amsterdam*, ed. R. J. van der Spek et al. Bethesda: CDL Press: 195–202.

Scurlock 2014 = J. Scurlock. *Sourcebook for Ancient Mesopotamian Medicine*. Writings from the Ancient World 36. Atlanta, Georgia: Society of Biblical Literature.

Scurlock 2017 = J. Scurlock. Medical Texts. In *The Context of Scripture 4. Supplements*, ed. K. L. Younger Jr. Leiden and Bosto: Brill: 275–312.

Scurlock and Andersen 2005 = J. Scurlock and B.R. Andersen. *Diagnoses in Assyrian and Babylonian Medicine. Ancient Sources, Translations, and Modern Medical Analyses*. Urbana: University of Illinois Press.

Searight, Reade, and Finkel 2008 = A. Searight, J. Reade, and I.L. Finkel. *Assyrian Stone vessels and related material in the British Museum*. Oxford: Oxbow Books.

Spencer 1989 = W.G. Spencer. *De medicina by Aulus Cornelius Celsus*. Loeb classical library 304. London: Heinemann.

Stadhouders 2011 = H. Stadhouders. The Pharmacopoeial Handbook *Šammu šikinšu* – An Edition. *Le Journal des Médecines Cunéiformes* 18: 3–50.

Stadhouders 2012 = H. Stadhouders. The Pharmacopoeial Handbook *Šammu šikinšu* – A Translation. *Le Journal des Médecines Cunéiformes* 19: 1–21.
Stadhouders 2018 = H. Stadhouders. The *mirišmarû*-Plant: Orthographic Novelties and a Consecratory Spell. *Die Welt des Orients* 48: 116–127.
Steinert 2015 = U. Steinert. "Tested" Remedies in Mesopotamian Medical Texts: A Label for Efficacy Based on Empirical Observation? In *In the Wake of the Compendia. Infrastructural Contexts and the Licensing of Empiricism in Ancient and Medieval Mesopotamia*, ed. J. C. Johnson. Boston and Berlin: Walter de Gruyter: 103–145.
Steinert, Panayotov, Geller, Schmidtchen and Johnson 2018 = U. Steinert, S.V. Panayotov, M.J. Geller, E. Schmidtchen, and J.C. Johnson. AMC Text Edition. In *Assyrian and Babylonian Scholarly Text Catalogues: Medicine, Magic and Divination*, ed. U. Steinert. Die babylonisch-assyrische Medizin in Texten und Untersuchungen 9. Boston and Berlin: Walter de Gruyter: 209–219.
Sternitzke 2012 = K. Sternitzke. Spatel, Sonde und Skalpell. Medizinische Instrumente im Archäologischen Befund. In *Stories of long ago. Festschrift für Michael D. Roaf*, eds. H. Baker, K. Kaniuth und A. Otto. Alter Orient und Altes Testament 397. Münster: Ugarit: 649–666.
Stol 1979a = M. Stol. *On Trees, mountains and millstones in the ancient Near East. With a chapter by K. van Lerberghe*. Mededelingen en verhandelingen van het Vooraziatisch-egyptisch Genootschap "Ex Oriente Lux" 21. Leiden: Ex oriente lux.
Stol 1979a = M. Stol. Review of Early Old Babylonian Documents by Stephen D. Simmons. *Journal of Cuneiform Studies* 31: 177–183.
Stol 1985 = M. Stol. The Cucurbitaceae in Cuneiform Texts. *Bulletin of Sumerian Agriculture* 3: 81–92.
Stol 1986 = M. Stol. Blindness and Night-Blindness in Akkadian. *Journal of Near Eastern Studies* 45: 295–299.
Stol 1989a = M. Stol. Old Babylonian Ophthalmology. In *Reflets des deux fleuves: volume de mélanges offerts à André Finet*, eds. M. Lebeau and P. Talon. Akkadica Supplementum 6. Leuven: Peeters: 163–166.
Stol 1989b = M. Stol. Malz. *Reallexikon der Assyriologie und Vorderasiatischen Archäologie* 7: 322–329.
Stol 1991/92 = M. Stol. Diagnosis and Therapy in Babylonian medicine. *Jaarbericht Ex Oriente Lux* 32: 42–65.
Stol 1993a = M. Stol. *Epilepsy in Babylonia*. Cuneiform Monographs 2. Groningen: Styx.
Stol 1993b = M. Stol. Milk, Butter, and cheese. *Bulletin on Sumerian Agriculture* 7: 99–113.
Stol 1994 = M. Stol. Beer in Neo-Babylonian Times. In *Drinking in Ancient Societies: History and Culture of Drinks in the Ancient Near East: Papers of a Symposium Held in Rome, May 17–19, 1990*, ed. L. Milano. History of the Ancient Near East, Studies 6. Padova: Sargon: 155–183.
Stol 1998 = M. Stol. Einige kurze Wortstudien. In *Festschrift für Rykle Borger zu seinem 65. Geburtstag am 24. Mai 1994: tikip santakki mala bašmu*, ed. S. Maul. Cuneiform Monographs 10. Groningen: Styx Publications: 343–352.
Stol 2007a = M. Stol. Fevers in Babylonia In *Disease in Babylonia*, eds. I. L. Finkel and M. J. Geller. Cuneiform Monographs 36. Leiden and Boston: Brill: 1–39.
Stol 2007b = M. Stol. Remarks on some Sumerograms and Akkadian. In *From the workshop of the Chicago Assyrian Dictionary, volume 2: Studies presented to Robert D. Biggs, June 4, 2004*, eds. M.T. Roth, et al. Chicago: The Oriental Institute: 233–242.
Stol 2012 = M. Stol. Bitumen in Ancient Mesopotamia. The Textual Evidence. *Bibliotheca Orientalis* 69: 48–60.
Stol 2014 = M. Stol. Trüffel. *Reallexikon der Assyriologie und Vorderasiatischen Archäologie* 14: 149–150.
Stol 2016a = M. Stol. Review of Borger, R. *Mesopotamisches Zeichenlexikon. Zweite, revidierte und aktualisierte Auflage. Orientalistische Literaturzeitung* 111: 119–134.

Stol 2016b = M. Stol. *Women in the Ancient Near East*. Boston and Berlin: Walter de Gruyter.

Stol, Cadelli, and Milano 2001 = M. Stol, D. Cadelli, D. and L. Milano. Vicino Oriente antico. La cura del corpo, in Storia della Scienza, <http://www.treccani.it/enciclopedia/vicino-oriente-antico-la-cura-del-corpo_%28Storia_della_Scienza%29/>.

Tecusan 2004 = M. Tecusan. *The Fragments of the Methodists, Methodism outside Soranus*. Leiden and Boston: Brill.

Thompson 1923 = R.C. Thompson. *Assyrian Medical Texts from the Originals in the British Museum*. London et. al.: AMS Pr.

Thompson 1924 = R.C. Thompson. Assyrian Medical Texts. *Proceedings of the Royal Society of Medicine* 17: 1–34.

Thompson 1926 = R.C. Thompson. Assyrian Medical Texts II. *Proceedings of the Royal Society of Medicine* 19 (*Section of the history of Medicine*): 29–78.

Thompson 1937a = R.C. Thompson. Assyrian Prescriptions for the Head. *The American Journal of Semitic Languages and Literatures* 53: 217–238.

Thompson 1937b = R.C. Thompson. Assyrian Prescriptions for the Head (Concluded). *The American Journal of Semitic Languages and Literatures* 54: 12–40.

Thompson 1949 = R.C. Thompson. *A Dictionary of Assyrian Botany*. London: The British Academy.

Townsend and Guest 1980 = C.C. Townsend and E. Guest. (eds.). *Cornaceae to Rubiaceae*. Flora of Iraq 4/1. Baghdad.

Van Dijk 1983 = J.J.A. van Dijk. *Lugal ud me-lám-bi Nir-gál: le récit épique et didactique des Travaux de Ninurta, du Déluge et de la Nouvelle Création: texte, traduction et introduction*. Leiden: Brill.

Van Dijk and Geller 2003 = J.J.A. van Dijk and M.J. Geller. *Ur III Incantations from the Frau Professor Hilprecht-Collection, Jena*. Texte und Materialien der Frau Professor Hilprecht Collection of Babylonian Antiquities im Eigentum der Universität Jena, Bd. 6. Wiesbaden: Harrassowitz.

Viano 2016 = M. Viano. *The Reception of Sumerian Literature in the Western Periphery*. Antichistica: Studi Orientali 9/4. Venezia: Edizioni Ca' Foscari.

Vodenicharov and Petrov 2001: *Otrovni rastenija i otravjanija s tjah* (Воденичаров, Д.Г. и А. Петров. Отровни растения и отравяния с тях). Sofia: Pensoft.

von Soden 1971 = W. von Soden. Der große Hymnus an Nabû. *Zeitschrift für Assyriologie und Vorderasiatische Archäologie* 61: 44–71.

von Soden 1995 = W. von Soden. *Grundriss der akkadischen Grammatik*. 3., ergänzte Auflage unter Mitarbeit von Werner R. Mayer. Roma: Pontificium Inst. Biblicum.

von Weiher 1983 = E. von Weiher. *Spätbabylonische Texte aus Uruk, Teil 2*. Ausgrabungen der Deutschen Forschungsgemeinschaft in Uruk-Warka 10. Berlin: Gebr. Mann Verlag.

von Weiher 1988 = E. von Weiher. *Spätbabylonische Texte aus Uruk, Teil 3*. Ausgrabungen der Deutschen Forschungsgemeinschaft in Uruk-Warka 12. Berlin: Gebr. Mann Verlag.

Wang and Carey 2014 = D.Q-H. Wang and M.C. Carey. Therapeutic Uses of animal biles in traditional Chinese medicine: An ethnopharmacological, biophysical chemical and medicinal review. *World Journal of Gastroenterology* 20. 9952–9975.

Wasserman 2007 = N. Wasserman. Between Magic and Medicine – Apropos of an Old Babylonian Therapeutic Text against the Kurārum Disease. In *Disease in Babylonia*, eds. I. L. Finkel and M. J. Geller. Cuneiform Monographs 36. Leiden and Boston: Brill: 40–61.

Wasserman 2010 = N. Wasserman. From the Notebook of a Professional Exorcist. In *Von Göttern und Menschen: Beiträge zu Literatur und Geschichte des Alten Orients. Festschrift für Brigitte Groneberg*, eds. D. Shehata, F. Weiershäuser, and K. Zand. Cuneiform Monographs 41. Leiden-Boston: Brill: 329–349.

Wasserman 2015 = N. Wasserman. Piercing the Eyes: an Old Babylonian love incantation and the preparation of kohl. *Bibliotheca Orientalis* 72: 601–612.

Weeden 2009 = M. Weeden. The Akkadian Words for "Grain" and the God Ḫaya. *Die Welt des Orients* 39: 77–107.
Westendorf 1999 = W. Westendorf. *Handbuch der altägyptischen Medizin 1. und 2. Band.* Handbuch der Orientalistik 36. Leiden: Brill.
Westenholz 2010 = J.G. Westenholz. Ninkarrak – an Akkadian goddess in Sumerian guise. In *Von Göttern und Menschen: Beiträge zu Literatur und Geschichte des Alten Orients. Festschrift für Brigitte Groneberg*, eds. D. Shehata, F. Weiershäuser, and K. Zand. Cuneiform Monographs 41. Leiden-Boston: Brill: 377–405
Westenholz and Sigrist 2006 = J.G. Westenholz and M. Sigrist. The Brain, the Marrow and the Seat of Cognition in Mesopotamian Tradition. *Le Journal des Médecines Cunéiformes* 7: 1–10.
Wiggermann 1992 = F.A.M. Wiggermann. *Mesopotamian Protective Spirits: The Ritual Texts.* Cuneiform Monographs 1. Groningen: Styx.
Wiggermann 2000 = F.A.M. Wiggermann. 'Lamaštu, Daughter of Anu. A Profile.' In *Birth in Babylonia and the Bible. Its Mediterranean Setting*, M. Stol. Cuneiform Monographs 14. Groningen: Styx: 217–52.
Wiseman and Black 1996 = D.J. Wiseman and J.A. Black. 1996. *Literary Texts from the Temple of Nabû.* Cuneiform Texts from Nimrud 4. Oxford: British School of Archaeology in Iraq.
Worthington 2005 = M. Worthington. Edition of UGU 1 (=BAM 480 etc.). *Le Journal des Médecines Cunéiformes* 5: 6–43.
Worthington 2006 = M. Worthington. Edition of BAM 3. *Le Journal des Médecines Cunéiformes* 7. 18–48.
Worthington 2007 = M. Worthington. Addenda and Corrigenda to "Edition of UGU 1 (=BAM 480 etc.)" and "Edition of BAM 3". *Le Journal des Médecines Cunéiformes* 9: 43–48.
Zaccagnini 1983 = C. Zaccagnini. Patterns of Mobility among Ancient near Eastern Craftsmen. *Journal of Near Eastern Studies* 42: 245–264.
Ziegler 2005 = N. Ziegler. Les vaisseaux sanguins et Enûma eliš VI: 5. *Le Journal des Médecines Cunéiformes* 5: 4–5.
Zomer 2015 = E. Zomer. Review of Böck. 2014. *The Healing Goddess Gula. Towards an Understanding of Ancient Babylonian Medicine. Bibliotheca Orientalis* 72: 106–110.
Zomer 2018 = E. Zomer. 'The Physician is the Judge!'— A Remarkable Divine Dialogue in the Incantation: ÉN ur-saĝ ^{d}asal-lú-ḫi igi-bé ḫé-pà saĝ-ḫul-ḫa-za ḫé-pà. *Le Journal des Médecines Cunéiformes* 31: 38–42.

Indices

Subject Index

https://doi.org/10.1515/9781501506550-015

Index of Divine Names

See also Divine Names in the Glossary

Index of Personal Names

Index of Geographical Names

Index of Texts

Obverse

col. i

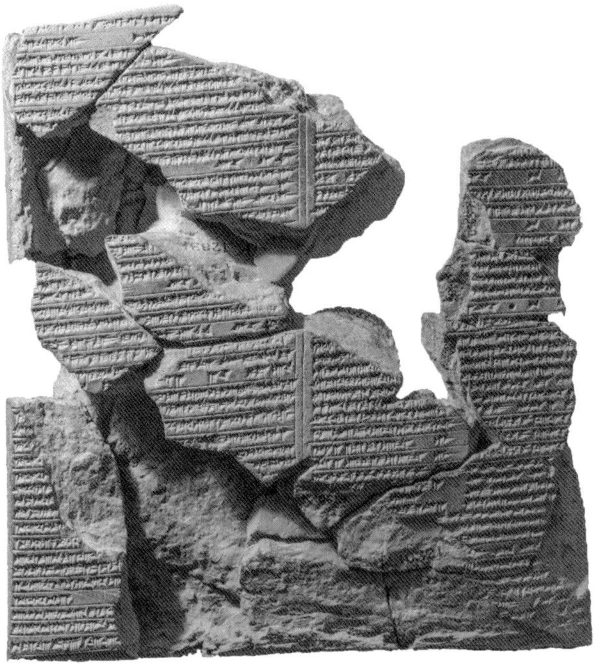

col. ii

Reverse

col. iv

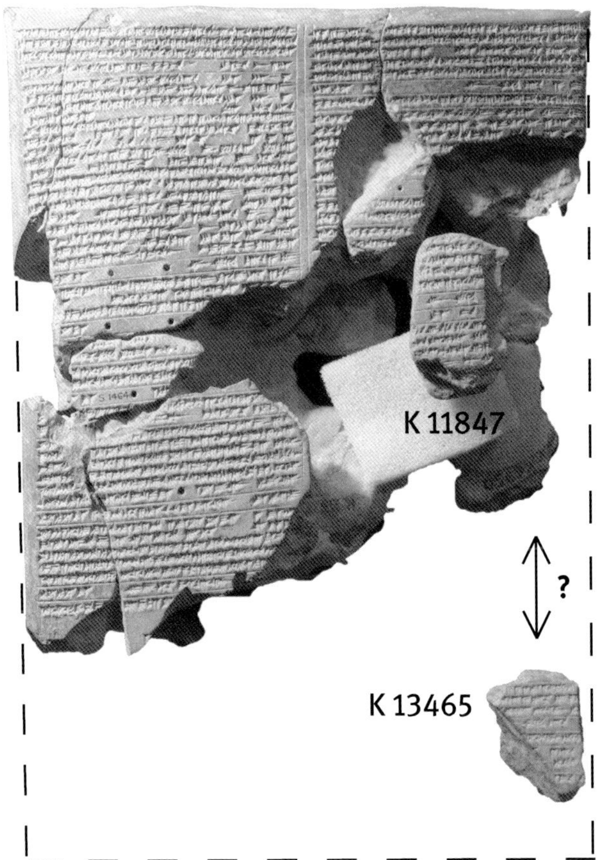

col. iii

Photos S.V.Panayotov

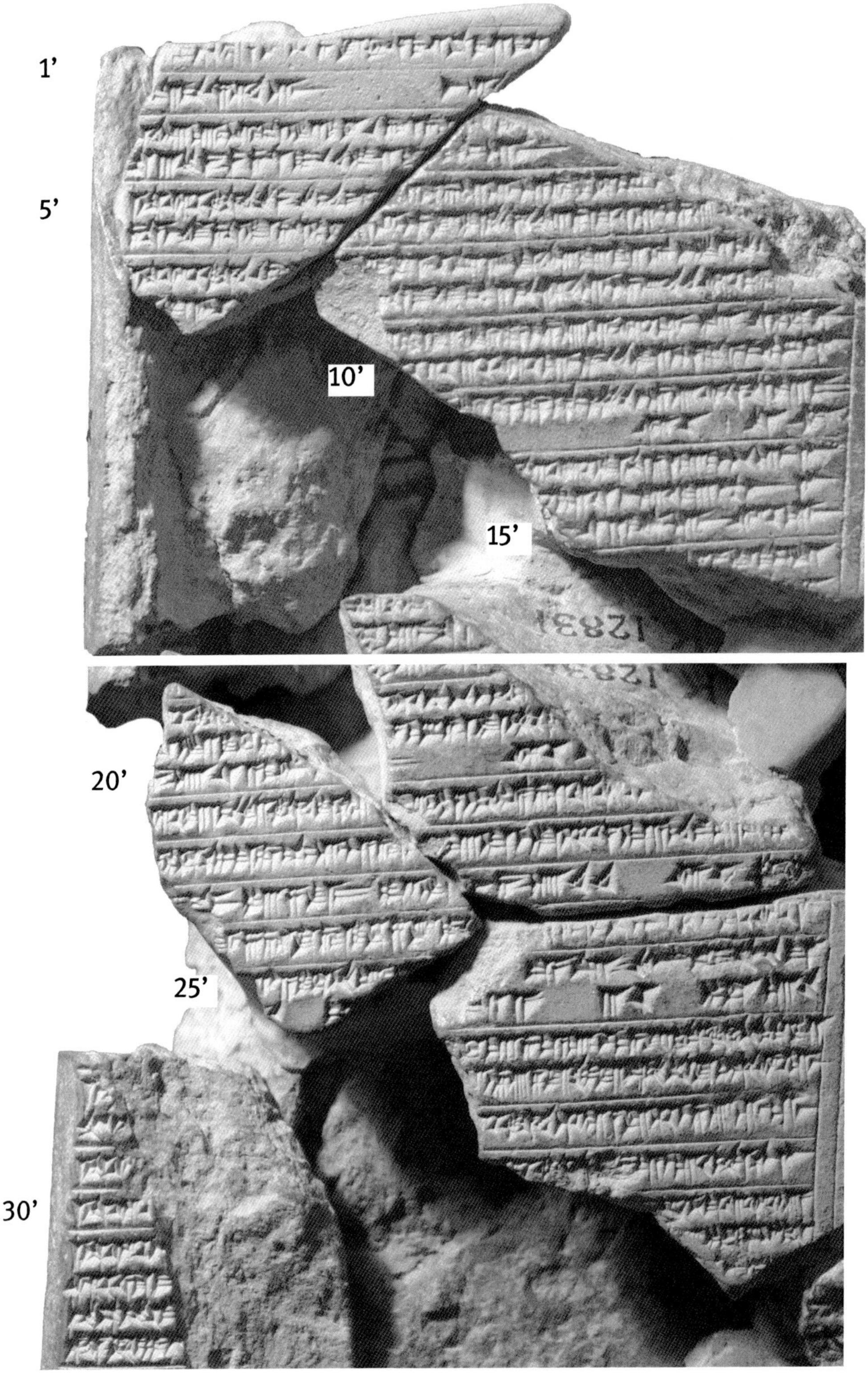

Photos S.V.Panayotov

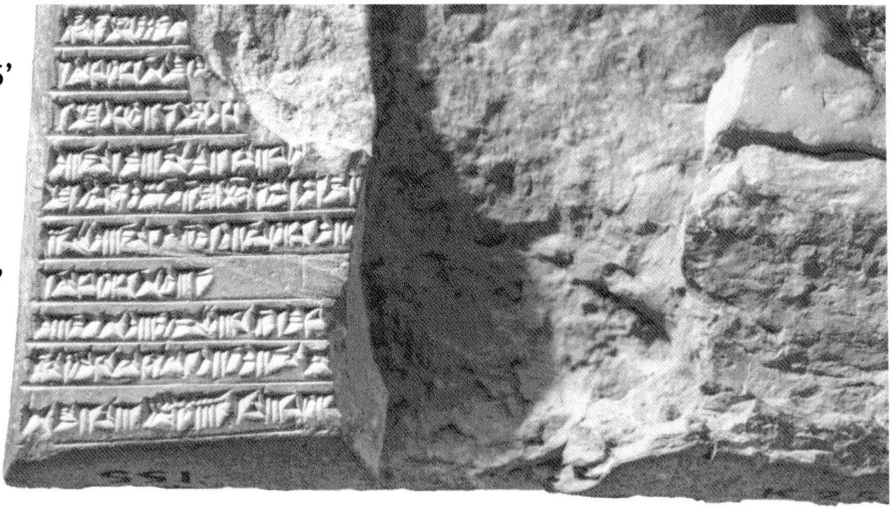

col. ii

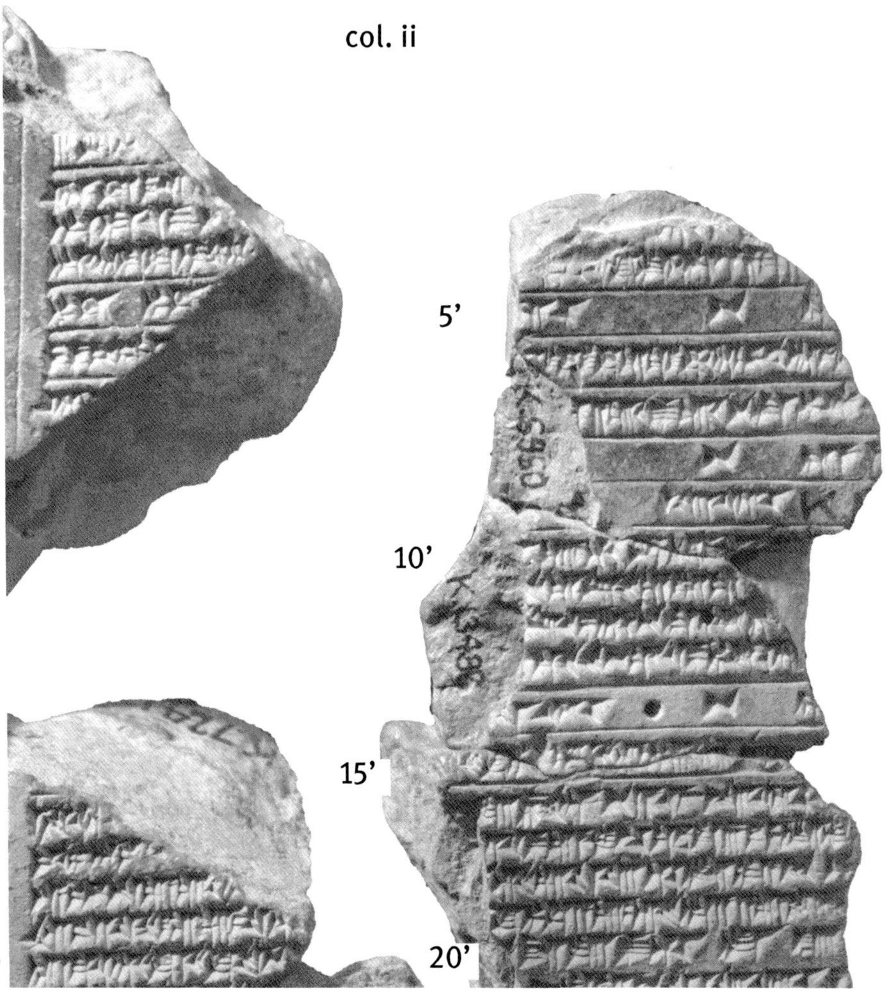

Photos S.V.Panayotov

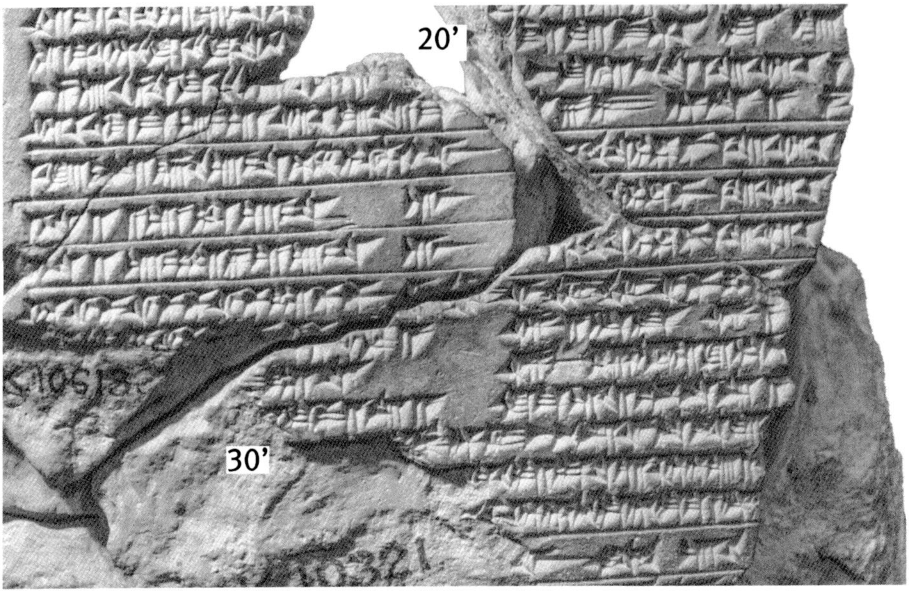

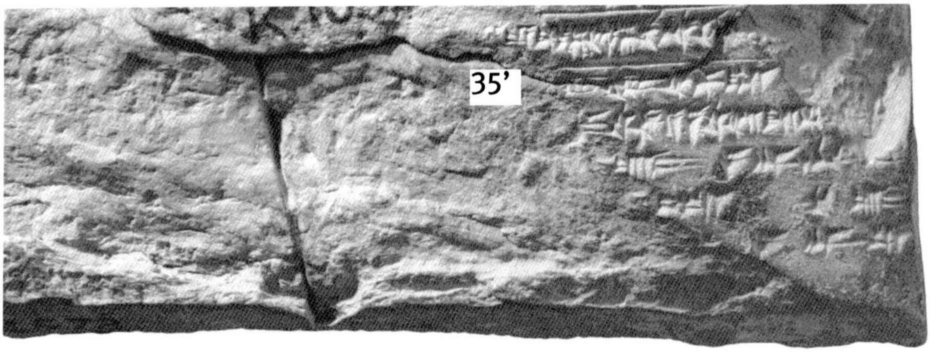

col. iii

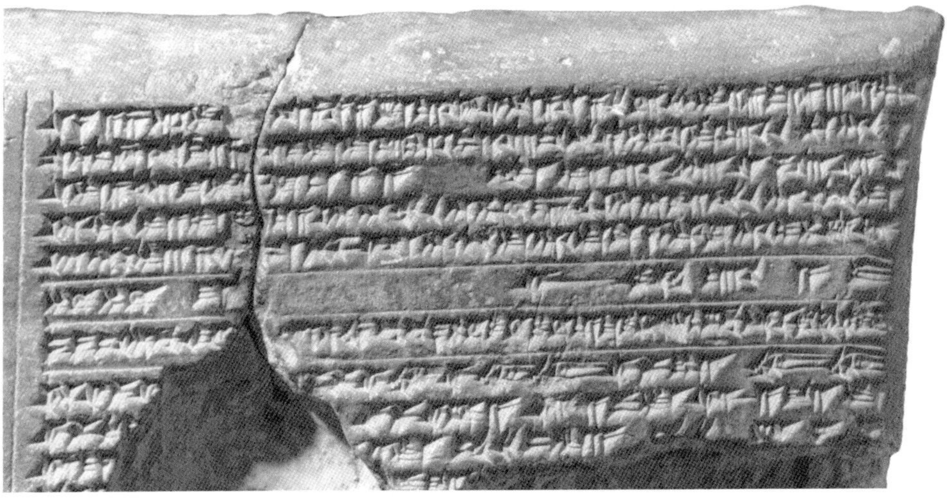

Photos S.V.Panayotov

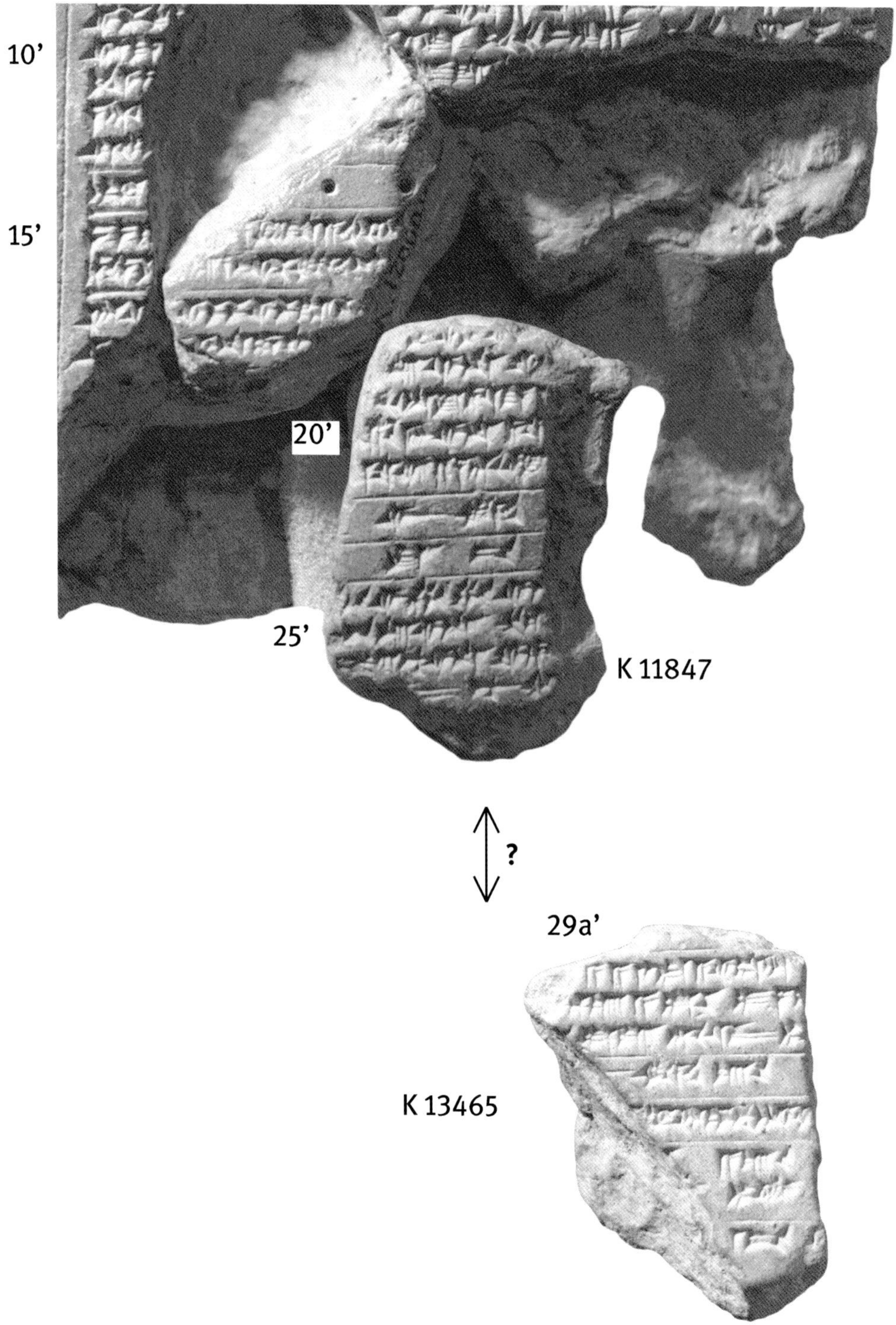

Photos S.V.Panayotov

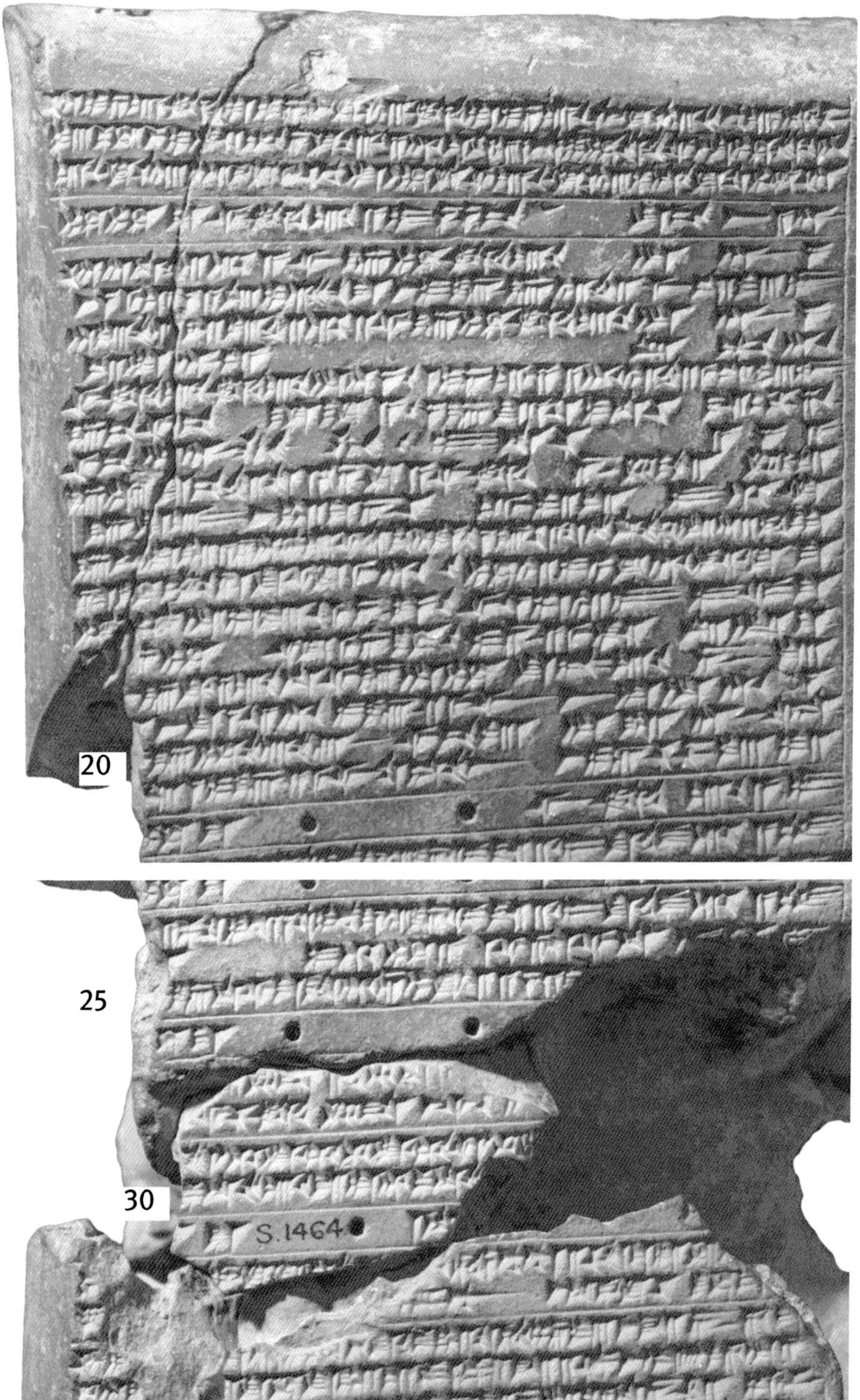

Photos S.V.Panayotov

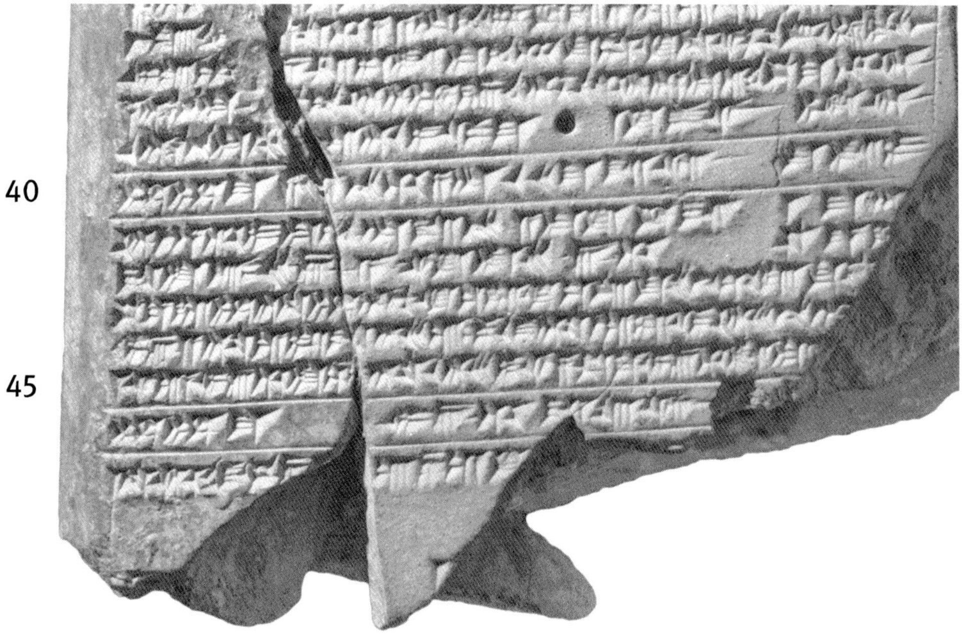

IGI Tablet I Manuscript NB (BAM 513) Overview Obverse

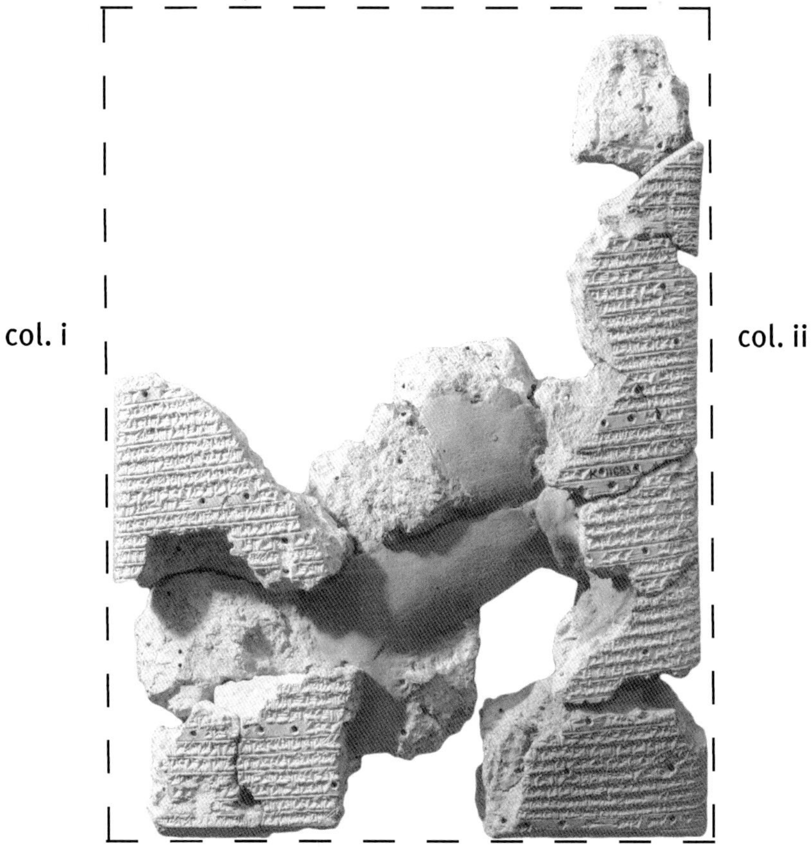

Photos S.V.Panayotov

Plate 8 — IGI Tablet I Manuscript NB (BAM 513) Col. i

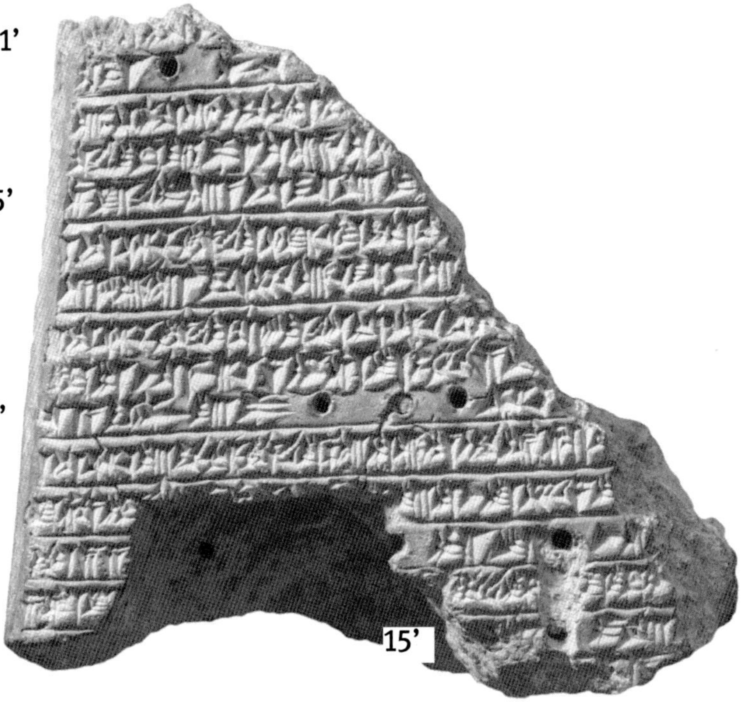

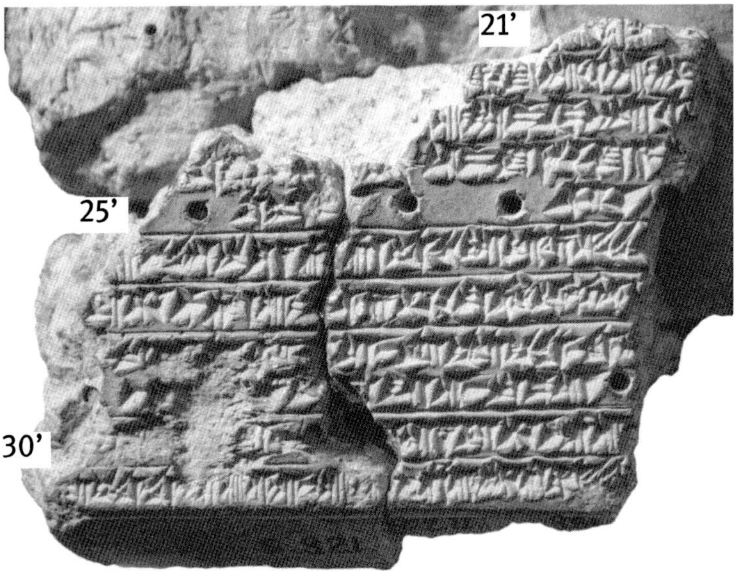

Photos S.V.Panayotov

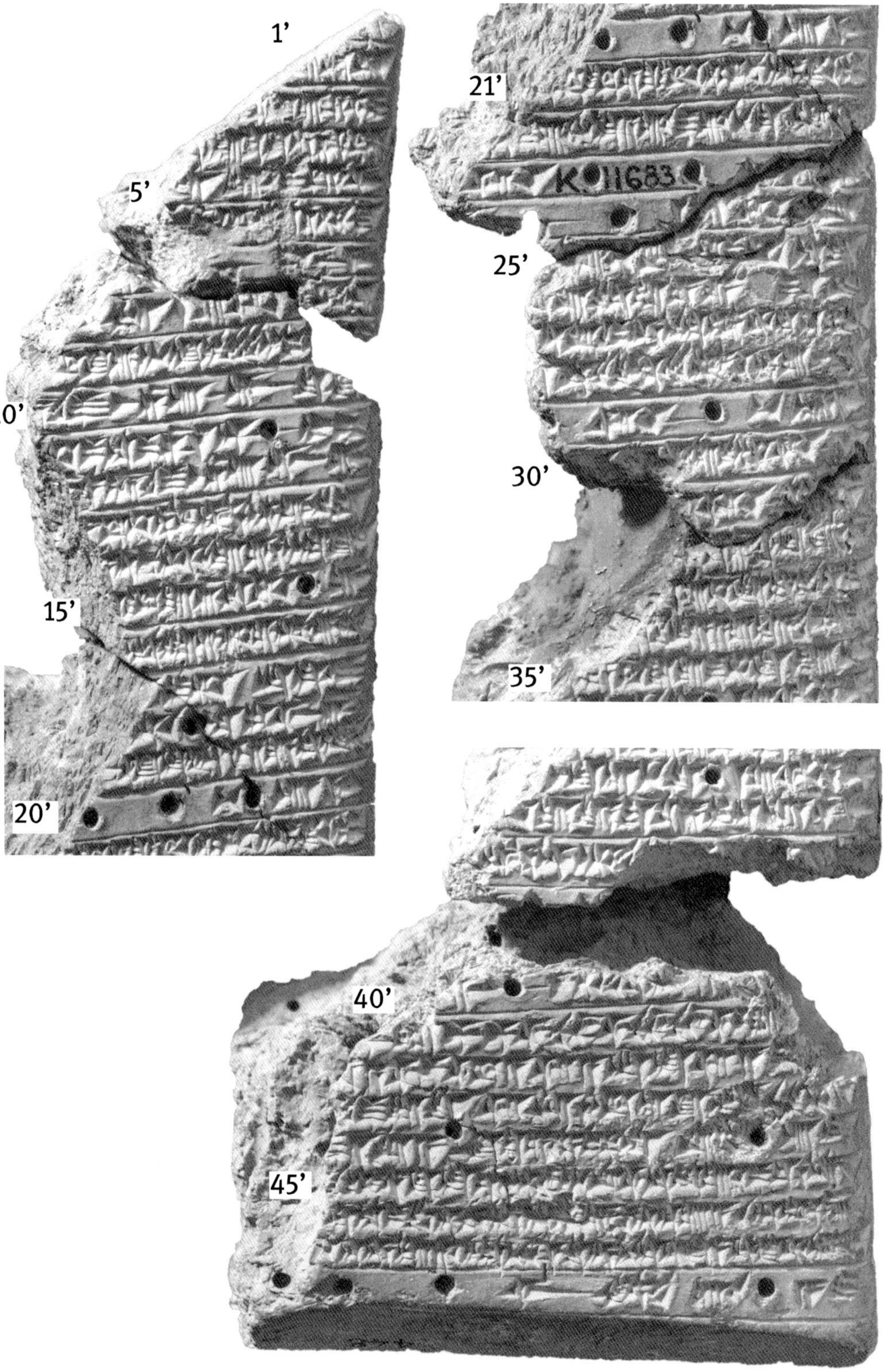

Photos S.V.Panayotov

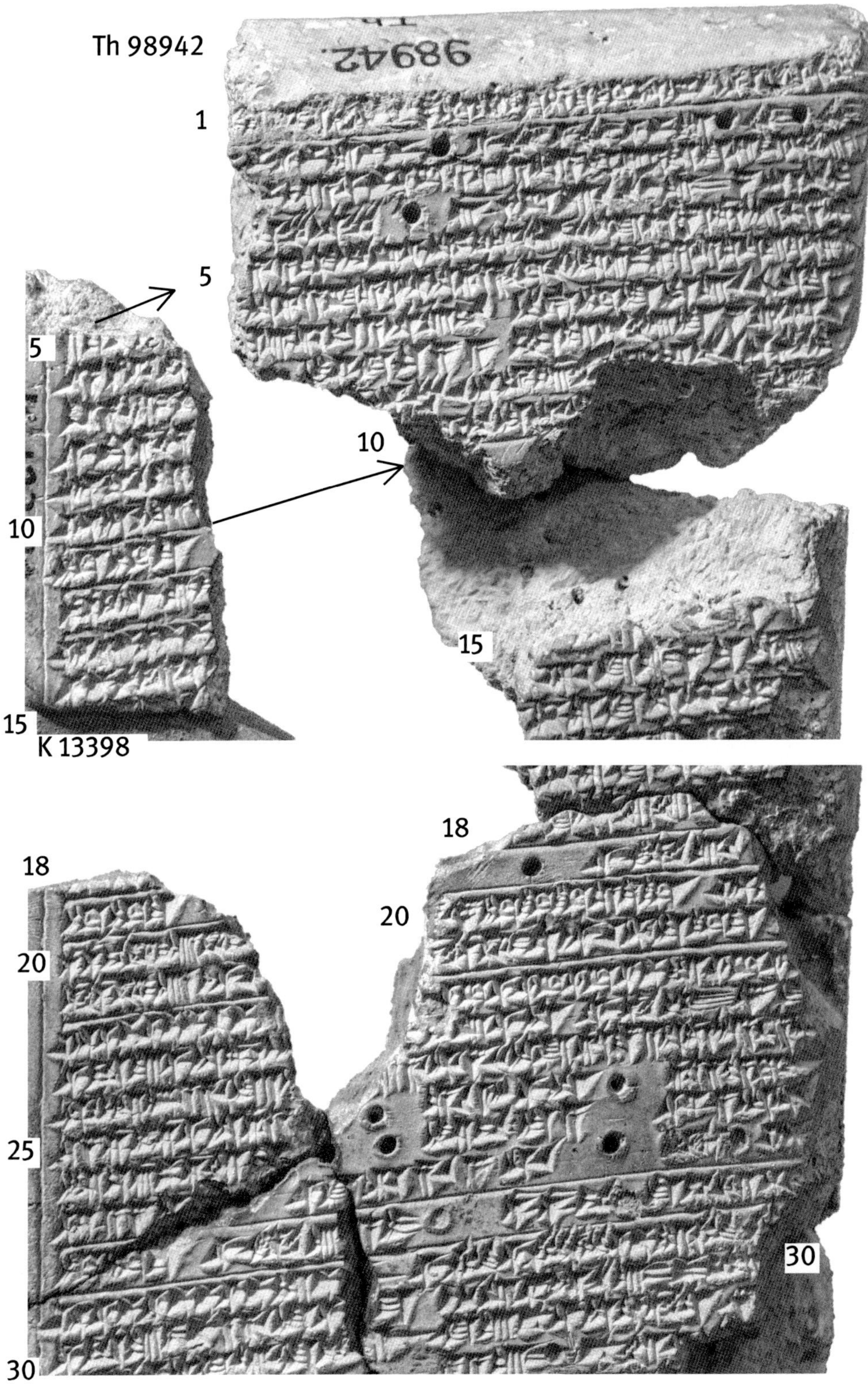

Photos S.V.Panayotov

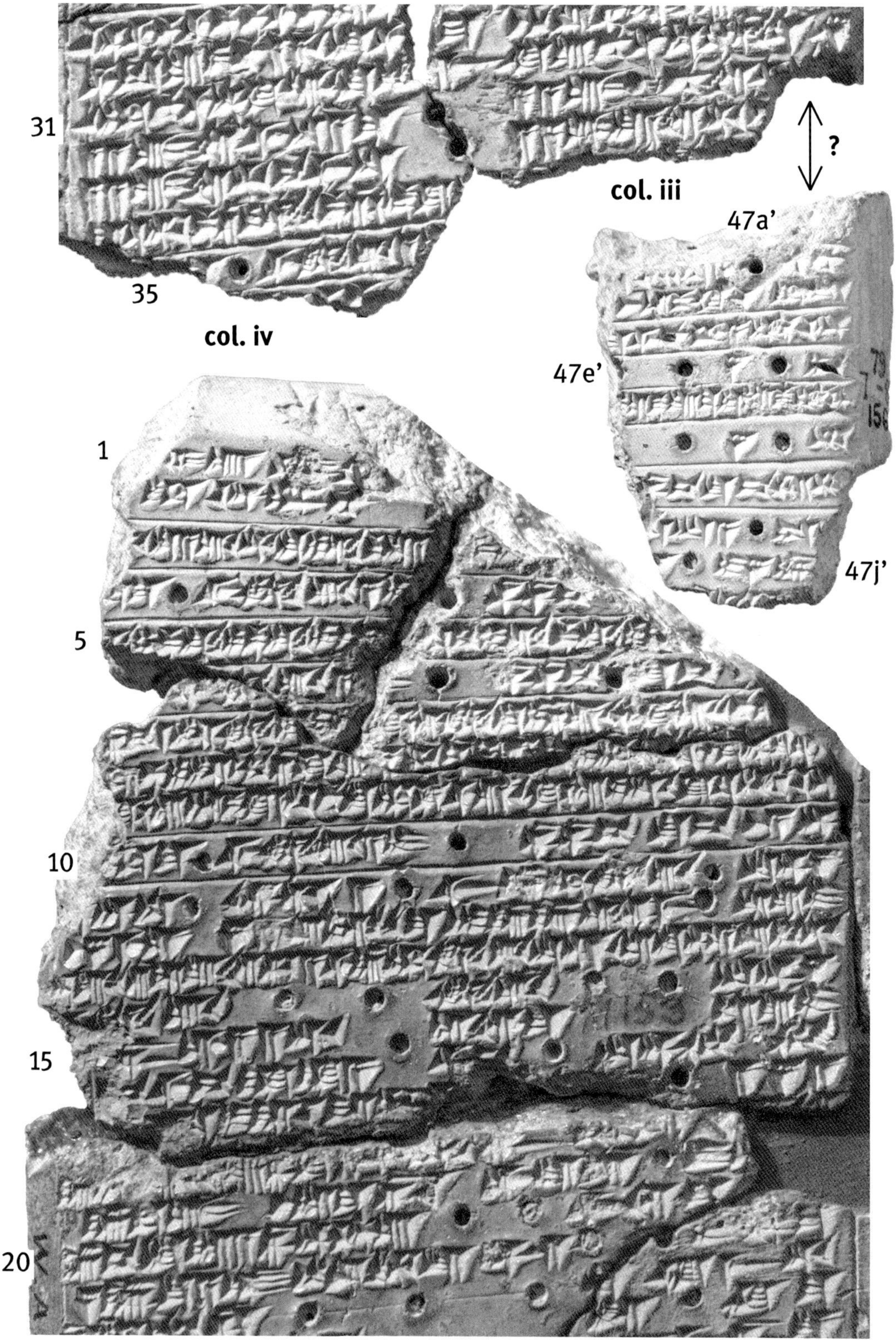

Photos S.V.Panayotov

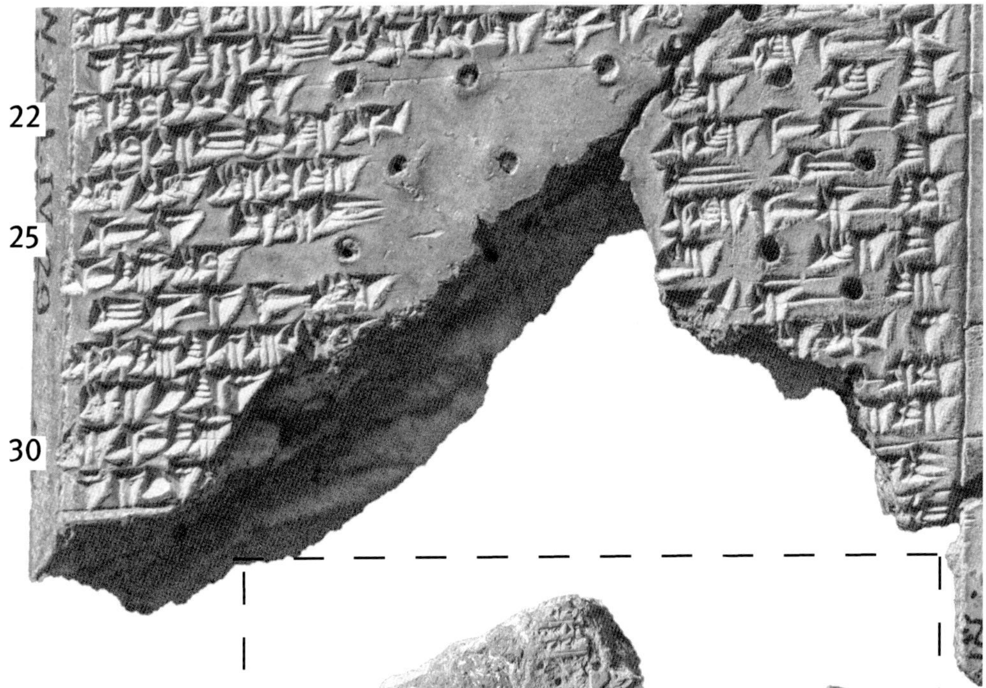

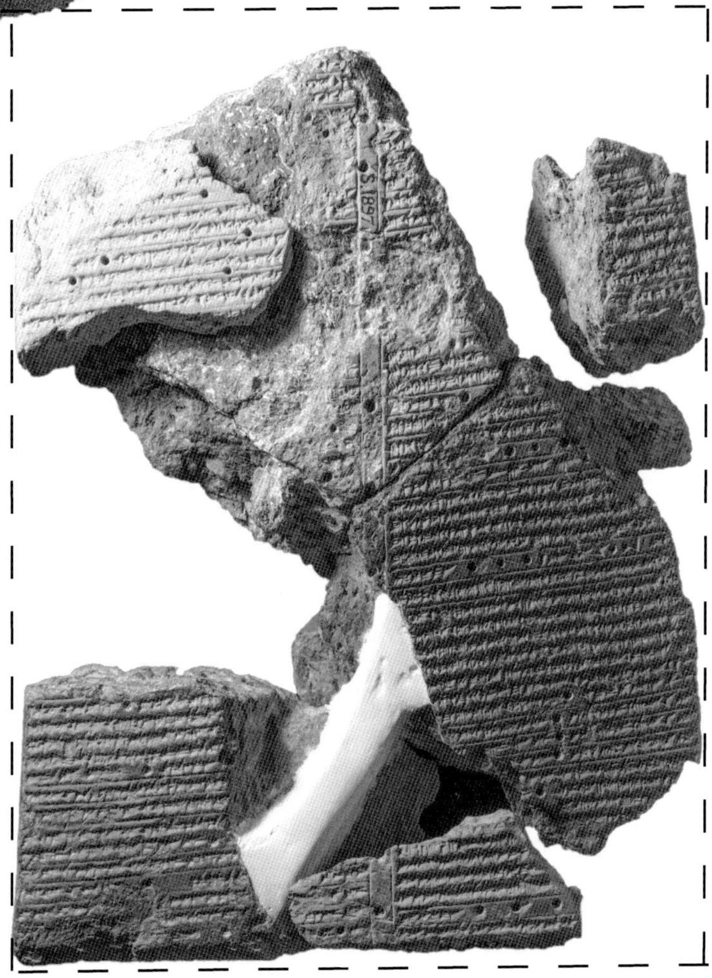

**IGI Tablet I
Manuscript NC
(BAM 514)
Overview
Obverse**

Photos S.V.Panayotov

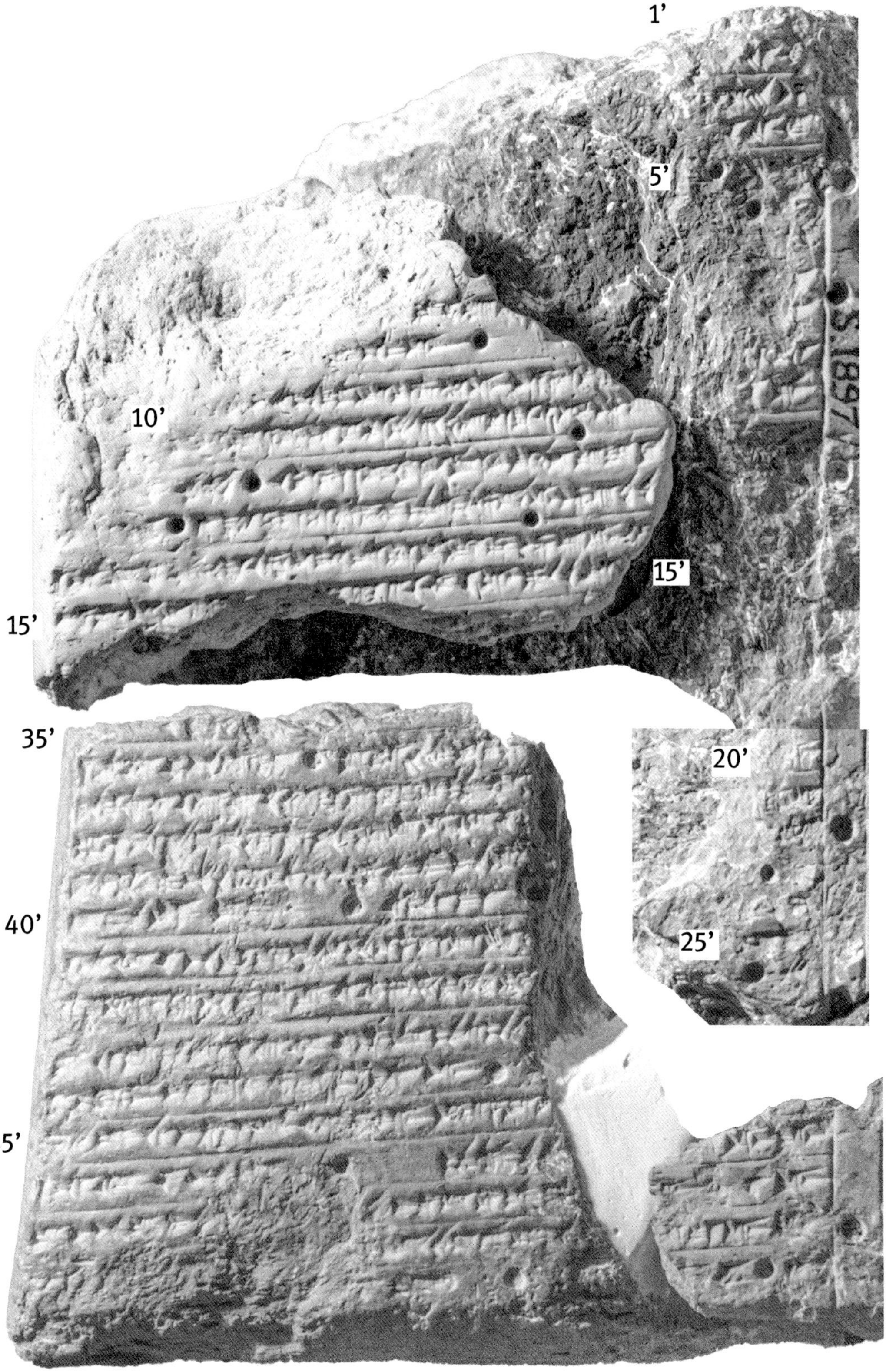

Photos S.V.Panayotov

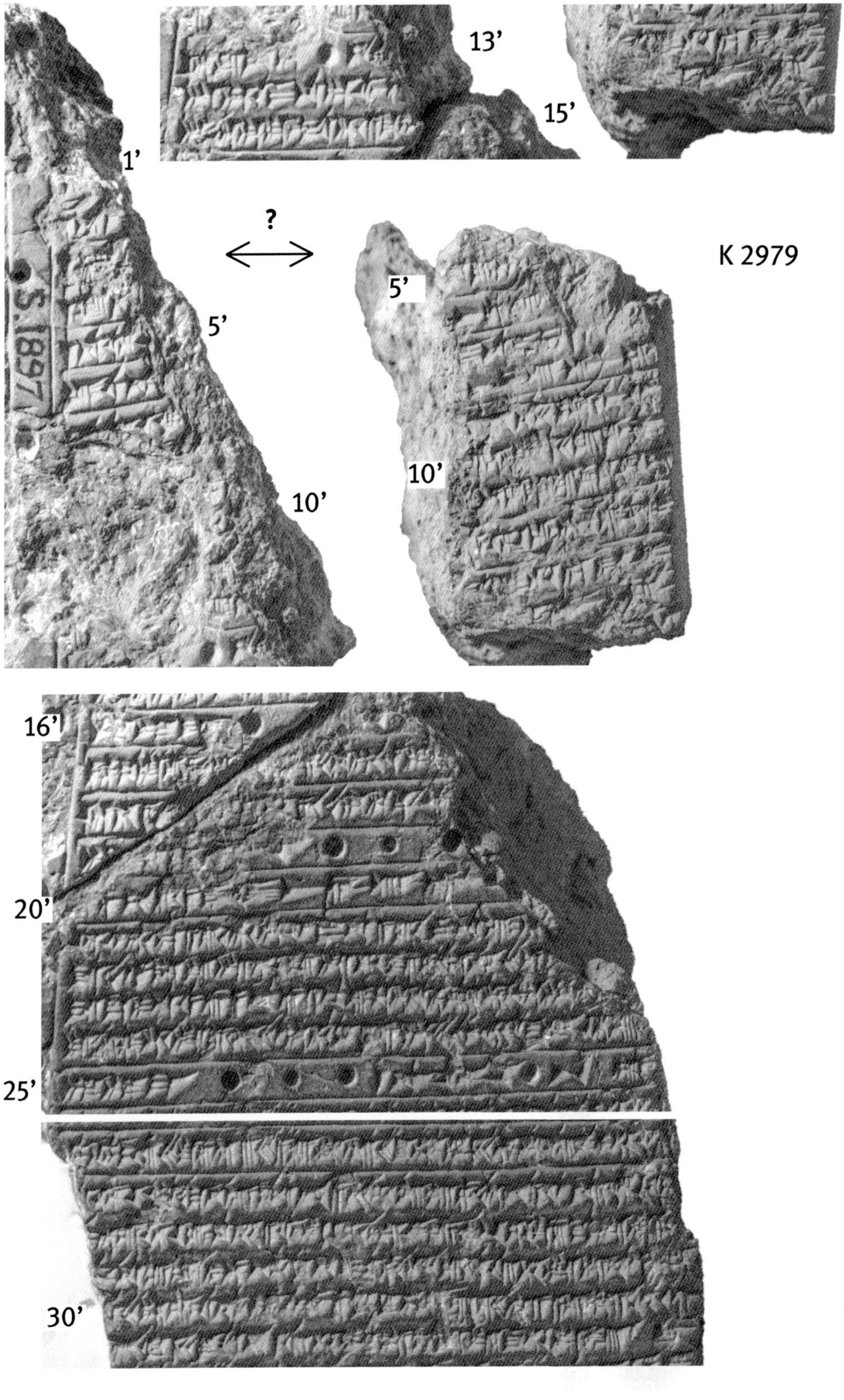

Photos S.V.Panayotov

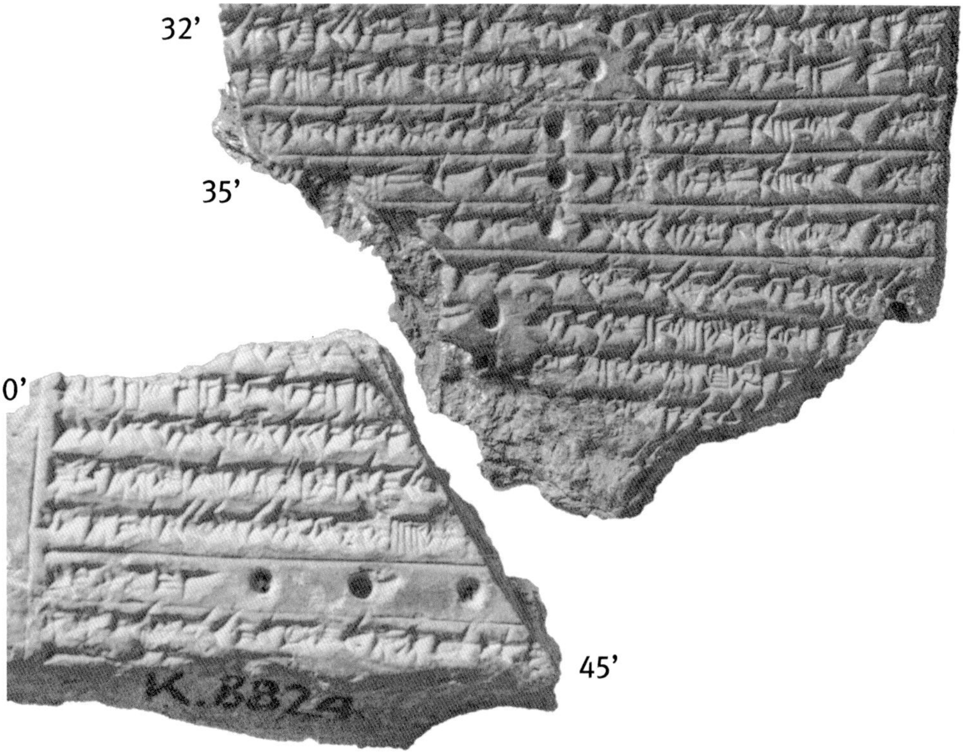

col. iii

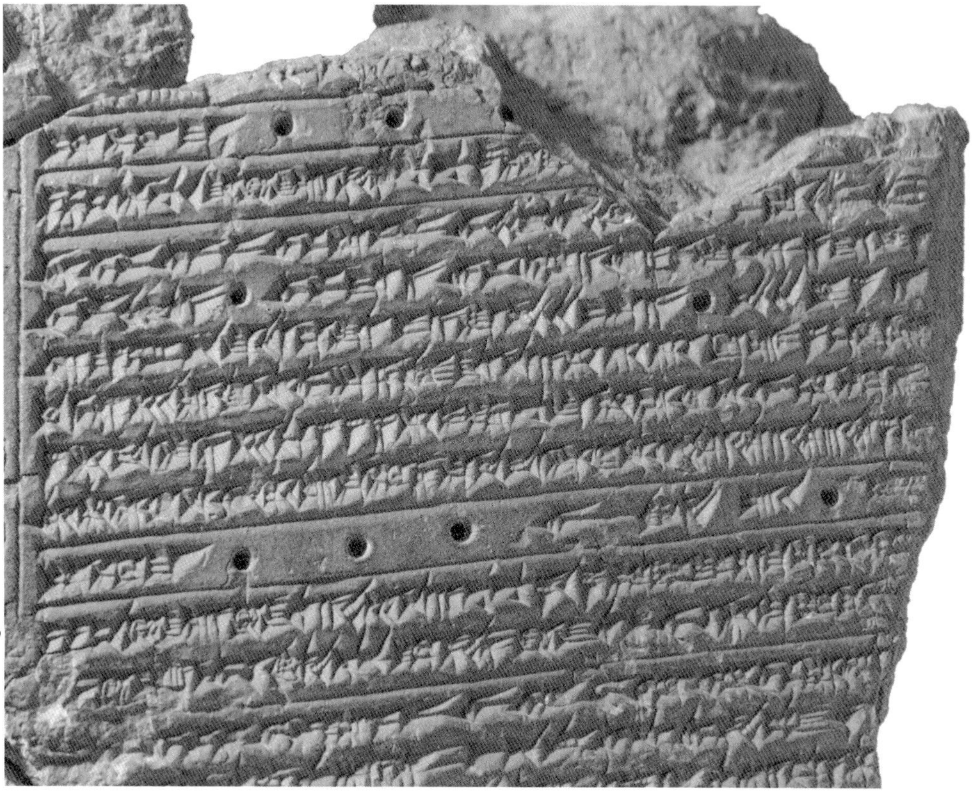

Photos S.V.Panayotov

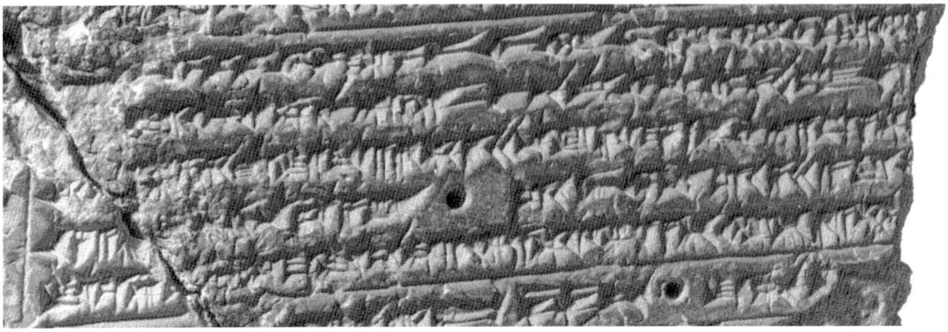

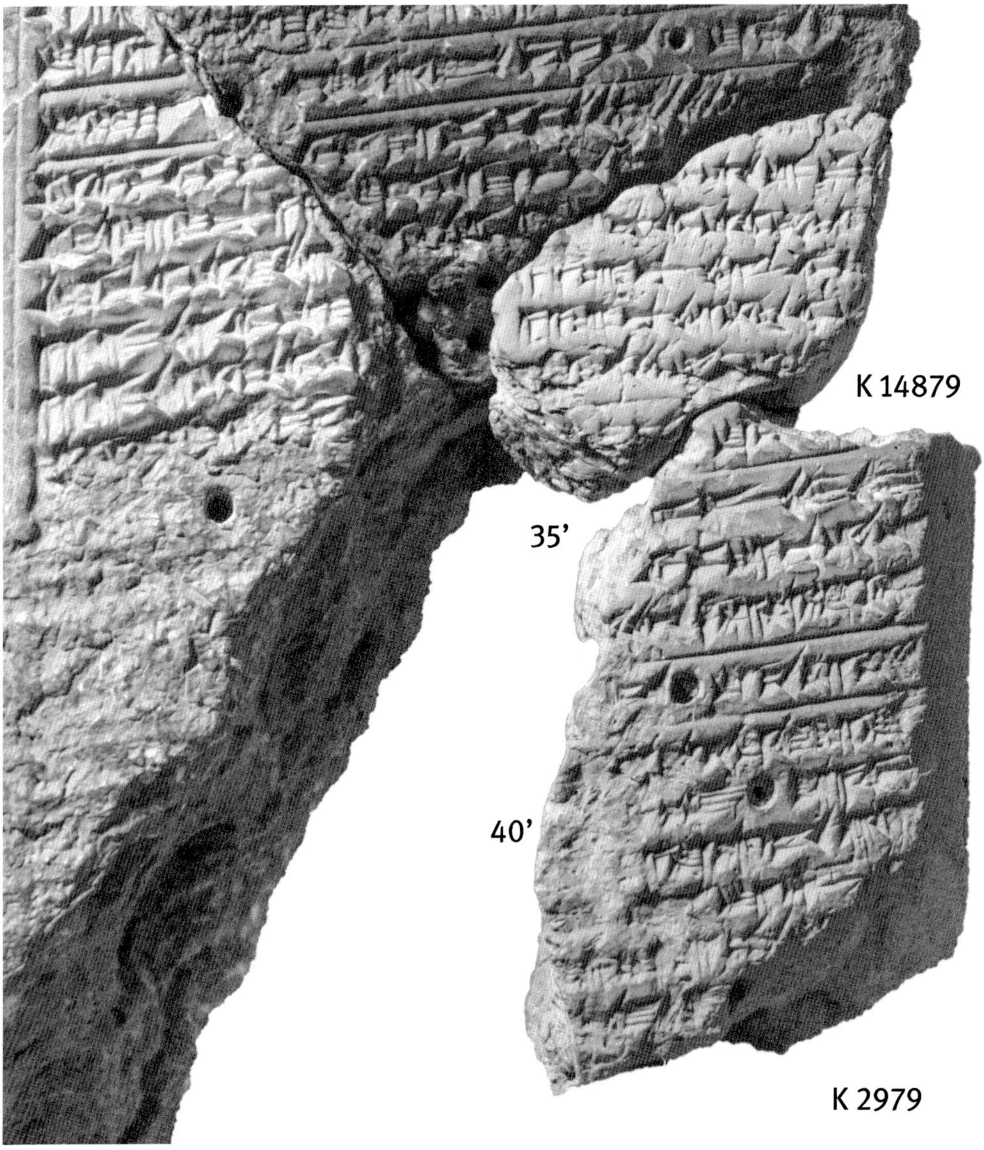

Photos S.V.Panayotov

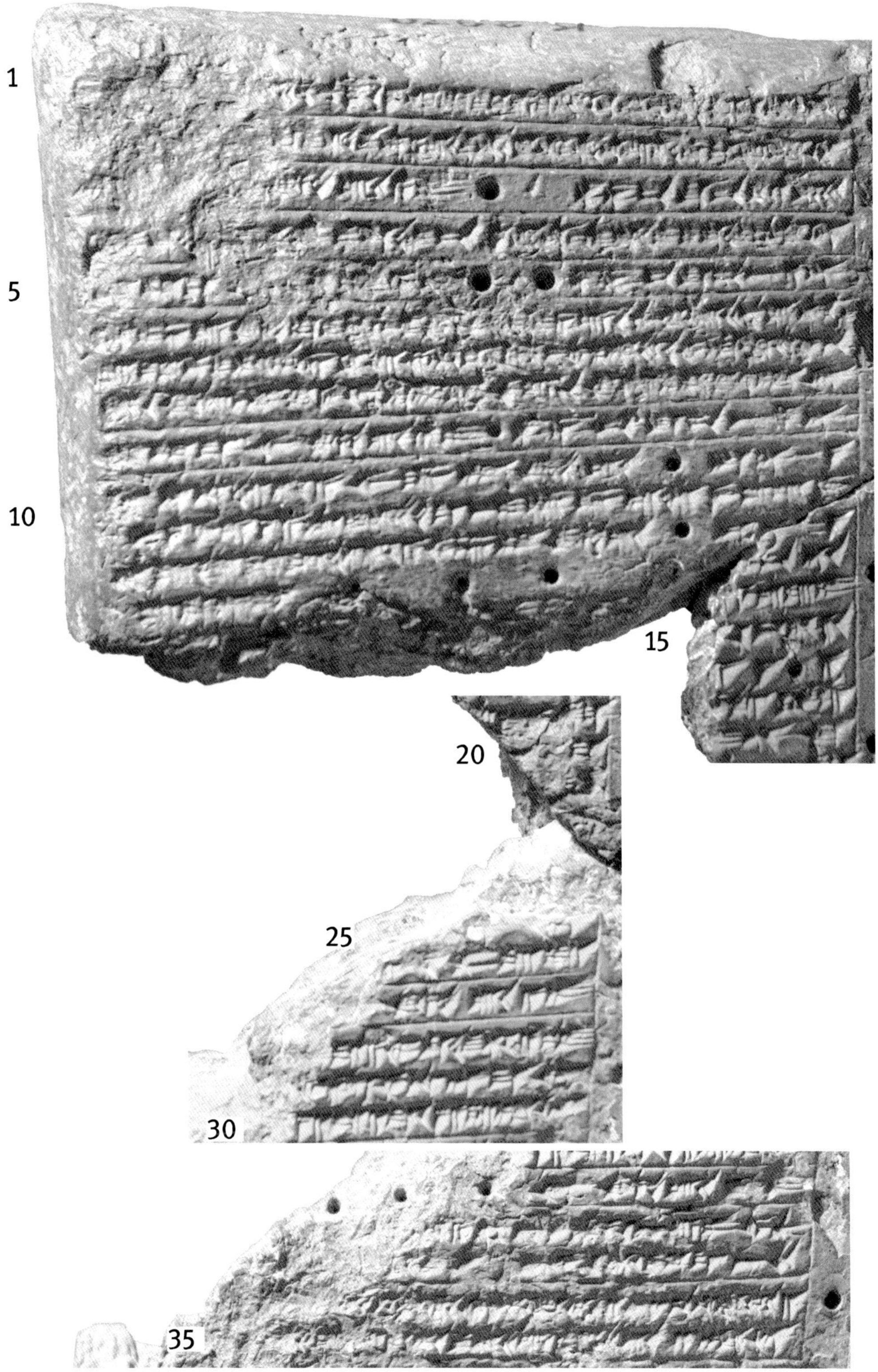

Photos S.V.Panayotov

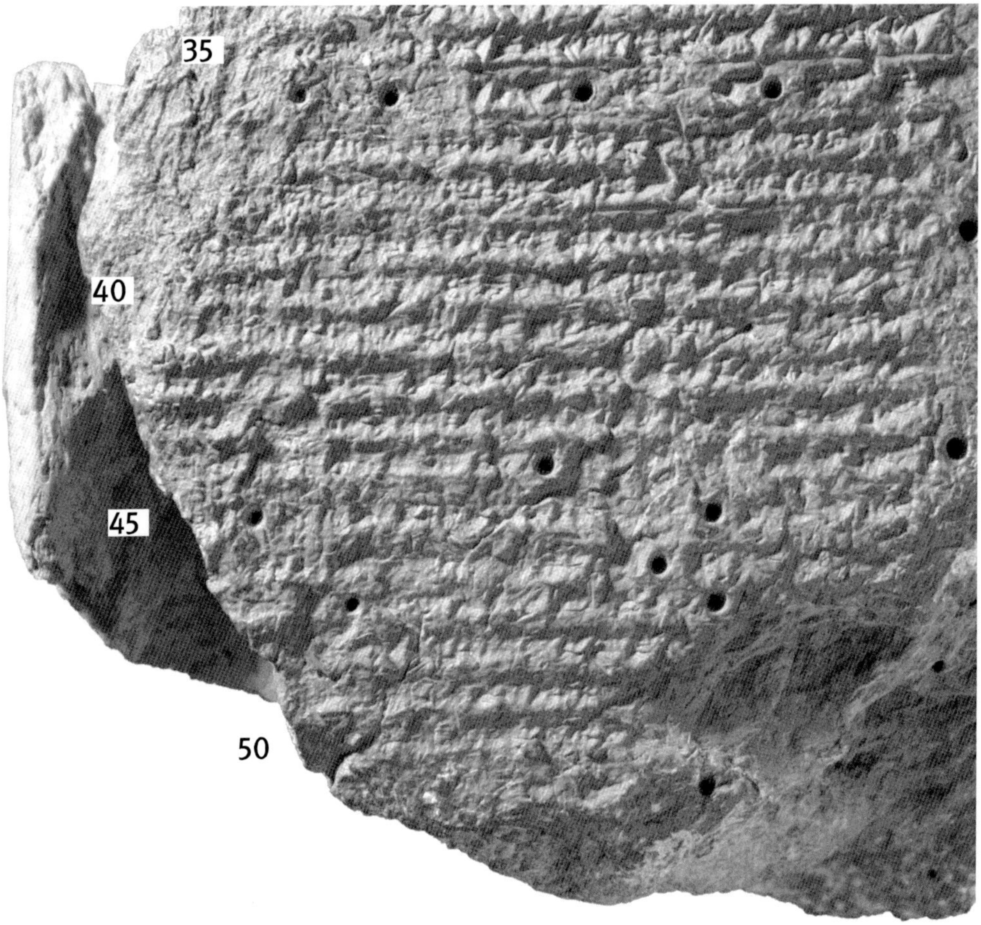

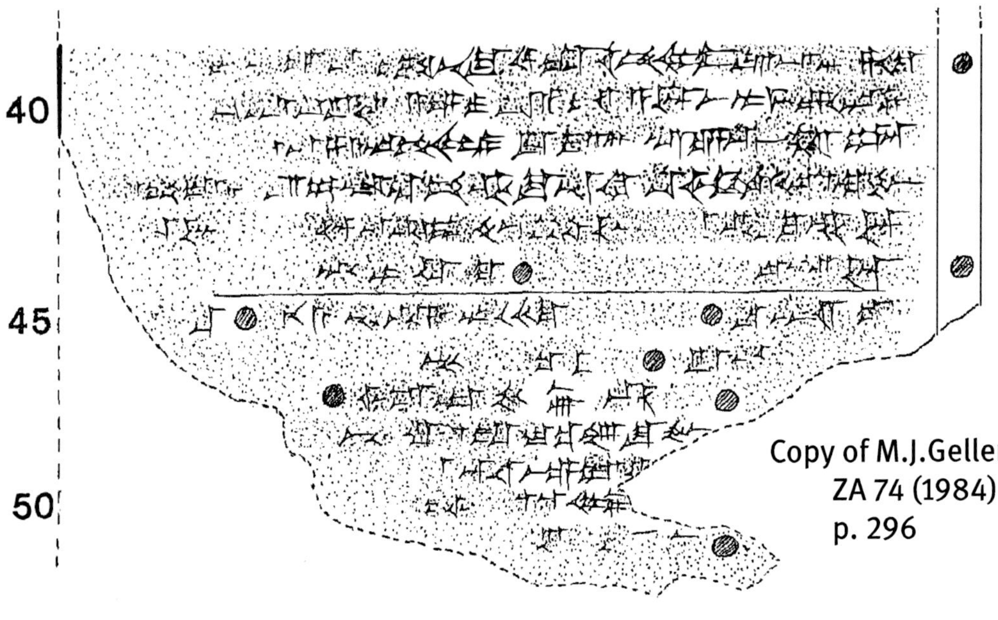

Copy of M.J.Geller
ZA 74 (1984)
p. 296

Photos S.V.Panayotov

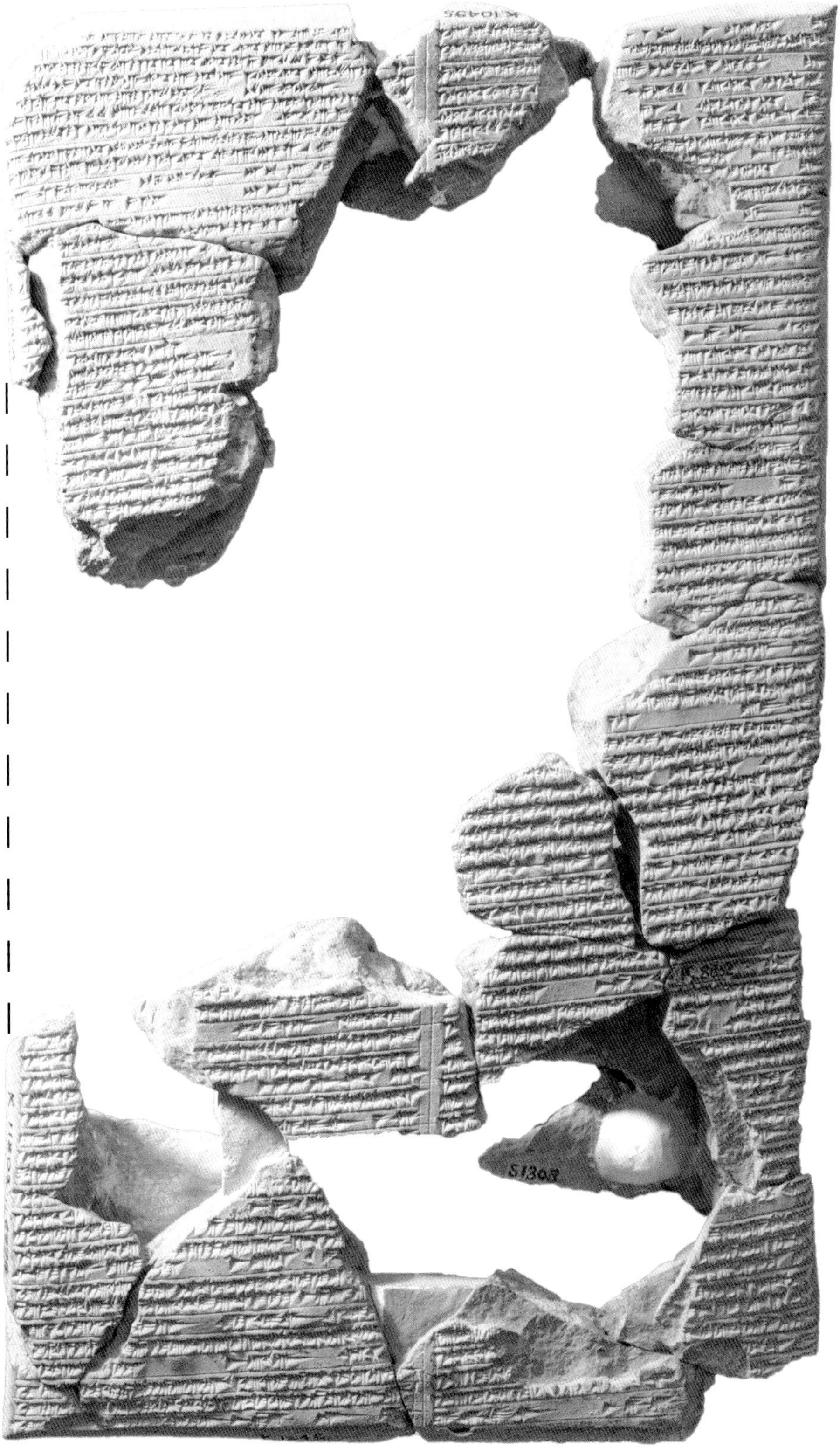

Photos S.V.Panayotov

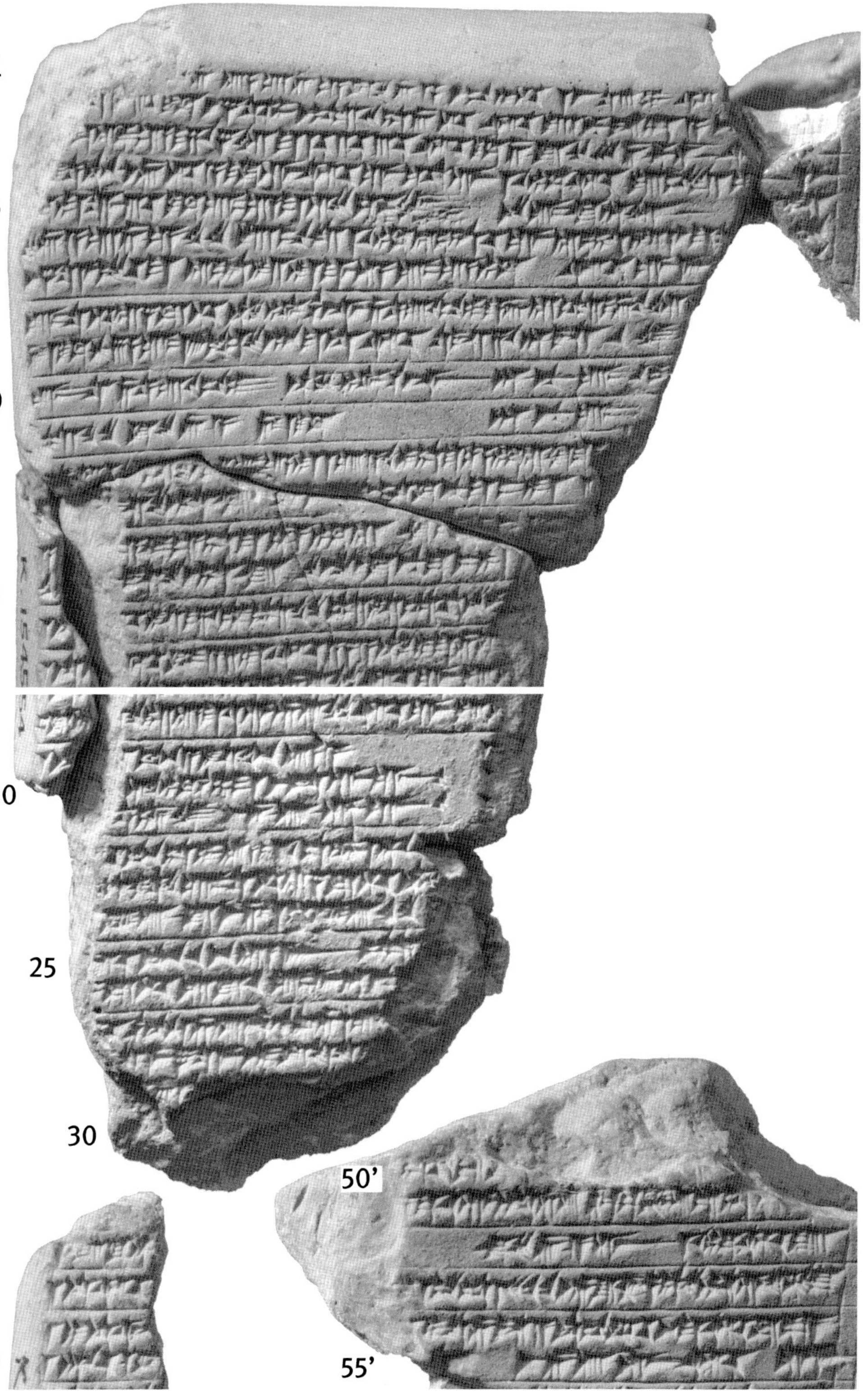

Photos S.V.Panayotov

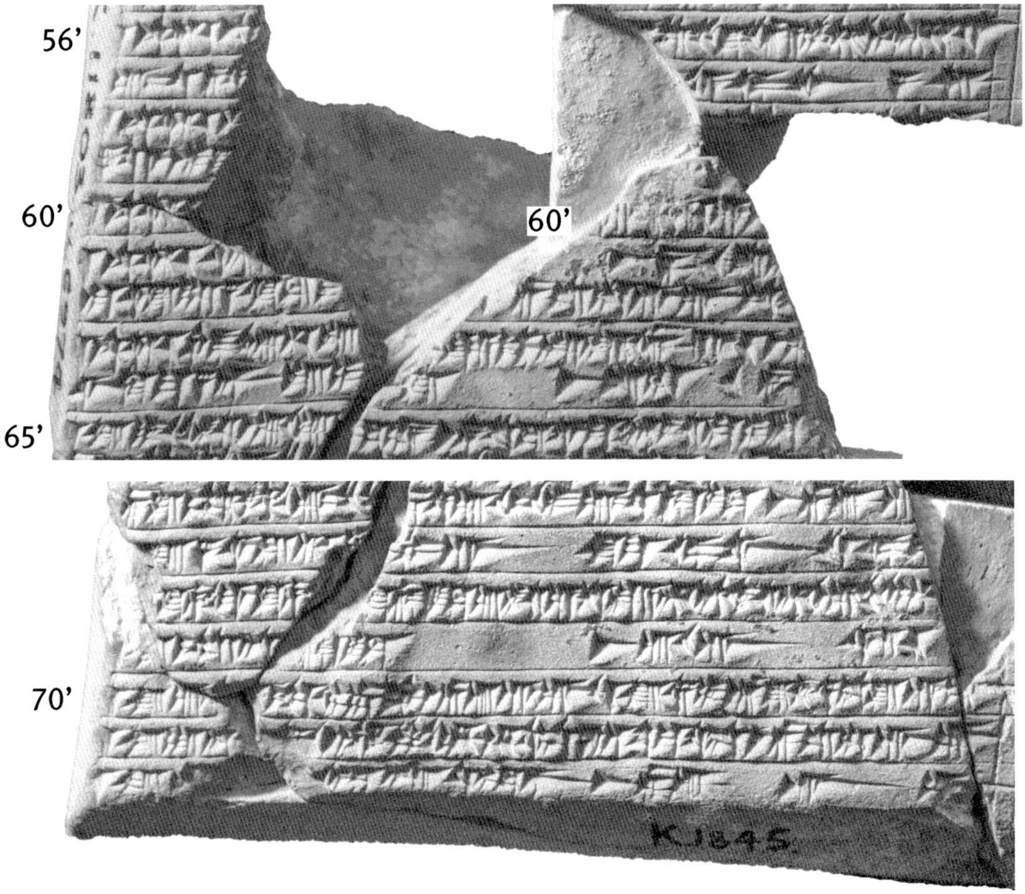

col. ii

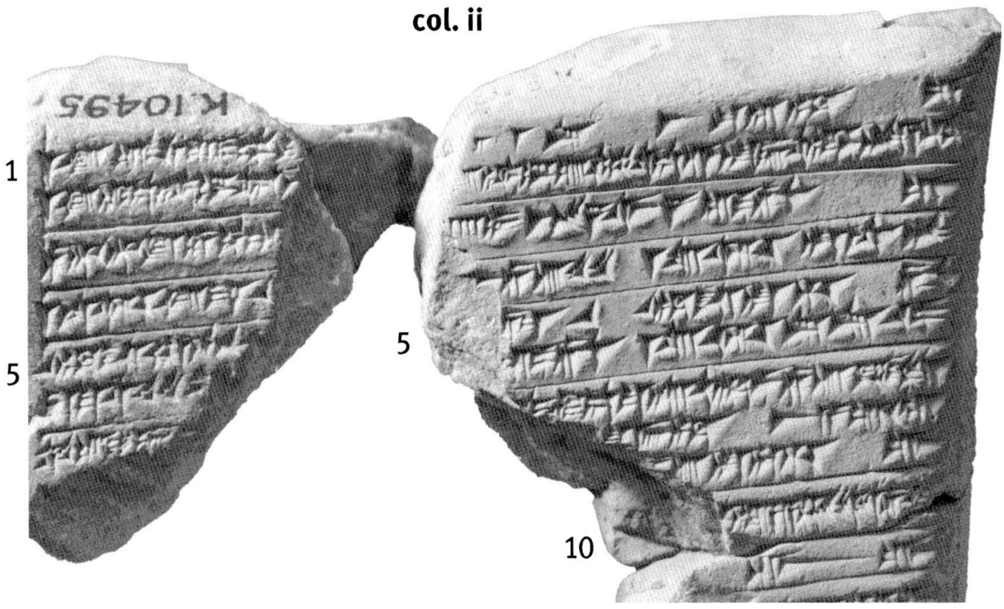

Photos S.V.Panayotov

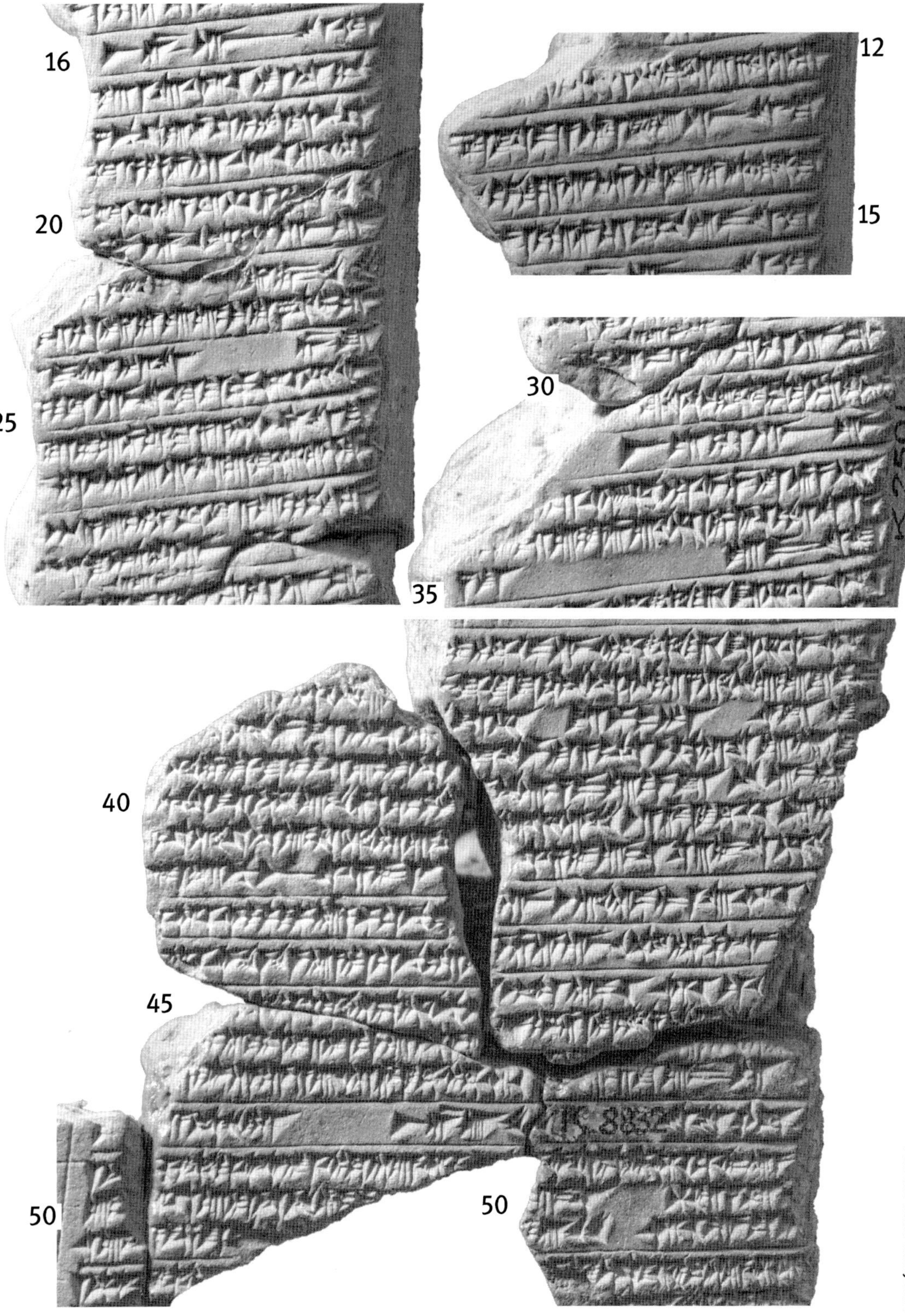

Photos S.V.Panayotov

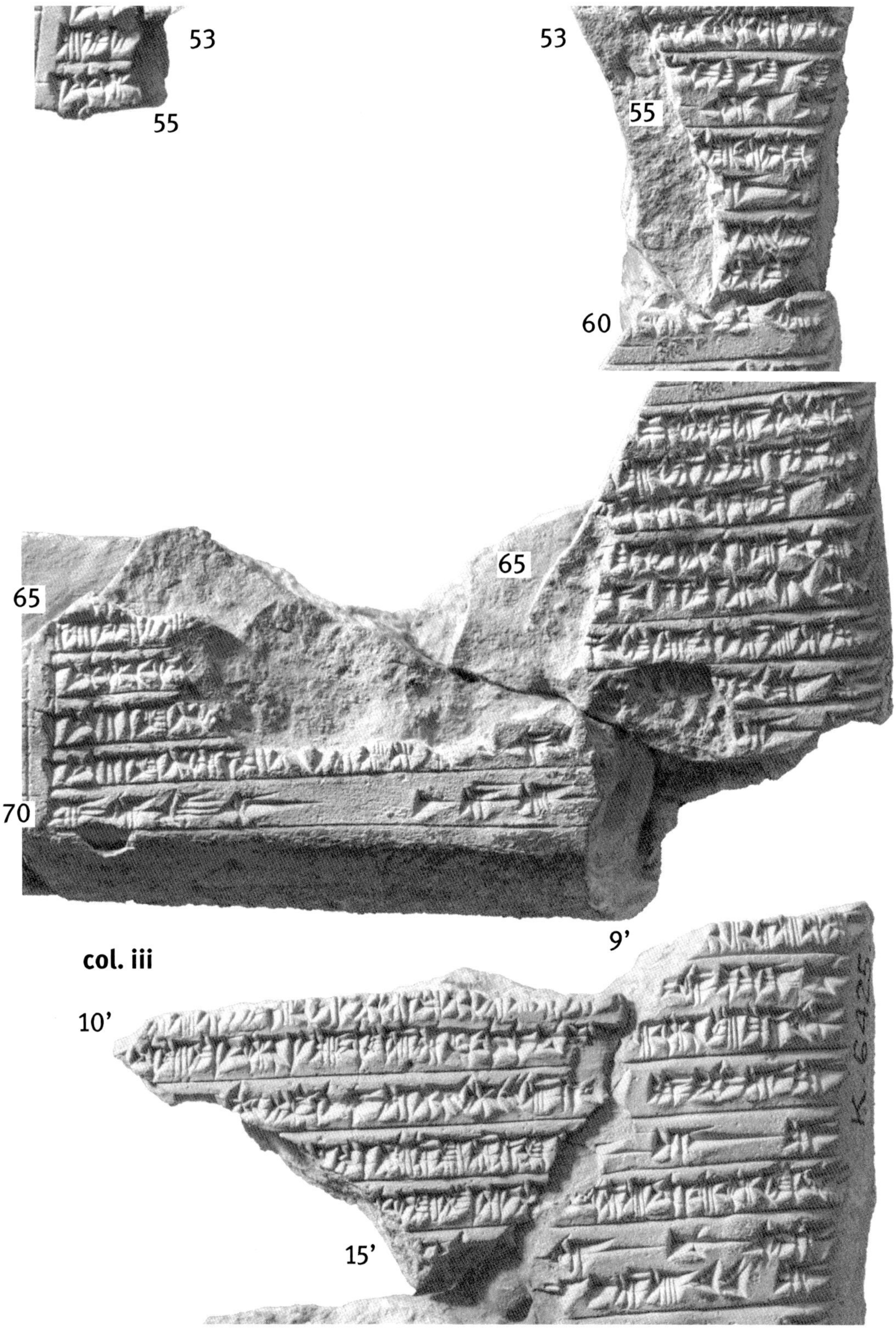

Photos S.V.Panayotov

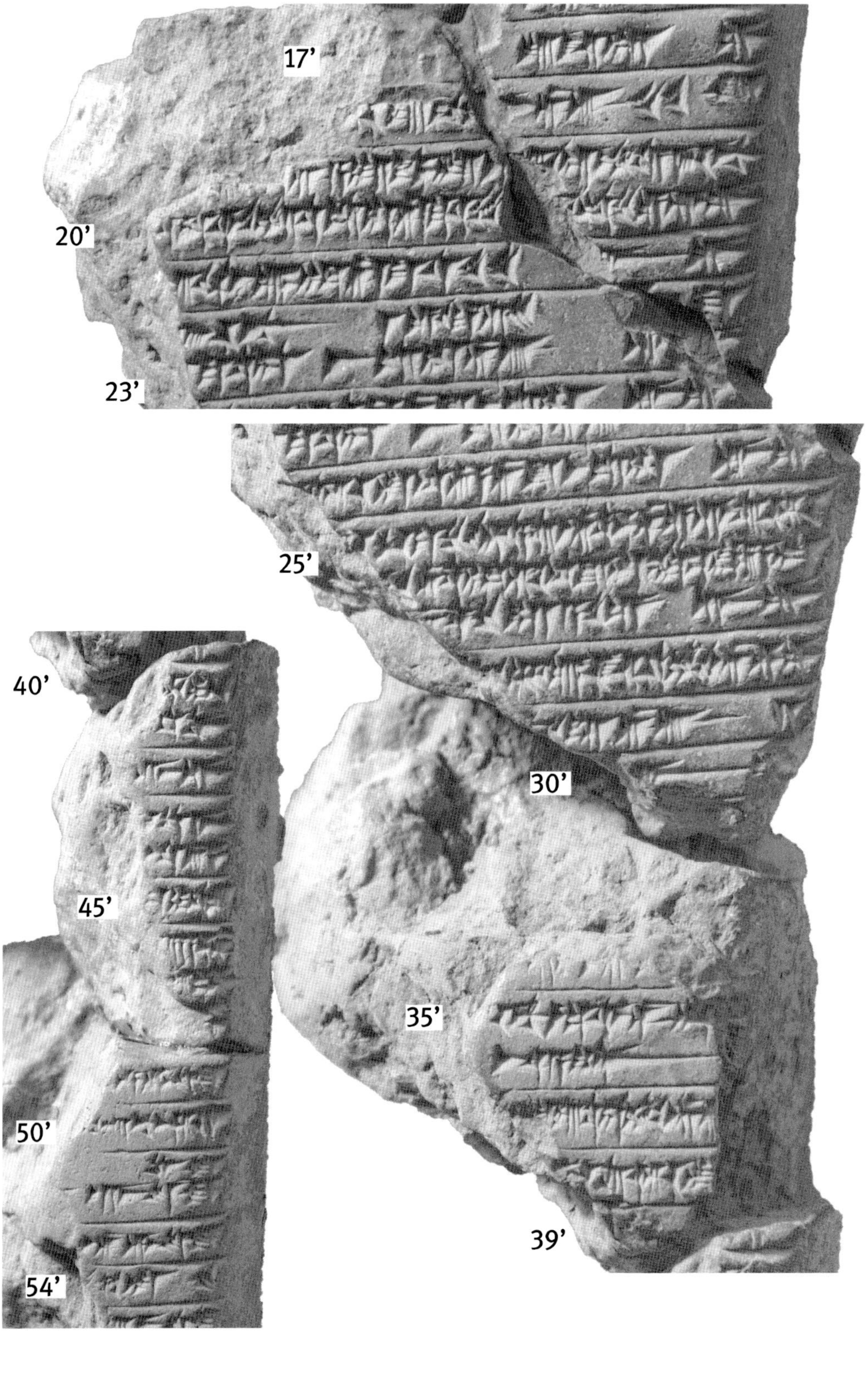
17’
20’
23’
25’
30’
35’
39’
40’
45’
50’
54’

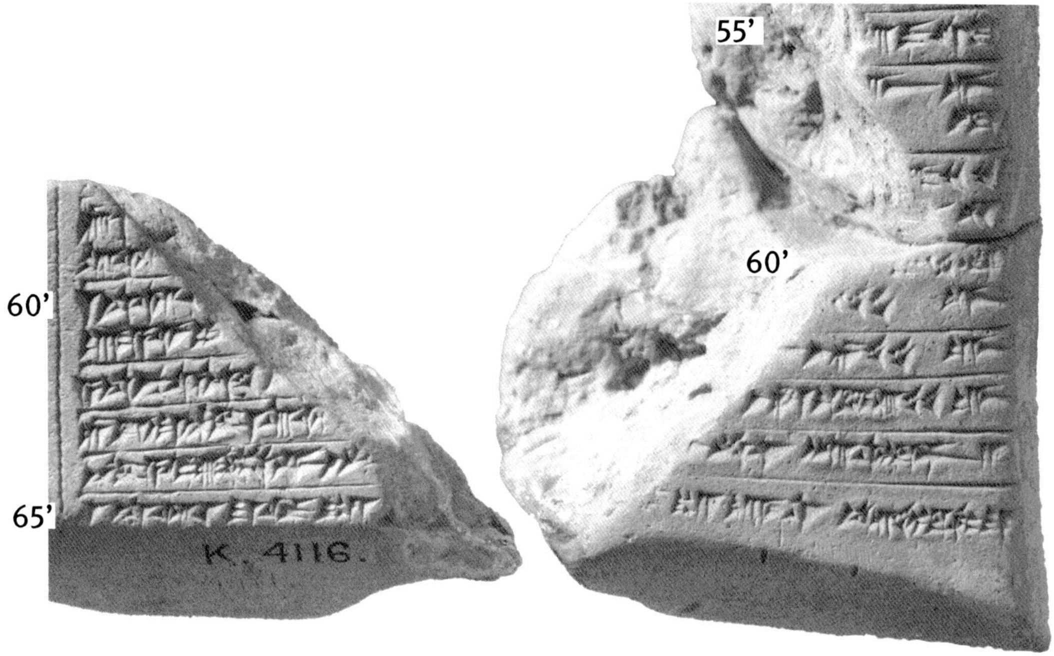

col. iv

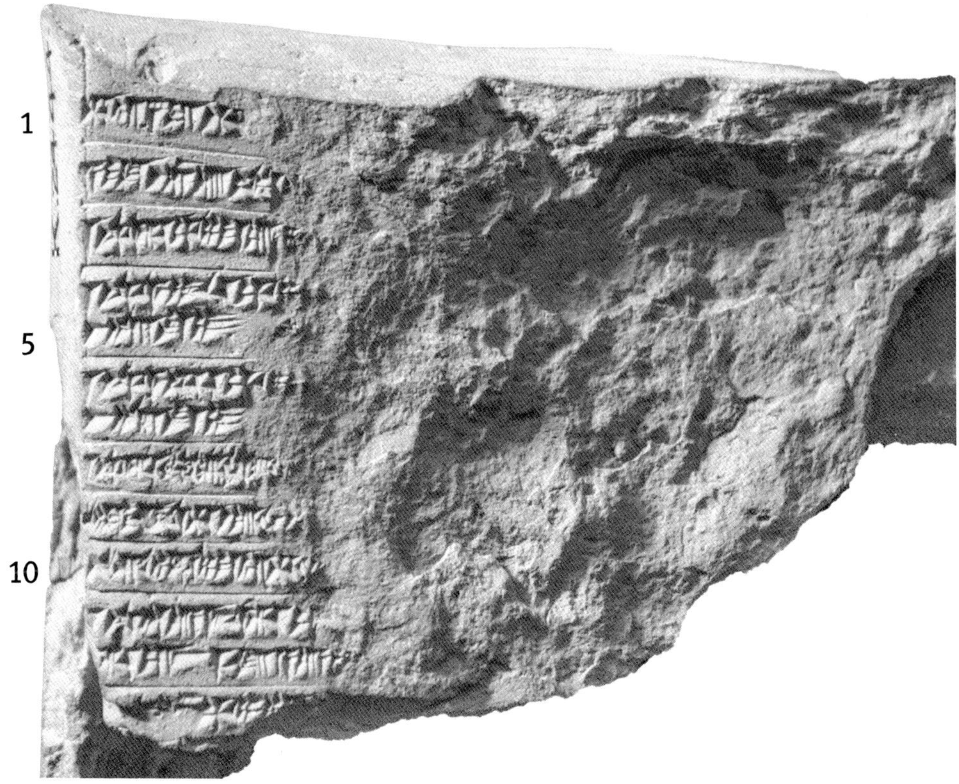

Photos S.V.Panayotov

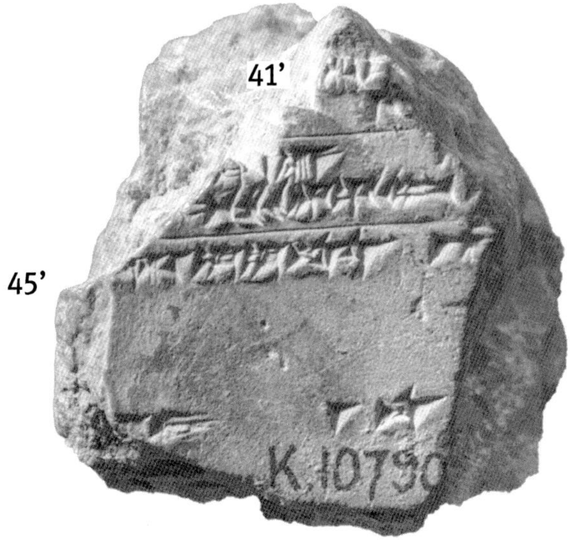

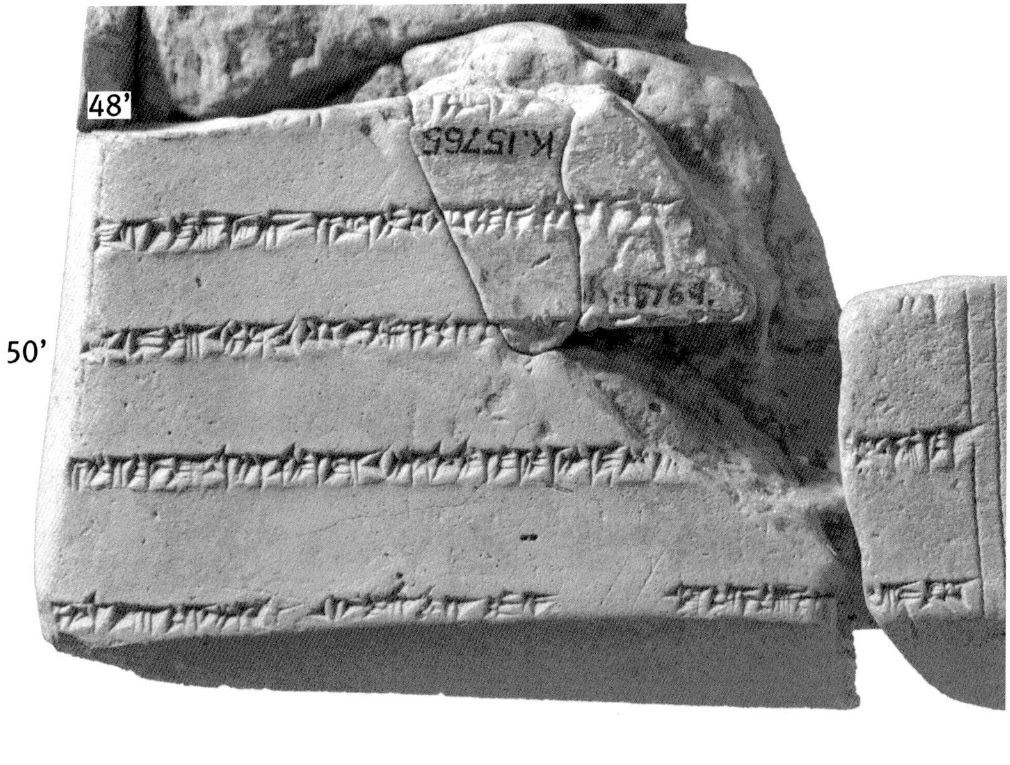

Assurbanipal's Colophon, BAK no. 329

Photos S.V.Panayotov

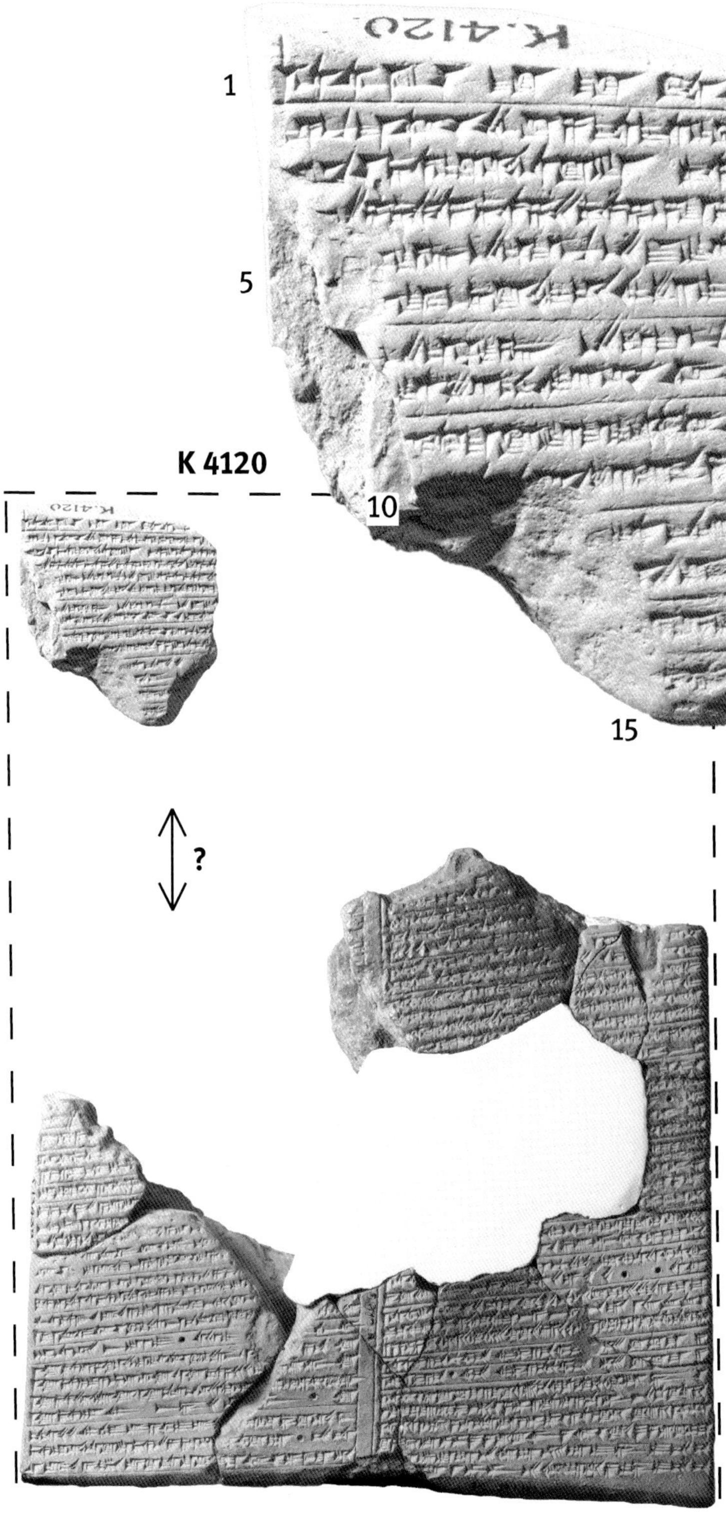

**IGI Tablet III
Manuscript NE
(BAM 516)
Overview
Obverse**

Photos S.V.Panayotov

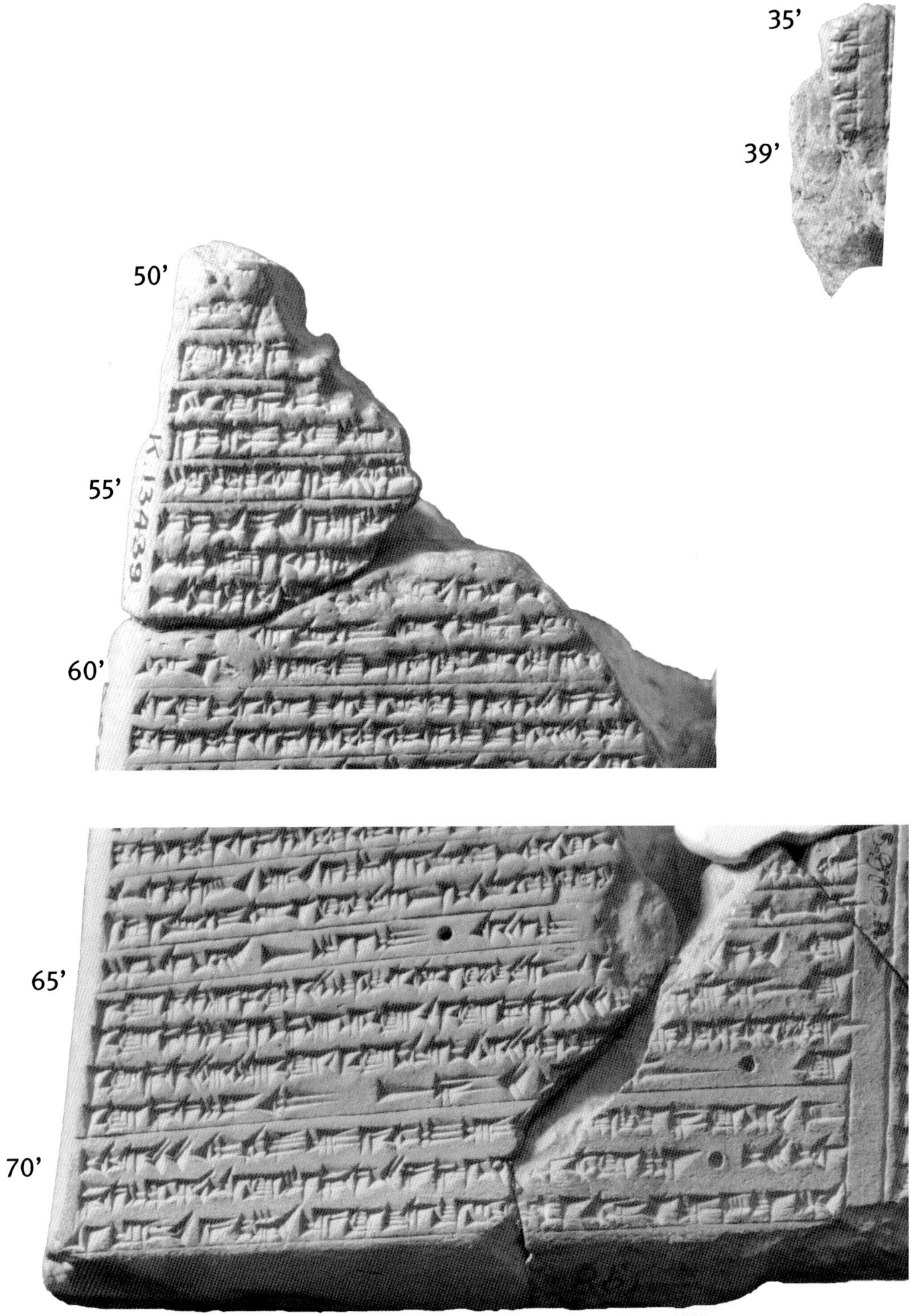

Photos S.V.Panayotov

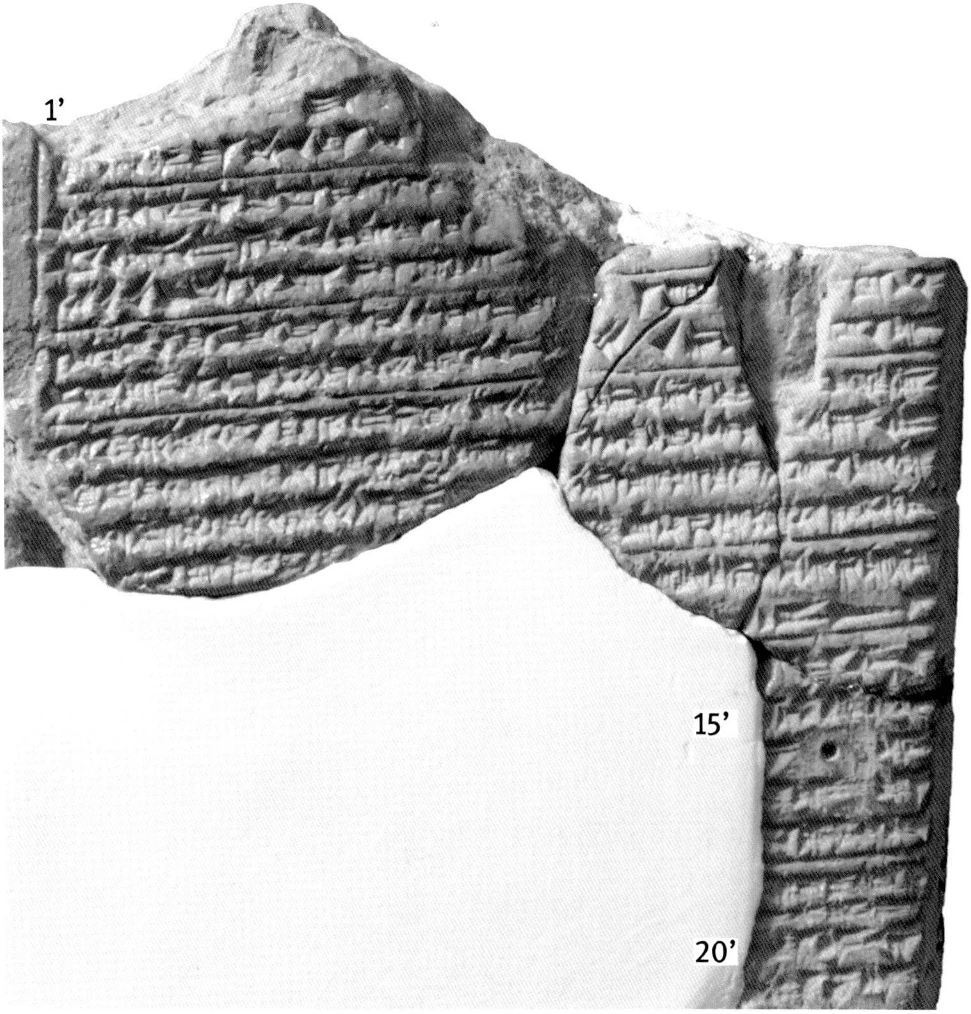

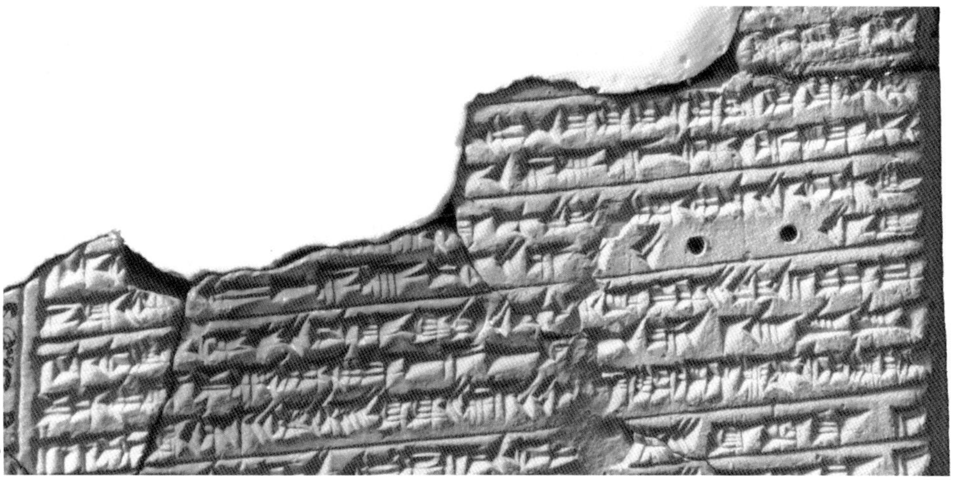

Photos S.V.Panayotov

col. ii

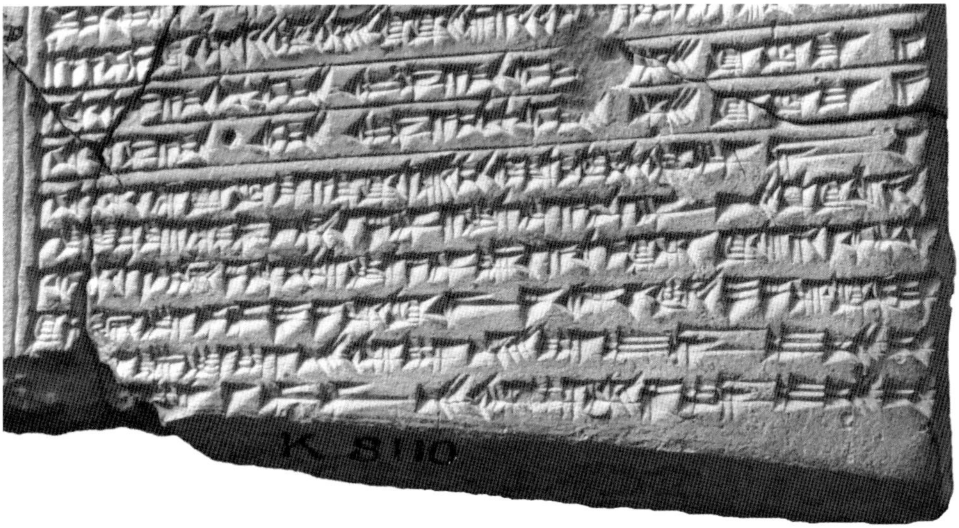

col. iii

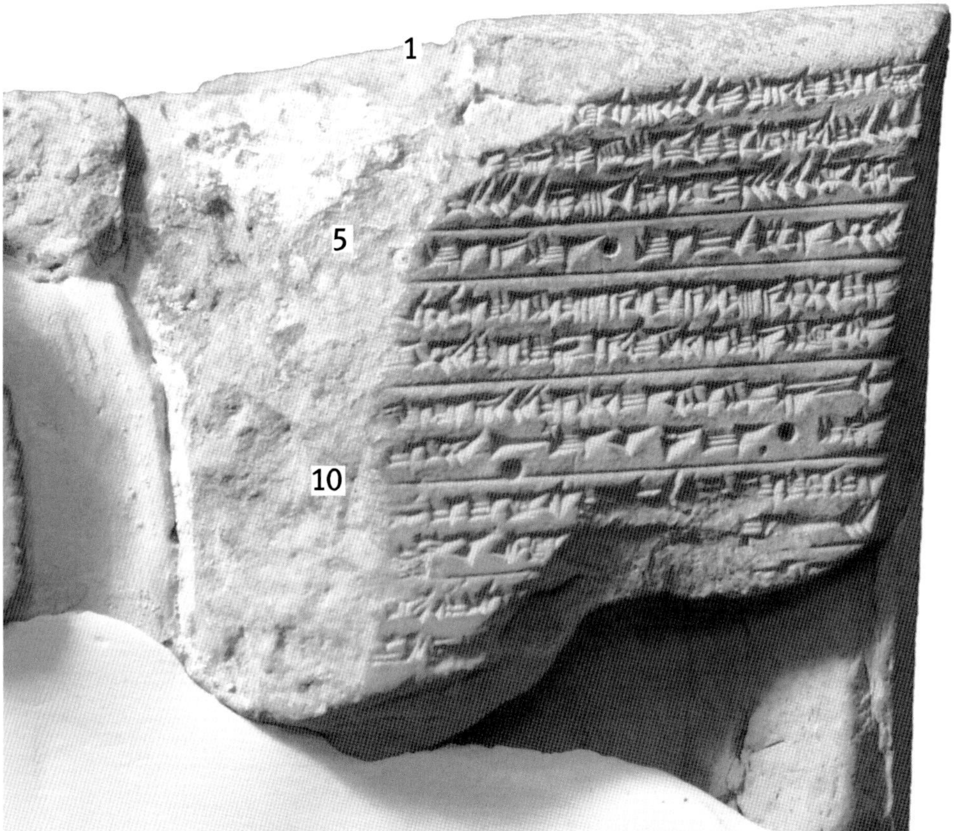

Photos S.V.Panayotov

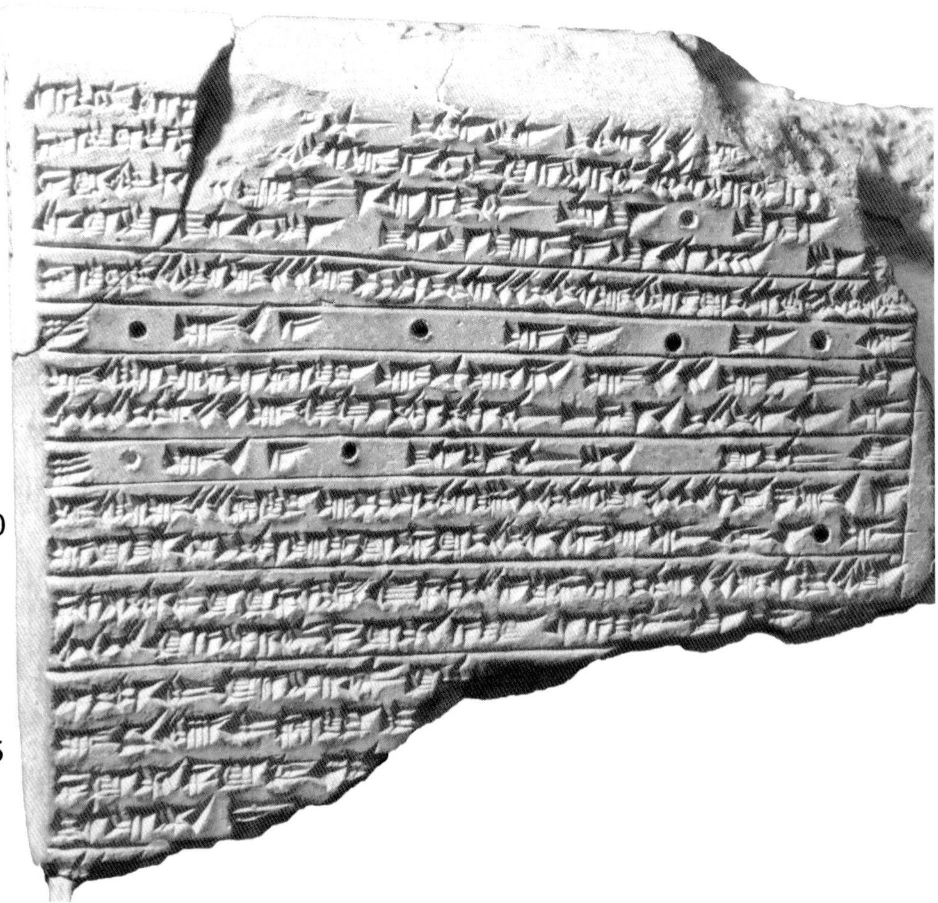

Photo S.V.Panayotov

Manuscript NF (BAM 520 + K 8784 (+) AMT 14/2) Overview

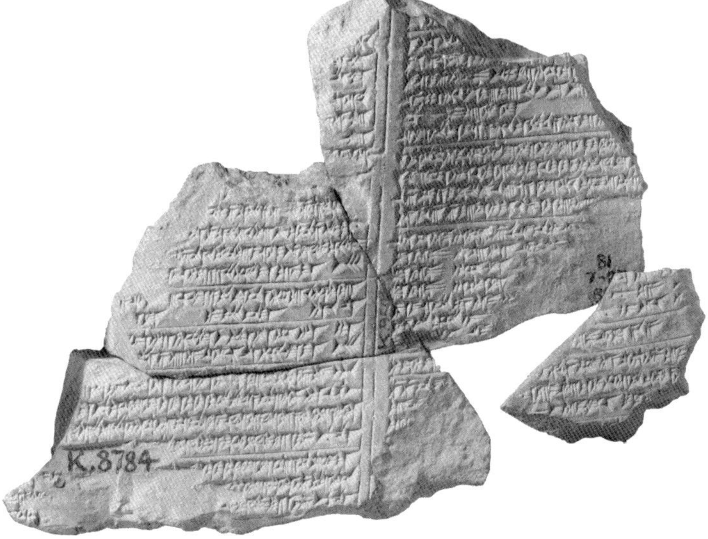

Photo Alberto Giannese

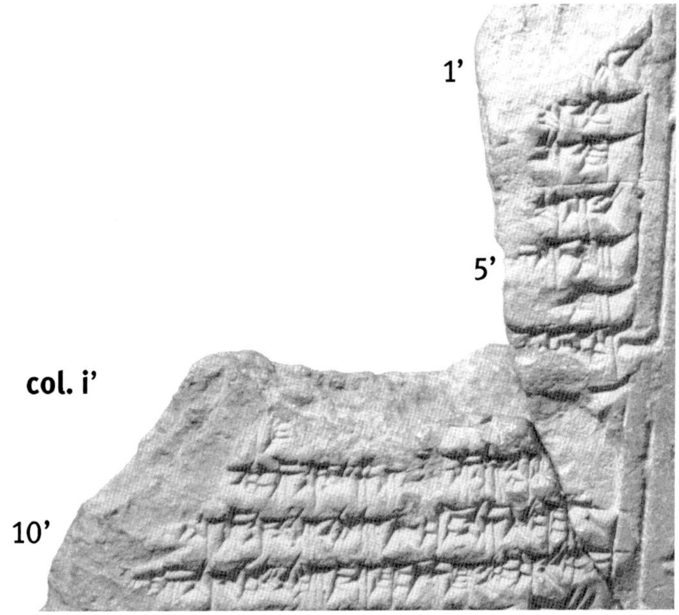

Photo S.V.Panayotov

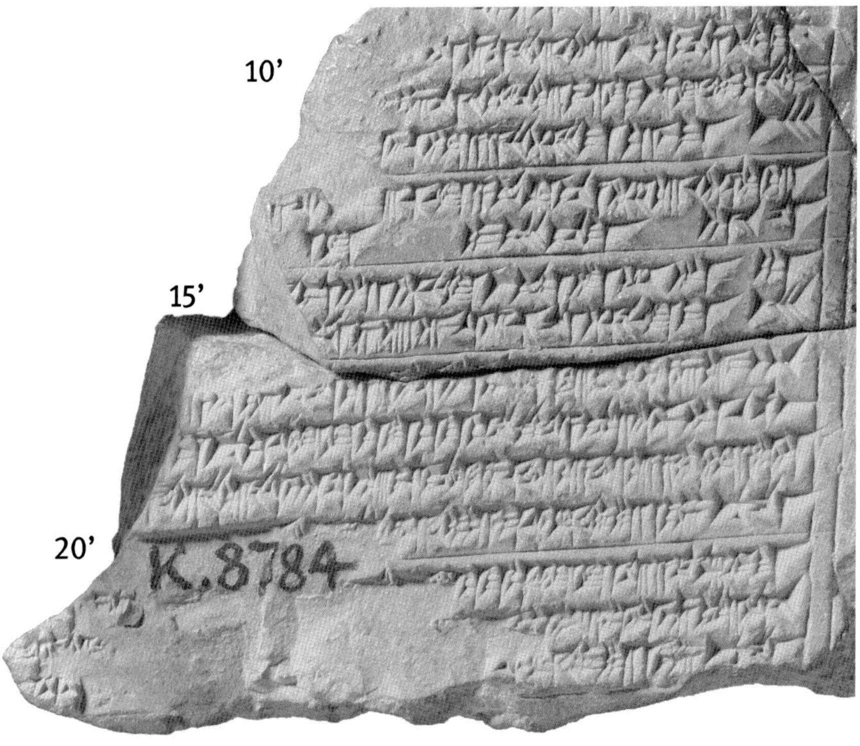

Photo Alberto Giannese

col. ii'

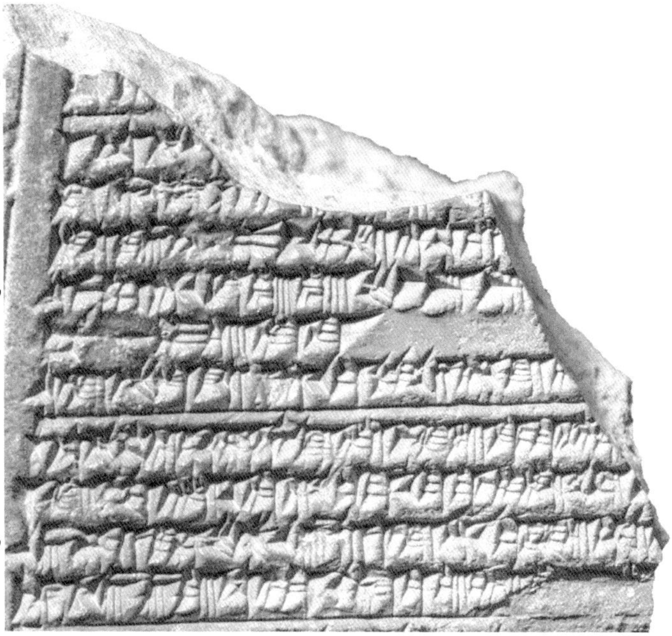

Photo S.V.Panayotov

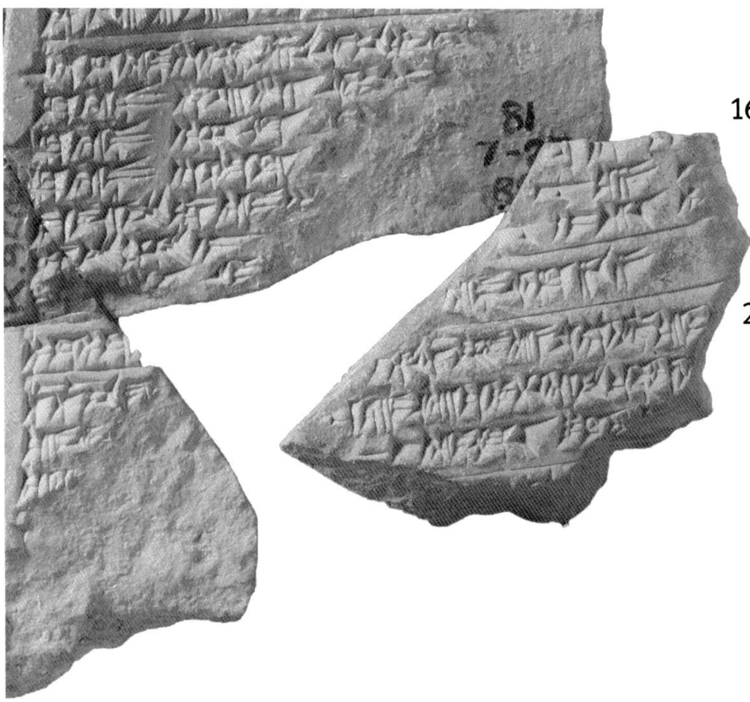

Photo Alberto Giannese

NK (BAM 518)

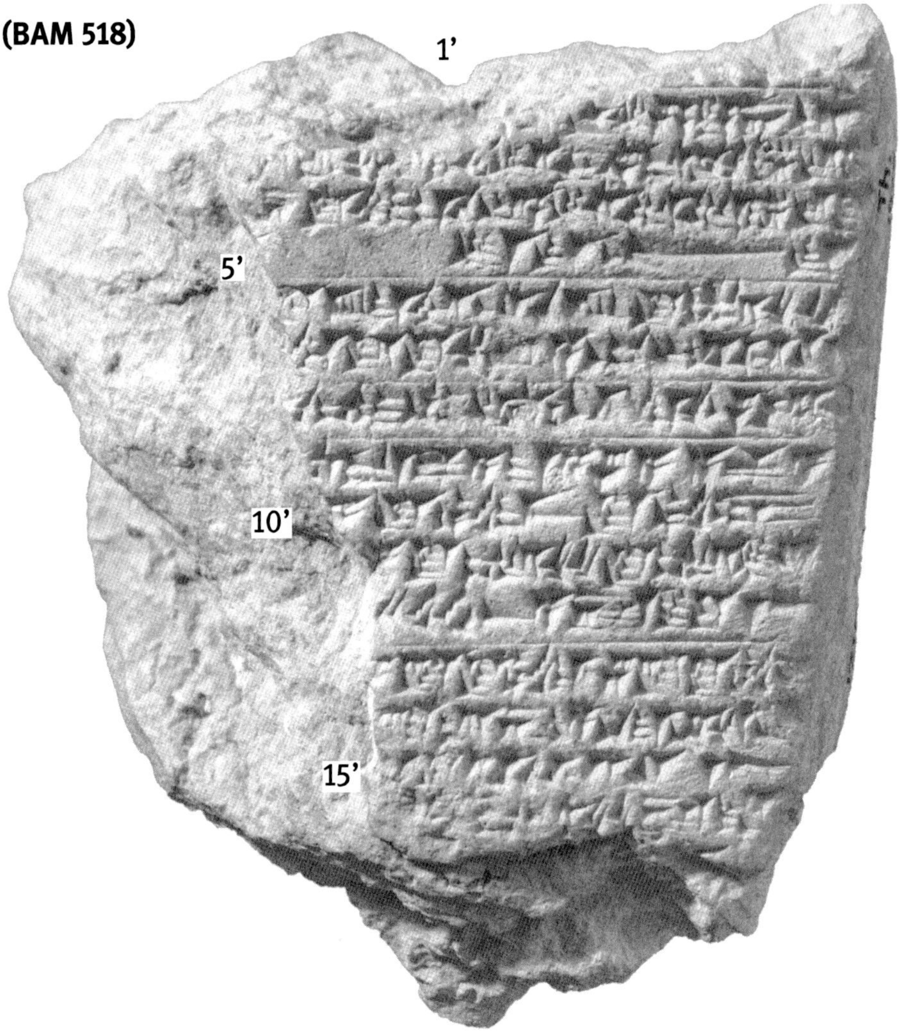

NP (BAM 517)

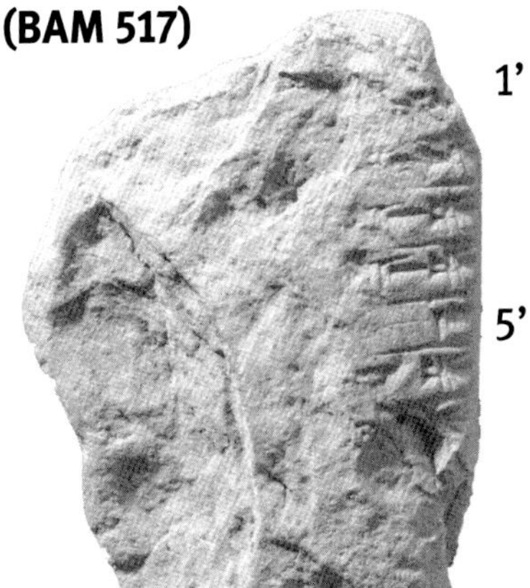

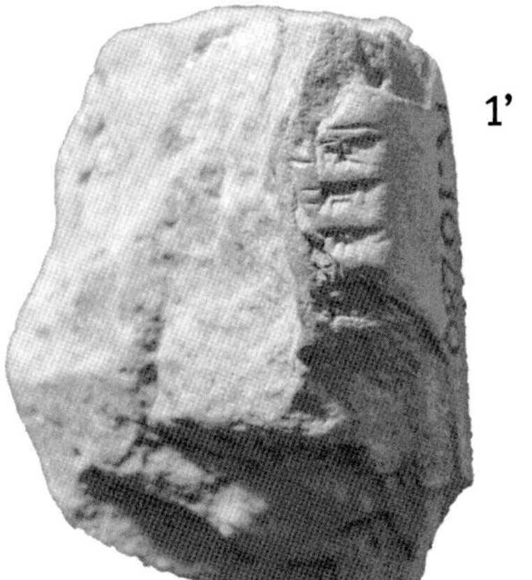

Obverse?

Reverse?

Photos S.V.Panayotov

NT (AMT 85/2)

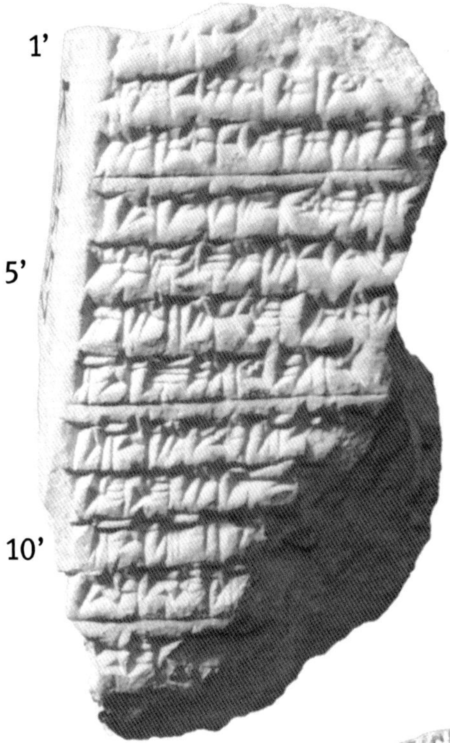

NS (AMT 18/4)

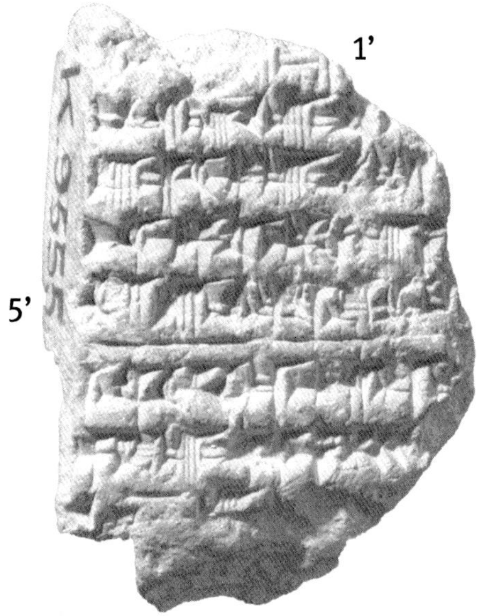

NR (BAM 522)

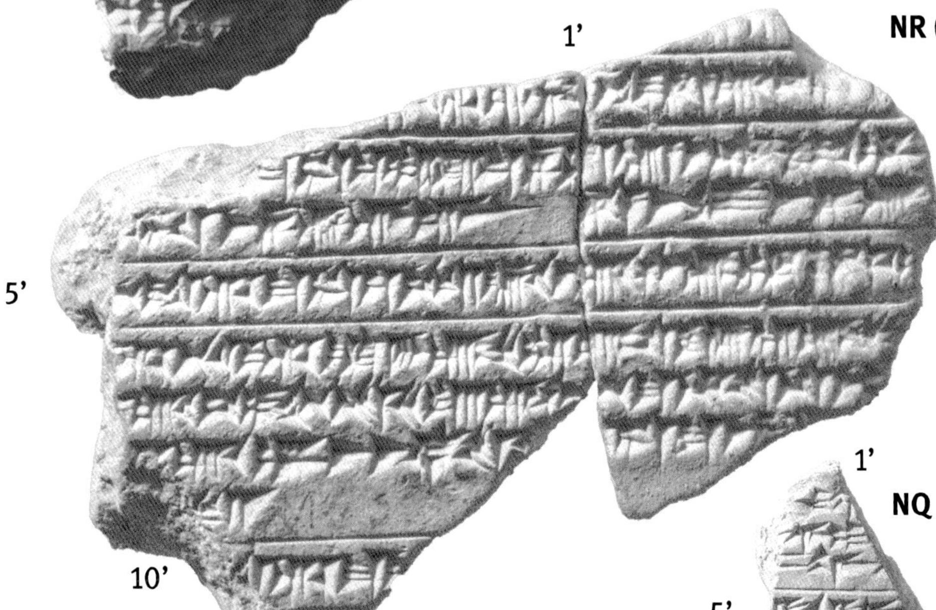

NQ (BAM 521)

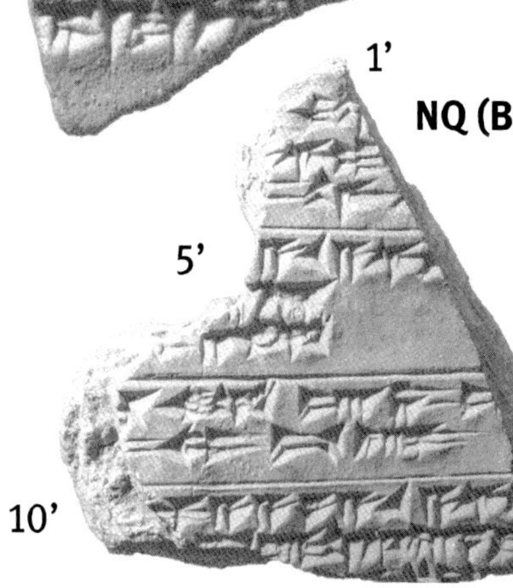

Photos S.V.Panayotov

NU (AMT 14/3)

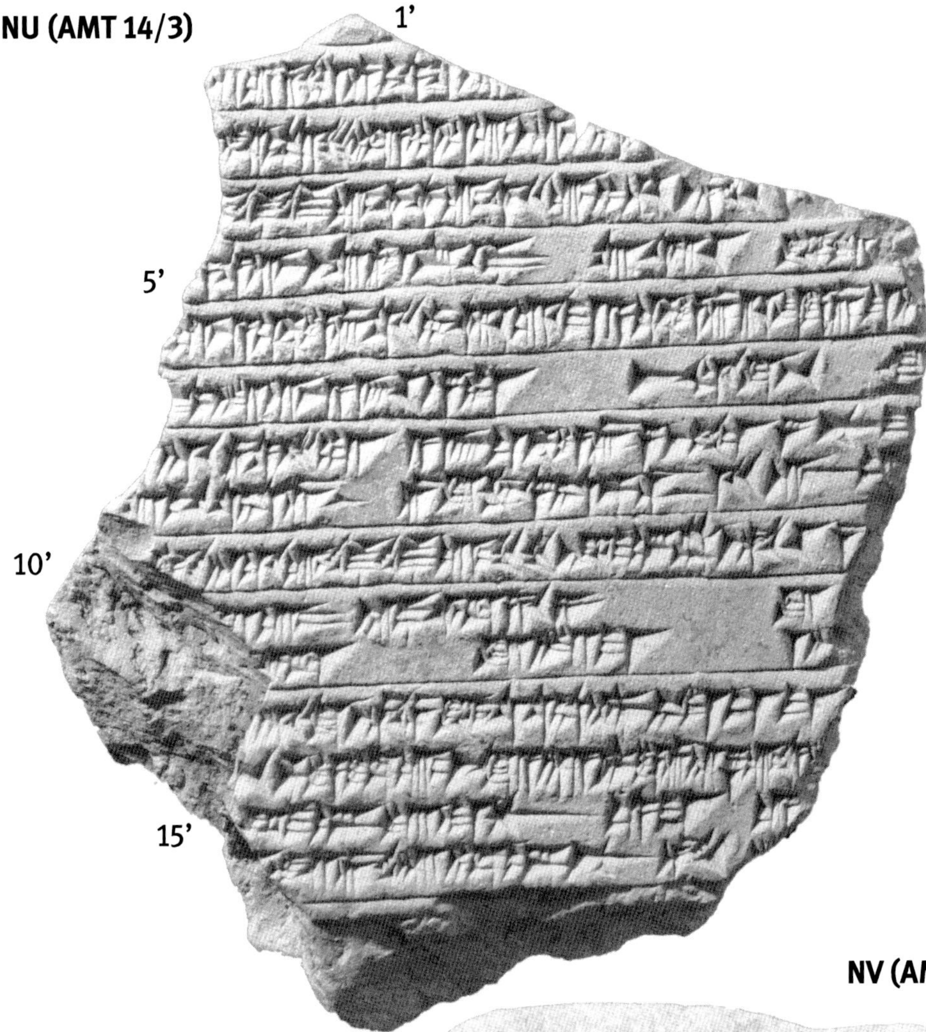

NV (AMT 18/3)

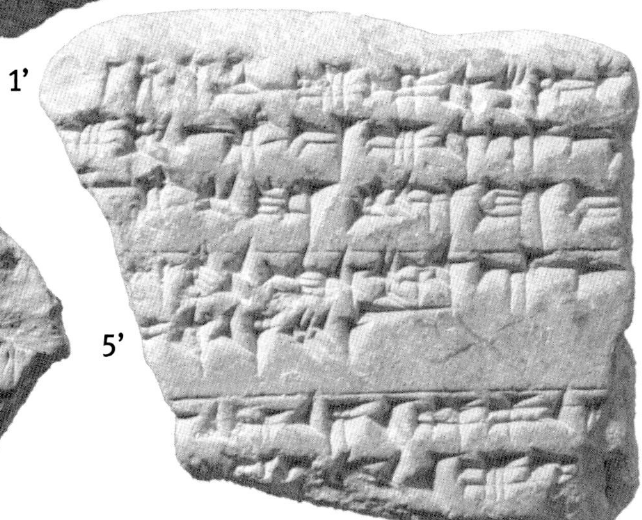

NW (BAM 439)

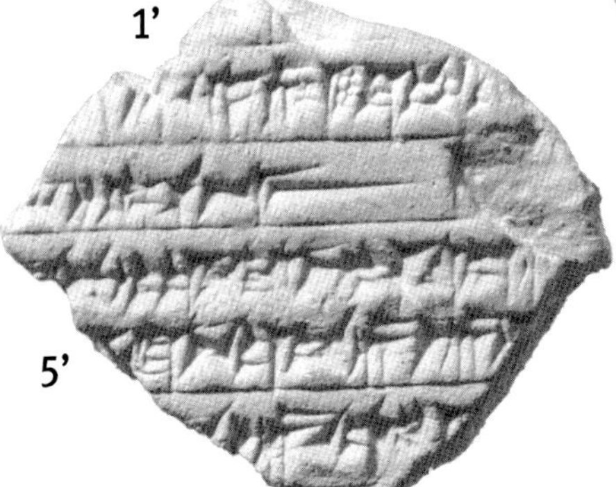

NZb (AMT 17/2)

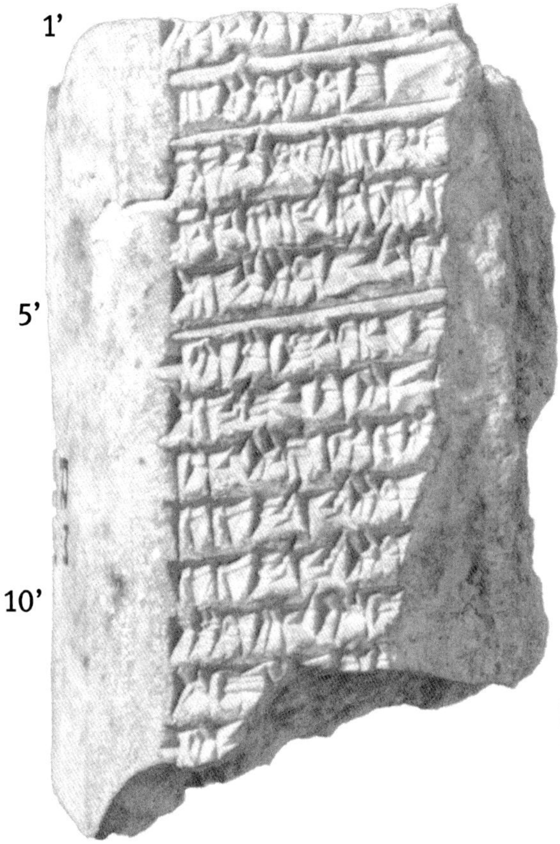

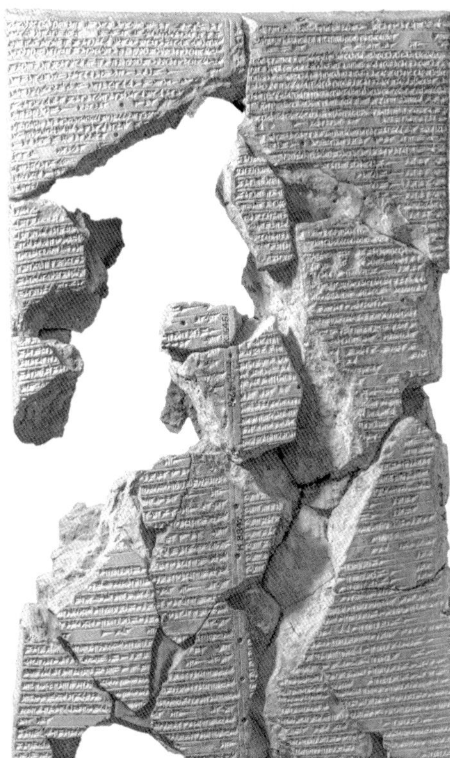

UGU Tablet I
Manuscript NI (BAM 480)
Overview Obverse

Photos S.V.Panayotov

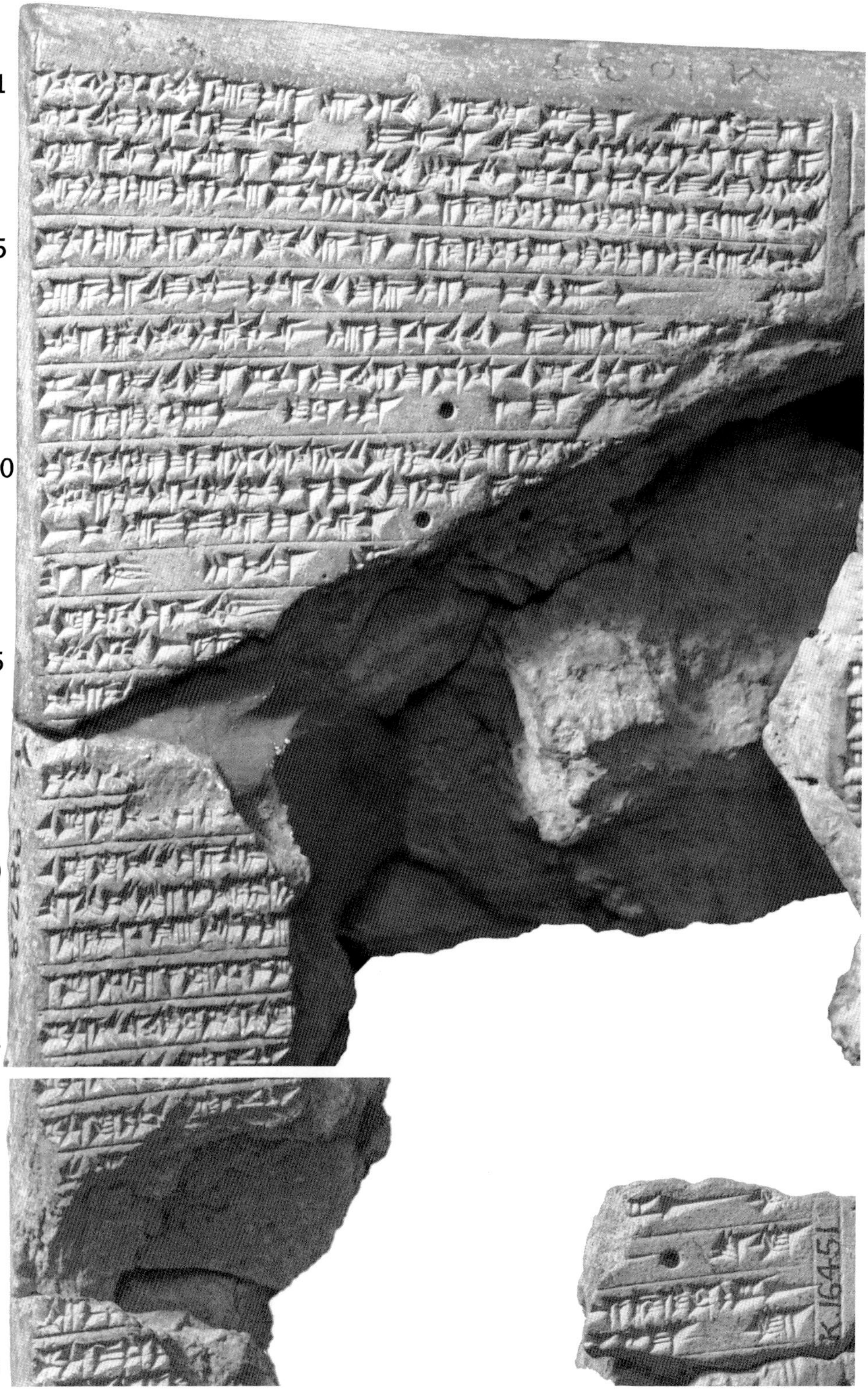

Photos S.V.Panayotov

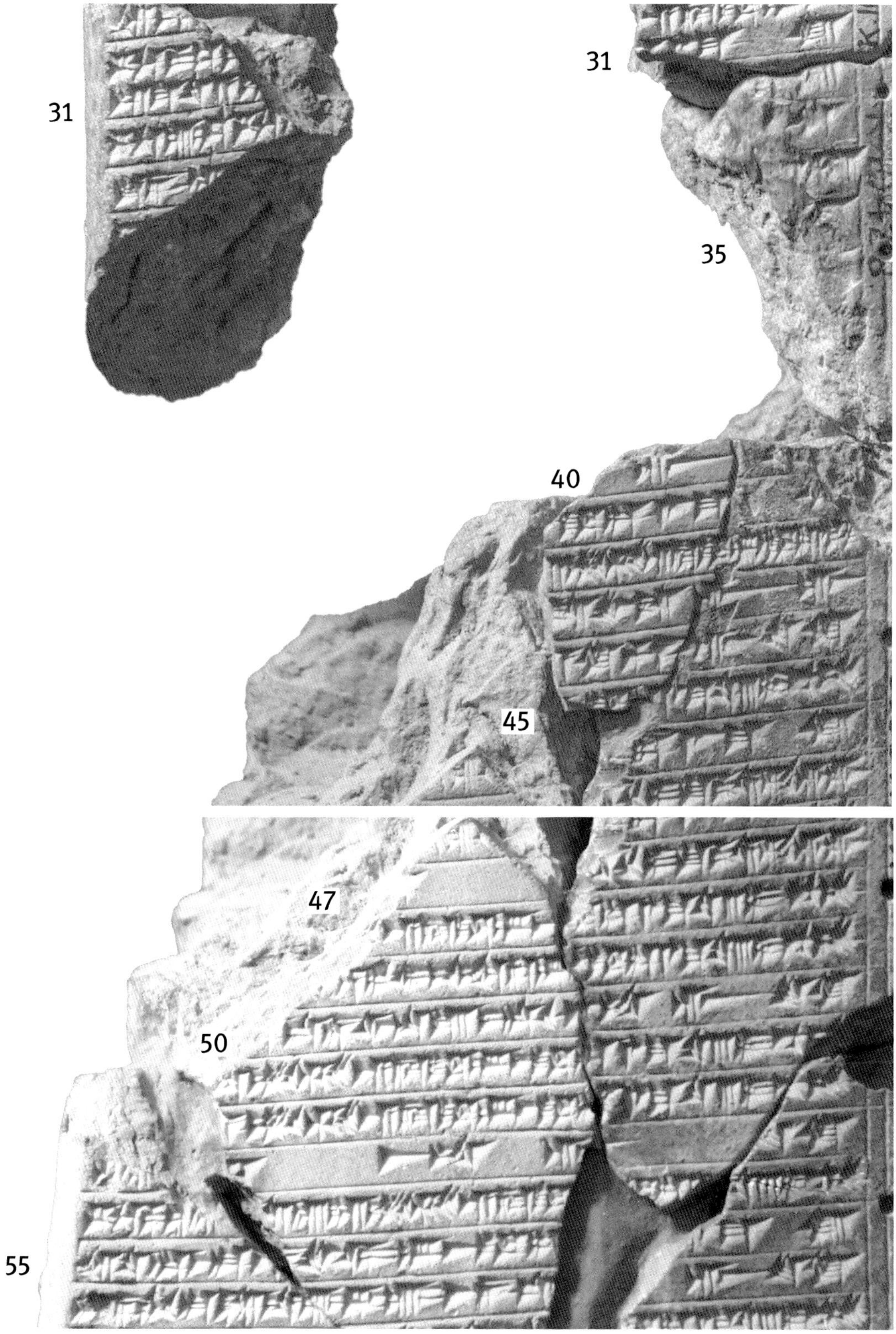

Photos S.V.Panayotov

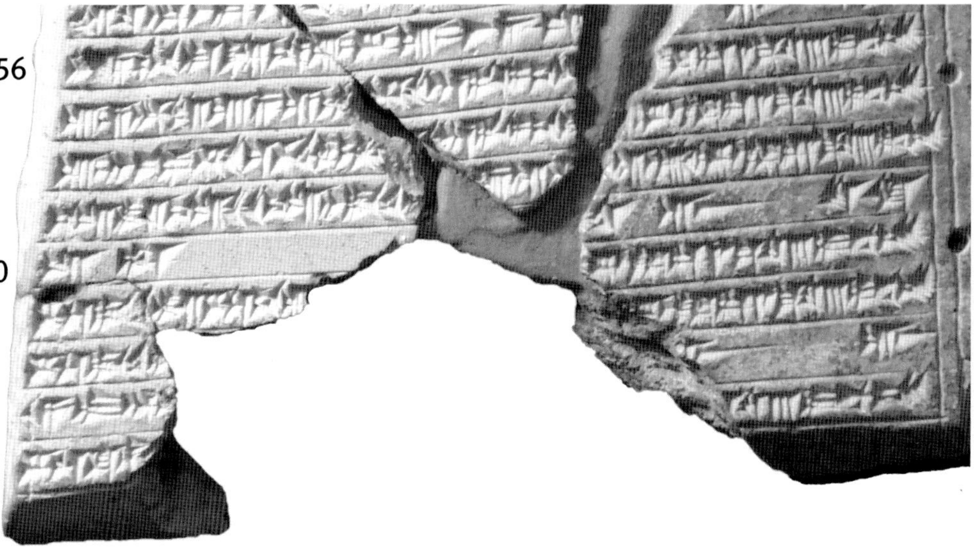

col. ii

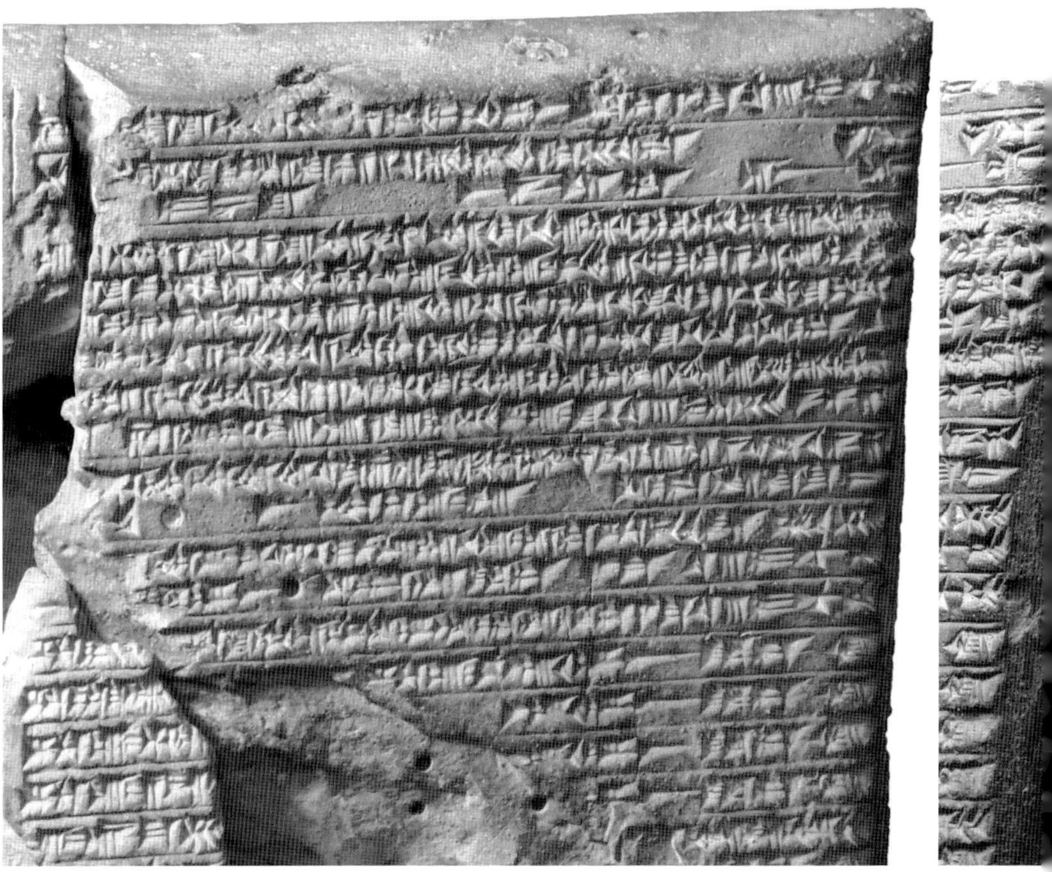

col. ii

col. i

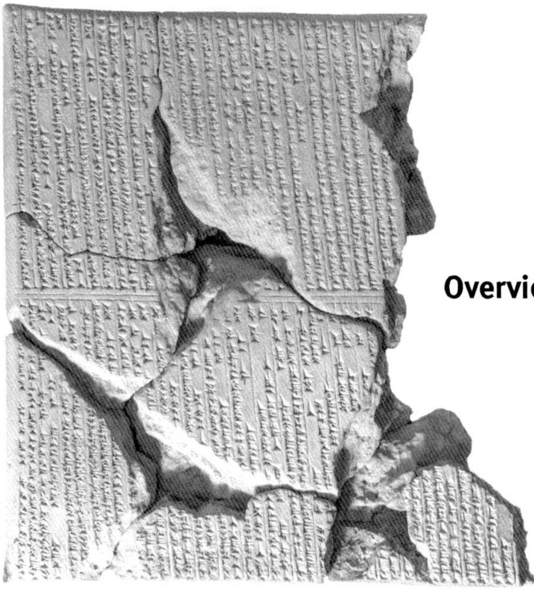

Overview Obverse

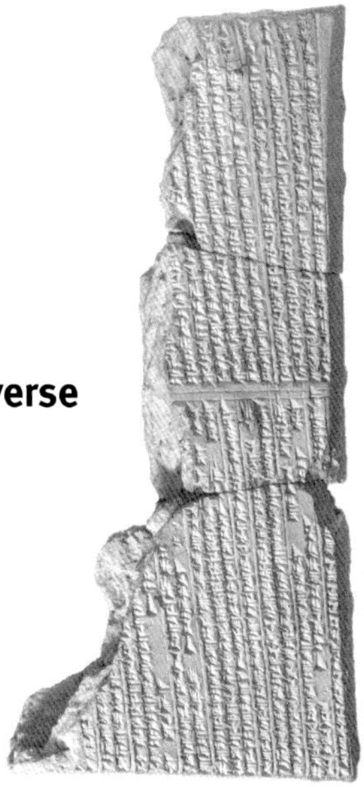

K 2611

col. ii

20

25

29

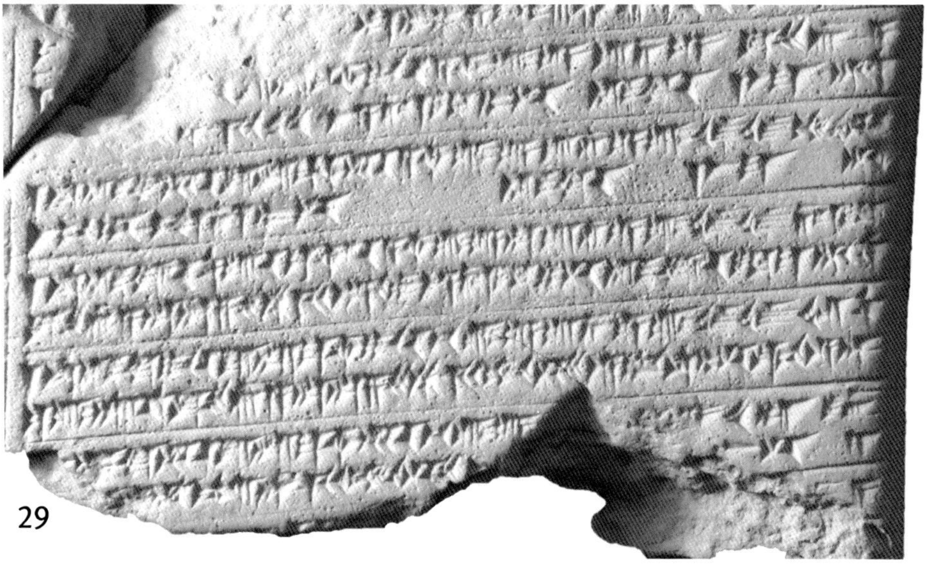

62'

65'

Photos S.V.Panayotov

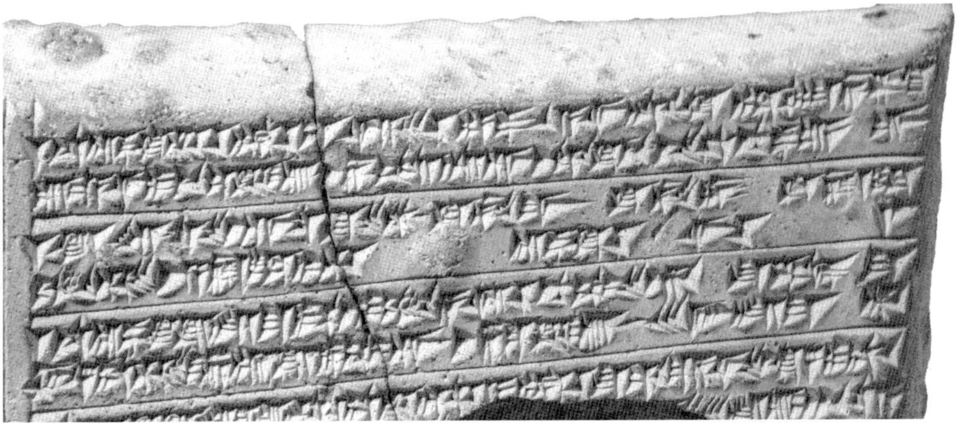

NY (AMT 25/8)

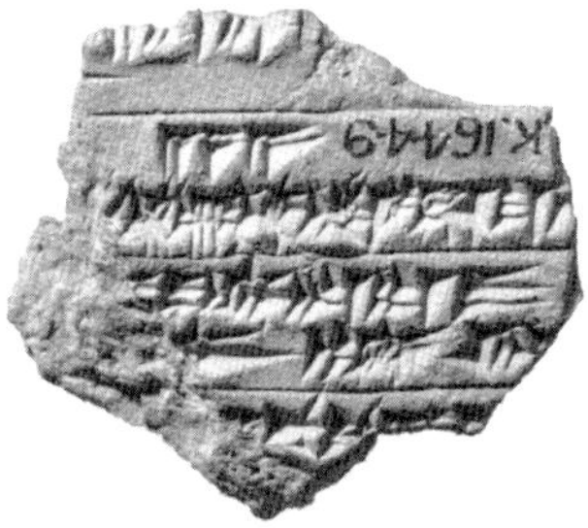

NZ (AMT 5/3)

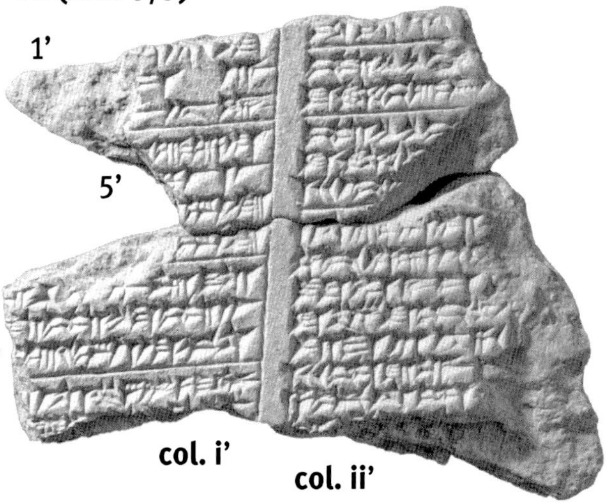

NZa (AMT 13/5 + 14/5)

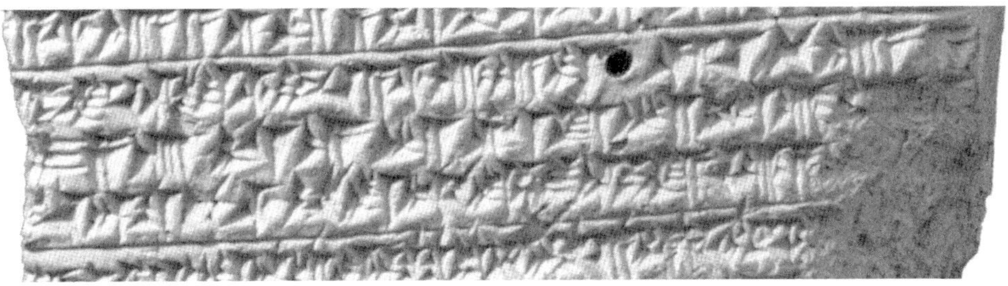

Photos S.V.Panayotov

Diagnostic Medical Omens, BM 121063

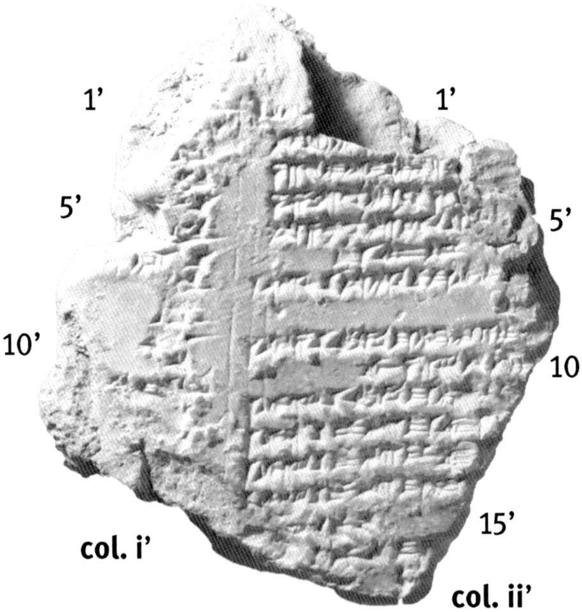

NJ (AMT 12/5)

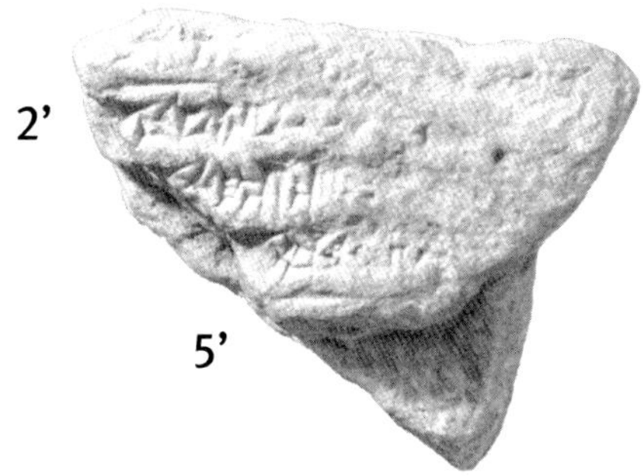

Photos BM 121063 and NJ S.V.Panayotov

AB (BAM 159) Overview

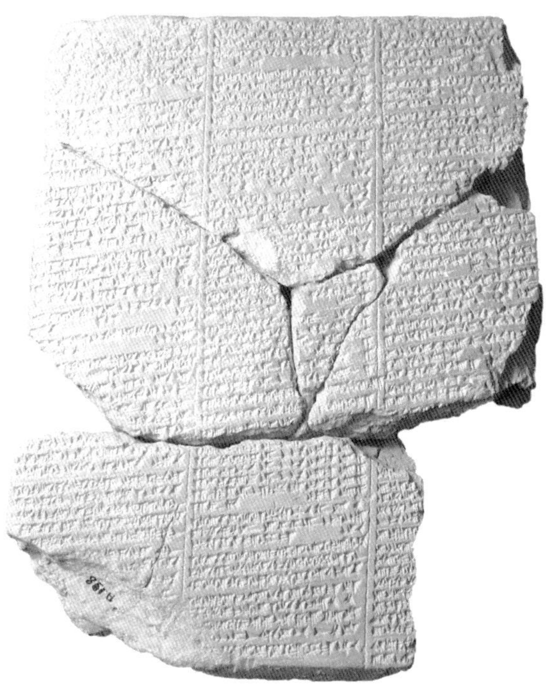

Obverse

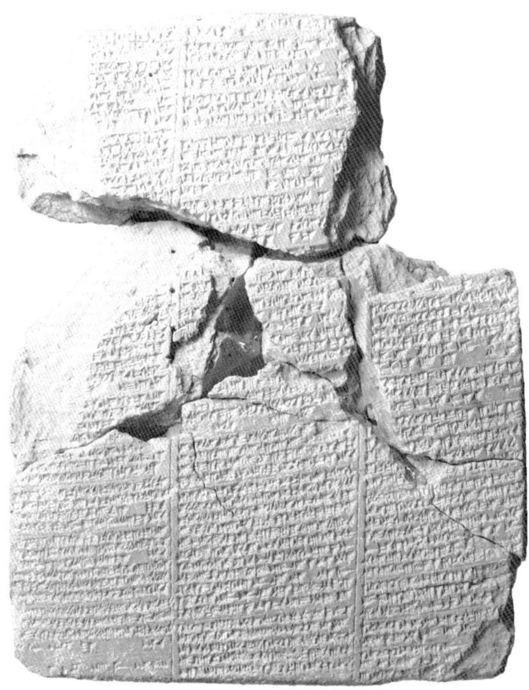

Reverse

Photos AB F. Badalanova-Geller

col. iv

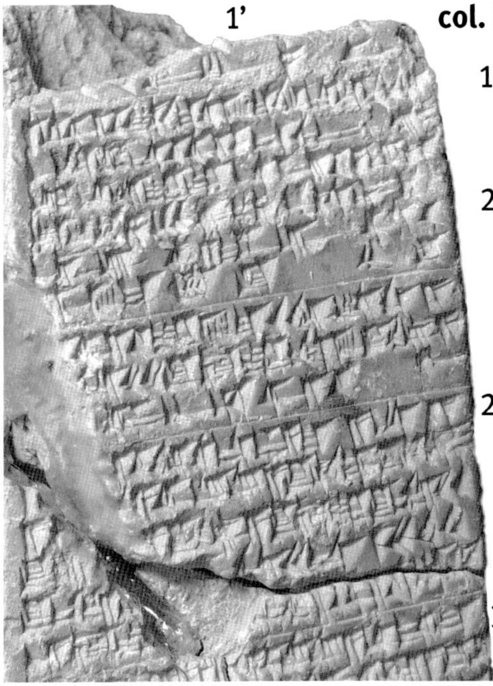

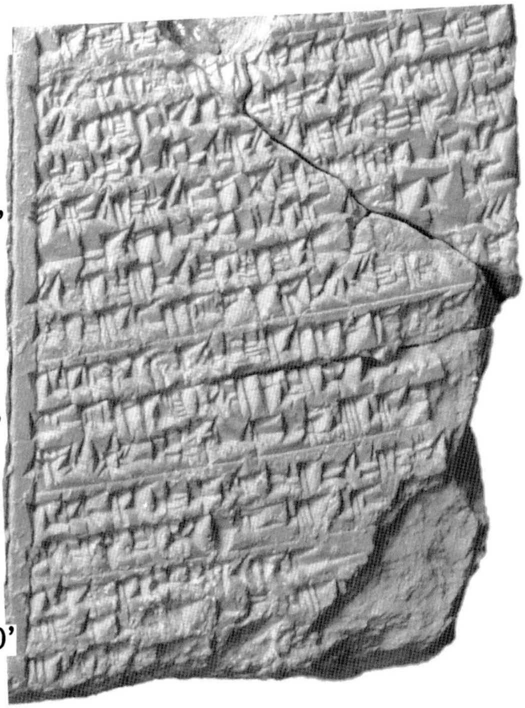

Photos AB F. Badalanova-Geller

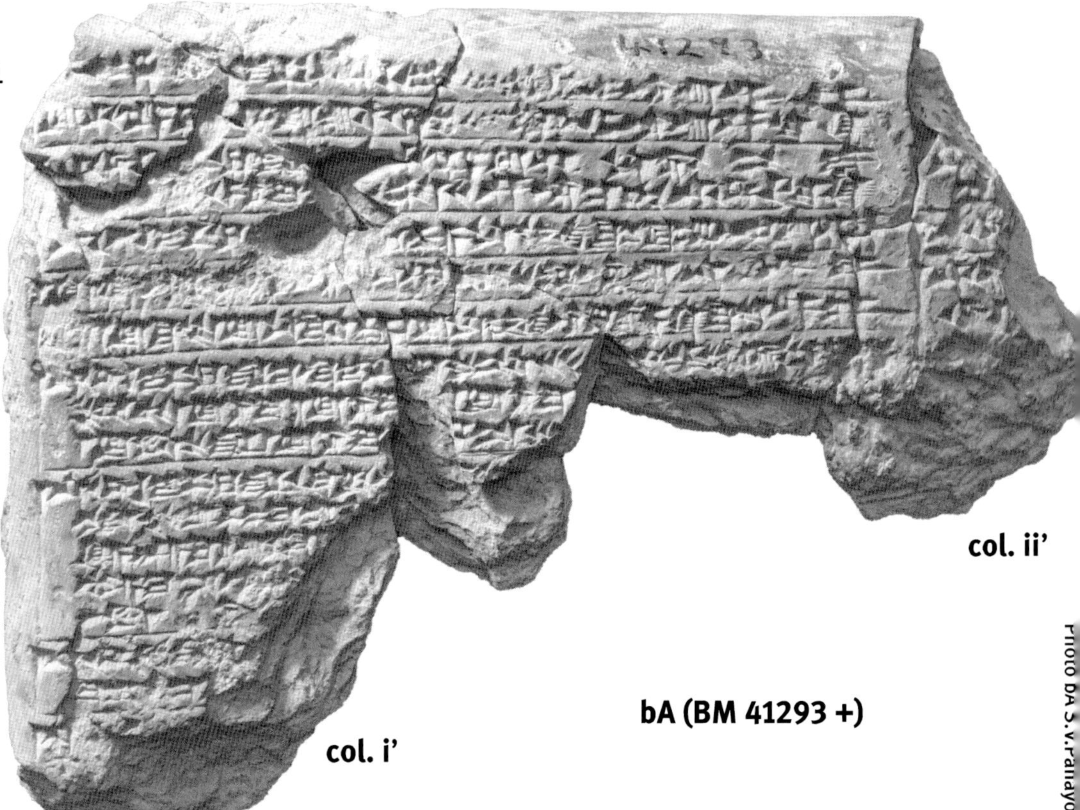

col. i'

col. ii'

bA (BM 41293 +)

Photo bA S.V. Panayotov

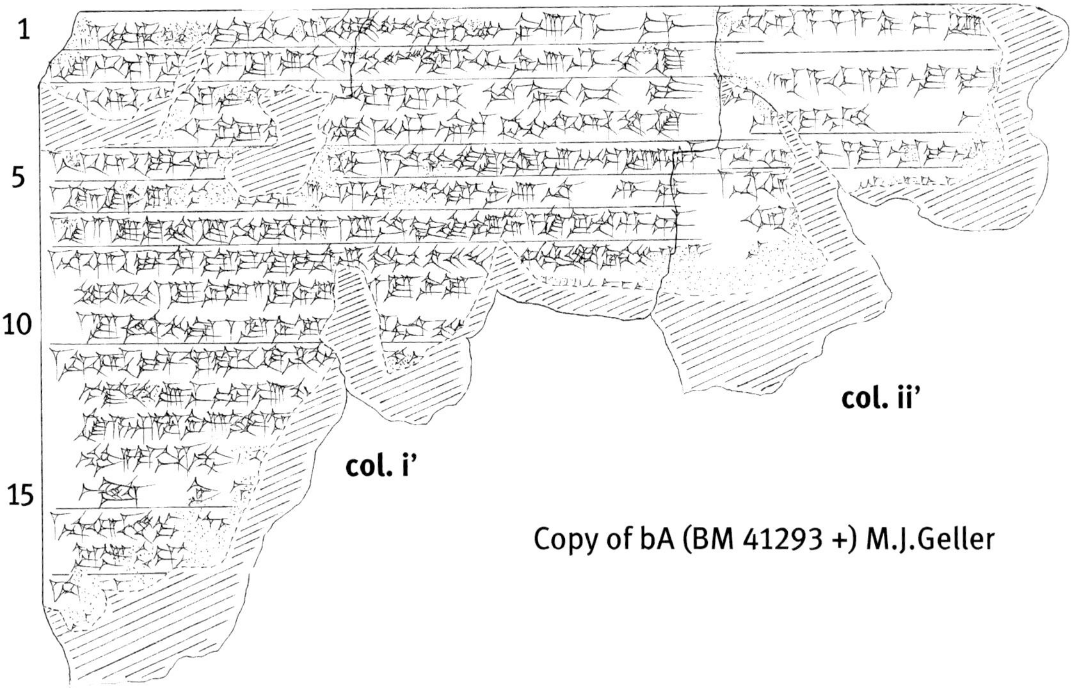

Copy of bA (BM 41293 +) M.J.Geller

NM (BAM 489 + 508) Obverse

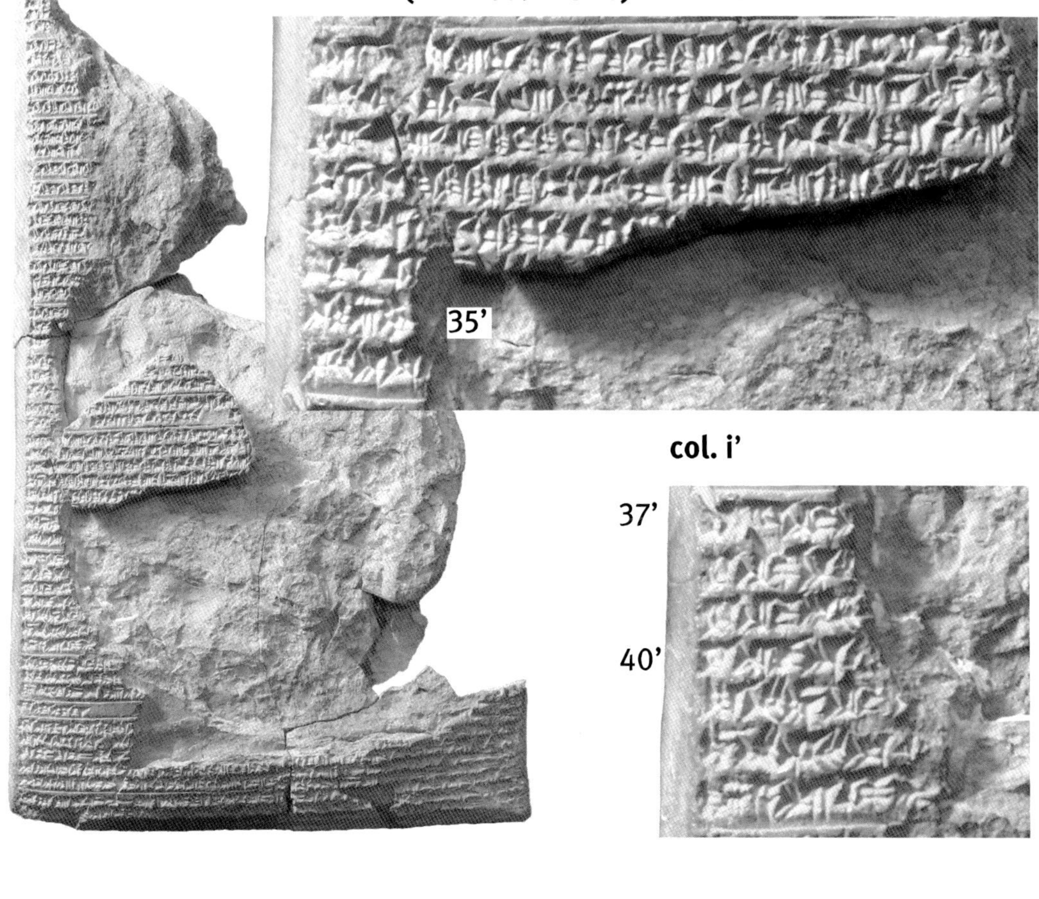

Photos S.V.Panayotov

NN (K 6329)

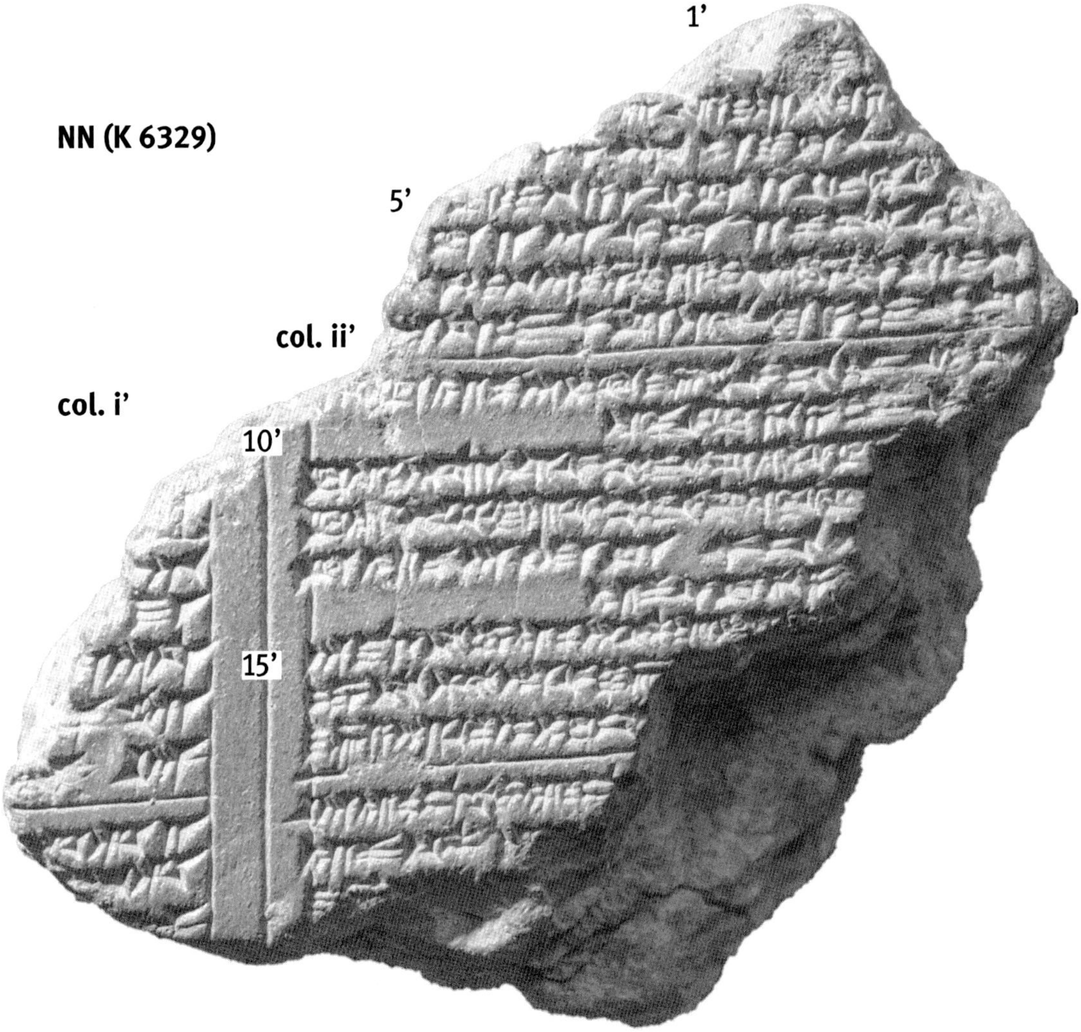

NO (K 8211+... (+) BM 98589 + ...) Overview

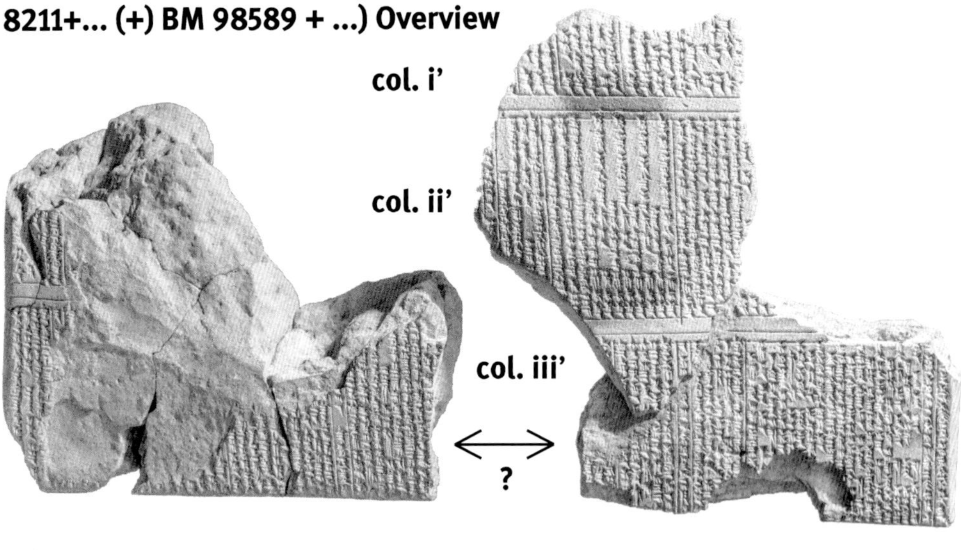

NO (K 8211+... (+) BM 98589+ ...) col. ii'

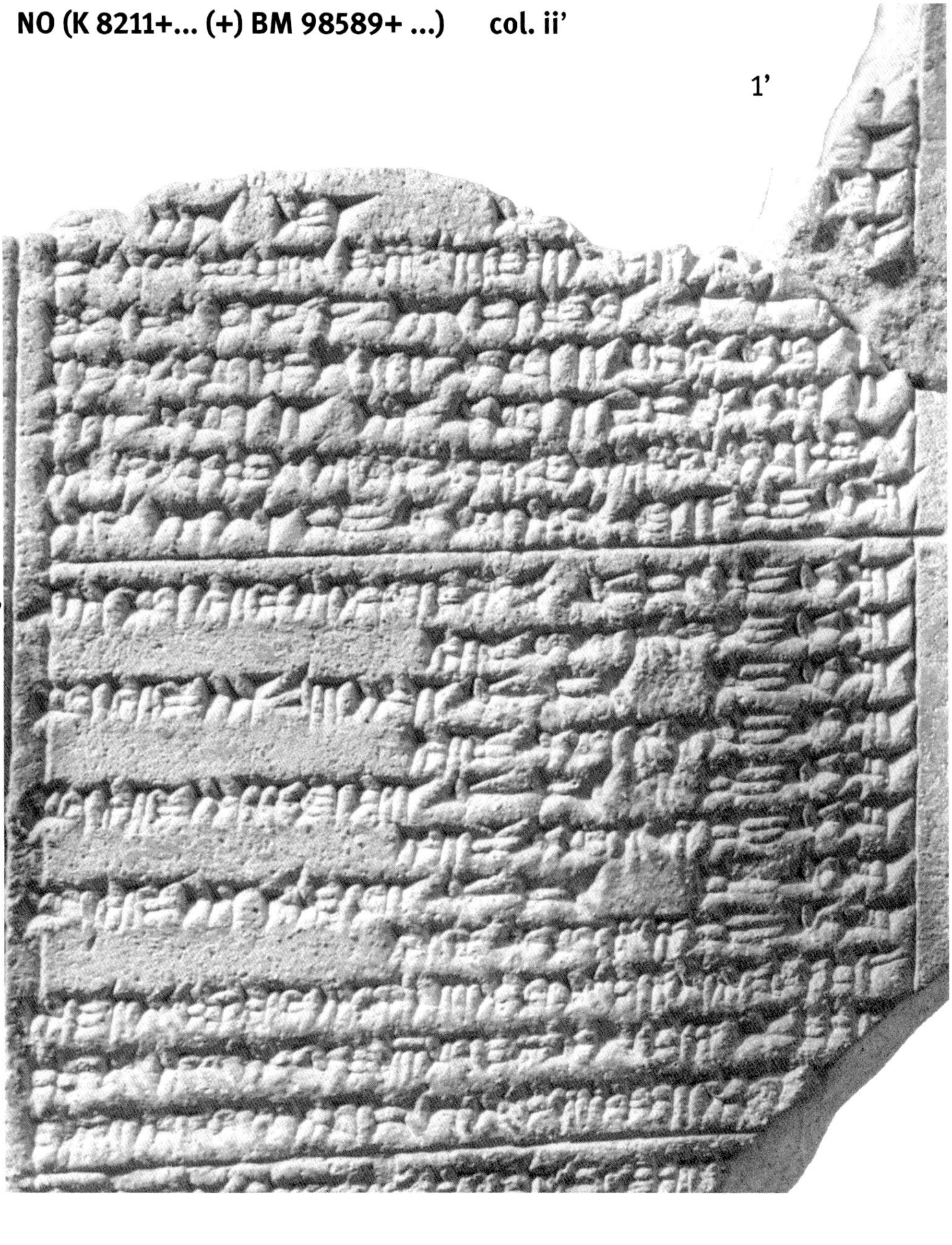

Photos S.V.Panayotov

XA (BM 123362)

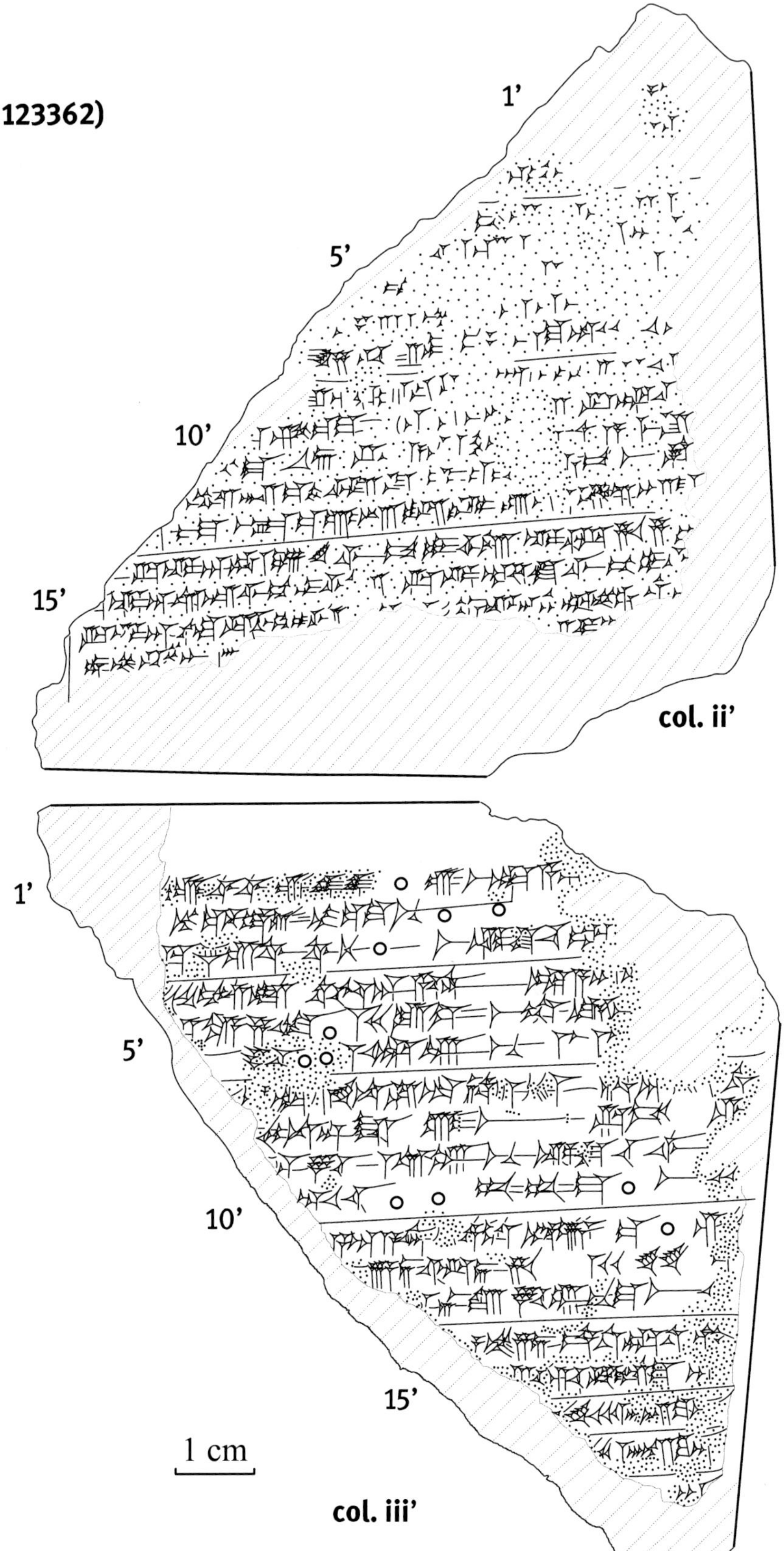

Copy S.V.Panayotov

XA (BM 123362)

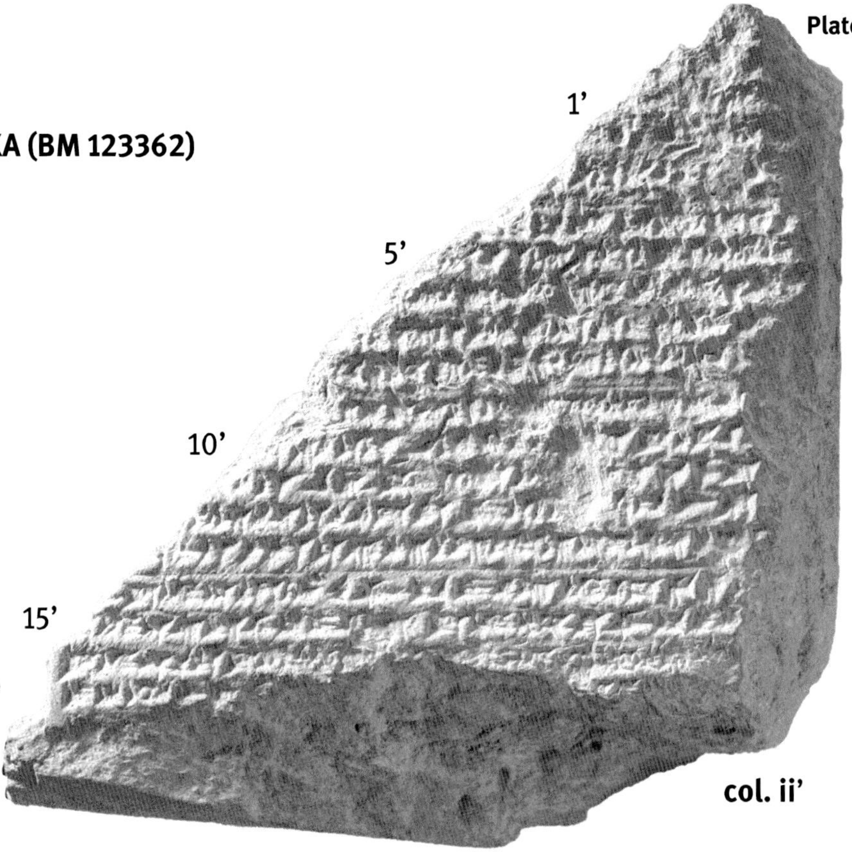

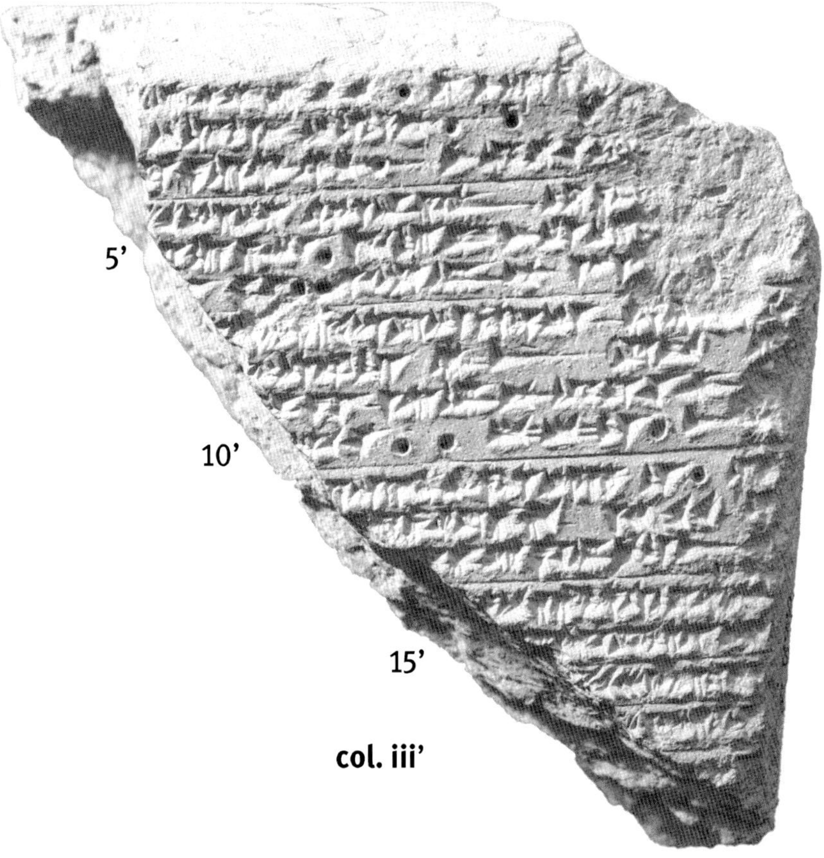

Photos S.V.Panayotov

AC (BAM 19)

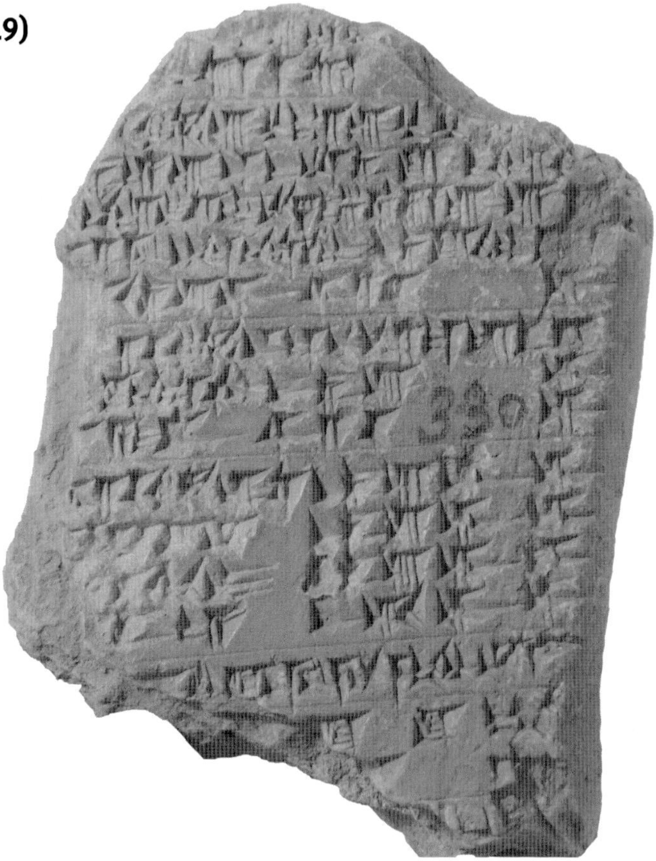

Photo M. Guichard